Manual of Clinical Procedures in the Horse

Manual of Clinical Procedures in the Horse

Edited by

Lais R.R. Costa

William Pritchard Veterinary Medical Teaching Hospital
School of Veterinary Medicine
University of California - Davis
Davis, CA, USA

and

Mary Rose Paradis

Department of Clinical Sciences
Cummings Veterinary School
Tufts University
North Grafton, MA, USA

WILEY Blackwell

Registered Office(s)
John Wiley & Sons, Inc., 111 River Street, Hoboken, NJ 07030, USA

Editorial Office
John Wiley & Sons, Inc., 111 River Street, Hoboken, NJ 07030, USA

For details of our global editorial offices, customer services, and more information about Wiley products visit us at www.wiley.com.

Wiley also publishes its books in a variety of electronic formats and by print-on-demand. Some content that appears in standard print versions of this book may not be available in other formats.

Library of Congress Cataloging-in-Publication Data

Names: Costa, Lais R.R., 1965- editor. | Paradis, Mary Rose, editor.
Title: Manual of clinical procedures in the horse / edited by Lais R.R. Costa,
    Mary Rose Paradis.
Description: Hoboken, NJ : John Wiley and Sons, Inc., 2017. | Includes
    bibliographical references and index.
Identifiers: LCCN 2016056642| ISBN 9780470959275 (pbk.) | ISBN 9781118701010
    (ePub) | ISBN 9781118700662 (Adobe PDF)
Subjects: LCSH: Horses—Diseases—Diagnosis. | MESH: Horse
    Diseases—diagnosis | Horse Diseases—surgery | Surgical Procedures,
    Operative—veterinary | Horses—surgery | Physical Examination
Classification: LCC SF951 .M346 2017 | NLM SF 951 | DDC 636.1/089—dc23 LC record available at https://lccn.loc
.gov/2016056642

Cover images: Courtesy of Lais R.R. Costa
Cover design by Wiley

Set in 10 pt and Warnock Pro by Aptara Inc., New Delhi, India

10 9 8 7 6 5 4 3 2 1

We dedicate this book to the veterinary students that throughout the years have taught us how to teach.

Finally, we want to dedicate this book to our families for their love and support.

Contents

List of Contributors

Antonio José de Araujo Aguiar, Med.Vet., MSc, PhD
Departamento de Cirurgia e Anestesiologia
Veterinária
Faculdade de Medicina Veterinária e Zootecnia
Universidade Estadual Paulista
Botucatu, SP, Brazil

Frank M. Andrews, DVM, MS, Diplomate ACVIM (LAIM)
Department of Veterinary Clinical Sciences
School of Veterinary Medicine
Louisiana State University
Baton Rouge, LA, USA

Ashley G. Boyle, BA, DVM, Diplomate ACVIM (LAIM)
Department of Clinical Studies
New Bolton Center
University of Pennsylvania
Kennett Square, PA, USA

Daniel J. Burba, DVM, Diplomate ACVS
Center for Veterinary Health Sciences
Department of Veterinary Clinical Sciences
Oklahoma State University
Stillwater, OK, USA

Renee Carter, DVM, Diplomate ACVO
Department of Veterinary Clinical Sciences
School of Veterinary Medicine
Louisiana State University
Baton Rouge, LA, USA

Joshua A. Cartmill, PhD
Equine Health Studies Program
School of Veterinary Medicine
Louisiana State University
Baton Rouge, LA, USA

Ann Chapman, DVM, MS, Diplomate ACVIM (LAIM)
Department of Veterinary Clinical Sciences
School of Veterinary Medicine
Louisiana State University
Baton Rouge, LA, USA

Lais R.R. Costa, Med.Vet., MS, PhD, Diplomate ACVIM (LAIM), Diplomate ABVP (Eq)
William Pritchard Veterinary Medical Teaching Hospital
School of Veterinary Medicine
University of California - Davis
Davis, CA, USA

Travis Henry, DVM, Diplomate AVDC (NSS), Diplomate AVDC (Eq)
Midwest Veterinary Dental Services
Elkhorn, WI, USA

Christine Heraud-Ridgway
PO Box 128
Montmorenci, SC, USA

Jill R. Johnson, DVM, MS, Diplomate ACVIM (LAIM), Diplomate ABVP (EQ)
Department of Veterinary Clinical Sciences
School of Veterinary Medicine
Louisiana State University
Baton Rouge, LA, USA

Patrick Loftin, DVM, MS, Diplomate ACVS (LA)
Equine Surgery and Sports Medicine
Tryon Equine Hospital
Columbus, NC, USA

K. Gary Magdesian, DVM, Diplomate ACVIM (LAIM), Diplomate ACVECC, Diplomate ACVCP, CVA
Department of Medicine and Epidemiology
School of Veterinary Medicine
University of California – Davis
Davis, CA, USA

Mustajab H. Mirza, DVM, MS, Diplomate ACVS
Department of Veterinary Clinical Sciences
School of Veterinary Medicine
Louisiana State University
Baton Rouge, LA, USA

Colin Mitchell, DVM, Diplomate ACVS
Department of Veterinary Clinical Sciences
School of Veterinary Medicine
Louisiana State University
Baton Rouge, LA, USA

Nóra Nógrádi, DVM, MS, Diplomate ACVIM (LAIM), CVA
Dubai Equine Hospital
Zabeel 2, Dubai
PO Box 9373

Mary Rose Paradis, DVM, MS, Diplomate ACVIM (LAIM)
Department of Clinical Sciences
Cummings Veterinary School
Tufts University
North Grafton, MA, USA

Carlos R. F. Pinto, Med.Vet., PhD, Diplomate ACT
Department of Veterinary Clinical Sciences
School of Veterinary Medicine
Louisiana State University
Baton Rouge, LA, USA

Cherie Pucheu-Haston, DVM, PhD, DACVD
Department of Veterinary Clinical Sciences
School of Veterinary Medicine
Louisiana State University
Baton Rouge, LA, USA

Catherine Renaudin, DVM, Diplomate ECAR
William Pritchard Veterinary Medical Teaching Hospital
School of Veterinary Medicine
University of California - Davis
Davis, CA, USA

Molly Rice, DVM
Midwest Veterinary Dental Services
Elkhorn, WI, USA

Kerry Ridgway, DVM, CVA
(Deceased)

Alfredo Sanchez Londoño, DVM, MS, Diplomate ACVIM (LAIM)
Tufts Ambulatory Service
Woodstock, CT, USA

Beatrice Sponseller, Dr. med. vet., Diplomate ABVP (Eq)
Lloyd Veterinary Medical Center
College of Veterinary Medicine
Iowa State University
Ames, IA, USA

Brett Sponseller, DVM, PhD, Diplomate ACVIM (LAIM)
Department of Veterinary Clinical Sciences
College of Veterinary Medicine
Iowa State University
Ames, IA, USA

Michelle Woodward, DVM, MS, Diplomate ACVD
Department of Veterinary Clinical Sciences
School of Veterinary Medicine
Louisiana State University
Baton Rouge, LA, USA

Preface

Our goal was to publish a well-illustrated procedural guide specifically aimed at equine and mixed practice veterinary practitioners, veterinary students, interns, residents and veterinary technicians.

During our careers as equine internists and educators we found ourselves reaching out to find detailed guidelines for clinical procedures that we taught our students, interns and residents. We envisioned this manual to serve as a source for common clinical procedures in the horse, and our idea was well received. So, we got to work gathering the information to describe the procedures step-by-step and illustrate them with colored photographs. We were able to count on the contributions of several clinical veterinarians who shared the same ideal. This book is a compilation of many teachers' time, effort and experience. We thank them for sharing their knowledge with us.

The book is organized by procedures pertaining to the body systems. We selected the procedures that are relatively common in clinical equine practice. Each procedure is described step-by-step (Technical Action segment) and concurrently explained how and why (Rationale segment). All chapters are illustrated with photographs and several chapters include tables and charts to aid in the understanding of the procedures.

We hope you will find this manual to be a useful guide for yourself and those you teach.

Lais R.R. Costa
Mary Rose Paradis

Acknowledgements

We would like to thank our contributors: Drs. Jill R. Johnson, Daniel J. Burba, Antonio J. A. Aguiar, Renee Carter, Ann Chapman, Mustajab H. Mirza, Colin Mitchell, Gary Magdesian, Nóra Nógrádi, Travis Henry, Molly Rice, Carlos Pinto, Catherine Renaudin, Cherie Pucheu-Haston, Michelle Woodward, Kerry Ridgway, Brett and Beatrice Sponseller, Alfredo Sanchez, Ashley G. Boyle, Frank M. Andrews, Patrick Loftin, Joshua A. Cartmill, and Mrs. Christine Heraud-Ridgway for their contributions, their patience and dedication. We also want to thank Drs. Carol Foil, Aloisio Bueno, Jose Garcia-Lopez, Eileen Johnson, Ghislaine A. Dujovne, Maria Masri, Cathleen Mochal, Jackie Bowser, Dale Paccamonti, Thomas R. Klei and others for providing images to illustrate this book.

We want to show our appreciation for the commitment and support by the Blackwell editors and staff, especially Erica Judisch, Nancy Turner, Catriona Cooper, Purvi Patel, Audrey Koh, Shalini Sharma, Susan Engelken as well as Lesley Montford that have worked with us to make this book materialize.

We also want to acknowledge the photographic contributions of Andy Cunningham, Daniel Cristian Ornelas de Oliveira, Lezlie Sterling, and Drs. Matthew E. Baur, Jill R. Johnson and Ashlee Oliver. And we thank Dr. Joel Figeroa for his insights in revising this manual.

We would like to mention the loss of Kerry Ridgway, an amazing veterinarian, great educator and a very dear friend. Equine practice has lost an extraordinary practitioner. We all share the sadness with his wife.

Lais R.R. Costa
Mary Rose Paradis

Part I
General Clinical Examinations and Routine Procedures

1

Principles of Horse Handling for Veterinarians: Horse Handling Versus Horse Restraint

Kerry Ridgway and Christine Heraud-Ridgway

We should recognize and think of good handling as psychological restraint, in contrast to our tendency to think of the term "restraint" as a means of physical application of force or chemicals to control the horse. Without question, restraint in order to accomplish a procedure, as well as for the safety of the veterinarian and the person holding the horse, is of utmost importance. However, the very least amount of physical restraint required is always the best level of physical restraint, and this will vary from no restraint to full chemical restraint.

Think of physical and chemical restraint as your second option. Good horse handling and psychological restraint starts before we even touch the horse. Start with things in your favor. Make it easy for the horse to do the right thing. For example, select an examination site where the horse will not be tempted by grass and other distractions.

Realize that we reach out to the world with our hands, that we may examine and evaluate what we see. The horse reaches out to the world with its nose and sense of smell to evaluate and check out its world. With this in mind, stand near the horse while taking the history and let it check you out. Pause periodically to give the horse a gentle scratch or stroke on its forehead or in the hollow behind the withers. When turning your attention to the horse, maintain a soft eye, do not stare it in the eye with a hard-focused look.

There is a contrasting principle for humans vs. horses in their behavior when they come very close to each other. If you walk up to a person and place your face about six inches from them, he or she becomes very tense or embarrassed and wants to back away from you. The horse has just the opposite, hard-wired, behavior. For the horse, your, or the handler's, closeness, or the closeness of another horse, is an invitation to examine and nuzzle or play.

Use this to your advantage, but also realize its disadvantages. When your handler stands right at the horse's face and is trying to help you by having a short and tight hold on the halter, the horse wants to push, be mouthy and play with the handler, or may attempt to free itself of the tight restraint. This can certainly make your examination more difficult. You want the horse be focused so that you can see its responses to palpation and handling.

Horses are very in tune with the body language of predators (humans are often seen as predators by the horse) and so they are in tune with the body language of the person holding the horse for you. This means that powerful signals and behavioral control can best be created while the handler is about three or four feet from the horse. Encourage your clients to learn appropriate techniques to teach the horse to stand quietly for examination by using appropriate body language and signals while standing back from the horse. With that, both you and the person holding the horse will be much happier and your examination will progress much more easily. You need to recognize when to have the handler hold onto the halter and when to control only with the lead rope.

Manual of Clinical Procedures in the Horse, First Edition. Edited by Lais R.R. Costa and Mary Rose Paradis.
© 2018 John Wiley & Sons, Inc. Published 2018 by John Wiley & Sons, Inc.

At this point, the handler is the alpha animal. There are very few horses that are truly "alpha" and that want to be in charge. They would far rather follow than lead. However, they commonly sense a threat when they are approached by multiple persons. Thus, with a tense or fearful horse it helps if you take the lead rope from the client and move the horse around by yourself. Walk in straight lines and ask the horse to turn in both directions and stop when asked. A few moments spent doing this will often let the horse accept you as being in charge.

If, in the process of your examination you need to move the horse's head via the halter, use a gentle "give and take" motion, avoiding force. There is value in turning the head and asking at the same time for a lower head position. The flight reaction is partially dependent on the horse markedly elevating its head and keeping it pointed straight ahead. The simple act of gently bringing the head around and downward using a gentle "give and take" pull on the halter will help extinguish the flight posture and reactivity. To get the horse to lower its head, it can be very helpful to place your free hand on the muscles overlying the first to third cervical vertebrae, that is, C-1 through C-3, called the cranialis group. The hand is simply laying on the muscle area - *no weight or pushing action is applied*. Give the horse a couple of minutes to respond. It will likely prove to be worth the time spent.

Next, move rearward to a position just at the back of the horse's shoulder. Good trainers often refer to this position as being in the "heart space." It tends to be a position of comfort and trust for the horse. You can evoke a beneficial parasympathetic calming effect by gently rubbing or scratching in the wither pocket area that the saddle would occupy. You can do this, for example, while listening to heart and lung sounds.

Do not start your physical examination with an area that you expect to be sore. Touch and palpate areas where you do *not* expect to elicit pain. This is a good general rule, but is particularly valuable when palpating the limb structures, that is, tendons, ligaments, and joints. If the horse has become accustomed to your handling of its normal limb(s), it gains confidence and becomes more accepting.

Prior to picking up a leg for examination, be sure the horse is balanced in such a way that it will be easy for it to stand on three legs. Lean your body slightly into the shoulder to encourage the horse to balance on its opposite side. This applies to both front and rear limbs. Next, on the front limbs, if you touch the horse lightly on the palmar aspect just distal to the accessory carpal bone, over 90% of horses will give you the leg. Sometimes a light touch is most effective (think of the horse's response to a fly on its leg). If the horse is still reluctant to lift the leg, squeeze moderately on the chestnut while asking for the leg.

In summary, remember that there are very few horses who are actually "mean." They have pain, tension or fear. They are flight animals who when not able to flee may try to fight back. Listen to the message that the horse is sending and forgive the action it takes.

A final point: our favorite saying is "if at first you don't succeed, the hell with it." That sounds facetious, but what it really means is you may have to abandon the process that you are using and select another way of achieving your goal. That will save both you and the horse a lot of time and frustration, or even a battle. Good horse handling is a good way to build up your practice. No one wants to see his or her horse "roughed up." If good horse handling is not sufficient to accomplish the examination or procedure, the client will probably accept that other restraint techniques need to be employed. Many of these techniques are described in Chapter 2.

2

Physical Restraint of the Horse for Clinical Procedures

Mustajab H. Mirza and Lais R.R. Costa

2.1 Purpose

- To allow completion of tasks safely with no injury to the patient, the person performing the examination or procedure, or the handler. Some guidelines for approaching a horse are as follows:
    - Approach the horse cautiously but with confidence. Horses can sense nervousness and become more difficult to handle.
    - Approach the horse by its left side (also called the near side) as this is the side most horses are used to being approached from, although most horses are workable from both sides.
    - Never position yourself in front of the horse because you are likely to be struck by the front feet or the head. Instead, position yourself beside and close to the horse's shoulder.
    - Stay close to the horse, letting the horse know what you intend to do. Make sure you never stand directly behind the horse. If you have to work around the horse's hind limbs, position yourself next to the flank and thigh, and stay close to the horse, so if the horse kicks you will not receive the full impact of the kick.

    - Effective restraint often requires a person familiar with horse handling and a combination of equipment such as halter, lead rope, twitch, chain, and rope.
    - The methods of physical restraint discussed in this chapter include halter placement, tying the horse, neck roll, ear hold, lip chain, lip rope, modified lip rope, nose or lip twitch, lifting and holding the front foot, lifting and holding the hind foot, lifting a front leg to prevent the horse from kicking, and restraining the horse in stocks.

2.2 Complications

- Injury to the patient, the person performing the examination/procedure, or the handler.
- Failure to complete the task (e.g., examination or procedure).
- Damage to the patient from restraint.
- Escape of patient to a dangerous situation.

2.3 Procedure: Halter Placement

Purpose: To restrain, lead and control the horse's movement.
Equipment: Halter (Figure 2.1a) and lead rope (Figure 2.1b).

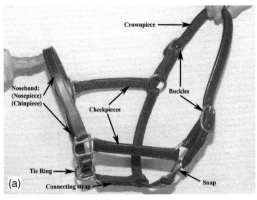

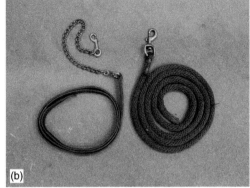

Figure 2.1 Parts of a halter. (a) The parts of the halter (halter with jaw snap). (b) Lead rope and lead shank.

Technical action	Rationale
Select a halter of appropriate size for the horse.	This is important. If the halter is too small, it may not be secured properly and the horse may escape, or, if able to secure the halter, the nose and chin strap might injure the horse. If the halter is too big, it might be removed unexpectedly.
Approach from the horse's left side at a 45° angle (Figure 2.2).	Position yourself beside the horse, next to the left side of the neck/shoulder. Never stand in front of the horse.
Secure the horse with the lead rope around the neck while putting on the halter (Figure 2.3).	Although the rope around the neck will not restrain the horse, and the horse can still escape, most horses give in to the procedure, allowing the halter to be placed properly. Many horses are very cooperative and allow the handler to place the halter properly without placement of the rope around the neck.
If the halter has a jaw snap, open the snap, slide the noseband over the muzzle, and place the crownpiece behind the ears, then clip the jaw snap (Figure 2.4). Snap the lead rope onto the tie ring.	If the halter does not have a jaw snap, open the left buckle, slide the noseband over the muzzle, place the crownpiece behind the ears, and secure the buckle (Figure 2.5).

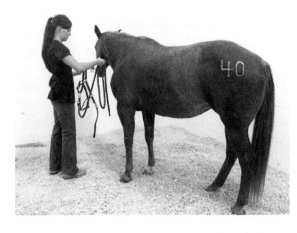

Figure 2.2 Approach the horse by the left side, by positioning yourself beside and close to the horse's left neck /shoulder.

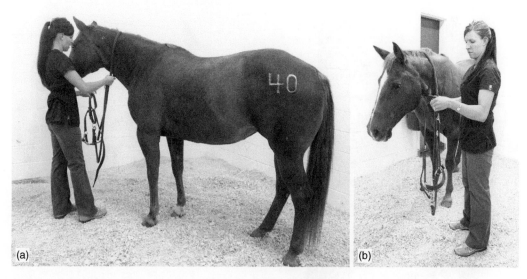

Figure 2.3 The horse can be secured with the lead rope around the neck.

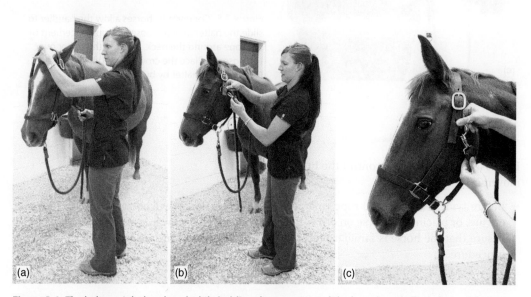

Figure 2.4 The halter might be placed while holding the rope around the horse's neck. For halters with a jaw snap, (a) place the noseband on the horse's muzzle, moving the crownpiece towards the poll, (b) place the crownpiece behind the ears, and (c) clip the jaw snap.

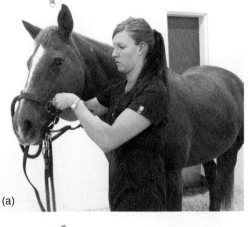

(a)

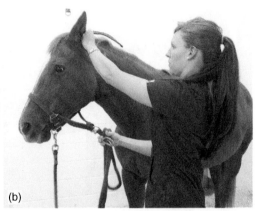

(b)

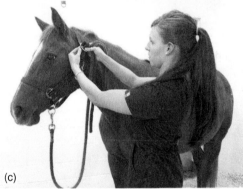

(c)

Figure 2.5 Cooperative horses allow the handler to slide the halter over the nose without placement of the rope around the neck. (a) Slide the halter over the nose. (b) Place the crownpiece behind the ears. (c) Secure the halter by buckling it.

2.4 Procedure: Tying the Lead Rope

Purpose: To restrain and control the horse's movement.

- Before tying a horse's lead rope to a post or ring, or placing the horse on cross-ties, ensure that the horse is familiar with this procedure.

- Some horses will not accept being tied and will pull backwards until they are released.
- Most horses are tolerant to cross-ties.

Equipment: Halter and lead rope, or cross-ties.

Technical action	Rationale
When tying a haltered horse, adjust the slack in the lead rope.	Prevent the horse from lowering its head and stepping on/over the rope. Stepping on the rope is likely to startle the horse and make him panic.
Tie the rope to a post or ring using a quick-release knot. Figure 2.6 details the steps for performing a quick-release knot.	The quick-release knot can be easily released in the case of an emergency (Figure 2.7). Alternatively, use cross-ties, which will also restrict the horse's movements (Figure 2.8).

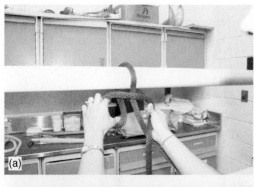

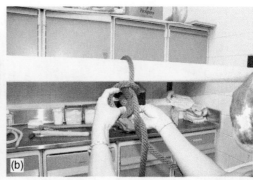

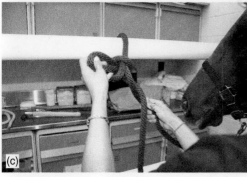

Figure 2.6 When tying a haltered horse, use a quick-release knot. (a) Wrap the rope around itself, making a loop. (b) Insert the rope through the loop. (c) Pull through the loop.

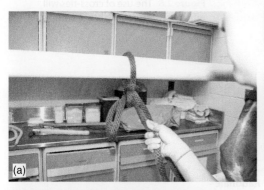

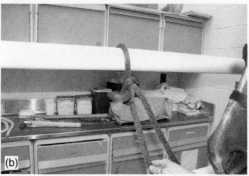

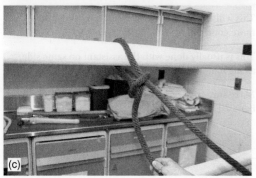

Figure 2.7 Release a quick-release knot by pulling the free end of the rope, (a) to (c).

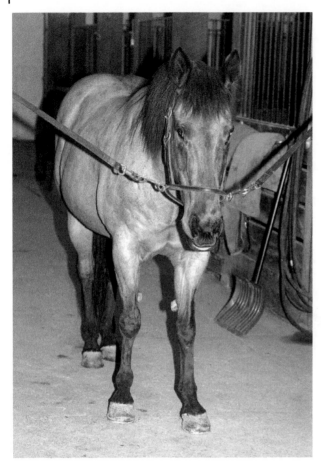

Figure 2.8 The use of cross-ties will effectively restrict the horse's movements.

2.5 Procedure: Neck Roll or Neck Skin Twitch

Purpose: To divert the attention of the patient from an examination or non-painful procedure for a short period of time.
Equipment: None.

Technical action	Rationale
Stand by the horse's shoulder and slide your hand over the horse's shoulder (Figure 2.9a).	This will warn the horse of your intention to take more control.
Grasp the loose skin in front of shoulder at the base of neck (Figure 2.9b).	This is usually done with the assistant on same side as the handler.
Apply a rolling motion to pull skin taut (Figure 2.9c).	Make sure to maintain a tight grip with one or two hands (Figure 2.9d,e).
Additional restraint can be accomplished by shaking the skin while holding it.	

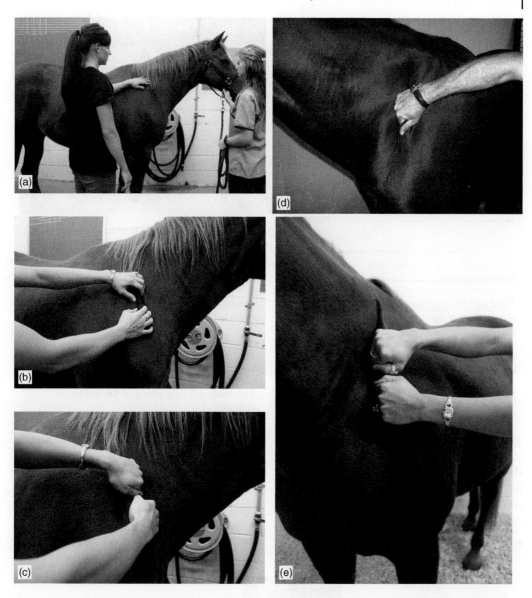

Figure 2.9 Applying a neck roll. (a) Stand by the horse's chest and slide your hands over the horse's shoulder. (b) Grasp the loose skin in front of shoulder at the base of the neck. (c) Apply a rolling motion to pull the skin taut. (d) Apply a neck roll with one hand. (e) Apply a neck roll with two hands.

2.6 Procedure: Ear Hold

Purpose: To provide short-term restraint.

- Used commonly in animals of small stature, such as ponies, miniature horses and foals, or used in conjunction with a nose twitch. *Warning*: Applying a twitch to the ear can result in permanent damage and is not recommended.

Equipment: None.

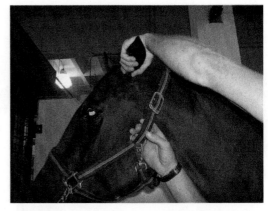

Figure 2.10 Applying an ear hold (also referred to as a manual ear twitch).

Technical action	Rationale
Stand to the side of horse near the shoulder. Slide your hand over the side of the horse's face towards the base of the ear.	This will warn the horse that you are about to approach the horse's head.
Reach forward and grasp the base of the ear between the index finger and the thumb (Figure 2.10).	Hold firmly so as not to lose your grip.
Squeeze the base of the ear.	A little twist will help your grip. Do not twist excessively.

2.7 Procedure: Lip Chain

Purpose: To restrain and control the horse's movement more forcefully, providing reward and negative reinforcement when needed.

- This method is commonly used in stallions and nervous horses.

- The use of the chain provides more rigorous restraint than halter and lead rope alone.

Equipment: Halter, lead shank (Figure 2.11a) or chain (Figure 2.11b), lead rope. Disinfectant (e.g., 0.05% chlorhexidine) should be used to clean the lip chain after use.

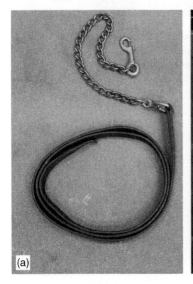

(a)

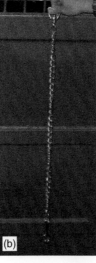

(b)

Figure 2.11 (a) The lead shank and (b) the chain that is attached to the snap of a lead rope.

Technical action	Rationale
Pass the chain end of the lead shank through the rostral ring on the left side of the halter from outside toward the horse (Figure 2.12a).	
Pass chain over the bridge of the nose (Figure 2.12b) and through the rostral ring on the right side of the halter from inside to outside (Figure 2.12c).	
Attach the snap on the chain to the upper right ring of the halter (Figure 2.12d).	
Slide the chain slack between the two rostral rings under the upper lip (Figure 2.12e).	The chain might be placed over the bridge of the nose (Figure 2.13), around the nose band (Figure 2.14) or under the chin to provide less severe restraint than the lip chain.
Apply slight tension to the chain to keep it properly positioned (Figure 2.12f).	Do not pull hard on the chain to avoid hurting the horse's gums unnecessarily. Only pull on the chain in jerky movements when negative reinforcement is needed.
Do not tie the horse with the chain in place.	Warning: Lip chain should only be used by experienced handler.

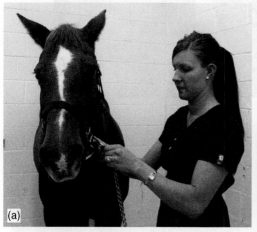 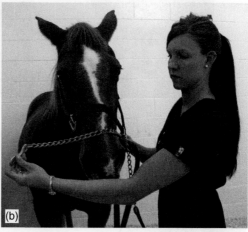

Figure 2.12 Placement of the lip chain. (a) Pass the chain end of the lead shank through the rostral ring on left side of halter from outside toward the horse. (b) Advance the chain over the bridge of the nose. (c) Pass the chain through the rostral ring on the right side from inside toward the outside. (d) Attach the snap on the chain to the upper ring on the right side of the halter. (e) Slide the chain slack between the two rostral rings under the upper lip. (f) Apply gentle tension to the chain to keep it properly positioned over the gum of the upper incisors.

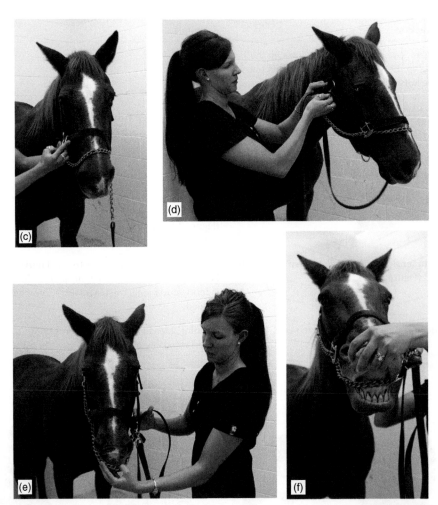

Figure 2.12 (*Continued*)

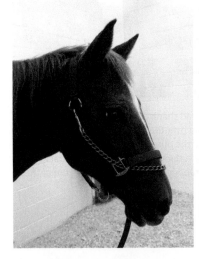

Figure 2.13 The chain might be placed over the bridge of the nose to give gentler restraint than the lip chain.

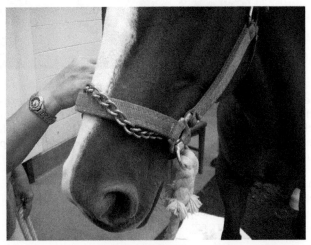

Figure 2.14 The chain might be placed around the nose band to give gentler restraint than the lip chain.

2.8 Procedure: Lip Rope

Purpose: To restrain and control the horse's movement and provide reward and negative reinforcement when needed.

- This method is commonly used as a training aid for fearful and nervous horses.

Equipment: Small diameter cotton rope (~7 mm) tied to the halter.

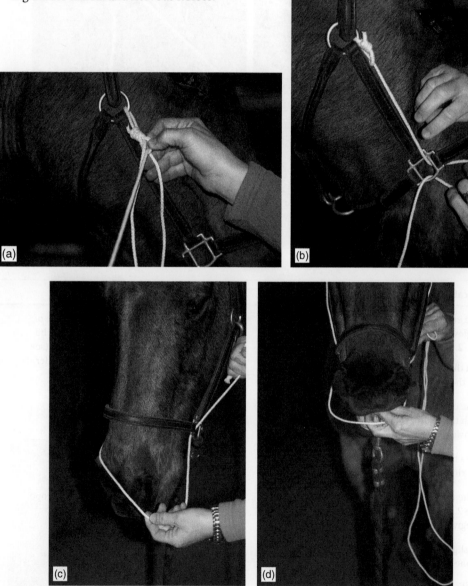

Figure 2.15 Restraint by a lip rope. (a) One end of a cotton rope is tied to the halter ring below the base of the ear on the right side. (b) The free end of the cotton rope is threaded through the rostral ring of the halter on the right side. (c) The rope is passed over the bridge of the nose and through the rostral ring on the left side of the halter from inside to outside, with the slack spanning the two rostral rings. (d) The slack of rope between the two rostral rings is placed under the upper lip. (e) The rope slack is placed under the upper lip to attain placement just above the gingiva at the dorsal aspect. (f) Maintain gentle pressure on the rope, and apply forceful pressure (punishment) and remove pressure (reward) from the rope as a tool to enforce the horse's compliance with the desired procedure.

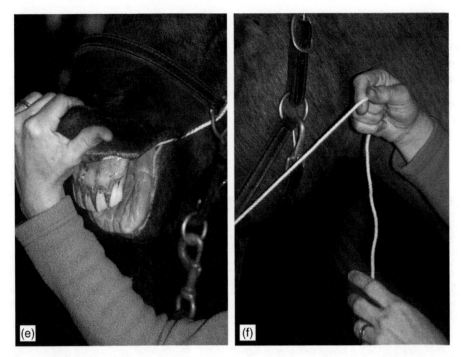

Figure 2.15 (*Continued*)

Technical action	Rationale
Tie one end of the cotton rope to the halter ring below the base of the ear on the right side (Figure 2.15a).	The way the lip rope is used is similar to use of the lip chain. The placement can, therefore, be performed in the same way as the lip chain (see above) or it can be performed in reverse order.
Thread the free end of the rope through the rostral ring of the halter on the right side (Figure 2.15b).	
Pass the cotton rope over the bridge of the nose and through the rostral ring on left side of the halter from inside to outside.	
Create a bit of slack in the rope spanning the two rostral rings (Figure 2.15c).	
Slide the rope slack under the upper lip (Figure 2.15d) to attain placement just above the gingiva at the dorsal aspect (Figure 2.15e).	The lip rope is kept separate from the lead rope.
Apply slight tension to the rope to keep it properly positioned (Figure 2.15f).	Caution:
Maintain gentle pressure on the rope.	• Avoid excessive force to prevent injury.
Apply forceful pressure (punishment) and remove pressure (reward) from the rope as a tool to enforce the horse's compliance with the desired procedure.	• Do not lead the horse by the lip rope. • The efficacy of this tool depends on proper application of pressure with the undesired behavior and withdrawal of the pressure as the horse complies.

2.9 Procedure: Modified Lip Rope

Purpose: To restrain and control the horse's movement.

- This method is effective in horses that resist application of a nose twitch, or strike when a nose twitch is applied. It is also effective in horses that tend to raise and shake their heads when approached for administration of oral medication and other ordinary maneuvers.

Equipment: Equine restraint and training system (Stableizer®).

Technical action	Rationale
Apply the equine restraint and training system according to the manufacturer's instructions (Figure 2.16a,b).	Position the system next to the horse such that the plastic tubing will be positioned under the horse's lip, the bottom pulley next to the left lip and the top pulley, and snap next to the left ear.
Unlock the button next to the handle to open it to the maximum.	
Place the system around the horse's neck by fitting the loop over the horse's head.	If unable to slide the loop over the horse's head, snap the hook open, put it around the horse's neck, and snap the hook back.
Place the top of the snap on the depression behind the ear.	Make sure the plastic tubing is intact (no cracks) and place it up against the aluminum ferrule and the bottom pulley.
Place the section of the rope protected by the plastic tubing under the lip, swiftly pulling the handle at the free end of the rope at the same time.	After placing the section with the plastic tubing under the lip, switch hands and unlock the button next to the handle.
Slide the button away from the handle up to the pulley, locking the rope in that position to take the slack, but not tightening it.	The device should remain properly placed under the upper lip by itself.
Wait a couple of minutes then adjust the length by sliding the tension-release button further away from the handle, thus tightening the hold under the lip.	Initially, just keep the rope snug so it won't slip out from under the lip, and let the horse get used to the device.

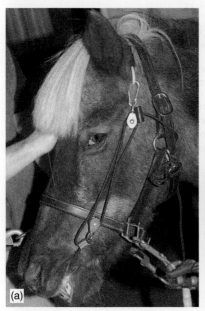
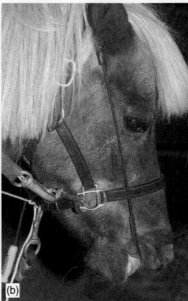

(a) (b)

Figure 2.16 Restraint by use of a modified lip rope. (a) Left view of the equine restraint and training system (Stableizer®, by Udderly (EZ) and Humbolt (IA)) placed correctly. (b) Right view of the equine restraint and training system place correctly. Note the plastic tubing is placed under the lip.

2.10 Procedure: Nose or Lip Twitch

Purpose: To restrain and divert the attention of the patient from other procedures, including those that involve mild discomfort (e.g., injections).

Equipment: Rope twitch or chain twitch or humane (aka Kendal or self-retained) twitch (Figure 2.17).

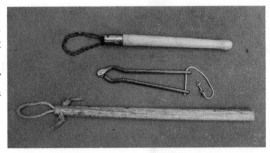

Figure 2.17 Types of nose twitch: rope (bottom), Kendal (middle), and chain (top).

Technical action	Rationale
Hold the handle of the twitch with one hand and place the fingers of the other hand through the chain or rope loop (Figure 2.18a). In order to prevent the chain or rope from sliding down to the wrist, leave one of the fingers over the chain or rope (Figure 2.18b).	If using the humane twitch, open it by separating the two handles (Figure 2.19a).
Position the hand securing the loop of the twitch in front of the horse's upper lip (Figure 2.18c). Grasp the upper lip with the hand securing the loop of the twitch, while keeping a hold on the handle of the twitch with the other hand.	Firm grasp is critical. If the horse tosses its head, make sure the handle of the twitch is held securely and does not dangle, as it can cause injuries.
Apply the twitch by sliding the chain or rope over the hand onto the upper lip (Figure 2.18d).	If using the humane twitch, surround the upper lip with the two sides of the twitch and squeeze it (Figure 2.19b,c).
Tighten the twitch by turning the handle (Figure 2.18e).	If using the humane twitch, tie the rope around the two handles (Figure 2.19d).
Use the twitch to control the horse rather than the lead rope, but do not lead the horse by the twitch.	Once in position, the lead rope may be wrapped around the twitch handle.
If applied for longer than 15 minutes, loosen the twitch slightly intermittently and re-apply to allow blood flow to the horse's lip.	Pay attention to the horse's behavior. If the twitch is too tight for too long, causing severe numbness and purple discoloration of the upper lip, the horse can become uncooperative.
When possible, remove the twitch promptly and massage the muzzle.	

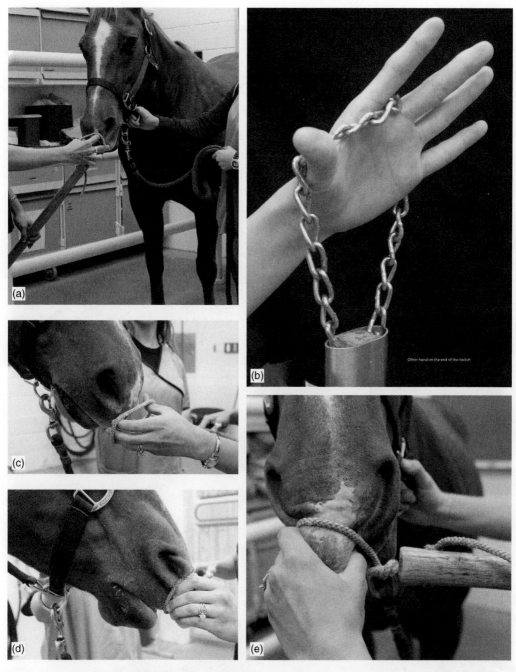

Figure 2.18 Use of the lip twitch. (a) Hold the chain or rope twitch with both hands, one hand holding on to the handle, and place the fingers of the other hand through the chain or rope loop. (b) Leaving one finger out will prevent the chain or rope from sliding down to the wrist. (c) Grasp the horse's upper lip. (d) Apply the twitch by sliding the rope (or chain) loop over the fingers and onto the upper lip. (e) Twist the wood handle, thus tightening the twitch, making sure to keep the fingers out of the way.

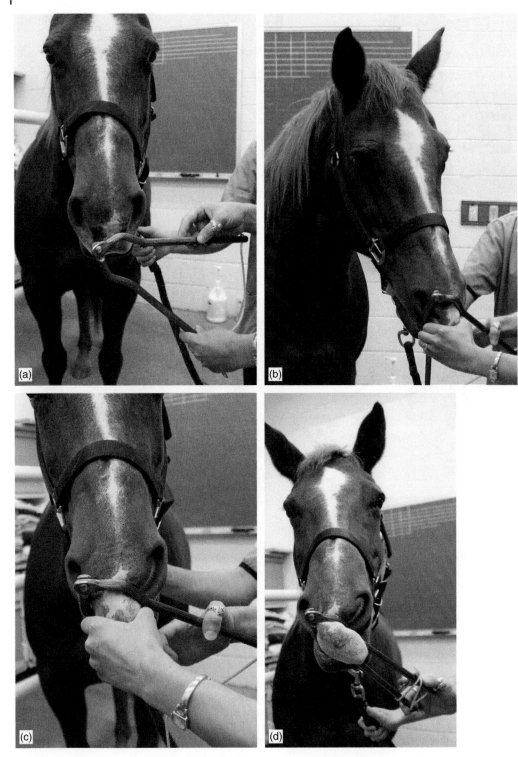

Figure 2.19 Placement of a Kendal nose twitch. (a) Open the Kendal twitch by separating the two aluminum bar handles. (b) Grasp the upper lip while sliding the flared part of the aluminum bars, encircling the upper lip. (c) Bring the two aluminum bar handles together, pinching the upper lip. (d) Secure the twitch bar by fastening the cord around the aluminum bar handles.

2.11 Procedure: Lifting and Holding Front Foot Safely

Purpose: To examine each front limb while off the ground.
Equipment: None.

Technical action	Rationale
Stand by the horse's side, with your shoulder against the horse's shoulder, and facing the horse's rump (Figure 2.20a)	This will warn the horse that you are about to approach the horse's foreleg.
Bend forward and slide one hand distally down the leg (Figure 2.20b), until you reach the carpi.	This will warn the horse that you intend to pick up that limb. Many horses are very cooperative and will pick the leg off the ground when you slide your hand down the limb.
Push with your shoulder against the horse's shoulder/forearm.	Only push gently to let the horse know you want it to shift the weight off that limb because you are about to pick it up.
Gently squeeze the flexor tendons or the chestnut (Figure 2.20c)	The goal is to ask the horse to give you the foot. Some horses are very sensitive to the squeeze of the chestnut. Do not engage in a wrestling match with the horse.
Pick the leg up as soon as the horse pulls the foot off the ground, holding on by the cannon bone (Figure 2.20d).	Make sure you do not hold the foot by the palmar aspect as this will traumatize the flexor tendons. Keep the limb aligned under the horse.
Use the other hand to support the foot by holding the front part of the hoof (Figure 2.20e).	Hold firmly so as not to lose your grip.
Hold the foot up by supporting the leg flexed with one hand (Figure 2.20f) and move your leg to place the foot between your knees (Figure 2.20g).	
The leg is held by the knees at the pastern in order to free up both hands (Figure 2.20h).	To clean and examine the sole of the hoof, and to apply hoof testers.
When you are done, pick up the limb by the pastern and place the limb on the ground. Avoid just letting the foot drop to the ground carelessly.	Make sure you show the horse that you have control of the situation and that the horse can put the limb down because you are done.

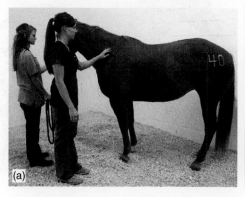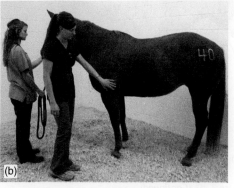

(a)　　(b)

Figure 2.20 Lifting and holding the front foot. (a) Place a hand on the horse's shoulder and face the horse's rump. (b) Bend forward, pushing with your shoulder against the horse's shoulder/forearm, and slide one hand distally down the leg until you reach the carpi. (c) Slide your hand further down and gently squeeze the flexor tendons or the chestnut. (d) Pick the leg up as soon as the horse pulls the foot off the ground, holding on by the cannon bone. (e) Use the other hand to support the foot by holding the front part of the pastern/hoof. (f) Support the leg flexed by holding on to the dorsal aspect of the pastern with one hand. (g) Move your leg to place the foot between your knees. (h) Hold the leg with your knees at the pastern to free up both hands.

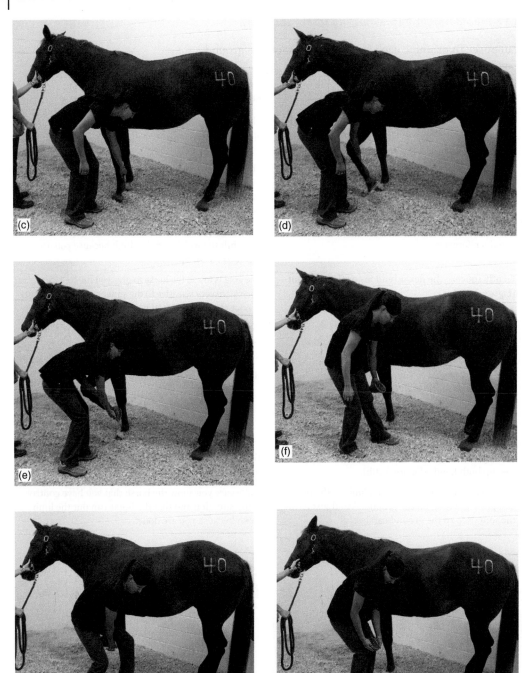

Figure 2.20 (*Continued*)

2.12 Procedure: Lifting and Holding the Hind Foot Limb Safely

Purpose: To examine each hind foot while off the ground.
Equipment: None.

Technical action	Rationale
Stand by the horse's torso, facing the rear of the horse and touching the horse's flank and thigh (Figure 2.21a).	This will warn the horse that you are about to approach its hind limb. You may tie the tail into a knot to prevent the tail hairs from being in your face.
Bend gradually and slide one hand distally down the leg until you reach the fetlock. If it is a cooperative horse, you may stand with your shoulder next to the thigh of the horse (Figure 2.21b) and pick the hind limb up as soon as the horse lifts the foot off the ground. If you do not know how cooperative the horse is, the safest way to pick up a hind foot is to face the horse's thigh, keeping one hand over the tuber coxae while sliding the other hand distally down the leg and bending down gradually.	This will warn the horse that you intend to pick up that limb, while making sure you protect yourself in case the horse wants to kick. Most horses are familiar with this maneuver and cooperate by readily lifting the foot off the ground. This way, you can sense if the horse's weight shifts as it prepares to kick, and if the horse kicks out you can push against the horse's hip and get yourself out of the way towards the horse's torso.
Pick the leg off the ground holding the dorsal aspect of the pastern with one hand while the other hand supports the dorsal aspect of the cannon bone (Figure 2.21c).	Many horses are very cooperative and will pick the leg off the ground when you slide your hand down the limb. Hold the dorsal aspect of the pastern or the cannon bone firmly so as not to lose your grip.
Once the horse appears comfortable standing on three legs, take a step toward the tail of the horse, bringing the limb with you (Figure 2.21d).	Hold the limb with one hand by supporting the dorsal aspect of the foot and pastern. A hoofpick or hoofknife can be used with the other hand.
The leg of the horses may be placed over your leg, such that the distal cannon bone and fetlock lay over your thigh, in order to free up both hands (Figure 2.21e).	This way, with two free hands the sole of the hoof can be examined and hoof testers applied.

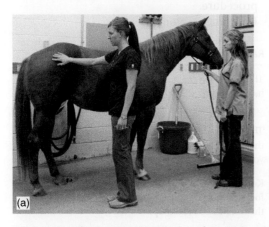 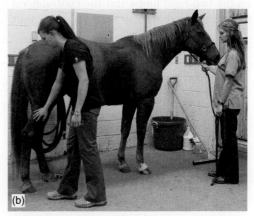

(a)　　(b)

Figure 2.21 Lifting and holding the hind foot. (a) Stand by the horse's torso, facing the rear of the horse and touching the horse's rump. (b) Bend gradually and slide one hand distally down the leg. (c) Bend down further, sliding your hand down to the fetlock, pick the hind limb up when the horse lifts it off the ground, and hold the limb with both hands (one supporting the dorsal aspect of the pastern and hoof and the other the dorsal aspect of the cannon bone). (d) Take a step caudally, so that the leg is moderately extended. (e) Place the fetlock over your thigh to support the leg and free up both hands.

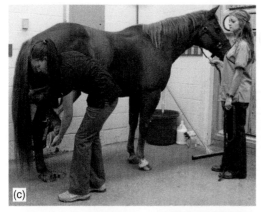

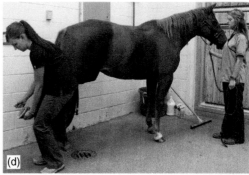

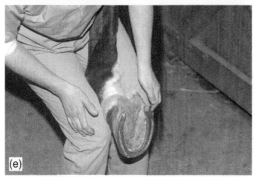

Figure 2.21 (*Continued*)

2.13 Procedure: Lifting a Front Leg to Prevent the Horse from Kicking

Purpose: To provide short-term minor distraction by forcing the horse to bear weight on the two hind limbs and the contralateral front limb so the horse is less able to shift body position quickly and less likely to kick the person performing an examination or procedure.

Equipment: None.

Technical action	Rationale
Approach the horse at the level of the shoulder, facing the rear of the horse, and touch the horse's shoulder.	This will warn the horse of your intention in handling him.
Lean gently on the horse, pushing against the horse's shoulder.	This will lead the horse to position itself, distributing the weight to the other limbs and allowing the limb you intend to lift to be non-weight bearing.
Slide your hand down the limb and hold the pastern.	Keep the shoulder pressed against the horse's forearm to maintain the weight shifted away from the limb to be picked up.
Pick up the limb and hold it with the carpus flexed (Figure 2.22). Do not press on the flexor tendons.	This allows the examiner to work around the hind limbs of the horse (e.g., palpating the hind limbs in a weight-bearing position, taking rectal temperature, examining the rump, tail and perineal area, examining the prepuce, inguinal area and mammary glands, etc.)

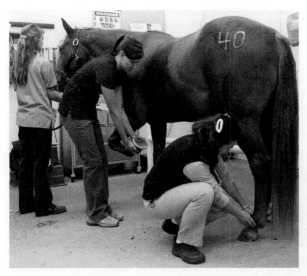

Figure 2.22 Lift and hold a front foot to prevent the horse from kicking while an examination or procedure is performed near the ipsilateral hind limb.

2.14 Procedure: Restraining the Horse in the Stocks

Purpose: To provide more forceful restraint of the horse's movement for examination or implementation of standing procedures with or without concomitant sedation or tranquilization.

Equipment: Stocks.

Technical action	Rationale
Lead the horse to the back gate of the stocks (Figure 2.23a).	Make sure both front and back gates are completely open and no one is standing behind the gates.
Walk through the back gate assertively, into the stocks and through the front gate (Figure 2.23b).	Some horses like to smell the bars to the stocks. Do not fight with the horse but try to avoid the horse taking control of the situation.
Alternatively, the horse may be lead into the stocks while the handler walks outside the stocks.	Less trusting horses may find this suspicious and refuse to walk into the stocks. If the horse pulls back, the arm of the handler could bang against the side post of the stocks and get hurt.
Once the horse has its entire body in the stocks, calmly close the back gate (Figure 2.23c). The front gate can then be closed carefully (Figure 2.23d). When closing the back gate, make sure to not position yourself at risk of being hit by the gate in case the horses backs up.	Try to move swiftly but calmly so as not to startle the horse. If scared, many horses will try to run through the front or back gates, and this is likely to cause injuries to people and the horse itself.

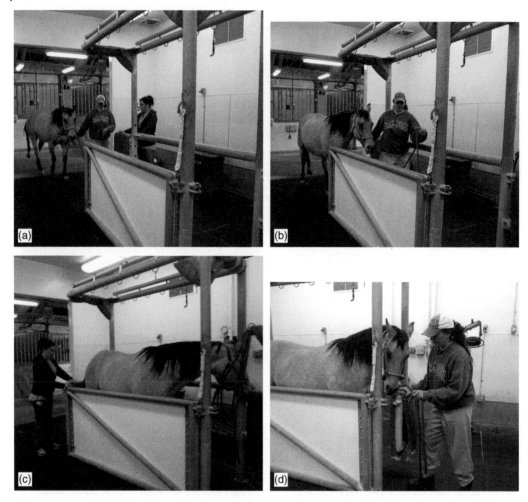

Figure 2.23 Restraint of the horse in the stocks. (a) The horse is led to the back gate of the stocks, with the handler walking in front of the horse. (b) The handler walks through the back gate in front of the horse, towards the front gate. (c) The back gate of the stocks should be closed quietly and calmly once the horse is completely in the stocks and after it has settled. (d) Lastly the front gate is closed.

Bibliography and Further Reading

Evans, J.W. (1989) Handling and training, in *Horses – A guide to selection, care and enjoyment*, 2nd edn. W.H. Freeman Company, New York, pp. 207–222.

Rose, R.J. and Hodgson, D.R. (2002) Physical examination, in *Manual of Equine Practice*, 2nd edn (eds R.J. Rose and D.R. Hodgson), W.B. Saunders, Philadelphia, pp. 16–23.

3

History and Physical Examination of the Horse

Lais R.R. Costa

3.1 Purpose

Accurate medical history and thorough physical examination are crucial procedures in equine practice, and constitute the foundation of clinical assessment of medical problem(s). Obtaining a concise, but complete, medical history (i.e., anamnesis) will guide the veterinarian's approach to the physical examination. The ability to obtain accurate information requires practice to avoid leading questions to which the respondent is likely to give a positive, but inaccurate, answer. The examination should be thorough, but expeditious, and it must be completed even after an abnormality is discovered.

The goals of obtaining a thorough and detailed history and physical examination include:

- to collect information regarding the medical status of the patient
- to address the concerns of the owner relating to the animal and to identify specific or predisposing problems
- to help develop a course of action to diagnose, manage, and treat problem(s)
- to try to prevent future liability problems by thorough anamnesis and physical examination, and help the veterinarian's defense if litigation does occur
- to perform complete wellness, performance and pre-purchase examinations.

3.2 Equipment Required

- Stethoscope
- Watch with second hand
- Source of bright light (e.g., penlight)
- Ophthalmoscope (optional)
- Microchip reader (optional)
- Examination gloves (optional)
- Hoof pick
- Hoof testers (optional)
- Means to record information and findings, as outlined below.
  - Identification:
  - History:
  - Physical Exam Findings:
    - General:
    - Integument:
    - Eye-Ear-Nose-Throat (EENT):
    - Lymph node:
    - Cardio-Vascular:
    - Respiratory:
    - Digestive:
    - Genito-Urinary:
    - Muscle-Skeletal:
    - Neurologic:

Manual of Clinical Procedures in the Horse, First Edition. Edited by Lais R.R. Costa and Mary Rose Paradis.
© 2018 John Wiley & Sons, Inc. Published 2018 by John Wiley & Sons, Inc.

3.3 Procedure: Obtaining Accurate and Complete History/Anamnesis

Technical action	Rationale
Record accurate information about the client (name and address) and patient (animal's name, age, breed, sex, color, and identification such as microchip, tattoo, etc.).	Proper identification of the animal is critical for medical and legal purposes.
Verify the breed, sex, color, age, and purpose or use of the horse.	Some conditions are more likely depending on the signalment of the animal. Knowing the age, breed, sex, color, and use of the horse will help to rank differential diagnoses.
Identify the respondent (indicate if it is the owner, agent, trainer, RDVM, etc.) and the duration of contact with the animal.	Frequency of observation and level of expertise may affect interpretation of the information obtained.
Inquire about insurance status and, if applicable, clarify whether the insurer is aware of the problem.	It is important to have an idea about the insurance coverage of the animal.
Inquire about equine infectious anemia (EIA) status. Try to obtain the specific date when the last test was done.	EIA testing is mandatory. In most places, animals infected with EIA virus are subjected to euthanasia regardless of other conditions.
Inquire about the previous, present, and intended use of the animal.	Identify predisposing conditions, as well as the owner's expectation for future performance.
Inquire about the presenting complaint and ask questions that focus on recent events. Identify who is responsible for the day to day care of the horse.	Formulate your questions carefully to avoid leading the respondent to providing an affirmative answer, which might be incorrect.
Ask details about treatments administered and current management practices that might impact on the horse's health.	It is not uncommon that the respondent has his/her mind made up about what the medical problem is, which might result in obtaining a misleading history.
Inquire about the duration of the current problem(s) or the date the problem(s) was/were noted, and if it has changed.	This helps to determine if the signs are static, regressing, recurrent or progressing over time.
Inquire about all currently administered medications, including those that are apparently unrelated to the presenting problem.	Administration of certain medications may contribute to or mask the current problem.
Inquire about previous illness(es) as well as previously administered medications.	Previous illness(es) or administration of certain medications may contribute to the current problem.
Ask about any other concerns pertaining to the health of the animal. List all the problems identified by the respondent, and attempt to get an outline of their priorities.	The owner's specific concern(s) may direct the diagnostic testing and the treatment or management. This information will help communication and the probability of meeting the owner's expectations.
Inquire about the horse's diet, including supplements and treats.	Some diseases might be suspected based on deficiency, excess or exposure to potential toxins.
Attempt to obtain accurate information concerning the dietary components as well as amounts.	Dietary practices may predispose the horse to certain problems.

Technical action	Rationale
Inquire about the housing or confinement (stall, paddock, pasture, etc.) and current exercise or training schedule, if applicable. Ask when the horse was last worked, ridden or raced.	Some diseases are more likely in certain types of environment or management practices.
Inquire about vaccination and deworming programs. Attempt to get accurate information of what products were used and when.	The likelihood of some diseases might be increased or decreased based on this information. Ask specific questions to obtain details such as the exact products used and the dates given.
Inquire about dental prophylaxis and hoof care.	The likelihood of some diseases might be increased or decreased based on this information.

3.4 Procedure: Performing Thorough Physical Examination

Technical action	Rationale
While performing a physical examination, record all findings during or immediately after completion of the examination according to a systematic approach: • Examine the horse in an orderly manner. • Summarize the findings related to each body system: general, integument, lymph nodes, cardiovascular, respiratory, alimentary, urinary, reproductive, locomotor, and neurologic.	Following a strict routine will minimize the risk of overlooking components or missing relevant information. At the end of the examination you need to be able to group the findings related to each body system and compile a specific problem list.
If it is an emergency case: • *perform a brief assessment of the patient's condition by obtaining heart rate, respiratory rate, pulse quality, rectal temperature, mucous membrane color and moisture, capillary refill time (CRT), jugular filling time, and skin tent* • *auscult the thorax and abdomen: evaluate heart rhythm and presence of murmurs, respiratory sounds, and gut sounds.*	*In case of emergency, a brief examination should be performed to access the patient's status without delaying the commencement of immediate treatment.*

Perform the physical examination in two phases:
 	
1. General overview
 	
  • Inspection from a distance.
2. Regional examination
 	
  • Palpation, auscultation, percussion, etc. of specific areas.
	Remember:
	
	"Look for nothing yet see what is actually there. Develop a thorough systematic routine identical for each patient seen. Think of pathologic changes rather than specific diseases." Anonymous

General Overview • Perform a general inspection of the horse from a distance to obtain an overall assessment of the horse with respect to its mentation, attitude, posture, ambulation, and breathing (Figure 3.1a and b).	Gather this information prior to handling the horse because these aspects often change once the animal is approached.

(continued)

Technical action	Rationale
Observe the animal's mental attitude and awareness of its surroundings: • bright, quiet or lethargic • alert, indifferent or dull • responsive, sluggish or unresponsive.	A horse's mental attitude may help to understand if it has a localized problem or if it is systemically ill.
Note the horse's behavior and observe posture, ambulation, and head position. Attempt to determine if the horse is anxious or in pain.	This is relevant to assess the patient (in case of neurologic deficit, pain or lameness), as well as for you to determine if sedation might be necessary to perform parts of the examination.
Visually inspect animal for any asymmetry or any deviation of the normal anatomy or conformation (Figure 3.1c). Observe the horse from both sides, and front and back.	Asymmetry of the horse's muscles due to atrophy or hypertrophy may indicate a neurologic or muscular problem. Note conformational defects that might predispose the animal to certain types of lameness.
Obtain the respiratory rate and observe the breathing pattern from a distance. Visually evaluate: • the expansion/relaxation of the ribcage • the contraction of the abdominal muscles • the nostril flaring.	The respiratory rate and breathing pattern often change after the animal is approached. Visual evaluation of the breathing pattern allows you to estimate the respiratory effort (Figure 3.2).
Observe horse's general appearance: body condition, hair coat, hooves, presence of discharge, wounds, drainage, etc. Specifically inspect integument, noting hair coat quality, length, thickness (if appropriate for the season), presence of alopecia, crusts, scales, pruritus, scars, wounds, etc.	To identify potential problems and overall care the animal might be receiving.
At this point you should take a little time to interact with the horse and establish an acquaintance with it so the horse will cooperate with your examination.	Make sure the handler is in tune with you and the horse. Refer to Chapter 1.
Obtain body weight (BW) Attempt to obtain a nearly accurate measure of BW when a scale is available. If a scale is not available the BW should be estimated using weight tape. There are different kinds of weight tape calculations: • based on girth circumference (Figure 3.3); only accurate for adult horses • based on girth circumference and body length (Figure 3.4); there are formulas for adults, weanlings and yearlings, as well as for miniature horses.	Evaluation of BW and body condition score (BCS) is crucial in identifying problems of obesity or underweight/weight loss. Estimation of BW using weight tapes: • Regardless of the type, weight tapes should provide an estimation of weight with a smaller margin of error than rough eyeballing. • Weight tapes are invaluable when used serially in the evaluation of a horse's weight over time. • For weight tapes based on girth circumference and body length, use the following formulas: $$BW_{Adult} = (GC)^2 \times BL/330$$ $$BW_{Yearling} = (GC)^2 \times BL/331$$ $$BW_{Weanling} = (GC)^2 \times BL/280$$ $$BW_{Miniature} = (GC \times 9.36) \times (BL \times 5) - 348.5$$
If weight tape is not available, consider the appropriate average ranges for the breed (Table 3.1).	(GC, girth circumference; BL, body length measurement in inches; and BW, body weight in lbs).

Technical action	Rationale
Obtain the BCS BCS is estimated by palpating along the body areas and averaging the score of all areas: • for a BCS ranging from 1 to 9 palpate and score the neck, withers, ribs, back, tailhead, and behind the shoulders (Figure 3.5 Table 3.2) • for the scale from 0 to 5 palpate and score the neck, back, ribs, and pelvis.	Evaluation of BW and BCS is crucial in identifying problems of obesity or underweight/weight loss and regional adiposity. Palpate and average the score of each area using the appropriate scale: • from 1 to 9, where 1 = poor, 9 = extremely fat, and the ideal is 5/9 (Table 3.2). • from 0 to 5, where 0 = very poor, 5 = very fat, and the ideal is 3/5 (Table 3.3).

If assessment of regional adiposity is indicated additional evaluation may be indicated.

1. Obtain the mean neck circumference as described below and shown in Figure 3.6:

• Measure the distance along a straight line starting at the poll and ending at the cranial aspect of the withers while the head and neck are in a neutral, normal upright position. Divide this distance into four equidistant sections and measure the circumference of the neck at three positions: at the points between the first and second quarters, the second and third quarters, and the third and fourth quarters.
• Calculate the mean of these three measurements.

2. Score the crest of the neck according to the published scoring system (Table 3.4 and Figure 3.7).

Interpretation of mean neck circumference (median and range):

• average size, non-obese, metabolically normal horse 87.7 cm (85.3–95.7 cm)
• average size, obese horse (likely to be insulin-resistant) 105.8 cm (94.3–110.3 cm).

Scoring of the neck crest adiposity ranges from 0 (no apparent crest) to 5 (large crest that droops to one side).

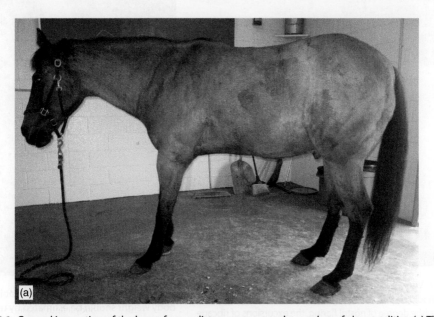

(a)

Figure 3.1 General inspection of the horse from a distance may reveal a number of abnormalities. (a) This horse has a high body condition score, the head position is low and the horse has its weight center towards the hindlimbs (slightly camped out). When walking, the horse shifts its weight to the hindlimbs, suggesting discomfort/pain the in the front limbs. (b) This horse has a noticeable head tilt. (c) This horse has muscle asymmetry (severe atrophy of the left gluteal musculature).

(continued)

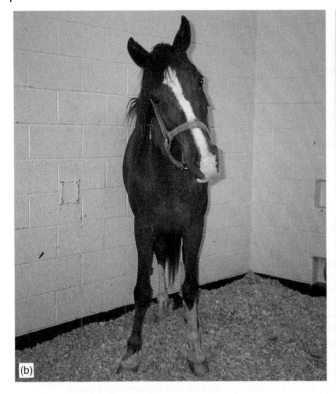

(b)

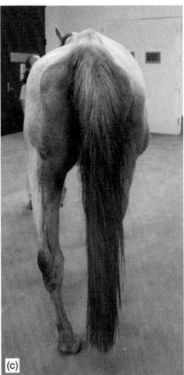

(c)

Figure 3.1 *(continued)*

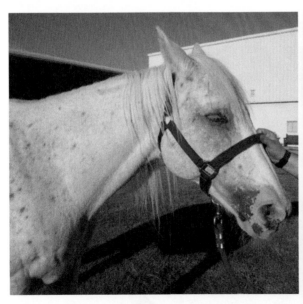

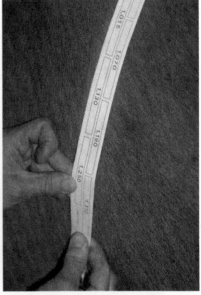

Figure 3.2 Visual evaluation of the respiration and the breathing pattern should be performed to assess the horse's respiratory rate and effort (the degree of nostril flaring, the excursions of ribcage and the degree of contraction of the abdominal muscles) without the interference of anxiety associated with being approached. This is an example of a horse with increased respiratory effort characterized by flaring of the nostrils at rest.

Figure 3.3 When a scale is not available, the body weight should be estimated by using a weight tape. This weight tape provides direct estimation of weight based on girth circumference. This weight tape is only recommended for the estimation of the weight of adult horses.

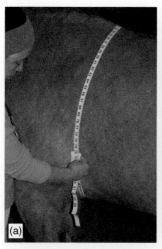
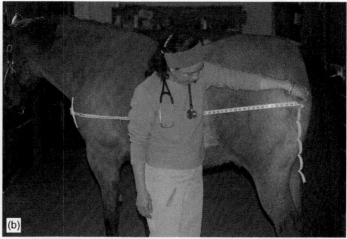

Figure 3.4 Body weight (BW in lbs) can be estimated by a calculation based on (a) girth circumference (GC in inches) and (b) body length (BL in inches). Calculations are performed by using the following formulas: $BW_{Adult} = (GC)^2 \times BL/330$; $BW_{Yearling} = (GC)^2 \times BL/331$; $BW_{Weanling} = (GC)^2 \times BL/280$; and $BW_{Miniature} = (GC \times 9.36) \times (BL \times 5) - 348.5$.

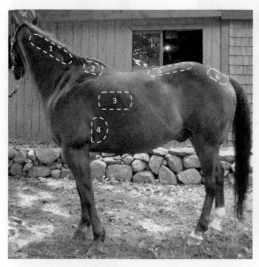
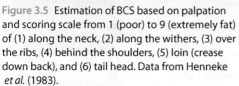

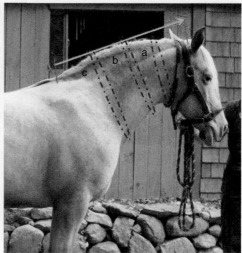

Figure 3.5 Estimation of BCS based on palpation and scoring scale from 1 (poor) to 9 (extremely fat) of (1) along the neck, (2) along the withers, (3) over the ribs, (4) behind the shoulders, (5) loin (crease down back), and (6) tail head. Data from Henneke et al. (1983).

Figure 3.6 Morphometric evaluation of neck circumference to assess regional adiposity. With the head and neck at neutral (i.e., normal upright position), measure the distance along a straight line (green arrow) starting at the poll (cranial orange line) and ending at the cranial aspect of the withers (caudal orange line). Divide this distance into four equidistant sections and measure the circumference of the neck at three positions: a = at the point between the first and second quarters, b = at the point between the second and third quarters, and c = at the point between the third and fourth quarters. Calculate the average of these three measurements to obtain the mean neck circumference. Data from Frank et al. (2006).

(continued)

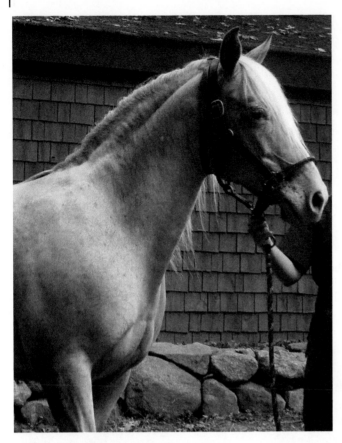

Figure 3.7 Horse with regional adiposity. Note the neck crest score of 3 to 4, according to the scoring system given in Table 3.4.

Table 3.1 Average body weight ranges for various equine breeds at ideal BCS.

	Breed	Age	BW (kg)
Light breeds	THB	Adult	500–600
		Newborn foal	50
	Arab, Morgan, etc.	Adult	450
		Newborn foal	40
	QH	Adult	450–550
		Newborn foal	45
Draft breeds		Adult	700–900
		Newborn foal	80
Pony		Adult	200–350
		Newborn foal	20–35
Miniature	AMH	Adult 30–34″	32–55
		Adult 35–40″	55–92
		Newborn foal	4–9

Table 3.2 Body condition scoring using scale from 1 to 9 (adapted from Henneke *et al.* 1983). The score is calculated by averaging the score for each area. Each area should be palpated, not just visually inspected to more accurately estimate its score.

Condition	Neck	Withers	Shoulder	Ribs	Loin*	Tail head
1 Poor	Bone structure easily noticeable	Bone structure easily noticeable	Bone structure easily noticeable	Ribs protruding prominently	Spinous processes projecting prominently	Tail head, tuber ischii and tuber coxae projecting prominently
2 Very thin	Bone structure faintly discernible	Bone structure faintly discernible	Bone structure faintly discernible	Ribs prominent	Slight fat covering over base of spinous processes; Transverse processes of lumbar vertebrae feel rounded; Spinous processes are prominent	Tail head prominent
3 Thin	Neck accentuated	Withers accentuated	Shoulder accentuated	Slight fat over ribs; Ribs easily discernible	Fat buildup halfway on spinous processes, but easily discernible; Traverse processes cannot be felt	Tail head prominent but individual vertebrae cannot be visually identified; Tuber coxae appear rounded, but are still easily discernible; Tuber ischii not distinguishable
4 Moderately thin	Neck not obviously thin	Withers not obviously thin	Shoulder not obviously thin	Faint outline of ribs discernible	Negative crease (peaked appearance) along back	Prominence depends on conformation; Fat can be felt. Tuber coxae not discernible
5 Moderate (ideal weight)	Neck blends smoothly into body	Withers rounded over spinous processes	Shoulder blends smoothly into body	Ribs cannot be visually distinguished, but can be easily felt	Back is level	Fat around tail head beginning to feel soft
6 Moderately fleshy	Fat beginning to be deposited	Fat beginning to be deposited	Fat beginning to be deposited	Fat over ribs feels spongy	May have a slight positive crease (a groove) down back	Fat around tail head feels soft
7 Fleshy	Fat deposited along neck	Fat deposited along withers	Fat deposited behind shoulder	Individual ribs can be felt with pressure, but there is noticeable fat filling between ribs	May have a positive crease down the back	Fat around tail head is soft
8 Fat	Noticeable thickening of neck	Area along withers filled with fat	Area behind shoulder filled in flush with body	Difficult to feel ribs	Positive crease down the back	Fat around tail head very soft
9 Extremely fat	Bulging fat	Bulging fat	Bulging fat	Patchy fat appearing over ribs	Obvious crease down the back	Bulging fat around tail head

*(Thoracolumbar epaxial muscles)

Table 3.3 Alternative body condition score, scale 0 to 5. Calculate BCS by averaging the score for each area.

	Neck	Back and ribs	Pelvis
0 Very poor	Markedly thin neck with a concave arch Narrow and slack at base	Skin tight over visible ribs Spinous processes sharp and easily seen	Angular pelvis, skin tight Deep cavity under tail and either side of croup
1 Poor	Thin neck with a concave arch Narrow and slack at base	Ribs easily visible Skin sunken either side of backbone Spinous processes well defined	Rump sunken, but skin supple Pelvis and croup well defined Deep depression under tail
2 Moderate	Narrow but firm	Ribs just visible Backbone well covered Spinous processes felt	Rump flat either side of backbone Croup well defined with some fat Slight cavity under tail
3 Good	No crest (except stallions) Firm neck	Ribs just covered but easily felt No "gutter" along back Spinous processes covered but can be felt	Covered by fat and rounded No "gutter" Pelvis easily felt
4 Fat	Slight crest Wide and firm	Ribs well covered, need firm pressure to feel them "Gutter" along backbone	"Gutter" to root of tail Pelvis covered by soft fat Pelvis felt only with firm pressure
5 Very fat	Marked crest Very wide and firm folds of fat	Ribs buried, cannot feel them Deep "gutter" Back broad and flat	Deep "gutter" to root of tail Skin distended Pelvis buried, cannot feel it

The scores can be adjusted by 0.5 points if they correspond to a description between the scores outlined.
Adapted from Leighton-Hardman (1988) *Equine Veterinary Journal*, **20** (1), 41–45.

Table 3.4 Evaluation of regional adiposity by standardized scoring of neck crest (Carter *et al.* 2009).

Score	Appearance of the crest	Palpation
0	No noticeable crest	No palpable crest
1	No noticeable crest	Slight filling felt
2	Noticeable appearance of crest Fat deposit evenly from poll to withers	Crest easily cupped in one hand and can be moved side to side easily
3	Enlarged and thickened crest, so that fat deposits more heavily in the middle of the neck than towards the poll and withers, giving a mounded appearance	Crest fills cupped hand, not as easily moved from side to side
4	Grossly enlarged and thickened crest, so that fat deposits have a wrinkles appearance	Crest no longer fits into a cupped hand Crest is not easily moved from side to side
5	Very large wrinkled crest that permanently droops to one side	Wrinkled and lumpy feel

Technical action	Rationale
It is generally easier to approach the horse by its left side, positioning yourself next to the shoulder. Start examining the horse in a non-threatening, easy, and quiet way.	Always let the horse know what you intend to do. Take this opportunity to auscult the heart carefully and quietly, while stroking the horse's withers (Figure 3.8).
Regional examination Proceed by examining each section of the animal, and as you do so try to determine how comfortable the horse is with your presence, and how the horse responds to your maneuvers. Areas to be evaluated include: • head, eyes, ears, nose, and throat • neck, torso, and back • thorax (cardiac and pulmonary assessments) and abdomen (gastrointestinal assessment) • external genitalia and perineum • limbs. During the examination, obtain a rectal temperature. At the end of the examination observe the horse's movements with respect to the locomotor and neurologic systems. Detailed explanation of regional examination are described below (next 6 pages).	If you are able to gain the horse's cooperation, the examination will be greatly facilitated. Gather visual, tactile, auditory, and olfactory information for the entire animal, including head, neck, thorax, abdomen, limbs, and tail. The exact order of examination may vary amongst clinicians, but make sure to consistently perform the examination following a pattern that suits you, for example starting front to back working around the animal on the left side and the right side. Do not narrow your focus prematurely on any particular area. Avoid areas that are likely to be sore or cause the horse discomfort. Leave those areas to be evaluated last. Start in areas that are going to help you gain the trust of the horse.
Once the horse is accustomed to being touched, move towards the head and proceed with the examination, touching the horse's neck and head as you move.	You can palpate the submandibular area as you move towards the head of the horse (Figure 3.9).

Once at the head of the horse:
 	
• Observe for the presence and character of discharge from eyes, nose, and ears.
• Evaluate the nostrils for:
  – evidence of discharge and appearance of discharge
  – airflow, bilaterally (Figure 3.10a)
	Make sure to not place yourself in a vulnerable position if the horse moves its head or front legs.
	
	Note the amount and character of discharge, and if it is unilateral or bilateral.
	
	Clear nasal discharge is often seen after exercise, trailering or in respiratory viral infections.
	
	Mucopurulent nasal discharge is often seen with suppurative inflammation such as in bacterial infections.
	
	Ocular discharge might indicate a blocked nasolacrimal duct.

• Air movement should be equal from both nostrils (Figure 3.10a). • Observe nostril dilation or flaring (Figure 3.10b) and how it changes during the respiratory cycle. • Check for any abnormal odor (be careful when placing your face near the horse's head to smell the horse's nose and breath).	Unequal air movement between nostrils suggests obstruction of nasal passages. Abnormal smell is common in infections of the nasal conchae, sinuses, teeth, and guttural pouches. Avoid getting hit on the face by the horse's head.
Observe symmetry or any deviation from the normal anatomy of the head, nose, eyes, ears, and throat. If asymmetry is noted, try to determine which side is normal (whether there is swelling or atrophy).	Presence of swellings or depressions may indicate current or past injuries. Examples of asymmetries include: • swelling over the paranasal sinuses • atrophy of masseter or temporal muscles • deviation of the muzzle (droopy nose and lip), droopy ear and eyelid • phthisis bulbi (shrunken and often non-functional eye) as a result of chronic ocular diseases (Figure 3.11).

(continued)

Technical action	Rationale
Evaluate the horse's vision: • Menace: by moving a hand towards the eye, without creating air current or touching the hair, and eliciting the blink reflex (Figure 3.12a). • Pupillary light responses, direct and consensual: by shining a bright light while in a darkened environment and observing constriction of the pupils (Figure 3.12b,c).	Evaluation of vision is part of the ocular as well as neurologic examinations. Abnormal responses warrant further evaluation (for ocular and neurologic examination, see Chapters 62 and 74, respectively).
Examine the eyes briefly, evaluating for any obvious deviation from the normal appearance of ocular structures such as changes in size, asymmetries, the presence of scars, opacities, and cloudiness (Figure 3.13). Evaluate each structure: • globe and orbit for asymmetries and changes in size • eyelids and adnexa • conjunctiva and third eyelid • cornea should be transparent, smooth, and glistening • anterior chamber: aqueous humor should be clear, note any cloudiness or other abnormalities • iris and pupil for size and position • lens: should be clear	Identify any abnormality, such as: • tearing (epiphora) • squinting (blepharospasm) • shrinkage of the globe (phthisis bulbi), often from severe trauma or intraocular inflammation • enlargement of the globe (buphthalmos), as in glaucoma • protrusion of the globe (exophthalmos), usually from enlarged structures in the retrobulbar space • entropion, presence of growths, protrusion of the third eyelid, and other lid abnormalities • corneal irregularities, opacities, pigmentation, vascularization, and scarring • aqueous flare (protein), hypopyon (accumulation of inflammatory cells), hyphema (hemorrhage) in the anterior chamber • abnormalities of the iris (such as anterior and posterior synechia). • opacity of lenses (cataracts) Detection of ocular abnormalities warrants further evaluation. Comprehensive ocular examination is discussed in Chapter 62.
Lift the upper lid while turning the head up slightly in order to evaluate the color of the sclera (Figure 3.14).	The sclera should be white and any abnormalities should be noted: • yellow tinged (jaundice) • presence of injected blood vessels.

Palpate the peripheral arterial pulse to determine pulse quality (character/amplitude and regularity). The peripheral arteries that are usually used are:
 	
• the facial arteries at the ventral aspect of the body of the mandibles (Figure 3.15a)
• the transverse facial arteries just caudal to the lateral canthus of the eye (Figure 3.15b)
• the median arteries in the medial aspect of the proximal antebrachium.
	The pulse quality of peripheral arteries reflects cardiac activity (heart rate and rhythm) and hemodynamic states:
	
	• pulse regularity reflects heart rhythm
	• pulse character might be qualified as normal, weak, bounding or variable
	• pulse amplitude is indicative of arterial blood pressure, estimated as the difference of pressure exerted by the fingers to occlude and then reopen the arterial pulse:
	  – waterhammer arterial pulse might indicate cardiac valvular disease
	  – variable pulse quality and irregularity result from cardiac arrhythmias.

Evaluate skin turgor by tenting the skin (Figure 3.16): • Pinch the skin over the shoulder or neck (with thumb and forefinger) and release it, then count the time it takes for the skin to get back to normal (it should take <1 second).	Care must be taken in evaluating skin tenting in older horses as decreased skin elasticity associated with ageing will result in prolonged skin tenting. Subcutaneous fat affects skin retraction time.

Technical action	Rationale

• Prolonged duration of skin tenting categories:
  – Mild: 1–3 seconds
  – Moderate: 3–5 seconds
  – Severe: >5 seconds.
• Prolongation of skin tenting indicates decreased skin turgor and, although subjective and imprecise, suggests some degree of dehydration (especially if considered in conjunction with moistness of mucous membranes and CRT).
	• Skin turgor varies depending on the anatomical site (e.g., upper eyelid, neck, over the shoulder), so in dehydrated horses the duration of skin tenting is not the same in different sites. Therefore, perform the skin tenting consistently on the same anatomical locations in order to minimize imprecision.

Evaluate and palpate both jugular veins (Figure 3.17), assessing: • symmetry • the patency of the jugular veins by evaluating jugular distension after occlusion and presence of firmness in the jugular groove	When evaluating the jugular vein patency, the lack of jugular distension on digital pressure to occlude the venous return, often accompanied by firmness in the jugular groove, is an indication of partial or complete jugular obstruction secondary to phlebitis or thrombophlebitis.
• the extent of distension without digital occlusion • the extent of distension after digital occlusion at the base of the neck	Jugular distension when the head is lowered is normal because the vein is ventral to the right atrium. When the head in the erect position, jugular distension results from impaired venous return, which can be secondary to jugular obstruction, increased central venous pressure and volume overload secondary to right-sided heart failure, mass in thorax, or severe pleural effusion. Further evaluation is warranted.
• jugular filling by measuring the time taken for the vein to fill completely after digital occlusion of venous return: if only one vein is occluded it should take less than 4-5 seconds; if both veins are occluded it should take less than 2-3 seconds	Jugular filling time is a crude and subjective estimation of cardiac output. Delayed jugular filling time occurs with hypovolemia and severe cardiac disease.
• the presence/extent of jugular pulsation. Normally, pulsation is present when the horse has its head lower than its heart, and disappears when the head is raised. Slight pulsation of the distal third of the jugular, while the horse has an erect head position is normal. Note the presence of jugular pulsation extending beyond the distal third of the neck.	If jugular pulsation extends beyond the distal third of the neck, while the head is held erect, further evaluation is warranted.
Part the lips to expose the oral mucous membrane (Figure 3.18a) and evaluate for: • Moistness • Color: can range from pale pink (normal) to brick red (injected), purple (congested), bluish (cyanotic), or yellowish to orange (icteric); note if presence of dark "bluish" line near the gum line • Presence of petechial hemorrhages, vesicles, ulcers, etc. • Obtain CRT by applying digital pressure to blanch the mucous membrane above the incisors and recording the time it takes for the color to return (Figure 3.18c).	Oral mucous membranes should be pale pink, glistening/moist, and CRT <2 seconds (Figure 3.18b). Color might be affected by lighting. CRT is an indicator of tissue perfusion and cardiovascular function: • prolonged CRT indicates hypoperfusion due to hypovolemia, poor cardiac output or peripheral vasoconstriction • shortened CRT indicates peripheral vasodilation. Be attentive for the presence of petechial hemorrhages and/or increased reddening of the mucous membranes as these might be signs systemic inflammation.

(continued)

Technical action	Rationale
Determine if the horse is receptive to have its mouth examined before proceeding with the oral/dental examination.	If the horse is uncooperative and resents having its mouth examined, forgo oral/dental examination.
If the horse seems cooperative, open the mouth and evaluate:	If able to perform brief oral and dental examination:
• tongue, labial, gingival, lingual, and buccal mucosa for lesions • dental age, dentition (particularly evaluating for malocclusions) • smell for abnormal odor.	• evaluate mucosa for the presence of lesions such as ulcers and vesicles • evaluate teeth for enamel points, hooks, overgrown crowns, missing teeth and other malocclusions. • malodorous breath suggests dental disease.
Comprehensive oral/dental examination is discussed in Chapter 11.	
Percuss the area of the frontal and maxillary sinuses while the mouth is partially open (Figure 3.19). Percussion of sinuses should elicit a "hollow" sound. Identify if a "dull" sound or pain are elicited.	Percussing the sinuses while the mouth is slightly open will increase the resonance and make sounds more distinctive. Eliciting a "dull" sound indicates the sinuses are filled, as in cases of sinusitis. Percussion might cause discomfort.
Palpate between the rami of the mandibles and locate the mandibular (aka submandibular) lymph nodes, evaluating their size and consistency (Figure 3.9). Normally, the mandibular lymph nodes are small and round. They may be difficult to find in a healthy adult horse, whereas young horses normally have fairly noticeable lymph nodes.	Note any enlargement of these lymph nodes and swelling in the throatlatch area. If enlargement is noted, consider the possibility of strangles and take precautions to avoid spreading contagious agents.
Palpate the throatlatch area (Figure 3.20). Feel the laryngeal cartilages and muscles to check for asymmetry. Note any scarring or thickening of the skin. Palpate the region of the Viborg's triangle (guttural pouch and retropharyngeal area) to determine any distortion or enlargement. Press gently on the larynx, normally this will not elicit cough.	Note any prominence or asymmetry in the throat area. Scars in this area might suggest previous surgery such as laringoplasty. Distortion in the area of Viborg's triangle suggests disease of the guttural pouch or retropharyngeal lymphoadenopathy.
Slide the hands caudally and palpate the thyroid gland with one lobe adjacent to each side of the trachea. Evaluate symmetry and size.	The thyroid glands in the horse are very movable between a more superficial and a deeper location. Note any enlargement.
Evaluate the neck for symmetry, anatomical deviations, and sign of pain (Figure 3.21).	The presence of swellings or depressions in the neck suggests current or past injury.
Place one hand on each side of the cervical column, palpating the transverse processes of the cervical vertebrae.	Pain and decreased range of motion of the cervical column are seen in cervical vertebral disease and warrant further evaluation (see Chapter 74).
Maneuver the neck and ask the horse to flex the neck ventrally, turning to the left and right to check the range of motion and pain, if indicated.	
Palpate the trachea.	Note any asymmetries, distortion or narrowing of the trachea.

Technical action	Rationale
Slide your hands over the shoulders, down the thoracic limb (Figure 3.22a) to the foot, feel changes in the skin and hoof temperature, and palpate the digital pulses (Figure 3.22b) of the each of the front feet, comparing them.	Note if there is an increase in warmth as you move your hand distally and over the hooves. Note any increased pulse of the digital artery. Warmth and increased digital pulse suggest inflammation, as in laminitis or hoof abscesses. Conversely, note if the extremities are cold.
Observe the position of the neck and elbow to evaluate possible discomfort in the chest.	A stretched neck and abducted elbow are abnormal positions that suggest pain in the thorax.

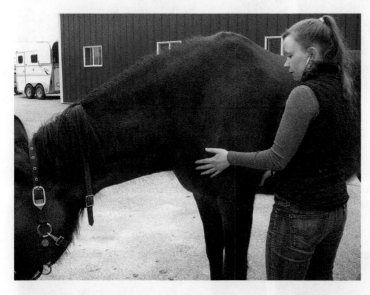

Figure 3.8 Approach the horse by its left side, positioning yourself next to the horse's left shoulder. Start with auscultation of the heart as this is a way to start examining the horse in a non-threatening, easy, and quiet way. Take this opportunity to stroke the horse.

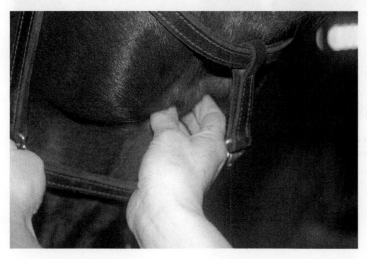

Figure 3.9 Palpate the submandibular area, between the rami of mandibles, feeling for the size and consistency of the left and right mandibular (aka submandibular) lymph nodes. The mandibular lymph nodes may be difficult to find in a normal adult horse. Note in this horse both left (between the fingers) and right lymph nodes are enlarged.

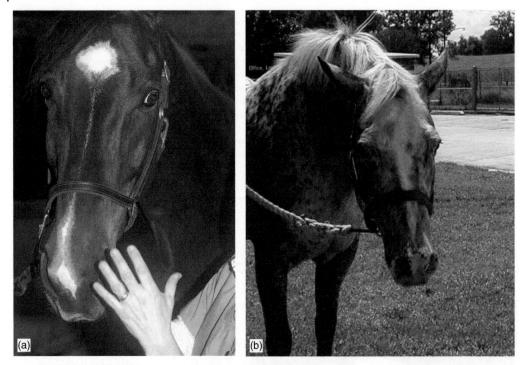

Figure 3.10 Evaluate the nostrils for (a) the presence airflow bilaterally, as air movement should be equal from both nostrils, and (b) nostril flaring while at rest, which suggests dyspnea.

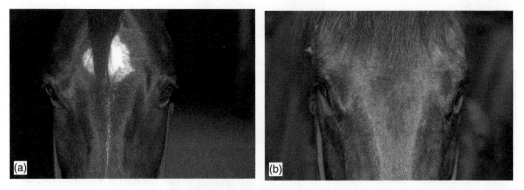

Figure 3.11 Observe symmetry or any deviation from the normal anatomy of the head, nose, eyes, ears, and throat. (a) Normal symmetrical eyes and (b) symmetrically abnormal eyes (phthisis bulbi bilaterally).

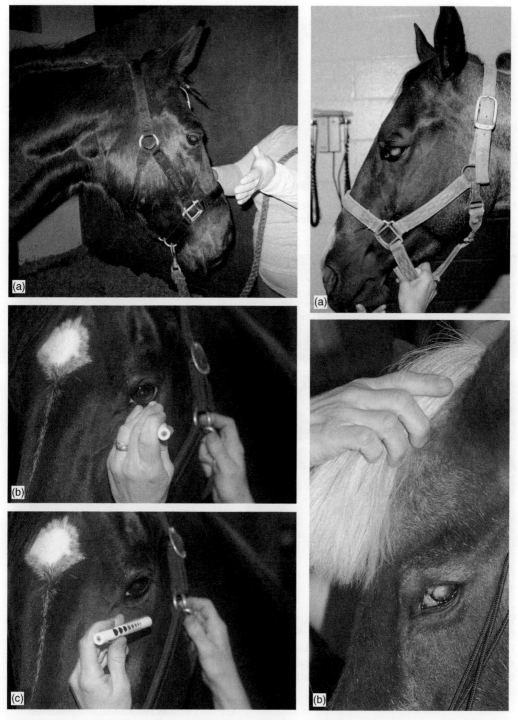

Figure 3.12 Evaluate the horse's vision. (a) Test the menace by moving a hand towards the eye, without creating an air current or touching the hair, and eliciting blink reflex. (b and c) Test the pupillary light responses by shinning a bright light, while in a darkened environment, and observing constriction of the pupils, direct and consensual, respectively.

Figure 3.13 Examine the eyes, noting any obvious deviation from the normal appearance of ocular structures. (a) Corneal edema causing severe opacity. (b) Phthisis bulbi and cloudiness.

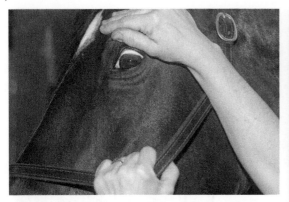

Figure 3.14 Lift the upper lid while turning the head up slightly in order to evaluate the color of the sclera and check for the presence of scleral injection.

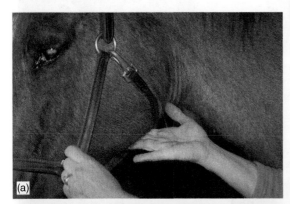

(a)

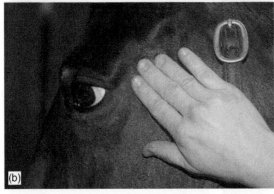

(b)

Figure 3.15 Evaluate the peripheral arterial pulse by palpating (a) the facial artery at the ventral aspect of the body of the mandible and (b) the transverse facial artery lateral to the lateral canthus.

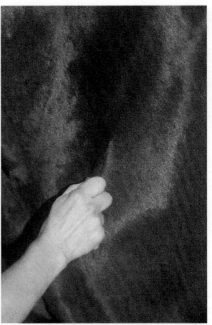

Figure 3.16 Evaluate skin turgor by pinching the skin over the shoulder (with thumb and forefinger) and releasing it, then count the time it takes for the skin to get back to normal.

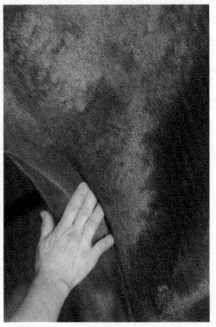

Figure 3.17 Evaluate and palpate each jugular vein, assessing them for patency, symmetry, and extent of distension without digital occlusion, and determining the jugular filling by measuring the time taken for the vein to fill completely after digital occlusion of venous return.

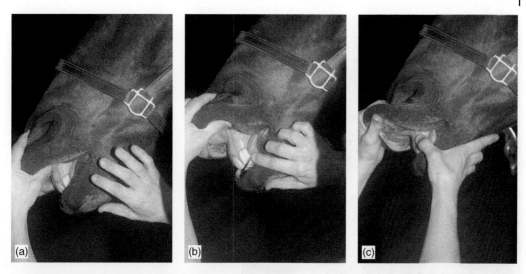

Figure 3.18 (a) Part the lips to expose the oral mucous membrane. (b) Evaluate for moistness and color, which normally should be pale pink. (c) Determine the CRT by applying digital pressure to blanch out the mucous membrane above the incisors and counting the seconds it takes for the mucous membrane to regain its color.

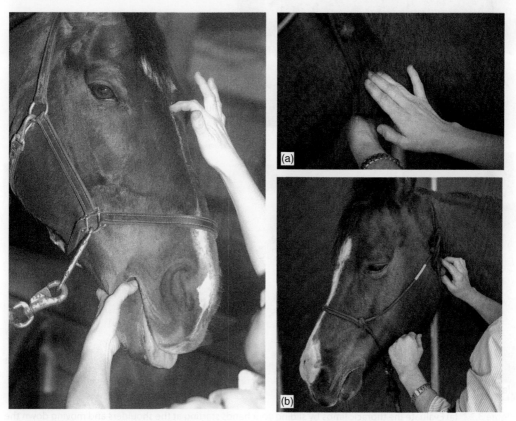

Figure 3.19 Percuss the area of the frontal and maxillary sinuses while the mouth is partially open. Percussion of normal sinuses should elicit a "hollow" sound.

Figure 3.20 Evaluate the cranial cervical area. (a) Palpate the throatlatch area and feel the laryngeal cartilages and muscles to check for asymmetry, scarring or thickening of the skin. (b) Palpate the region of Viborg's triangle (guttural pouch and retropharyngeal area) to determine any distortion or enlargement.

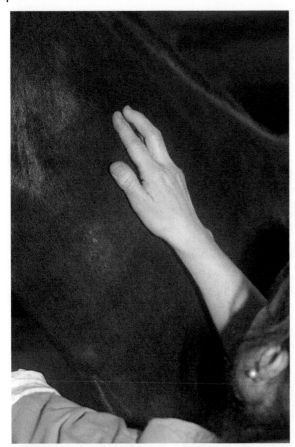

Figure 3.21 Palpate the neck along the cervical vertebrae with one hand on each side of the cervical column, palpating the transverse processes of the cervical vertebrae, and evaluate for symmetry, anatomical deviations, and sign of pain.

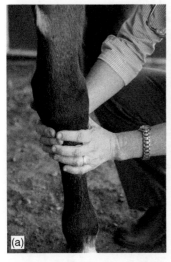

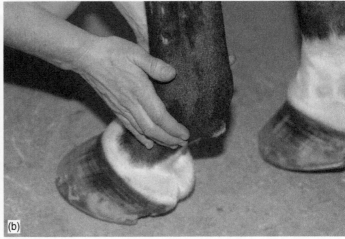

(a)

(b)

Figure 3.22 (a) Evaluate the thoracic limbs by sliding your hands starting at the shoulders and moving down the limb to the foot, feeling for changes in temperature towards the extremities (down to the hoof wall). (b) Palpate the digital arteries in the front feet on the palmar lateral and medial aspects distal to the proximal sesamoid bones.

Technical action	Rationale
Proceed with evaluation of the chest, assessing the heart and lungs. Start by placing your left hand flat over the chest underneath the triceps and feeling the apex beat (Figure 3.23).	The order in which you perform thoracic examination is a personal preference. Regardless of the order, conduct the auscultation in a quiet area.
Perform careful auscultation of the heart on both sides of the chest. The heart sounds are summarized in Table 3.5. Start with the stethoscope placed on the left side of the thorax under the triceps muscle at the level dorsal to the elbow (Figure 3.24). Identify the heart sounds (Table 3.5). Move the stethoscope bell one or two intercostal spaces dorsally and cranially to the level just ventral to the point of the shoulder, listening for at least 2 minutes. Obtain the HR and listen for rhythm. Obtain the HR over 60, 30, and 15 seconds. Alterations in rhythm can result in variable bpm over different evaluation times. If an alteration in rhythm is noted, determine the regularity of the arrhythmia Palpate the pulse at the facial artery and verify if the HR matches the pulse. Note any abnormalities in rhythm. Evaluate each of the four valve areas for at least 1 minute in each location, noting the presence of murmurs. • First, on the left side at the level dorsal to the elbow to focus on the mitral valve region. • Second, move cranially and dorsally (well under the triceps muscle) to listen to the aortic valve sounds. • Third, move slightly cranial and ventral (again deeper under the triceps muscle) for the pulmonic valve sounds. • Lastly, move to the right side of the chest, at approximately a hand's width dorsal to the point of the elbow for the tricuspid valve region. If presence of murmur(s), is noted, attempt to characterize it: • the timing of the murmur (Table 3.6): palpate the pulse on the facial artery while ausculting the heart: – systolic begins with or after S1 and ends before or with S2 – diastolic begins with or after S2 and ends with or before S1 of the next cycle • the grade of the murmur, ranging from 1 to 6 (Table 3.7)	Cardiac evaluation includes the rate, rhythm, and the presence of murmurs. First evaluate the rate and rhythm. The normal resting heart rate (HR) of adult horses ranges from 28 to 40 beats per minute (bpm). If the horse appears anxious or nervous with the examination or excited, allow some time then recheck the HR. Note if there are any pulse deficits. A combination of two to four heart sounds might be heard on the normal horse. Note any deviation from a regular rhythm. Second-degree atrioventricular blocks are a common finding in horses and in most cases have little clinical significance, disappearing when the HR increases, as with exercise. Persistent abnormalities in HR and rhythm warrant further investigation. To interpret the murmur(s) you first need to characterize the murmur(s) with respect to timing, location, grade, quality, and shape. However, it is important to remember that generalizations concerning the interpretation of murmurs tend to lead to erroneous conclusions. Be cognizant that more than one murmur may be present. For instance, generally grade 1/6 or 2/6 systolic murmurs might be flow murmurs with little clinical significance. It is important to emphasize the words "generally" and "might" and remember that there will be exceptions. Similarly, grade 3/6 to 6/6 systolic murmurs and all diastolic murmurs should be considered pathologic until proven otherwise. The words "should be considered" must be emphasized. Moreover, the temporal relationship between the murmur and the heart sounds (if the murmur interferes with the normal sounds) should be determined. When a murmur is detected, further evaluation of its significance is warranted.

Technical action	Rationale

- the localization of the point of maximum intensity (PMI)
- the character of the murmur, including:
  - the quality of the murmur (soft, noisy, rumbling, musical)
  - the "shape" of the murmur (crescendo-decrescendo, band-shaped, crescendo, decrescendo).

See Table 3.8 for a summary of common cardiac murmurs.

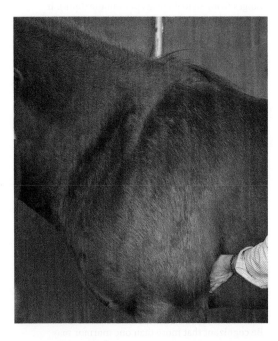

Figure 3.23 Place your left hand flat over the chest underneath the triceps and feel the apex beat.

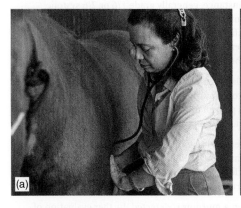
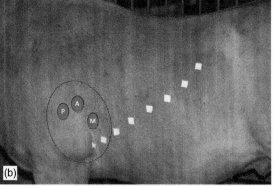

Figure 3.24 Perform careful auscultation of the heart. (a) Start with the stethoscope placed on the left side of the thorax under the triceps muscle at the level dorsal to the elbow. (b) Move the stethoscope bell in order to auscult the mitral(M), aortic(A), and pulmonic(P) valves on the left side of the horse's chest.

Table 3.5 Heart sounds in the horse

	Point of maximum intensity		Event in the Cardiac Cycle
S1	Left apex	Loud High frequency	AV valves closure; Semilunar valves opening; Ventricular contraction; Ejection of blood into great vessels.
S2	Left base	Loud High frequency	Semilunar valves closure; AV valves opening
S3	Left apex	Soft Low frequency	Deceleration of blood into the ventricles; Rapid ventricular filling
S4	Left base	Soft Low frequency	Atrial contraction

Table 3.6 Timing of murmurs in the horse

Systolic	Murmur begins with or after S1 and ends before or with S2	
	Pansystolic	Murmur begins with S1 and extends into S2
	Holosystolic	Extends between S1 and S2 but does not encroach on either
Diastolic	Murmur begins with or after S2 and ends with or before S1 of the next cycle	
	Holodiastolic	Extends between S2 and S1
Continuous	Murmur spans through systole and diastole	

Table 3.7 Intensity of murmurs

Grade 1	Softest, only audible after careful auscultation
Grade 2	Faint murmur, audible only when the stethoscope is placed over the PMI
Grade 3	Moderately loud, audible not only at the PMI
Grade 4	Loud murmur, audible over a wide area, but no palpable thrill is present
Grade 5	Loud murmur, audible over a wide area, and a palpable thrill is present
Grade 6	Loud murmur, audible even when the stethoscope is just lifted off the thoracic surface, and a palpable thrill is always present

PMI, point of maximum intensity.

Table 3.8 Types of murmurs in the horse

Side	Timing	Point of maximum intensity	Intensity	Duration	Quality	Murmur
Left	Systolic	M or M and A	2/6 to 6/6	Holosystolic or pansystolic	Mixed, plateau	Mitral regurgitation
		M or A	1/6 to 3/6	Early, mid, late or holosystolic	Low frequency	Physiologic or flow
		M	2/6 to 6/6	Mid or late	Crescendo	Mitral valve prolapse
		P	3/6 to 6/6	Holosystolic or pansystolic	Plateau	VSD (best heard on the right side)
	Diastolic	M, A or P	1/6 to 3/6	Early, mid, late	Low frequency	Physiologic or flow
		A	1/6 to 6/6	Holodiastolic	Low frequency, decrescendo, decrescendo musical	Aortic regurgitation
		P	1/6 to 6/6	Holodiastolic	Low frequency, decrescendo musical	Pulmonic regurgitation
Right	Diastolic	T	1/6 to 3/6	Early, mid, late	Low frequency	Physiologic or flow
	Systolic	T	2/6 to 6/6	Holosystolic or pansystolic	Mixed, Plateau	Tricuspid regurgitation
			3/6 to 6/6	Holosystolic or pansystolic	Plateau	VSD
			2/6 to 6/6	Mid to Late	Crescendo	Tricuspid valve prolapse
			1/6 to 2/6	Early, mid, late or holosystolic	Low frequency	Physiologic or flow

VSD = ventricular septal defect.

Technical action	Rationale
Evaluate the breathing pattern and respiratory rate (RR). Note any prolongation in expiration or inspiration. Note the abdominal component of expiration. Determine if the breathing pattern and RR have changed from your initial assessment at a distance.	The resting RR ranges from 8 to 16 breaths per minute. Normally, there should be limited chest wall excursion and minimal movement of the nostrils. Prolongation and increased abdominal component of expiration suggest lower respiratory disease. Increased abdominal effort at the end of expiration is seen with obstructive pulmonary disease.
Auscult the trachea (Figure 3.25a).	
Air movement through the trachea should sound like wind going through a clear pipe.	Note the presence of fluid (rattling with air movement) stridor or wheezes in the trachea.
Carefully auscult the lungs on both sides of the chest (Figure 3.25b).	Normal tidal (resting) breathing is quiet, so few sounds are detectable.
If breathing is effortless and quiet with minimal chest excursion, a rebreathing bag might be applied and auscultation repeated (Figure 3.26).	
Evaluate breath sounds throughout the entire lung field. Note: • if the bronchovesicular sounds are louder or quieter than normal • if there is radiation of heart sounds • the presence, character, and timing of adventitial sound, such as wheezes and crackles • the presence, frequency, and character of cough • the absence of or muffled sounds ventrally suggestive of effusion.	The application of a rebreathing bag induces more frequent and deeper respiration by recruiting airways and alveolar parenchyma, leading to air movement throughout the lungs and exacerbation and accentuation of abnormal sounds. Use of a rebreathing bag is contraindicated in horses with severe effort or dyspnea.

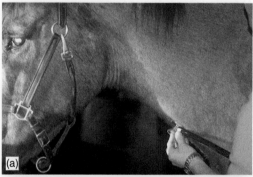

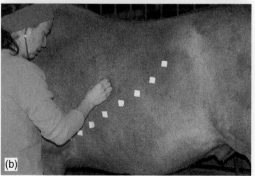

Figure 3.25 Assess the lower respiratory tract. (a) Auscult the trachea. The air movement through the trachea should sound like wind going through a clear pipe, whereas the presence of mucus or secretion in the trachea results in a gurgling sound. (b) Carefully perform auscultation of the lung on both sides of the chest, evaluating the breath sounds throughout the entire lung field on the left and right sides. The border is a line drawn from the 16th rib at the level of the tuber coxae to the 11th rib at the level of the point of the shoulder and ending ventrally near the elbow.

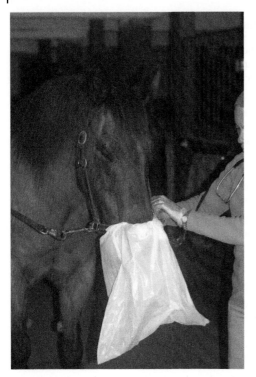

Figure 3.26 Where breathing is effortless and quiet with minimal chest excursion, auscultation of the lungs is repeated after application of a rebreathing bag. The application of a rebreathing bag induces more frequent and deeper respiration by recruiting airways and alveolar parenchyma, leading to air movement throughout the lungs, and exacerbation and accentuation of abnormal sounds. Continue auscultation after removal of the rebreathing bag because the breaths are often deepest right after the removal of the bag. Ensure bag does not close in on the nostrils.

Technical action	Rationale
Systematically auscult the abdomen on both sides (Figures 3.27a,b).	Abdominal auscultation and percussion are critical in the examination of a horse. Most abdominal abnormalities in the horse are associated with the digestive system and involve alteration of gastrointestinal motility.
Divide the abdomen into four quadrants:	
<ul><li>upper left = left paralumbar to midflank</li><li>lower left = left midflank to ventral abdomen</li><li>upper right = right paralumbar to midflank</li><li>lower right = right midflank to ventral abdomen.</li></ul>	Sounds originating from the large intestine tend to be of lower intensity and deeper than the sounds originating from the small intestine. Ausculatation of the right paralumbar area should reveal a high-pitch rumbling sound resembling water flush down a pipe (ileocecocolic sound); normally the ileocecocolic sound should occur once to three times per minute.
Listen to each quadrant for at least 1 to 2 minutes.	
Listen for the presence of borborygmi (rumbling, bubbling sounds), frequency, intensity, duration and character of the sounds.	
Percuss the dorsal quadrants (Figure 3.27c) to evaluate for the presence of tympany.	Lack of gut sounds for 4 to 5 minutes indicates marked abnormality.
	Assessment of the abdomen in horses is challenging and often requires rectal palpation (see Chapter 16).
Evaluate the contour of the thorax and abdomen, note the shape.	View the horse from each side, and front and back.
Note the presence of swelling of the pectoral area (Figure 3.28a), under the thorax (Figure 3.28b) and under the abdomen, and any dependent edema (Figure 3.28c). Note any abdominal distension.	

Technical action	Rationale
Evaluate the male external genitalia: • prepuce and penis, scrotum of castrated males (Figure 3.28d) • prepuce and penis, scrotum and testicles of intact males • palpate testicles for number, size and position.	If possible observe the horse urinating. Exposure of the penis may require sedation. Further evaluation of the stallion requires specific reproductive examination (see Chapter 35).
Assessment of the mare's external genitalia. Evaluate perineal conformation. Check for evidence of vaginal discharge and urine scalding. Observe the vulva and vaginal mucosa. Observe and palpate the mammary area, including the udder and teats for condition, secretion, edema and tumors.	Abnormal vulvar conformation can lead to vaginal and uterine infection. Further evaluation of the mare requires specific reproductive examination (see Chapter 36).

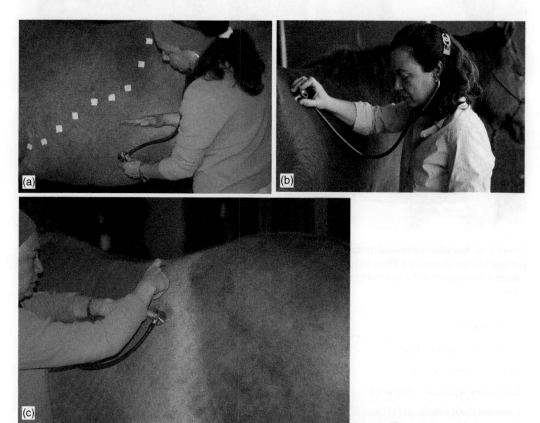

Figure 3.27 Systematically auscult the abdomen on both sides by dividing the abdomen into four quadrants: upper left = left paralumbar to midflank, lower left = left midflank to ventral abdominal region, upper right = right paralumbar to midflank, and lower right = right midflank to ventral abdominal region. (a) Note the white tape outlining the thorax, and the division of one side (left) of the abdomen into upper and lower quadrants as indicated by clinician's arm.(b) Auscult the right paralumbar fossa and carefully evaluate for the cecal contraction sounds. (c) Percuss the dorsal quadrants to evaluate for the presence of tympany (place the stethoscope on the flank region while flicking your finger on different regions of the abdomen around the stethoscope. Tympany will be noted as a high-pitched "pinging" sound.

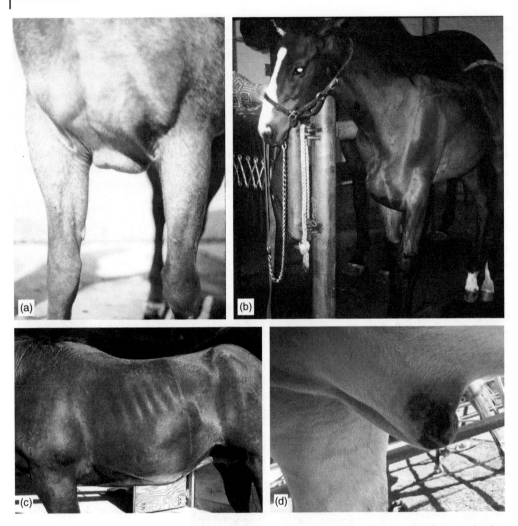

Figure 3.28 Evaluate the ventral thoracic and abdominal region. (a) This mare has ventral edema under the pectorals to the xiphoid. (b) This colt has enlargement in the pectoral area. (c) This mare has a plaque of ventral edema extending from the xiphoid to the mammary gland. (d) This gelding has an ulcerated lesion on the prepuce.

Technical action	Rationale
Evaluate perineum and tail.	Normal rectal temperature of an adult horse ranges between 99 and 101.5°F (i.e., 37.2 and 38.7°C).
Check anal and tail tone.	
Check for evidence of loose stool.	
Lubricate the thermometer (Figure 3.29a) and obtain rectal temperature (Figure 3.29b).	
Evaluate the thoracic limbs starting from the feet and proceeding proximally.	Look for any deviation from the normal anatomy (swellings, depressions, sweating). Decreased range of motion or pain on limb movement may indicate an injury.
Note any distortion of symmetry (comparing both limbs) and anatomical deviations.	

Technical action	Rationale
Palpate and move the limb, evaluating for range of motion (Figure 3.30).	If abnormalities are noted, further evaluation is warranted (see Lameness examination, Chapter 27, and Evaluation of foot conformation, Chapter 32).
Pick up each front foot, clean the bottom of it, and inspect it. Apply hoof testers (Figure 3.31) if indicated.	For details on applying the hoof testers using an 8-point evaluation, Figure 27.11 , page 269.
Observe and palpate the pelvis, hips, pelvic limbs, and feet for symmetry and anatomical deviations.	Note any asymmetry or any deviation from the normal anatomy and any deficits or evidence of discomfort.
Observe and palpate for abnormalities (Figure 3.32b) and evaluate range of motion.	If abnormalities are noted, further evaluation is warranted (see Lameness Examination, Chapter 27, and Evaluation of Foot Conformation, Chapter 32).
Palpate the digital pulses of the hind feet (Figure 3.33).	
Pick up each hind foot, clean the bottom of it, and inspect it (Figure 3.33).	
Briefly assess the locomotor and neurologic systems by observing the horse's movements and gait at walk and trot, both on straight line and in turns, and backing.	If lame, record what limb. Observe the stance of the animal (e.g., if pointing a limb, may be due to pain). If abnormalities are noted, further evaluation is warranted (see Chapter 27 for lameness examination and Chapter 74 for neurologic examination).

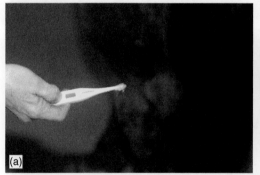
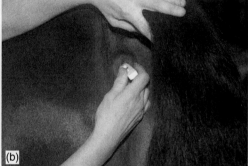

Figure 3.29 Obtain the rectal temperature. (a) Lubricate the thermometer. (b) Care should be taken to approach the horse from the side first and slowly work your way back to the tail. Lift the tail with one hand and insert the thermometer. One should not stand directly behind the horse when performing this function.

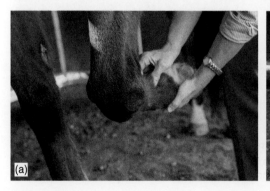
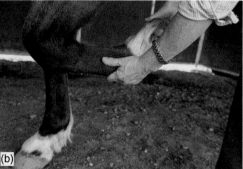

Figure 3.30 Evaluate the thoracic limbs. (a) Palpate along the limbs, noting any distortion of symmetry (comparing both limbs), anatomical deviations and reaction to palpation indicating pain. (b) Evaluate the range of motion.

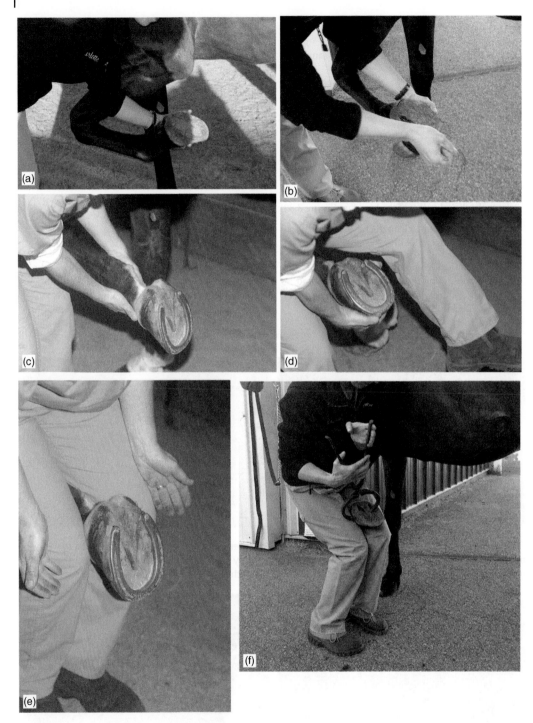

Figure 3.31 Evaluate each front foot off the ground. (a) Pick up the front foot. (b) Clean the bottom of it, if necessary, and inspect it. (c–e) Place the limb so you can hold it with your knees, allowing you to have both hands free. (f–h) If indicated, apply hoof testers along and across the sole, including at the toe.

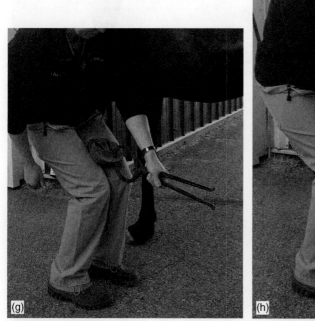
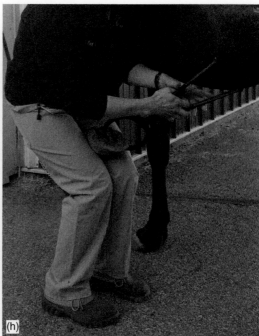

Figure 3.31 (*Continued*)

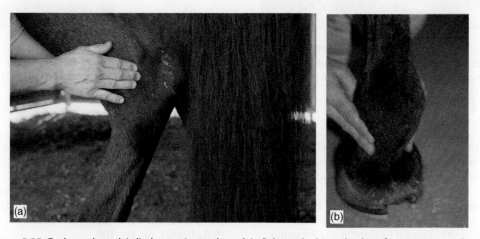

Figure 3.32 Evaluate the pelvic limbs starting at the pelvis. Palpate the hips, checking for symmetry and anatomical deviations, and proceed with the evaluation distally. (a) Evaluate the hock. (b) Palpate the digital pulses of the medial and lateral digital arteries of the hind limb.

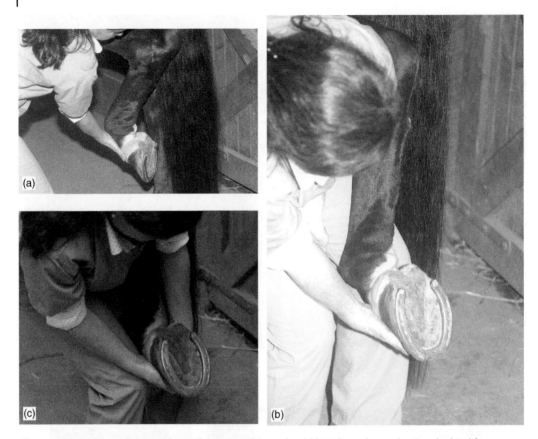

Figure 3.33 Evaluate each hind foot off the ground (care should be taken when palpating the hind feet to avoid being kicked). (a) Pick up the hind foot and inspect it. (b) Place the fetlock/pastern on your thigh while taking a step forward. (c) With the limb propped on your thigh use both hands to examine the foot and apply hoof testers if indicated.

Bibliography and Further Reading

Carroll, C.L. and Huntington, P.J. (1988) Body condition scoring and weight estimation of horses. *Equine Veterinary Journal*, **20** (1), 41–45.

Carter, R.A., Geor, R.J., Staniar, W.B., Cubitt, T.A., and Harris, P.A. (2009) Apparent adiposity assessed by standardized scoring systems and morphometric measurements in horses and ponies. *The Veterinary Journal*, **179**, 204–210.

Frank, N., Elliot S.B., Brandt L.E., and Keisler D.H. (2006) Physical characteristics, blood hormone concentrations, and plasma lipid concentrations in obese horses with insulin-resistance. *Journal of the American Veterinary Medical Association*, **228** (9), 1383–1390.

Henneke, D.R., Potter, G.D., Kreider, J.L., and Yeates, B.F. (1983) Relationship between condition score, physical measurements and body fat percentage in mares. *Equine Veterinary Journal*, **15** (4), 371–372.

Jesty, S.A. and Reef, V.B. (2008) Cardiovascular system, in *Equine Emergencies*, 3rd edn (eds J.A. Orsini and T.J. Divers), W.B. Saunders, Philadelphia, pp. 60–100.

Reef, V.B., Bonagura, J., Buhl, R., McGurrin, M.K.J., Schwarzwald, C.C., van Loon, G., and Young, L.E. (2014) Recommendations for management of equine athletes with cardiovascular abnormalities. *Journal of Veterinary Internal Medicine*, **28** (3), 749–761.

Rose, R.J. and Hodgson, D.R. (2000) *Manual of Equine Practice*, 2nd edn, W.B. Saunders, Philadelphia.

Speirs, V.C. (1997) *Clinical Examination of Horses*, W.B. Saunders, Philadelphia.

4

Venous Blood Collection

Lais R.R. Costa and Ann Chapman

4.1 Purpose

- To obtain venous blood samples via venipuncture, which is the placement of a needle into a vein.
- To obtain venous blood samples for diagnostic tests requiring whole blood, plasma or serum.
- The choice of the venipuncture site is based on the evaluation of the patient, the ease of access of the vein, and examination of the specific vein prior to the procedure.

- The most common sites of venipuncture in the horse include the jugular vein (Figure 4.1), the cephalic vein (Figure 4.2), the transverse facial vein/venous sinus (Figure 4.3), and occasionally the superficial/lateral thoracic vein (Figure 4.4). Certain conditions might affect venipuncture or preclude the use of a particular vein (Table 4.1). Knowledge of the anatomical location of the vein is crucial (Table 4.2).

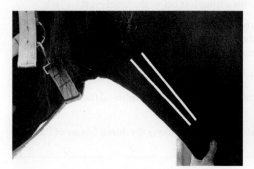

Figure 4.1 Location of the jugular vein in the jugular furrow. Drawn white lines indicate the location of the jugular vein.

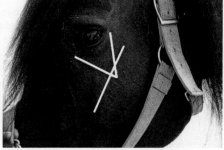

Figure 4.3 Location of the transverse facial vein/venous sinus.

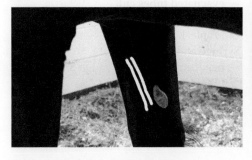

Figure 4.2 Location of the cephalic vein.

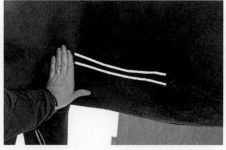

Figure 4.4 Location of the superficial/lateral thoracic vein.

Manual of Clinical Procedures in the Horse, First Edition. Edited by Lais R.R. Costa and Mary Rose Paradis.
© 2018 John Wiley & Sons, Inc. Published 2018 by John Wiley & Sons, Inc.

Table 4.1 Abnormal conditions that affect or preclude venipuncture

Abnormal conditions	Action/effect
Pre-existing phlebitis of the chosen vein	Do not obtain a sample from the affected vein, choose a different site
Severe dehydration and hypovolemia	Hamper visualization and localization of peripheral veins
Patients with endotoxemia	There is an increased risk of thrombophlebitis
Neonatal patients	There is an increased risk of septicemia, thus a strict aseptic technique is imperative

Table 4.2 Sites of venipuncture in horses

Vein	Anatomical descriptions
Jugular (Figure 4.1)	The right and left external jugular veins are large paired superficial veins located in the jugular groove of the cervical neck
	The cleidomastoideus muscle is located dorsal to the vein and the sternocephalicus muscle is located ventrally. Avoid venipuncture on the lower third of the neck
Cephalic (Figure 4.2)	This is a superficial vessel that courses medially in the proximal thoracic limb
	It is located in a small furrow on the medial radius
Transverse facial vein/sinus (Figure 4.3)	The transverse facial vein forms a sinus just below the facial crest
	The site of venipuncture corresponds to the apex of the intersection of two lines drawn from the medial canthus to the midpoint of the facial crest, and the lateral canthus and the midpoint of the facial crest
	The needle is positioned perpendicular to the skin
Superficial/lateral thoracic (Figure 4.4)	Also called the "spur vein", this is located on the ventrolateral thorax just caudal to the elbow
	It courses horizontally toward the olecranon along the dorsal border of the deep pectoral muscles

4.2 Complications

- Minor hemorrhages.
- Vascular trauma.
- Perivascular hematoma formation.
- Intravascular thrombi formation.
- Thrombophlebitis.

4.3 Equipment Required

- Gauze or cotton soaked with 70% alcohol.
- Vacuntainer® needles:
  - 20 or 22 gauge, 5/8–1.5"
  - evacuated tubes cuff
  - appropriate evacuated tubes (Table 4.3).
- Syringe and needles:
  - needles: 20, 22 or 25 gauge 5/8", 1–1.5" (Table 4.4)
  - syringe: tuberculin, 1, 3, 5 or 10 ml
  - appropriate evacuated tubes (Table 4.3).
- Exam gloves (optional).

Table 4.3 Types of evacuated tubes for blood collection (size of the tube will depend on the volume needed for the test, consult with the laboratory)

Top/stopper color of evacuated tube	Additive	Analysis possible
Red	No additive	Serum chemistry Serology
Red speckled or "tiger"	No additive and silica particles with separator (silica acts as clot activator)	Serum chemistry Serology
Lavender/purple	Sodium EDTA (binds calcium preventing clotting of blood and preserves cells)	Hematology studies (CBC with differential, platelet count, fibrionogen) Immunohematology Coombs' test Fluid cytology Cross-match
Pink	Potassium EDTA	Hematology studies (CBC with differential, platelet count, fibrionogen) Immunohematology Coombs' test Cross-match
Green	Heparin (sodium, lithium or ammonium)	Chemistry studies
Green and gray speckled or light green	Heparin with separator	Chemistry studies
Yellow	Acid citrate dextrose (ACD preserves RBC)	Cross-matching
Pale yellow	Sodium poly-anetholsulfonate or SPS (inhibits action of complement, phagocytes, antibiotics)	Blood culture
Light blue	Sodium citrate	Coagulation studies (fibrinogen, fibrin degradation products, PT, aPTT, AT III) Platelet count
Royal blue	Sodium EDTA or Sodium heparin (special stopper does not contain metals)	Trace metal determination (e.g., zinc, lead, cooper, mercury)
Gray	Sodium fluoride (antiglycolytic agent) and potassium oxalate (binds calcium)	Glucose, Lactate

CBC, complete cell count; PT, prothrombin time; aPTT, activated partial thromboplastin time; AT III, antithrombin III; EDTA, Ethylenediaminetetraacetic; RBC, red blood cells.

Table 4.4 Recommended needle size for blood collection

Location	Gauge	Length (")
Jugular vein	20–22	1½
Transverse facial sinus	22–25	5/8 or 1
Cephalic vein	20–22	1
Superficial/lateral thoracic vein	20–22	1½

4.4 Restraint and Positioning

- Physical restraint by a handler, properly positioned at the side of the horse.
- A chain across the bridge of the nose or a twitch may be required if the horse is uncooperative.

4.5 Procedure: Venipuncture of the Jugular or Cephalic Veins

Technical action	Rationale
Chose the vein for venipuncture, taking into consideration the patient and the conditions of the vein. Find the landmarks and locate the vein of choice.	For the landmarks see Table 4.2, and Figures 4.1–4.4.
Wash your hands and make sure the hair and skin around the site are free of dirt and debris. If necessary clean the area. If possible, wear exam gloves.	Ensure the site is clean before you handle the needle and other blood-collection supplies.
Hold the vein such that venous return is impaired. Press the vein between the site of venipuncture and the heart, and allow time for the vein to distend (Figure 4.5). Ensure vein patency.	Ensure you are able to see the vein, and that the vein does distend with blood. Many horses have had thrombi formation from previous venipunctures and the vein may not distend with blood when held. Do not proceed if you are unable to distend the vein. Procure another vein or site for the venipuncture.
Swab the area to be punctured with an alcohol swab. Do not place a needle through dirty skin and hair.	Besides being good practice to swab the skin and haircoat to ensure a clean procedure, swabbing the site will also help you see the vein more easily.
As the vein becomes distended with blood, insert the needle at a 45° angle to the skin (Figure 4.6a). If collecting blood directly into evacuated tubes, allow the blood to fill the tube completely (Figure 4.6b). If using a syringe and needle, pull the plunger of the syringe gently (Figure 4.7). If using a blood-collection set (or butterfly needle) attached to a syringe, keep the syringe upside down while pulling the plunger gently (Figure 4.8).	Be patient and allow the blood to flow out of the vessel and into the tube or syringe. Avoid excessive pressure on the plunger as this may damage the wall of the vessel and may cause hemolysis of the red blood cells. Collection from the cephalic is best performing using a blood-collection set because it allows better adjustment of needle position in case of movement.
If collecting blood directly into evacuated tubes, after the tube is filled completely disconnect the tube from the needle before pulling the needle from the vein.	This will minimize trauma, bleeding, and hematoma formation.
Apply moderate pressure to the puncture site after removal of the needle (Figure 4.9). If collection from the jugular vein, keep the horses' head and neck in the upright position for several minutes.	This helps to avoid bleeding and formation of hematomas at the puncture site.

Technical action	Rationale
If transferring blood from a syringe to an evacuated tube, fill the evacuated tube upside down such that the rubber stopper is in the most ventral portion (Figure 4.10).	This will minimize the impact of the cells against the walls of the glass tube and thus minimize damage to the blood cells.

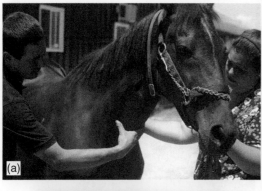

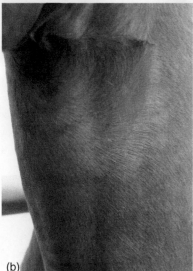

Figure 4.5 Preparation for venipuncture of the jugular vein. (a) Evaluation of the jugular vein for patency prior to venipuncture. (b) Distended jugular vein filling the jugular furrow.

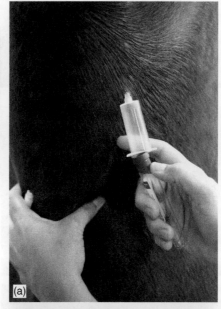

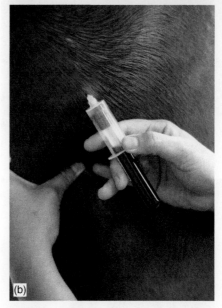

Figure 4.6 Collection of the venous blood from the left jugular vein of a horse. (a) Insertion of a needle attached to a cuff for collection of blood using an evacuated tube. (b) Blood filling the evacuated tube directly from the jugular vein.

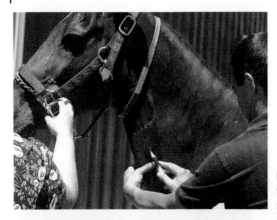

Figure 4.7 Collection of the venous blood from the left jugular vein of a horse using a needle and syringe.

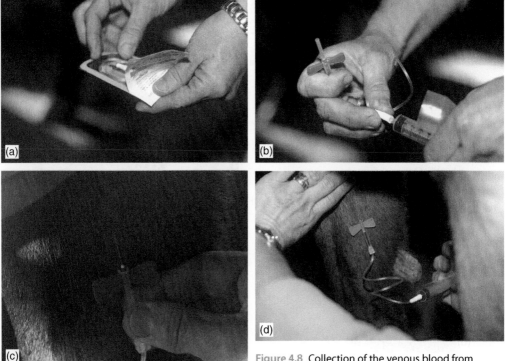

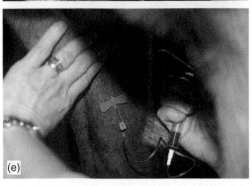

Figure 4.8 Collection of the venous blood from the right cephalic vein of a horse using a blood-collection set attached to a syringe. (a) Remove the blood-collection needle from its package. (b) Attach it to a syringe of appropriate size for the amount of blood to be taken. (c) Block the venous return of the cephalic vein with your non-dominant hand proximal to the point of needle insertion while holding the blood-collection needle between the thumb and index fingers, and keeping the syringe in the palm of the hand. (d) Insert the needle at a 45° angle into the distended vein; blood will appear. (e) Slowly aspirate the blood, keeping the syringe upside down and avoiding any motion of the needle insertion.

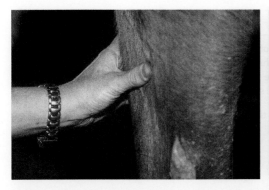

Figure 4.9 Holding off the vein after blood collection to allow hemostasis and diminish formation of hematoma.

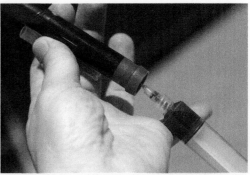

Figure 4.10 Filling an evacuated tube by injecting the needle into the rubber stopper and allowing the blood to be sucked into the tube. Note that tube is kept upside down to minimize the impact of the cells again the walls of the tube.

4.6 Procedure: Blood Collection from the Transverse Facial Vein/venous Sinus

Technical action	Rationale
If you chose to collect blood from the transverse facial vein/venous sinus, locate the landmarks:	This site is generally used for the collection of a small amount of blood.
• facial crest • midpoint between the medial and lateral canthus of the eye.	For the location of landmarks see Table 4.2 and Figure 4.3.
Wash hands and make sure the hair and skin around the site are free of dirt and debris. If necessary clean the area. If possible, wear exam gloves..	Ensure the site is clean before you handle the needle and other blood-collection supplies.
Carefully swab the area to be punctured with a swab slightly dampened with alcohol or another antiseptic. Avoid an excessive amount of alcohol as it might irritate the eye.	It is good practice to swab the skin and haircoat to ensure a clean procedure. Do not place a needle through dirty skin and hair.

(continued)

Technical action	Rationale
The site of venipuncture corresponds to the intersection of the apex of the two lines drawn from each of the medial canthus and the lateral canthus of the eye, and the midpoint of the facial crest. The needle is positioned perpendicular to the skin.	The transverse facial sinus cannot be palpated so accurate determination of the landmarks is necessary to locate the sinus.
Use a 25- or 22-gauge needle directed at a 90° angle to the skin. Introduce the needle until bone is felt. Blood from the transverse facial venous sinus can be withdrawn by use of: • a needle attached to a syringe (Figure 4.11) or • a needle attached to a cuff and evacuated tube (Figure 4.12).	Be patient, allowing the blood to flow out of the vessel and into the tube or syringe. Avoid excessive pressure on the plunger.
If using a a needle attached to a cuff and evacuated tube, after the evacuated tube is filled, disconnect the tube from the needle before pulling the needle from the venous sinus.	This will minimize trauma, bleeding, and hematoma formation.
Apply moderate pressure to the puncture site after removal of the needle. Keep the horse's head and neck in the upright position for several minutes.	This helps to avoid bleeding and formation of hematomas at the puncture site.

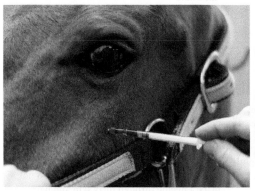

Figure 4.11 Collection of the venous blood from the transverse facial vein/venous sinus using a needle and syringe.

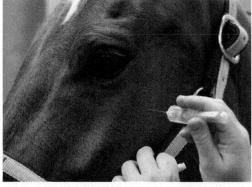

Figure 4.12 Collection of the venous blood from the transverse facial vein/venous sinus directly into an evacuated tube using a needle, cuff and evacuated tube.

Bibliography and Further Reading

Corley, K. (2008) Collection of blood samples and intravenous injection, in *The Equine Hospital Manual* (eds K.Corley and S Jennifer), Blackwell, Oxford, pp. 10-12.

Schaer, B.D. and Orsini, J.A. (2008) Blood collection, in *Equine Emergencies*, 3rd edn (eds J.A. Orsini and T.J. Divers), W.B. Saunders, pp. 2-5.

Schumacher, J. and Moll, H.D. (2006) Collection of blood from sites other than the jugular vein, in *Manual of Equine Diagnostic Procedures*, Teton New Media, pp. 25-28.

Walesby, H.A., Hillman, D.J., Blackmer, J.M. and Williams J. (2007) The transverse facial venous sinus: an alternative location for blood collection in the horse. *Equine Veterinary Education*, **19** (2), 100-102.

5

Arterial Blood Collection

Lais R.R. Costa

5.1 Purposes

- To obtain an arterial blood sample via an arteriopuncture, which is the placement of a needle into an artery.
- To collect an arterial blood sample for specific diagnostic tests such as arterial blood gas analysis and arterial blood ammonia.

- The arteries commonly used for arterial blood collection in the horse include the transverse facial artery (Figure 5.1), the facial artery (Figure 5.2), the common carotid artery (Figure 5.3), the dorsal metatarsal artery (Figure 5.4), and the brachial artery (Figure 5.5).

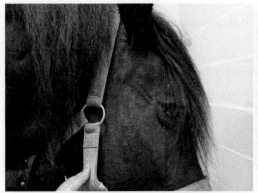

Figure 5.1 Location of transverse facial artery.

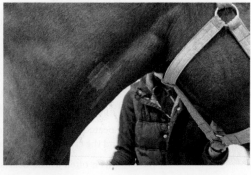

Figure 5.3 Location of common carotid artery.

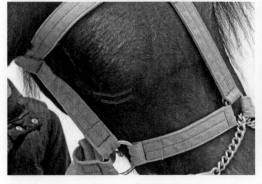

Figure 5.2 Location of facial artery.

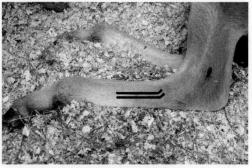

Figure 5.4 Location of dorsal metatarsal artery.

Manual of Clinical Procedures in the Horse, First Edition. Edited by Lais R.R. Costa and Mary Rose Paradis.
© 2018 John Wiley & Sons, Inc. Published 2018 by John Wiley & Sons, Inc.

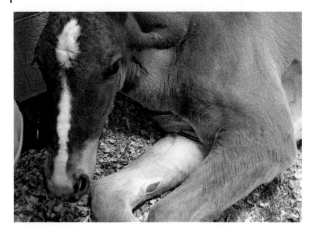

Figure 5.5 Location of brachial artery.

Table 5.1 Sites and anatomical descriptions of arteries commonly used for arteriopuncture in horses

Artery	Anatomical landmarks and descriptions
Transverse facial artery	Located caudal to the lateral canthus of the eye, ventral to the zygomatic arch (Figure 5.1)
Facial artery	The facial artery crosses the ventral border of the mandible at the level of the first/second molar (Figure 5.2)
	This artery is very "rolly" and for the most part it is only useful when the animal is anesthetized
Common carotid artery	Located medial and deep to the jugular vein in the ventral one half of the neck (Figure 5.3)
	The omohyoideus muscle is transposed between the carotid artery and the jugular vein in the upper one half of the neck
	The vagosympathetic trunk is located dorsal to the carotid artery and the recurrent laryngeal nerve is located ventral to the artery
Dorsal metatarsal artery	Located on the lateral aspect of the hind leg between the third metatarsal bone and the cranial ridge of the fourth metatarsal bone (Figure 5.4)
	This is often use in foals (see Chapter 49).
Brachial artery	Located at the level of the medial collateral ligament of the elbow
	It can be palpated between the elbow and shoulder (Figure 5.5)
	It is an alternative artery to use in foals

- The choice of the arteriopuncture site is based on the evaluation of the patient, the knowledge of the anatomical location of commonly used arteries, and the ease of access of the specific artery (Table 5.1).

5.2 Complications

- *Hematoma:* Arteries have a higher pressure and are more likely to have hematoma formation after puncture than are veins.

- *Trauma and laceration of the artery:* Vascular trauma may occur if multiple punctures are needed to obtain a sample. Laceration of the artery may ensue.
- *Hemorrhage:* Significant bleeding at the arterial puncture site may occur if a bleeding disorder is present.
- *Contamination and infection:* Contamination of the puncture site and surrounding tissue can lead to localized or generalized infection.

- *Inability to obtain sample:* Arterial pulses may be difficult to find in peripheral arteries in animals with circulatory compromise, such as low blood pressure and hypovolemia.

5.3 Equipment Required

- Gauze or cotton soaked with 70% alcohol.
- Needle: size 20, 22 or 25 gauge, length 5/8″ or 1–1.5″.
- Syringe, heparinized:
  - sizes: tuberculin, 1, 3 or 5 ml
  - specific blood gas syringe.
- Exam gloves (optional).

5.4 Restraint and Positioning

- Physical restraint by a handler, properly positioned at the side of the horse.
- A chain across the bridge of the nose or a twitch may be required if the horse is uncooperative.
- In a foal the handler may need to stabilize the limb to prevent motion during the procedure.
- Subcutaneous 2% lidocaine over the proposed site of puncture may also help prevent motion during arterial blood collection.

5.5 Procedure: Arterial Blood Collection

Technical action	Rationale
Find the landmarks to locate the chosen artery. Figures 5.1–5.5 illustrate the location of the arteries commonly used in horses for arterial blood collection. Table 5.1 describes their anatomical locations.	Ensure you are able to visualize/feel the artery otherwise you may obtain a mixed arterial/venous sample.
Wash hands and make sure the hair and skin around the site are free of dirt and debris. If necessary clean the area. Wear exam gloves (optional).	Do not place a needle through dirty skin and hair as this could result in infection.
Carefully palpate the pulse to identify the point for puncture (Figure 5.6a).	Press the fingertips gently against the skin and wait until you can feel the pulse.
Swab the area to be punctured with an alcohol swab (70% alcohol) or another skin antiseptic (Figure 5.6b). Avoid an excessive amount of alcohol as it might irritate the eye.	Besides being good practice to swab the skin and haircoat to ensure a clean procedure, swabbing the site will also help you visualize the artery more easily.
Feel the arterial pulse (Figure 5.6c) and insert the needle at a 45° angle to the skin (Figure 5.6d). Note the blood at the hub of the needle (Figure 5.6e). Allow the blood to fill the syringe by its own pressure (Figure 5.6f,g).	Be patient and allow the proper blood flow out the vessel. Spontaneous filling of the syringe is a good sign that you have punctured the artery and not a vein.
Hold the site of the puncture after removal of the needle for 3 minutes. Keep the horse's head and neck in the upright position.	This avoids bleeding and formation of hematomas at the puncture site.
	If the need for multiple samples is anticipated, an indwelling arterial catheter should be placed.
Turn the syringe upright and promptly remove air bubbles (Figure 5.7a). Immediately seal the syringe (Figure 5.7b). Tilt the syringe gently to ensure mixing of blood and heparin.	It is important to prepare the arterial blood sample properly by removing bubbles, avoiding contact with air and homogenizing with heparin. Placing a seal (stopper at the end of the syringe/needle) will prevent air from contaminating the sample.
Perform arterial blood analysis immediately.	If the sample is not analyzed immediately, store the sample in ice (2–4 °C). Analyze iced samples within 2 hours.

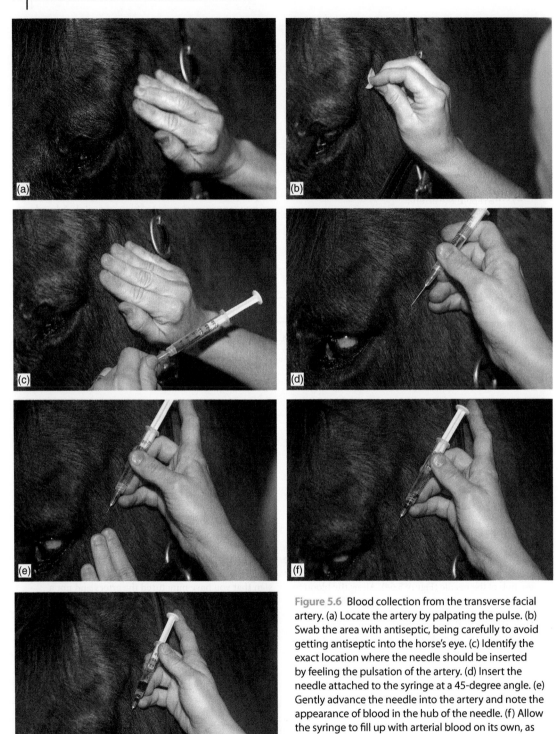

Figure 5.6 Blood collection from the transverse facial artery. (a) Locate the artery by palpating the pulse. (b) Swab the area with antiseptic, being carefully to avoid getting antiseptic into the horse's eye. (c) Identify the exact location where the needle should be inserted by feeling the pulsation of the artery. (d) Insert the needle attached to the syringe at a 45-degree angle. (e) Gently advance the needle into the artery and note the appearance of blood in the hub of the needle. (f) Allow the syringe to fill up with arterial blood on its own, as the arterial pressure pulsates blood. (g) Monitor the progression of the blood flow and ensure the amount of blood will suffice for the test required.

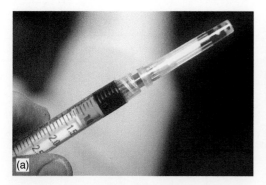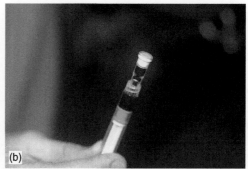

Figure 5.7 Prepare the arterial blood sample. (a) Turn the syringe upright and promptly remove air bubbles. (b) Immediately seal the syringe to prevent air contamination of the sample (alternatively a rubber stopper from an evacuated tube can be used to seal the end of the needle).

Bibliography and Further Reading

Bedenice, D. (2006) Foal with septic pneumonia, in *Equine Neonatal Medicine: A Case Based Approach* (ed. M.R. Paradis), Elsevier Saunders, Philadelphia, pp. 99-111.

Mair, T.S. (2006) Arterial blood collection, in *Diagnostic Techniques in Equine Medicine*,

2nd edn (eds F.G.R.Taylor, T.J.Brazil, and M.H. Hillyer), W.B. Saunders, pp. 241-242.

Schaer, B.D. and Orsini, J.A. (2008) Blood collection, in *Equine Emergencies*, 3rd edn (eds J.A. Orsini and T.J. Divers), W.B. Saunders, pp. 2-5.

6

Injection Techniques

Ann Chapman

6.1 Purpose

- To administer approved injectable medications, biological agents or testing substances according to the approved route for the injectable solution that will be administered.
- To utilize the appropriate technique for injecting solutions in horses: intravenous (IV), intramuscular (IM), subcutaneous (SC), and intradermal (ID).

6.2 Complications

- Adverse drug reaction.
- Anaphylactoid reaction and anaphylaxis.
- Accidental intra-arterial injection.
- Tissue damage (e.g., neuropathy).
- Hemorrhage.
- Hematoma formation.
- Iatrogenic infection.
- Venous air embolism.

6.3 Contraindications and Concerns

- Always administer the injectable solution by the correct route and dose that is recommended by the manufacturer.
- Do not use any injectable solutions that are past the expiration date given by the manufacturer.
- Owners should be warned that adverse drug reactions can occur whenever a horse receives an injectable product, despite having received that agent safely in the past.
- Horses with a history of adverse drug reaction to a particular substance should

not receive that injectable agent again without weighing the risks versus the benefits and discussing it with the owner.
- Horses with a known sensitivity to silicone may require special needles that do not have a silicone coating.

6.4 Equipment Required

- Injectable solution
- Sterile syringe
- Sterile needle
- Gauze sponge, 4″ × 4″
- 70% alcohol
- Biohazard container
- Optional: clippers with a #40 blade
- Exam gloves (optional)
- Halter
- Lead rope
- Optional: rope or chain twitch

6.5 Restraint and Positioning

- The patient should be properly restrained during the procedure to prevent excessive movement and avoid accidental improper injection.
- The minimum requirement for all horses receiving an injection is a handler who holds the head using a halter and lead rope.
- Fractious horses or horses that are sensitive to needle injections will require additional forms of humane restraint, including nose or lip twitch, neck roll or skin twitch, lip rope, manual ear twitch (see Chapter 2).

Manual of Clinical Procedures in the Horse, First Edition. Edited by Lais R.R. Costa and Mary Rose Paradis.
© 2018 John Wiley & Sons, Inc. Published 2018 by John Wiley & Sons, Inc.

6.6 Procedure: General Preparation

Technical action	Rationale/amplification
Clean hands with alcohol gel or foam.	Cleaning hands helps to reduce the spread of nosocomial infection.
Verify the following: • correct patient • correct medication • correct route • correct dosage • correct timing • the expiration date of the medication • the medication has been correctly stored.	This step is important to avoid inaccuracies in the administration of an injectable medication. It is important to choose the correct route as some drugs can result in tissue reaction if given by an inappropriate route (Table 6.1).
Select an appropriate needle and syringe.	The needle size will be determined based on the route of administration, the location of the injection, and the age of the patient (see IV, IM, SQ, and ID sections). The volume of medication to be administered will determine the size of the syringe.
Carefully attach the needle to the syringe without contaminating the hub of the needle or the tip of the syringe (Figure 6.1).	Maintaining a closed aseptic system is ideal for injections.
Disinfect the rubber stopper on the medication bottle by wiping with gauze soaked in 70% alcohol (Figure 6.2).	In multidose vials, the surface of the injection port can become contaminated with organic debris and bacteria. Disinfection prior to withdrawing medication may help to reduce the chance of contamination.
Carefully remove the needle cover and aseptically insert the needle into the bottle.	Take care to avoid touching the needle during insertion into the bottle. If the rubber stopper has become damaged, consider using a new bottle of medication since the integrity of the medication may be compromised.
Invert the bottle and aspirate the appropriate volume of medication (Figure 6.3).	It may be helpful to aspirate a small additional amount of medication because air may be aspirated into the syringe as well.
Hold the needle/syringe vertically and tap on the syringe to allow air bubbles to move to the tip of the syringe (Figure 6.4).	It has been demonstrated that horses can tolerate 0.25 ml/kg of air before showing any clinical signs. However, removing excessive air bubbles from injection solution reduces the chance of air embolism, especially during IV injection.
Depress the plunger to force the air back into the bottle. Withdraw additional medication if necessary to obtain the desired volume.	Large volumes of air in the syringe can result in inaccurate drug dosing and therefore should be removed. Maintain the needle in the bottle when removing the air to avoid accidentally exposing anyone nearby to hazardous substances.
Remove the needle and syringe from the bottle.	Recapping needles is a hazard and can be avoided by laying the cap on a solid surface and sliding the needle into the cap. If at any time the needle becomes contaminated, it should be replaced with a new one.
Label the syringe with drug, concentration, date, time, patient.	Labeling the syringe with appropriate information will mitigate errors.

Table 6.1 Recommended routes of injection for commonly used injectable solutions (check manufacturer recommendations)

Type of injectable	Possible routes
Pharmacologic agents (antibiotics, sedatives, anti-inflammatories, hormones, supplements, etc.)	IV, IM, SQ
Vaccines and other biologicals	IM, IN
Local anesthetics	IM, SQ
Specialized test substances (e.g., allergens or epinephrine for testing)	ID

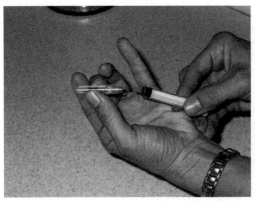

Figure 6.1 Attach the needle to the syringe without contaminating the hub of the needle or the tip of the syringe.

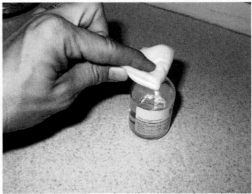

Figure 6.2 Disinfect the rubber stopper on the medication bottle by wiping with gauze soaked in 70% alcohol.

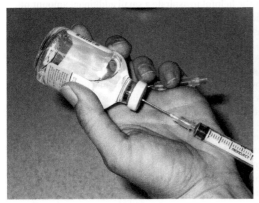

Figure 6.3 Invert the bottle and aspirate the appropriate volume of medication.

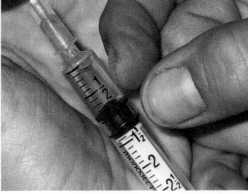

Figure 6.4 Hold the needle/syringe vertically and tap on the syringe to allow air bubbles to move to the tip of the syringe.

6.7 Procedure: Intravenous Injection

Technical action	Rationale
Prepare the needle and syringe, and prepare the patient for injection.	See the General Preparation section above. Select the correct size of needle (Table 6.2).
Verify the following: • correct patient • correct medication • correct route • correct dosage • correct timing.	This step is important to avoid inaccuracies in the administration of an injectable medication.
Apply a halter and lead rope to the patient. Have a handler hold the head using the lead rope. Use additional forms of humane restraint if necessary.	Proper restraint is necessary to reduce the risk of injury to the patient, handler, and veterinarian or veterinary technician.
Ensure that the horse is properly restrained by the handler to avoid perivascular injections.	Advise the handler on how you want the horse positioned and restrained. Handler should stand on the same side as the person performing the injection.
Select the vein and insertion site that will be used for injection. The three most common sites for IV injection include the jugular vein, the cephalic vein, and the superficial thoracic vein (Table 6.3, Figure 6.5).	Selection of the vein is based on multiple factors: patency of the vein, how well the vein can be seen, and how safely the vein can be accessed. Although many different veins can be used, it is important to consider all these factors and evaluate how cooperative the patient will be during the procedure. Remember, when using the jugular vein it is important to insert the needle in the cranial one half of the vein.
Swab the vein with a gauze sponge soaked in 70% alcohol (Figure 6.6).	Disinfection of the venipuncture site will reduce the bacterial contamination of the skin.
Distend the vein by occluding it distal to the insertion site (Figure 6.7).	The vein may be difficult to see in horses with very developed neck musculature or very long hair. Clipping the hair or wetting the area with disinfectant may allow better visibility of the vein.
Detach the needle from the syringe. Choose the direction of needle insertion: • directed toward the head (upward), against the flow of blood (Figure 6.8a) • directed toward the heart (downward), with the flow of blood (Figure 6.8b).	The direction of needle insertion is a personal preference. There is no clear consensus among experts which method is superior.
Hold the needle with the bevel facing towards you (Figure 6.9).	When the bevel is placed downward, it may contact the opposing side of the vein, obstructing the lumen of the needle.
Insert the needle into the skin at a 30° angle, mimicking the course of the vein.	Avoid sudden stabbing of the area, which can startle many horses. Rather, gently guide the needle into the skin. Most veins that are accessible for venipuncture are fairly superficial. Mimicking the course of the vein will result in more success than briskly inserting the needle and searching or "fishing" for the vein.

(continued)

Technical action	Rationale
Advance the needle into the vein until blood appears in the hub (Figure 6.10). Release the distension pressure from the vein. Verify the placement of the needle in the vein and not an artery by observing the pressure of blood flow.	It is important to seed the needle in the vein completely to stabilize it. If blood pulsates out of the needle hub with pressure, it is likely that an artery has been punctured. Remove the needle and hold slight pressure for a minute and repeat venipuncture in a different location if necessary.
Carefully attach the syringe to the needle (Figure 6.11).	When attaching the syringe, stabilize the needle with one hand to prevent it from advancing deeper through the vein, or withdrawing out of the vein.
Aspirate, watching for the appearance of blood in the syringe (Figure 6.12).	Aspirating blood helps to verify that the needle is within a blood vessel, but it does not indicate whether it is a vein or an artery. If blood does not appear in the syringe, disconnect the syringe and re-verify the needle placement.
Inject the solution slowly. Midway in the injection, aspirate blood to re-verify the placement.	Some solutions can be administered faster than others. For patient safety, inject all medications slowly and observe the vessel to ensure the medication is not being deposited perivascularly. The patient should also be observed for any adverse reactions. Periodically aspirating blood during the administration of the medication solution can help to identify if the needle has become displaced.
Once injection of the drug is complete, withdraw the needle from the vein and discard in an approved biohazard container.	Take care when removing the needle to avoid accidental needle stick. Re-capping syringes with hazardous substances can be dangerous.
Apply light pressure to the venipuncture site with a gauze sponge for 30 seconds (Figure 6.13).	Applying pressure to the injection site can reduce the chance of hemorrhage, hematoma or perivascular leakage of the medication.
Document the medication in the patient record.	Legally the generic name of the medication, the amount, the dose, and the time of administration should be recorded and initialed.

Table 6.2 Recommended needle size for IV injection

Type of drug	Gauge	Length (")
Most injectable solutions	18–22	1–1½
Irritating substances (e.g., NSAIDs, certain antibiotics, etc.)	18–20	1½
Drugs to give slowly (e.g., sedatives, certain antibiotics)	20–22	1–1½
Viscous substances (e.g., euthanasia solutions)	14	1½–2

Table 6.3 Description of sites commonly used for IV injection in horses

Site of injection	Anatomical location
Jugular vein: the cranial half of the jugular vein is preferable for IV injection (Figure 6.5a)	The right and left external jugular veins are large paired superficial veins located in the jugular groove of the cervical neck. The cleidomastoideus muscle is located dorsal to the vein and the sternocephalicus muscle is located ventrally. The common carotid artery is located deep to the jugular vein in the ventral half of the neck. The omohyoideus muscle is transposed between the carotid artery and the jugular vein in the upper half of the neck. The vagosypathetic trunk is located dorsal to the carotid artery and the recurrent laryngeal nerve is located ventral to the artery.
Cephalic vein (Figure 6.5b)	The cephalic vein is a superficial vessel that courses medially in the proximal thoracic limb. It originates from the external jugular vein and is located in a small furrow on the medial radius.
Superficial thoracic vein	The superficial thoracic vein ("spur vein") is located on the ventrolateral thorax just caudal to the elbow. It courses horizontally to the olecranon along the dorsal border of the deep pectoral muscles (see Chapter 4, Figure 4.4).

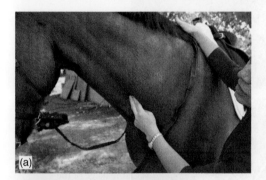

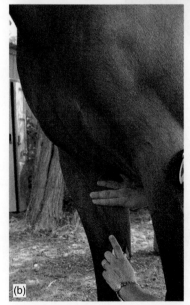

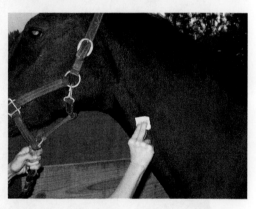

Figure 6.6 Swab the vein with a gauze sponge soaked in 70% alcohol.

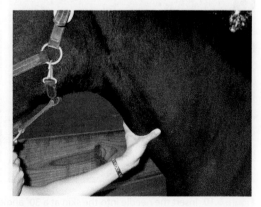

Figure 6.5 The two most common sites for IV injection are (a) the jugular vein and (b) the cephalic vein. Courtesy of Dr. Lais R.R. Costa.

Figure 6.7 Distend the vein by occluding it distal to the insertion site.

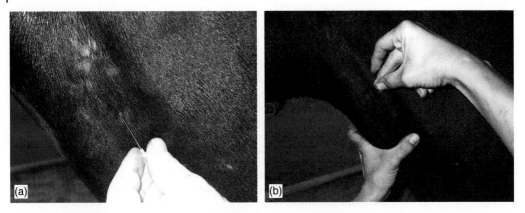

Figure 6.8 Choose the direction of needle insertion: (a) upward, directed toward the head, or (b) downward, directed toward the heart.

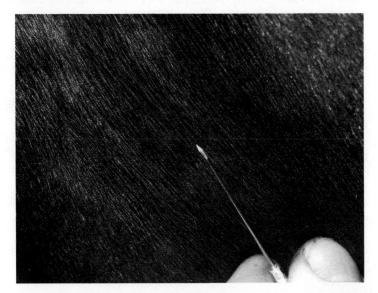

Figure 6.9 Hold the needle with the bevel facing towards you.

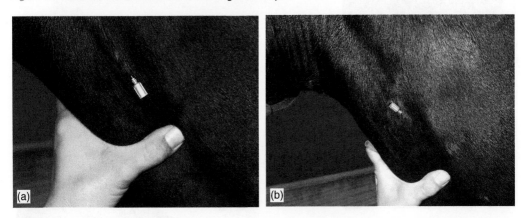

Figure 6.10 Insert the needle into the skin at a 30° angle, mimicking the course of the vein: (a) upward, which is against the flow of blood, or (b) downward, which is with the flow of blood. Gently guide the needle into the skin, avoiding sudden stabbing of the area.

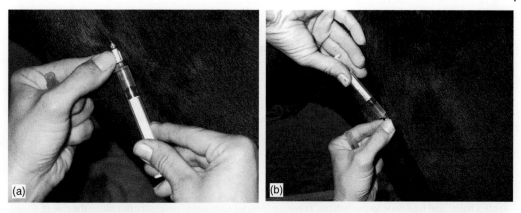

Figure 6.11 Attach the syringe to the needle carefully, stabilizing the needle with one hand to avoid needle displacement from the vein: (a) upward, (b) downward.

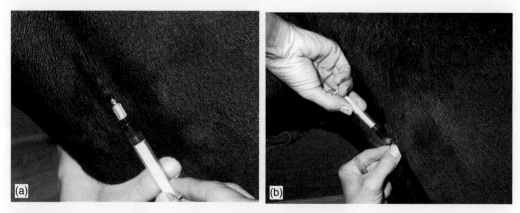

Figure 6.12 Aspirate, watching for the appearance of blood in the syringe to verify that the needle is within a blood vessel: (a) upward, (b) downward. Push the plunger to inject the medication. If a large volume is being injected, aspirate midway in order to verify that the needle is still in the vessel.

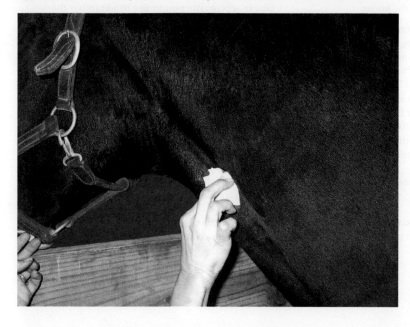

Figure 6.13 Apply light pressure to the venipuncture site with a gauze sponge for 30 seconds to reduce the chance of hemorrhage, hematoma or perivascular leakage of the medication.

6.8 Procedure: Intramuscular Injection

Technical action	Rationale
Prepare the needle and syringe for injection.	See the General Preparation section above.
Verify the following: • correct patient • correct medication • correct route • correct dosage • correct timing.	This step is important to avoid inaccuracies in the administration of an injectable medication.
Apply a halter and lead rope to the patient. Have a handler hold the head using the lead rope. Use additional forms of humane restraint if necessary.	Proper restraint is necessary to reduce the risk of injury to the patient, handler, and veterinarian or veterinary technician.
Ensure that the horse is properly restrained by the handler because intramuscular injections can be painful and the horse might react adversely.	Advise the handler on how you want the horse positioned and restrained.
Select the appropriate size of needle for the IM injection.	Table 6.4 provides guidelines for selection of needle size for IM injections.
There are multiple sites that can be used for IM injection in horses. The most common sites include: • the lateral cervical muscles (Figure 6.14a) • the semitendinosus muscles (Figure 6.14b) • the pectoral muscles (Figure 6.14c).	Selection of the muscle is based on multiple factors: the type of medication, the injection volume, and how safely the muscle site can be accessed. Although different muscles can be used, it is important to consider how cooperative the patient will be during the procedure.
Identify the landmarks to ensure administration of the medication to the proper site (Figure 6.15).	See Table 6.5 for landmarks for the sites of injection.
Position yourself next to the horse: • For cervical IM injection, stand next to the horse's shoulder (Figure 6.16a). • For pectoral IM injection, stand to one side and not directly in front of the horse (Figure 6.16b). • For semitendinosus IM injection it is preferable to restrain the horse in stocks. If stocks are unavailable, stand next to the pelvic limb and face caudally (Figure 6.16c). It may be preferable (safer) to reach across the hind end and inject the muscle in the contralateral limb (Figure 6.16d).	Ensure appropriate positioning to administer the injection safely.
Swab the area with a gauze sponge soaked in 70% alcohol.	Disinfection of the IM injection site will reduce the bacterial contamination of the skin.
Pinch the skin adjacent to the muscle injection site (Figure 6.17a). This is not possible when using the semitendinosus muscle.	Pinching the skin will help to distract some horses during the procedure. It may also serve to cover the muscle injection site with the skinfold.

Technical action	Rationale
Determine if it is best to detach the needle from the syringe as shown in Figure 6.16d. It may be preferable in some circumstances to leave the needle attached to the syringe during injection, as shown in Figure 6.17b.	It may be preferable in some circumstances to leave the needle attached to the syringe during injection. There is no clear consensus among experts which method is superior. However, when administering medications that could produce a severe reaction if inadvertently introduced into a blood vessel (e.g., procaine penicillin G), it is best to detach the needle prior to injecting.
Insert the needle perpendicular to the skin into the muscle (Figure 6.17b).	Avoid sudden stabbing of the area, which can startle many horses. Rather, gently guide the needle into the skin.
Advance the needle fully into the muscle.	If blood appears in the hub of the needle, remove it and repeat in an alternate location.
Attach the syringe to the needle. Aspirate to verify placement in muscle (Figure 6.17c) and not in a vessel.	When attaching the syringe, stabilize the needle with one hand. If blood appears when aspirating, remove the needle and syringe, and repeat in a different location using a new needle.
Inject the solution slowly (Figure 6.17d).	The maximum volume that should be injected in one site is 10–15 ml. For larger volumes, the needle should be removed and placed in an adjacent area. Always aspirate before injecting the medication to verify that no blood appears. Avoid injecting too rapidly because the excessive pressure may cause the syringe to become detached from the needle (if using a regular tip syringe rather than a screw tip syringe) and potentially spray those nearby.
Remove the needle and syringe from the muscle and discard in an approved biohazard container.	For biosafety reasons, used needles and syringes should not be left in publicly accessible places.
Release the pinch of skin.	The skin pinch can serve as a sticking plaster for the muscle injection.
Document the medication in the patient record.	Legally the generic name of the medication, the amount, the dose, and the time of administration should be recorded and initialed.

Table 6.4 Recommended needle size for IM injection

Location	Gauge	Length (")
Lateral cervical muscles	18–22	1½
Semitendinosus muscle	18–22	1½
Pectoral muscles	20–22	1

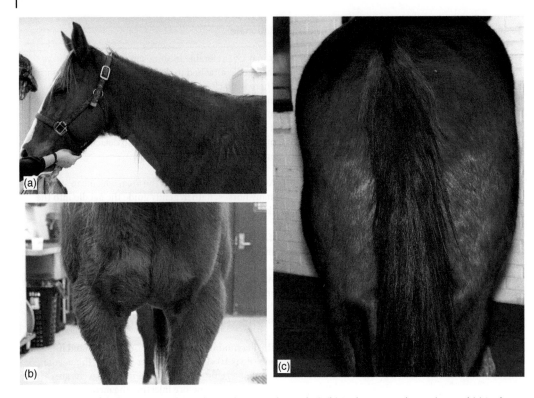

Figure 6.14 Site for IM injections: (a) in the neck (cervical muscles), (b) in the pectoral muscles, and (c) in the semimembranosus/semitendinosus muscles.

Table 6.5 Sites that can be used for IM injection in horses

Site of injection	Anatomical location	Comments
Lateral cervical muscles (Figure 6.14)	Located in either side of the neck The landmarks form a triangle 4″ above the dorsal border of the cervical vertebrae, 4″ cranial to the cranial border of the scapula, and 4″ below the border of the crest of the neck	Care must be taken to avoid injection directly over the cervical vertebrae or into the nuchal ligament For cervical IM injection, stand next to the horse's shoulder.
Petoral muscles	The pectoral muscles are located in the cranial most part of the chest, craniomedial to the thoracic limbs (Figure 6.16)	If using the pectoral muscles, stand to one side and not directly in front of the horse (Figure 6.18a)
Semitendinosus muscle	Located on either side of the tail, distal to the tuber ischii and medial to the sciatic groove of the thigh (Figures 6.17a,b)	If using the semitendinosus muscles, it is preferable to restrain the horse in stocks If stocks are unavailable, stand next to the pelvic limb and face caudally It may be preferable to reach across the hind and inject the muscle in the contralateral limb (Figure 6.17c)

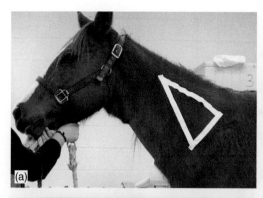

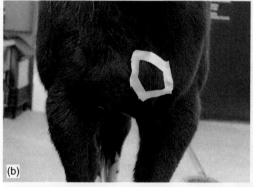

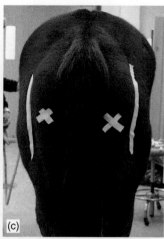

Figure 6.15 The landmarks for IM injections. (a) The lateral cervical muscles: a triangle formed 4″ above the dorsal border of the cervical vertebrae, 4″ cranial to the cranial border of the scapula, and 4″ below the border of the crest of the neck. (b) The pectoral muscles: the cranial-most part of the chest, craniomedial to the thoracic limbs. (c) The semitendinosus muscle is located on either side of the tail, distal to the tuber ischii and medial to the sciatic groove of the thigh.

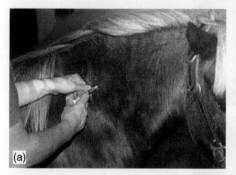

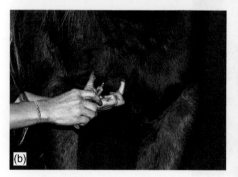

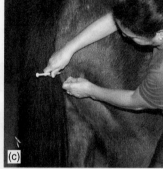

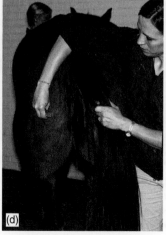

Figure 6.16 Proper positioning for IM injections. (a) Stand next to the horse's shoulder for cervical IM injection. Courtesy of Dr. Lais R.R. Costa. (b) Stand to one side and not directly in front of the horse for pectoral IM injection. (c) Stand next to the pelvic limb and face caudally and inject the same side for semitendinosus IM injection. Courtesy of Dr. Lais R.R. Costa. (d) Stand next to the pelvic limb and face caudally and reach across the hind end, injecting the muscle in the contralateral limb for safer IM injection into the semitendinosus.

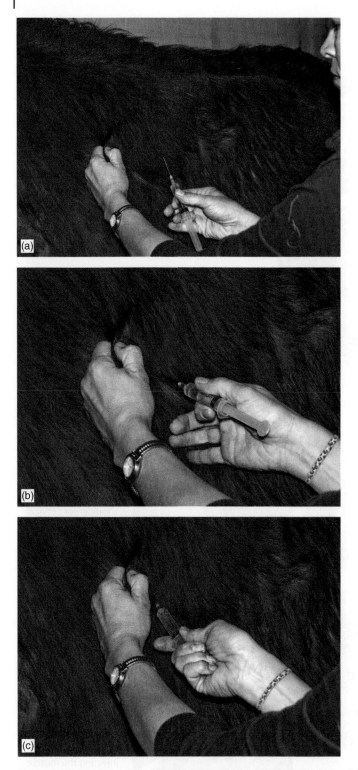

Figure 6.17 Administration of medication intramuscularly. (a) Pinch the skin adjacent to the muscle injection site to distract the horse (this is not possible when using the semitendinosus muscle). (b) Gently guide the needle perpendicularly into the skin and muscle. (c) Advance the needle fully into the muscle. Quickly aspirate to verify needle placement. (d) Once needle placement is ensured, inject the solution slowly.

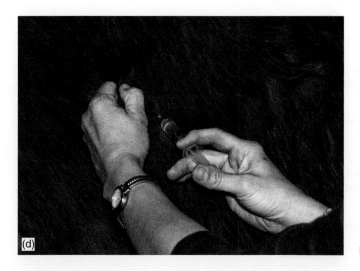

(d)

Figure 6.17 *Continued*

6.9 Procedure: Subcutaneous Injection

Technical action	Rationale/amplification
Prepare the needle and syringe for injection.	See the General Preparation section above.
Verify the following: • correct patient • correct medication • correct route • correct dosage • correct timing.	This step is important to avoid inaccuracies in the administration of an injectable medication.
Apply a halter and lead rope to the patient. Have a handler hold the head using the lead rope. Use additional forms of humane restraint if necessary.	Proper restraint is necessary to reduce the risk of injury to the patient, handler, and veterinarian or veterinary technician.
The most common location for SC injection is the lateral neck. Subcutaneous injection is also used to deposit local anesthetic for a variety of procedures (e.g., skin biopsy, transtracheal aspirate, organ biopsy, centesis, etc.).	Selection of the site is based on multiple factors: the purpose of the injection (administration of medication or local anesthesia), type of medication, and injection volume. Alternative locations for subcutaneous injections include the area in front of the shoulder blade and the axillary region.
Disinfect the skin for injection.	Disinfection of the injection site will reduce the bacterial contamination of the skin.
Pinch the loose skin and create a "tent".	Pinching the skin will help to distract some horses during the procedure. It creates a space in the subcutaneous tissue to deposit the solution.
Gently glide the needle into the fold of skin "tent".	It should be easy to advance the needle into the subcutaneous space. If the needle is located in the dermis, there will be some resistance.

(continued)

Technical action	Rationale/amplification
Release the skin and aspirate to verify needle placement. If blood appears in the hub of the needle, remove it and repeat in an alternate location.	The appearance of blood may indicate the needle is placed in a blood vessel. Certain medications may cause an anaphylactoid reaction if deposited intravascularly.
Inject the solution slowly, creating a bleb under the skin (Figure 6.18).	Unlike in companion animals, in horses only small volumes can be injected subcutaneously. A correctly deposited SC injection will create a bleb under the skin.
Remove the needle and syringe from the skin and discard in an approved biohazard container.	For biosafety reasons, used needles and syringes should not be left in publicly accessible places.
Document the medication in the patient record.	Legally the generic name of the medication, the amount, the dose, and the time of administration should be recorded and initialed.

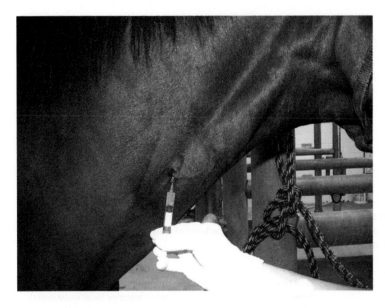

Figure 6.18 Subcutaneous injection of a drug such as a local anesthetic. After pinching the skin, the needle is inserted in the subcutaneous space and the solution is injected slowly, creating a bleb under the skin.

6.10 Procedure: Intradermal Injection

Technical action	Rationale/amplification
Prepare the needle and syringe for injection.	See the General Preparation section above.
Verify the following: • correct patient • correct medication • correct route • correct dosage • correct timing.	This step is important to avoid inaccuracies in the administration of an injectable medication.
Apply a halter and lead rope to the patient. Have a handler hold the head using the lead rope. Use additional forms of humane restraint if necessary.	Proper restraint is necessary to reduce the risk of injury to the patient, handler, and veterinarian or veterinary technician.

Technical action	Rationale/amplification
The most common location for ID injection is the lateral cervical region.	Allergy skin testing or sweat testing is typically performed on the lateral neck. Other sites of ID injection are based on the purpose of the procedure.
Prepare the skin for injection.	Disinfection of the injection site will reduce the bacterial contamination of the skin. However, in some instances minimal disinfection is indicated for subcutaneous injections.
Holding the syringe with the bevel upward, gently glide the tip of the needle into epidermis.	It is not necessary to advance the needle fully into the skin, since very small volumes are typically deposited.
Verify needle placement by lifting the needle slightly upward, and observe the outline of the needle.	If the needle is located in the subcutaneous space, the outline of the needle will be difficult to discern.
Inject the solution slowly, creating a bleb within the skin (Figure 6.19).	Small volumes (0.1–0.2 ml) are typically injected for skin testing. Larger volumes may be required for other procedures.
Remove the needle and syringe from the skin and discard in an approved biohazard container.	For biosafety reasons, used needles and syringes should not be left in publicly accessible places.
Document the medication in the patient record.	Legally the generic name of the medication, the amount, the dose, and the time of administration should be recorded and initialed.

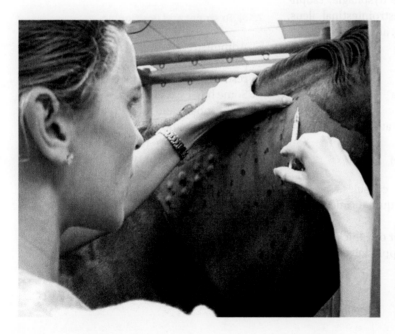

Figure 6.19 Intradermal injection. The needle is inserted into the epidermis and the solution is injected slowly, creating a bleb within the skin. Courtesy of Dr. Carol Foil.

Bibliography and Further Reading

Corley, K. (2009) Collection of blood samples and intravenous injections, in *The Equine Hospital Manual* (eds K.Corley and J.Stephen), Blackwell, Oxford, pp. 10.

Stephen, J. (2009) Intramuscular injections, in *The Equine Hospital Manual* (eds K.Corley and J. Stephen), Blackwell, Oxford, pp. 13.

7

Other Routes of Medication Administration

Ann Chapman

Medications, supplements or fluids that are not available in an injectable formulation, or that cannot be administered parenterally, require administration by oral or intra-rectal routes.

7.1 Oral Medication Administration

7.1.1 Purpose

- To administer formulation of medications or supplements by mouth.
- Contraindications to oral administration of medication include dysphagia, esophageal obstruction, gastrointestinal ileus, malabsorptive disease, and cleft palate.

7.1.2 Complications

- Aspiration pneumonia
- Dosing inaccuracies
- Oral ulceration or irritation

7.1.3 Equipment Required

- Medication (tablets, capsules, powder, paste, suspension or liquid formulations)
- Dosing syringe
- Dissolving agent: water or a thick, flavored fluid (e.g., molasses, applesauce or syrup)
- Small wooden dowel stick
- Coffee grinder or mortar and pestle
- Funnel (plastic or paper)

7.1.4 Restraint and Positioning

- Administration of oral medication can be performed in standing horses with basic restraint using halter and lead rope.
- Some horses are resentful of manipulation of the mouth and might require additional restraint methods such as neck roll (i.e., skin twitch), lip rope and modified lip rope, or manual ear twitch (see Chapter 2).
- Restraint methods that may interfere with swallowing, such as sedation or upper lip/nose twitch, are not recommended.
- Specialized medication halters are available for horses that resent oral dosing of medications.

Manual of Clinical Procedures in the Horse, First Edition. Edited by Lais R.R. Costa and Mary Rose Paradis.
© 2018 John Wiley & Sons, Inc. Published 2018 by John Wiley & Sons, Inc.

7.1.5 Procedure: Oral Medication Administration

Technical action	Rationale
Create an open-ended dosing syringe by removing the end of the syringe with a sharp instrument (Figure 7.1). Syringe size depends on the volume and amount of medication that will be administered. For larger volumes, use a 60 ml syringe and either cut off the entire end of the syringe (Figure 7.1) or shorten the tip of the catheter tip syringe.	The opening size should be at least the size of a dime. If using a catheter tip syringe for administration of oral medication, it is best to shorten the tip to avoid hurting the horse's mouth.
Prepare the dried powder medication. Count the correct number of tablets (Figure 7.2a) or capsules. *Capsules containing powdered drug*: Open the capsule, depositing the powder onto a folded piece of paper or a small funnel. *Tablets*: Crush tablets using a mortar and pestle (Figure 7.2b) or a small coffee grinder. *Powder*: Measure the correct volume. *Paste*: Measure out the correct weight or volume and place it in an appropriate size of syringe. Avoid using a multi-dose syringe for individual uses because of the risk of overdosing. *Suspension*: Aspirate the correct volume. Avoid aspirating air bubbles.	Because the particles of some medication can be hazardous to people (e.g., chloramphenicol), tablets should not be crushed, but instead allowed to dissolve in water. Some tablets dissolve very easily in tepid water. Make sure to add enough water in a syringe to make a paste, and avoid making it too watery. If the medication is in paste or suspension form, measure the correct volume.
Place the powder medication into the dosing syringe (Figure 7.2c).	To ensure all the powder is transferred to the syringe without spilling any, it is recommended that the powder is deposited onto a folded or rolled piece of paper, or a funnel.
After placing the powder medication into the dosing syringe, add a flavored liquid or syrup to the syringe. Add a small amount of the medication, followed by some of the flavored liquid or syrup, then the remaining medication, followed by more flavored liquid. Mix well with a wooden dowel stick (Figure 7.2d).	For dry medications some kind of flavored thick liquid is necessary to prepare a paste. Use flavored liquid or syrup such as apple sauce, molasses or corn syrup. If using a liquid formulation (suspension or syrup) aspirate it into the dosing syringe.
Verify the following: • correct patient • correct medication • correct route • correct dosage • correct timing.	This step is important to avoid inaccuracies in the administration of an injectable medication.
Apply a halter and lead rope to the patient. Restrain the horse's head (Figure 7.3a).	Proper restraint is necessary to reduce the risk of injury to the patient, handler, and veterinarian or veterinary technician.

(continued)

Technical action	Rationale
Make sure there is no residual hay or food material in the horse's mouth. Rinse horse's mouth, if needed.	If food is in the mouth then the medication may coat the food and be easily spat out by the horse.
Carefully part the lips at the lateral commissure using a thumb (Figure 7.3b,c).	Some horses shy from contact with the lips and mouth. Gentle parting of the upper lip at the commissure is better tolerated by most horses.
Insert the dosing syringe containing the mixed medication into the interdental space (Figure 7.3d).	The interdental space does not have teeth that could interfere with administration. Do not insert the syringe between the incisors since this could result in a bite or breakage of the syringe.
Direct the syringe caudally toward the base of the tongue (Figure 7.3e).	Placing the medication on the tongue increases the likelihood that it will be swallowed. Depositing the medication along the cheek may result in the horse refusing to swallow it.
Depress the plunger to deposit the medication between the cheek teeth and the tongue, while slightly lifting the head to stop the medication from falling out of the mouth (Figure 7.3f).	Use care when depressing the plunger to avoid contacting the teeth. If administering large volumes of medication, stop periodically and allow the patient to swallow, then repeat.
Massage the throat or elevate the head slightly to encourage the horse to swallow.	Use caution in elevating the head in horses that may be at risk for aspiration.
Observe the patient after completed oral dosing to ensure the medication is eaten.	Some horses may refuse to consume the medication or attempt to discharge the medication on the ground.
Record the medication in the patient record.	Legally the generic name of the medication, the amount, the dose, and the time of administration should be recorded and initialed.

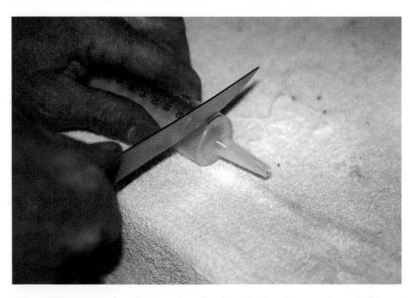

Figure 7.1 Make a dosing syringe for administration of oral medication. Remove the end of the syringe with a sharp instrument, making sure that the diameter of the opening is large enough (at least the size of a dime) and that there are no rough or sharp edges to avoid the tip hurting the horse's mouth.

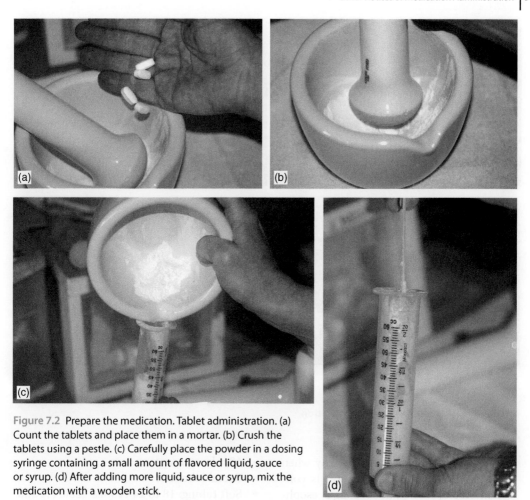

Figure 7.2 Prepare the medication. Tablet administration. (a) Count the tablets and place them in a mortar. (b) Crush the tablets using a pestle. (c) Carefully place the powder in a dosing syringe containing a small amount of flavored liquid, sauce or syrup. (d) After adding more liquid, sauce or syrup, mix the medication with a wooden stick.

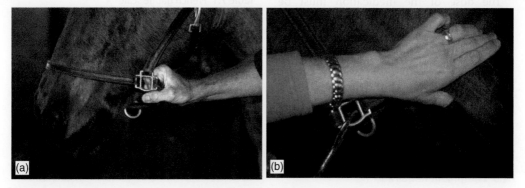

Figure 7.3 Oral administration. (a) Restrain the animal by holding onto the halter. (b) Separate the upper and lower lips at the lateral commissure using a thumb. (c) If necessary hold the noseband of the halter with three fingers while opening the lip with the thumb and index finger. (d) Insert the dosing syringe containing the mixed medication into the interdental space. (e) Advance the syringe, directing it caudally toward the base of the tongue. (f) Depress the plunger to deposit the medication between the cheek teeth and the tongue while lifting the head to prevent the medication falling out of the mouth.

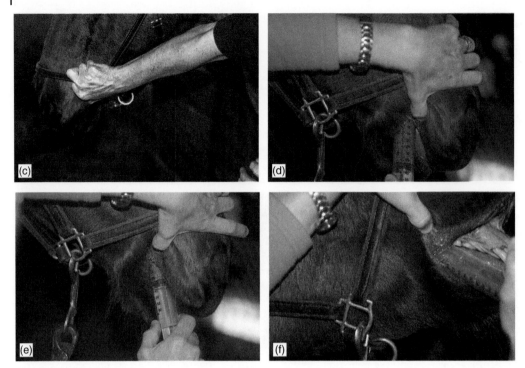

Figure 7.3 (*continued*)

7.2 Intra-rectal Medication Administration

7.2.1 Purpose

- To administer medications rectally when the oral route of administration is contraindicated, such as in dysphagia, esophageal obstruction, gastrointestinal ileus, malabsorptive disease, and cleft palate. The dose of the medication must be adjusted for this route of administration.

7.2.2 Complications

- Rectal trauma
- Rectal tear
- Defecation right after administration with loss of the medication and need for re-administration

7.2.3 Equipment Required

- Medication (tablets, capsules, powder or liquid formulation)
- 60 ml catheter tip syringe (at least two syringes)
- 60 ml warm water
- Rectal lubricant
- Soft tubing: 18 to 24 Fr (See Table 7.1 and Figure 7.4 for French gauge scale)

Table 7.1 French gauge scale

French gauge	External diameter (mm)
3	1
5	1.7
8	2.7
10	3.3
18	6
20	6.7
24	8
28	9.3
30	10

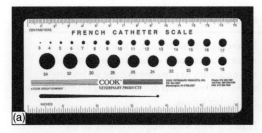 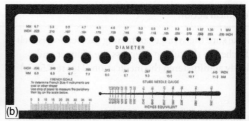

Figure 7.4 French size is the measure of the external diameter of a tube or catheter, one French gauge corresponds to a diameter of one third of a millimeter (1 Fr = 1/3 mm).

7.2.4 Restraint

- Administration of intra-rectal medication can be performed in standing horses with basic restraint using a halter and lead rope.
- Some horses might require additional restraint methods such as neck roll (i.e., skin twitch), lip rope or manual ear twitch (see Chapter 1).
- It may be preferable to perform intra-rectal medication administration in stocks if available.

7.2.5 Procedure: Intra-rectal Medication Administration

Technical action	Rationale
Prepare the medication by counting the correct number of tablets or measuring the correct volume. Crush tablets in a small coffee grinder or using a mortar and pestle.	Mix the medication with water not flavoring.
Add the medication to the catheter-tipped syringe.	Mix the medication with water not flavoring.
Verify the following: • correct patient • correct medication • correct route • correct dosage • correct timing.	This step is important to avoid inaccuracies in the administration of an injectable medication.
Apply a halter and lead rope to the patient. Have the handler restrain the horse.	Proper restraint is necessary to prevent injury from the horse to the patient, handler, and veterinarian or veterinary technician.
Stand next to the pelvic limb, facing caudally.	Horses that resent procedures such as rectal temperature may require additional restraint methods.
Apply rectal lubricant to the soft rubber tubing (Figure 7.5a).	Use care when inserting the soft rubber tubing to prevent trauma to the rectal mucosa.
Insert the tubing 2″ or 3″ into the rectum using gentle insertion pressure (Figure 7.5b).	If unable to advance the tube, reassess, redirect or gently move the tube in and out.

(continued)

Technical action	Rationale
Make sure the syringe containing medication is well attached to the tubing. Depress the plunger and slowly administered the medication (Figure 7.5c–e).	Following administration, if some of the medication remains within the tip of the syringe it is necessary to rinse the syringe with a small amount of water and deliver it rectally through the red rubber tubing.
Remove the empty syringe and flush the tubing with a syringe containing 60 ml of warm water.	Flushing with water helps to ensure all the medication is delivered to the rectum.
Carefully remove the red rubber tubing.	If the patient passes feces after intra-rectal administration of medication, the medication may be evacuated as well. Repeating the procedure may be indicated.
Record the medication in the patient record.	Proper record keeping is essential. Legally the generic name of the medication, the amount, the dose, and the time of administration should be recorded and initialed.

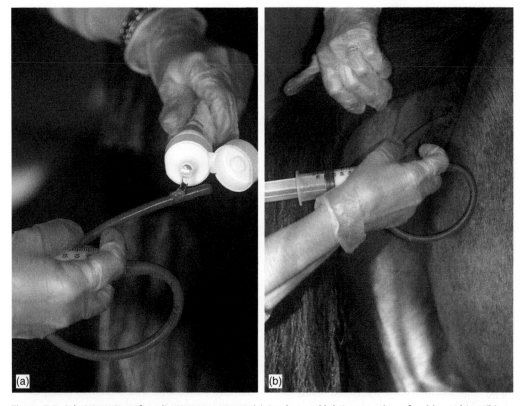

Figure 7.5 Administration of medication per rectum. (a) Apply rectal lubricant to the soft rubber tubing. (b) Standing next to the pelvic limb facing caudally, lift the tail to the side and insert the tubing in the rectum. (c) Advance the tubing 2″ or 3″ (5-8 cm). (d) Make sure the syringe containing the medication is well attached to the tubing and depress the plunger. (e) Slowly and steadily administer the medication.

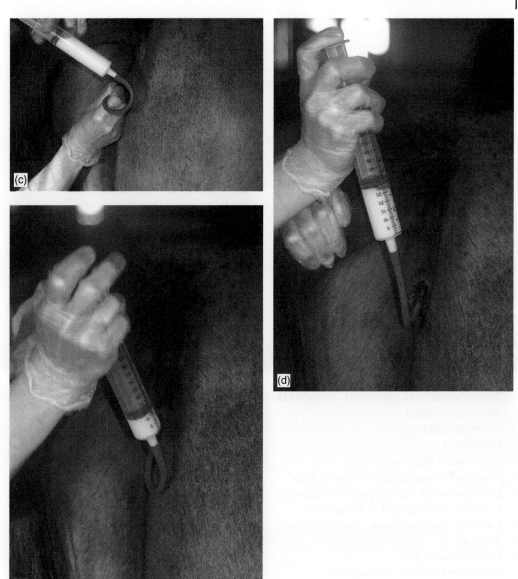

Figure 7.5 *Continued*

Bibliography and Further Reading

Schaer, B.D. and Orsini, J.A. (2008) Medication administration, in *Equine Emergencies*, 3rd edn (eds J.A. Orsini and T.J. Divers), W.B. Saunders, pp. 7–10.

8

Placement and Care of Intravenous Catheters

Ann Chapman

8.1 Purpose

- To administer injectable medications, blood products, fluids, and anesthetic agents intravenously.
- To allow venous access for repeated blood collection or rapid administration of therapeutic agents.
- To monitor central venous pressure.

8.2 Complications

- Thrombophlebitis, especially in patients with endotoxemia
- Phlebitis/cellulitis
- Hematoma
- Perivascular abscess
- Septicemia, especially in neonatal foals
- Embolism (air, thrombus, part of the catheter)
- Catheter breakage and dislodgement
- Catheter misplacement (subcutaneous, arterial)
- Catheter occlusion
- Recurrent laryngeal neuropathy
- Bacterial endocarditis secondary to thrombophlebitis

8.3 Equipment Required

- Intravenous catheter (see Table 8.1)
- Clipper with a #40 blade
- Gauze sponges, 4″ × 4″
- Skin antiseptics:
  - 0.5% triclosan surgical scrub, or
  - 2% chlorhexidine surgical scrub, or
  - 0.75% povidone-iodine surgical scrub
  - 70% ethyl alcohol
- Examination gloves
- Sterile gloves
- Syringe containing 3 ml of 2% lidocaine with a 25-gauge needle
- Syringe containing 10 ml of heparinized saline (2 IU heparin/ml)
- Extension tubing (see Table 8.2) or injection T-port
- Injection cap
- White porous tape
- 2-0 Nylon suture on a cutting needle
- Needle holders
- Suture scissors

Optional

- Cotton elastic adhesive tape
- Triple antibiotic ointment

Table 8.1 Types of intravenous catheter according to length of use

Use	Material	Type	Size
Short term (<24 hours)	Ethylene propylene or Teflon	Over the needle	10 or 12 gauge, 5.25″
Medium term (up to 3 days)	Teflon	Over the needle	14 gauge, 5.25″
Long term (up to 2 weeks)	Polyurethane	Over the needle	14 or 16 gauge, 5.25″
	Polyurethane ± antimicrobial coating	Over the wire	14 or 16 gauge, 6 or 8″
	Polyurethane ± antimicrobial coating	Through the needle	14 or 16 gauge, 6 or 8″

Manual of Clinical Procedures in the Horse, First Edition. Edited by Lais R.R. Costa and Mary Rose Paradis.
© 2018 John Wiley & Sons, Inc. Published 2018 by John Wiley & Sons, Inc.

Table 8.2 Types of extension set according to use

Use	Type	Size (gauge)	Length (″)
Emergency fluid resuscitation	High flow	13	7–18
Intravenous fluids	High flow	13	7–18
General use	Small bore	16	7

8.4 Restraint and Positioning

- Prior to intravenous catheterization, the patient should be appropriately restrained to avoid excessive neck and head motion.

- Atraumatic placement of the intravenous catheter is important to reduce the chances of complications (see above).

8.5 Procedure: Preparation for Intravenous Catheterization

Technical action	Rationale
Examine the patient carefully to determine if there are any special concerns with intravenous catheterization and care of the patient.	The poor jugular filling time in severely dehydrated and hypovolemic patients will make it more difficult to place the intravenous catheter.
Wash hands and disinfect with alcohol-based hand sanitizer.	Removing organic debris and disinfection of skin will reduce the chance of introducing bacteria.
Choose the location of the catheter site based on the accessibility of the vessel (Figure 8.1).	The jugular vein is the most commonly utilized site in horses. Alternatives include the cephalic vein and the superficial thoracic vein. For recumbent anesthetized horses, the medial saphenous can be catheterized.
Inspect the vein for patency.	Patients with pre-existing phlebitis should not be catheterized in the affected vein.
Clip the hair over a generous area surrounding the catheter site, about 8–10 cm × 8–10 cm (4″ × 4″) (Figure 8.2).	For an indwelling catheter, removing the hair is recommended because of the possibility that organic debris and bacteria may become trapped in the hair and eventually colonize the catheter. When rapid intravenous access is needed for emergency therapy, clipping may be omitted due to clinical priority.
Wearing examination gloves, aseptically prepare the catheter insertion site and the surrounding area (Figure 8.3). Ensure that all organic debris is removed and use 7 minutes of antiseptic contact time to reduce bacterial skin contamination.	Aseptic technique is recommended to disinfect the skin thoroughly and reduce the chance that foreign material or bacteria will be introduced. An abbreviated preparation may be necessary in emergency cases, where rapid intravenous access is necessary.
Inject approximately 1.5 ml of 2% lidocaine subcutaneously directly at the site of catheter placement. If using an extension set, inject an additional 1.5 ml of 2% lidocaine approximate 4–5 ml dorsal to the first injection (Figure 8.4).	Local anesthetic may reduce patient movement during placement of the catheter and reduce the chance of jugular vein trauma. A second deposit of local anesthetic at the location of the extension set will assist when securing this to the patient.

(continued)

Technical action	Rationale
Repeat aseptic skin preparation at the site of lidocaine injection.	Repeat antiseptic scrub because bacterial skin contamination may occur during lidocaine injection. This time the aseptic scrub step should be performed using sterile gloves.
Chose the appropriate catheter according to your specific needs (Table 8.1). Catheters vary in size, the specific material that they are made of, the number of lumens and the technique that is used to insert them.	Catheters that are made of propylene or Teflon tend to be more thrombogenic and should only be left in place for 1–3 days. Over-the-wire or through-the-needle catheters may be easier to place in patients that are hypovolemic.
Prepare a sterile field to aseptically open the intravenous catheter, extension set, and injection cap (Figure 8.5a).	Do not touch any portion of the catheter without sterile gloves.
Apply a new pair of sterile gloves and aseptically pre-load the catheter and extension set with heparinized saline (Figure 8.5b,c). You may need the help of an assistant.	Maintain strict sterile technique to reduce the chance of bacterial contamination. Pre-loading the catheter and extension set with heparinized saline helps to reduce clot formation in the lumen.

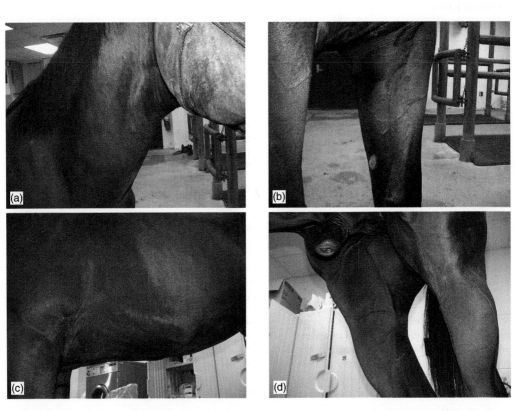

Figure 8.1 Choose the location of the catheter site: (a) the jugular vein, (b) the cephalic vein, (c) the superficial thoracic vein, and (d) the medial saphenous (only used when the horse is recumbent or under general anesthesia).

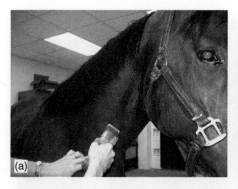
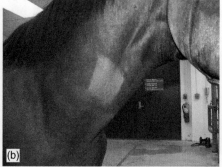

Figure 8.2 Remove the hair over a generous area surrounding the desired site for placement of the catheter. (a) Clip the hair using a #40 blade. (b) Make sure the clipped area is large enough over the desire location of catheter placement.

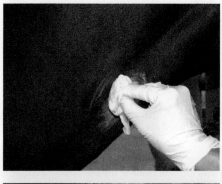

Figure 8.3 Aseptically prepare the catheter insertion site and the surrounding area by applying antiseptic scrub followed by 70% alcohol.

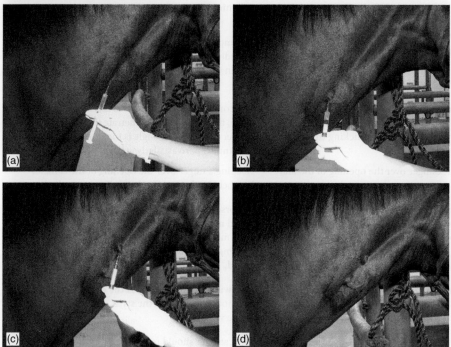

Figure 8.4 Perform subcutaneous anesthesia. (a) Inject 2% lidocaine subcutaneously. (b) Make a bleb directly at the site of catheter placement. (c) Make another bleb approximately 4–5 cm dorsal to the first injection if the extension set is to be sutured into the skin. (d) Double-check the location of the two sites of local anesthetic injection.

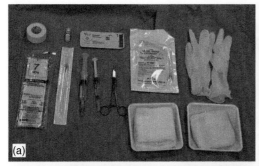

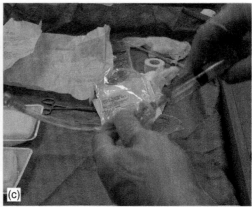

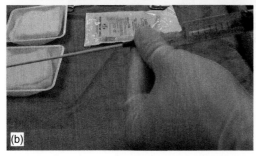

Figure 8.5 (a) Aseptically prepare the material for catheter insertion. Pre-load the catheter (b) and extension set (c) with heparinized saline.

8.6 Procedure: Insertion of an Over-the-needle Catheter

Technical action	Rationale
Prior to introduction of the catheter, a small stab incision with a #15 scalpel blade may be made at the chosen site of catheter insertion: tent the skin, guard the blade, leaving only 1 cm exposed, insert the blade through the tent of the skin. Occlude the vein distal to the insertion site using the back of the non-dominant hand.	A small stab incision made at the site of the insertion will minimize the drag of the catheter through the skin. It is important to avoid breaking sterile technique when occluding the vessel. An aseptically prepared wide area of skin will reduce risk of contamination.
While occluding the vein distal to the insertion site with the back of the non-dominant hand, hold the catheter at a 30° angle, mimicking the course of the vein.	The correct angle is important. If the angle is too steep, the catheter may penetrate through the vein to deeper tissues. If the angle is too shallow, the catheter may tunnel perivascularly and not enter the vein.
Keep the index finger over the opening of the hub (Figure 8.6).	Keeping a finger over the opening of the catheter hub helps to keep it filled with heparinized saline.
Insert the tip of the catheter through the skin and into the vein. Once the catheter is in the lumen of the vein, blood should begin to appear at the hub (Figure 8.7).	In horses with poor jugular fill, the appearance of blood may be slow. It may be helpful to check the placement by having an assistant aseptically attach a syringe with heparinized saline and aspirate for blood.
Decrease the angulation to be more parallel to the vein and advance the catheter 1–2″ (2–4 cm) further. Ensure that blood is still flowing freely from the hub.	This will help to ensure that the catheter and stylet, and not just the tip of the stylet, are inside the lumen of the vein.
Hold the stylet stationary with one hand and advance the catheter into the vein with the other hand (Figure 8.8).	The catheter should move smoothly. If there is excessive tissue drag, then the catheter may be located perivascularly and the placement should be re-verified.

Technical action	Rationale
Remove the stylet and confirm proper placement by occluding the vein and observing blood in the hub of the catheter.	In the event that the catheter is not placed in the vein, the stylet should not be replaced in the catheter. Replacement of the stylet could result in damage or breakage of the catheter. The catheter should be removed and the procedure repeated with a new catheter.
Attach an extension set or T-port with an injection cap to the hub of the catheter (Figure 8.9). Check again for blood to confirm proper placement of the catheter.	The type of extension set and the lumen size will be dictated by the function of the catheter. Alternatively, for short-term catheters, an injection cap alone may be attached to the catheter hub.
Flush the catheter with 5–10 ml of heparinized saline.	Flushing the catheter is recommended to prevent the formation of a clot in the catheter.
The catheter is secured to the skin promptly after insertion and flushing.	Steps to secure the catheter to the skin are described in procedure 8.10 and Figure 8.16.

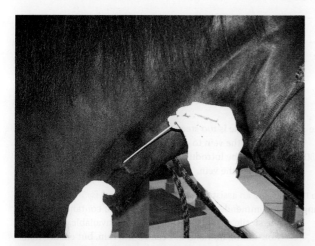

Figure 8.6 Hold the catheter at a 30° angle, mimicking the course of the vein with the index finger over the opening of the hub, and occlude the vein distal to the insertion site with the non-dominant hand, avoiding the use of the thumb and index finger to maintain aseptic technique.

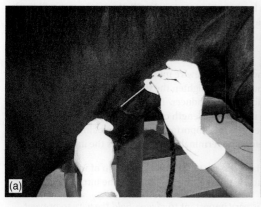
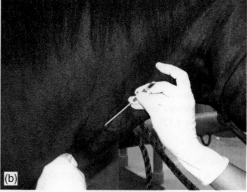

Figure 8.7 Insertion of the over-the-needle catheter. (a) Introduce the tip of the needle and catheter through the skin. (b) As the catheter is advanced into the vein, blood begins to appear at the hub when the catheter is in the lumen of the vein.

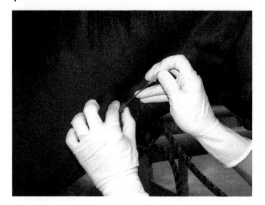

Figure 8.8 Hold the stylet stationary with one hand and advance the catheter into the vein with the other hand.

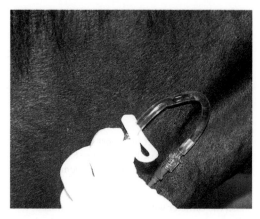

Figure 8.9 Attach an extension set with an injection cap to the hub of the catheter.

8.7 Procedure: Insertion of an Over-the-wire Catheter

Technical action	Rationale
Identify the components of the over-the-wire catheter kit (Figure 8.10). Open the over-the-wire catheter kit, ensuring strict aseptic technique.	The introducer is either a large needle or a short over-the-needle catheter. The introducer will guide the wire into the vein.
Make a small stab incision at the insertion site to minimize the drag of the catheter through the skin. Take the introducer and hold it at a 30° angle, mimicking the course of the vein.	If the angle is too steep, the introducer may penetrate through the vein to deeper tissues. If the angle is too shallow, the introducer may tunnel perivascularly and not enter the vein.
Have the vein distend by occluding it distal to the insertion site, preferably by an assistant holding the vein outside the sterile field.	Using an assistant to occlude the vessel is recommended to reduce the chance of contaminating the sterile gloves. If an assistant is unavailable, use the non-dominant hand to occlude the vein, but ensure that a wide area of skin has been surgically prepared.
Insert the introducer through the skin and into the vein (Figure 8.11). Once the introducer is in the lumen of the vein, blood should begin to appear at the hub.	In horses with poor jugular fill, the appearance of blood may be slow.
Using the thumb, retract the guidewire slightly into the plastic housing to straighten the tip. Attach the plastic housing to the introducer and pass the guidewire into the vein for approximately 20 cm (Figure 8.12).	The "J" tip guidewire must be retracted into the plastic housing to straighten the tip so that it will fit into the hub of the introducer. The guidewire will have markings to indicate the length of the wire that has passed into the vein. It is important to stop advancing the guidewire before the terminal end approaches the introducer.
Remove the plastic housing from the guidewire, leaving at least 10 cm of guidewire externally.	It is necessary to leave at least 10 cm of wire exposed outside the vein to safely remove the introducer.
Carefully remove the introducer from the vein, leaving just the guidewire in the vein. Be careful to always maintain a good hold on the guidewire.	It is very important to *always hold the wire* to prevent accidental contamination or possible dislodgement from the vessel or loss of the wire into the vessel.

Technical action	Rationale
Optional: Pass the vessel dilator over the guidewire and into the vein, then removed again carefully.	The vessel dilator, if provided, will enlarge the catheter opening and facilitate the passage of the catheter.
Insert the end of the guidewire into the tip of the catheter and feed the guidewire up through the catheter hub (Figure 8.13). Grasp the guidewire at the catheter hub.	It is important to maintain contact with the guidewire to prevent accidental contamination or embolization.
Advance the catheter through the skin and into the vein (Figure 8.14).	Because of tissue drag, it may be necessary to push the catheter into the vein with a slight twisting close to the skin. The catheter should be fully seated in the vein after insertion.
Carefully remove the guidewire (Figure 8.15).	Make sure to maintain the catheter all the way into the vein while pulling the wire.
Attach an extension set or T-port to the hub of the catheter, then attach an injection cap. Alternatively, if the extension set is integrated into the catheter, attach an injection cap alone.	Some catheter kits provide a one-way valve attachment that can be secured to the hub of the catheter after the guidewire is removed to protect against air embolism. An injection cap is necessary to seal the catheter and prevent bacterial contamination. If the catheter has more than 1 lumen, place an injection cap to seal each hub.
Check again for blood to confirm proper placement of the catheter. Flush the catheter with 10 ml of heparinized saline.	Flushing with heparinized saline will help prevent clot formation. If the catheter has more than 1 lumen, flush each port.
The catheter is secured to the skin promptly after insertion and flushing.	Steps to secure the catheter to the skin are described in procedure 8.9, and Figure 8.16.

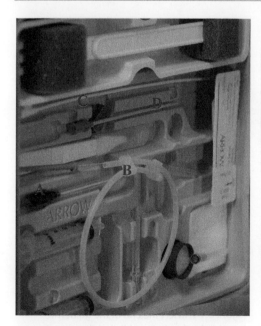

Figure 8.10 Identify the components of the over-the-wire catheter kit: A, introducer catheters; B, guidewire ("J" wire"); C, over-the-wire catheter; D, vessel dilator. Courtesy of Dr. Lais R.R. Costa.

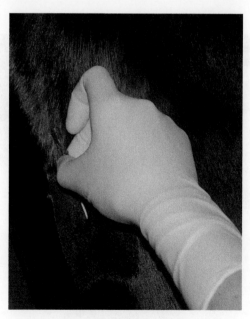

Figure 8.11 Insert the introducer through the skin and into the vein. Advance the introducer catheter and remove the stylet. Courtesy of Dr. Lais R.R. Costa.

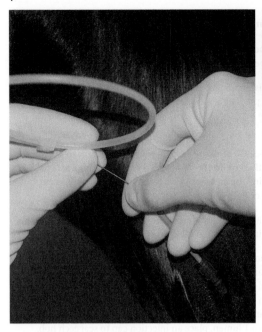

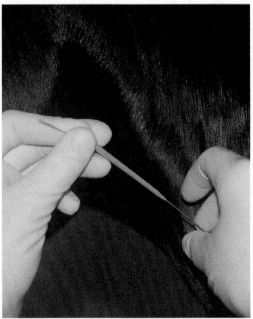

Figure 8.12 Attach the plastic housing of the guidewire to the hub of the introducer to pass the guidewire into the vein. Make sure to retract the guidewire slightly into the plastic housing to straighten the tip beforehand. Courtesy of Dr. Lais R.R. Costa.

Figure 8.13 Remove the guidewire plastic housing and the introduced, leaving at least 10 cm of guidewire out of the vein. Maintain a good hold on the guidewire at all times. Courtesy of Dr. Lais R.R. Costa.

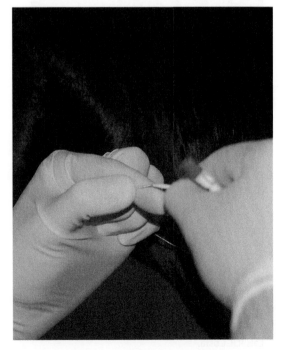

Figure 8.14 Insert the end of the guidewire into the tip of catheter while holding the wire in place. Pull out the wire while advancing the catheter, always holding the wire. Courtesy of Dr. Lais R.R. Costa.

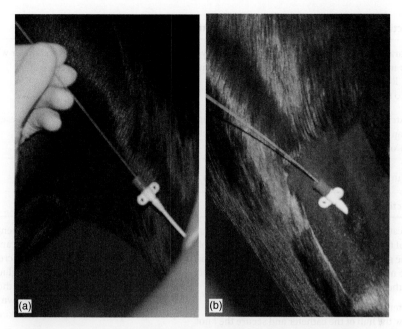

Figure 8.15 Advance the catheter through the skin and into the vein, while holding the wire in place (a) until the catheter is inserted completely into the vein and the hub of the catheter is lodged at the skin. (b) Remove the guide wire while the catheter remains fully seated in the vein. Courtesy of Dr. Lais R.R. Costa.

8.8 Procedure: Insertion of a Through-the-needle Intravenous Catheter

Technical action	Rationale
Remove the sterile peel-away introducer.	The introducer is usually a short peel-away catheter with a stylet.
Make a small stab incision at insertion site to minimize the drag of the catheter through the skin. Hold the introducer at a 30° angle, mimicking the course of the vein.	If the angle is too steep, the introducer may penetrate through the vein to deeper tissues. If the angle is too shallow, the introducer may tunnel perivascularly and not enter the vein.
Occlude the vein distal to the insertion site using the non-dominant hand or have an assistant distend the vein outside the sterile field.	Using an assistant to occlude the vessel is recommended to reduce the chance of contaminating the sterile gloves. If an assistant is unavailable, the non-dominant hand may occlude the vessel, but ensure that a wide area of skin has been surgically prepared.
Insert the introducer through the skin and into the vein. Once the introducer is in the lumen of the vein, blood should begin to appear at the hub.	In horses with poor jugular fill, the appearance of blood may be slow.
Remove the stylet.	The stylet must be removed so the catheter can be introduced into the vein.
Carefully insert the catheter into the hub of the peel-away introducer and advance it fully into the vein.	The catheter should be seated completely in the vein until it comes into contact with the hub of the peel-away introducer.
Pull the tabs of the peel-away introducer upward and outward away from the insertion site, causing them to separate completely.	To get the peel-away introducer to split at the level of the skin, it is important to maintain upward and outward motion.

(continued)

Technical action	Rationale
During separation of the peel-away introducer, the catheter may withdraw from the insertion site slightly. Re-insert the catheter through the skin and into the vein if necessary.	Try to minimize the withdraw of the catheter while removing the peel-away introducer.
Attach an extension set to the hub of the catheter, then attach an injection cap. The catheter is secured to the skin promptly after insertion and flushing.	Steps to secure the catheter to the skin are described in section 8.9.

8.9 Procedure: Securing the Intravenous Catheter

Technical action	Rationale
Secure the catheter to the skin by placing a suture on each wing of the butterfly (Figure 8.16a,b). Placement of a suture in the groove of the hub of the catheter is optional for over-the needle catheters, but recommended for over-the-wire catheters. If the catheter does not have butterfly wings place a suture below the hub of the catheter and secure the knot above the rim.	It is important to reduce the movement of the catheter since excessive movement can damage the endothelium of the vessel and increase the risk of thrombophlebitis. Adhesive glue is not recommended because it may bond the hub too tightly to the skin and has been known to cause breakage of the catheter below the skin surface.
In case of over-the-wire catheters, it is important to place the suture below the wings of the catheter, around the hub of the catheter, and positioned into the little grove midway through the hub of the catheter (Figure 8.16c).	This extra suture is important for proper placement of over-the-wire catheters.
Make a butterfly using adhesive tape and apply it to the distal portion of the extension set. Curve the extension set to relieve tension on the catheter and secure it to the neck with one or two sutures through the tape butterfly (Figure 8.17 and 8.18a). If using a T-port, place sutures immediately proximal to the T (Figure 8.18b).	Slight laxity in the extension set may help to reduce tension on the catheter with head and neck movement. Evaluate the placement of the sutures to ensure proper positioning of the catheter (Figure 8.18).
Again, flush the catheter with 10 ml of heparinized saline (Figure 8.19)	Flushing with heparinized saline will help prevent clot formation.

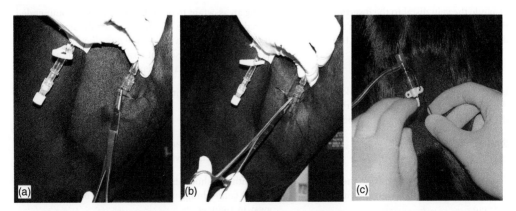

Figure 8.16 (a) Secure the over-the-needle catheter. (b) Place a suture on each wing of the butterfly. (c) Secure the over-the-wire catheter by placing the suture on each wing and an additional suture below the wings of the catheter around the hub and position it in the little grove midway along the hub of the catheter. Courtesy of Dr. Lais R.R. Costa.

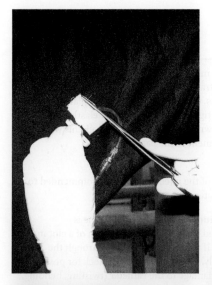

Figure 8.17 Suture the extension set to the skin. Make a butterfly using adhesive tape and apply it to the distal portion of the extension set, curve the extension set, and secure it to the neck with one or two sutures through the tape butterfly.

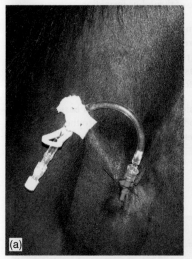

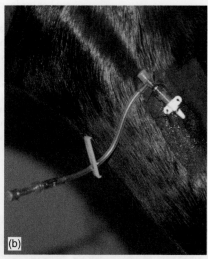

Figure 8.18 Evaluate the placement of the sutures to ensure proper position of the catheter: (a) over-the-needle catheter placement and (b) over-the-wire catheter placement showing the use of a T-Port, which is sutured to the skin just below the T..

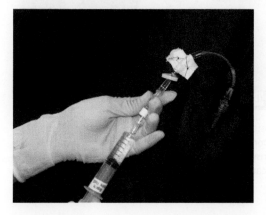

Figure 8.19 Flush the catheter with 5–10 ml of heparinized saline, preferably before placing the skin sutures rather than after.

8.10 Procedure: Catheter Care and Maintenance

Technical action	Rationale
Optional bandaging of the catheter. Place a small amount of antiseptic ointment on a small stack of gauze sponges (Figure 8.20a). Place the gauze sponges over the catheter insertion site to protect it (Figure 8.20b). Apply several layers of cotton elastic adhesive tape, ensuring the injection port of the catheter is visible (Figure 8.20c,d).	The catheter may be bandaged in horses with a tendency to traumatize the area (e.g., recumbent patients, foals, etc.). Make sure to avoid placing the bandage too tight. Unwrap the roll of elastic adhesive tape and re-wrap it loosely onto the roll; this will help proper placement of the bandage.
Wipe the injection cap with a disinfectant (e.g., 70% alcohol) prior to injecting any solutions.	Disinfection of the injection port is recommended to minimize bacterial contamination.
Flush the indwelling catheter every 6 hours with 6–10 ml of heparinized saline (the volume of heparinized saline will depend on the size of the extension set).	Periodic flushing with heparinized saline is recommended to prevent the formation of a clot in the catheter. If solutions do not flow through the catheter easily, do not force them. Check for possible mechanical damage to the catheter (twisting, bending, etc.) or evidence of thrombus formation.
Examine the catheter every 12 hours and palpate the vein for pain, warmth, swelling or discharge.	Pain, warmth, and swelling over the vein are signs suggestive of thrombophlebitis. The catheter should be immediately removed aseptically and the distal tip of the catheter aseptically placed in a plain blood-collection tube for bacterial culture and sensitivity.
Change the injection cap every 24–48 hours.	Replacing the injection cap on a regular basis helps to reduce the introduction of bacteria into the catheter and extension set.

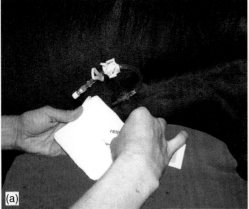 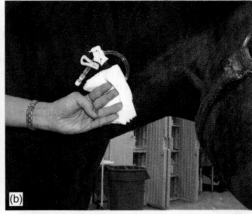

Figure 8.20 Apply a bandage over the intravenous catheter. (a) Place a small amount of antiseptic ointment on a small stack of gauze sponges. (b) Place the gauze sponges over the catheter insertion site to protect it. (c) Apply several layers of cotton elastic adhesive tape, ensuring the injection port of the catheter is visible. (d) Make sure the bandage extends at least 1½" cranial and caudal to the 4" × 4" gauze sponges.

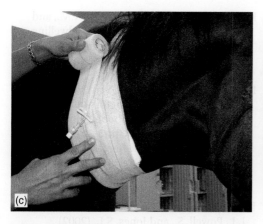
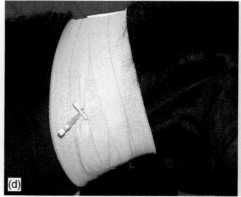

Figure 8.20 (continued)

8.11 Procedure: Removal of an Intravenous Catheter

Technical action	Rationale
The catheter should be removed by first removing the sutures.	Use caution when removing the sutures and do not cut the catheter itself.
Apply a clean gauze sponge with antiseptic ointment over the insertion site and remove the catheter (Figure 8.21).	Antiseptic ointments that can be used include triple antibiotic, chlorhexidine, povidone iodine or silver sulfadiazine.
Apply light pressure over the insertion site for 1–2 minutes.	Applying pressure after the catheter is removed will promote hemostasis and prevent hemorrhage or hematoma formation.
Inspect the catheter after removal; ensure the catheter is intact and it has been removed in its entirety.	If indicated submit the catheter for bacterial culture and sensitivity.

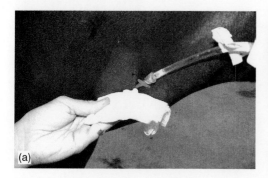
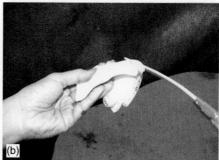

Figure 8.21 Removal of the intravenous catheter. (a) Apply a clean gauze sponge with antiseptic ointment over the insertion site once the sutures have been removed. (b) Pull out the catheter and apply light pressure over the insertion site for 1–2 minutes.

Acknowledgement

The author would like to acknowledge and thank Mila International, Inc. for generously providing catheter images.

Bibliography and Further Reading

Barakzai, S. and Chandler, K. (2003) Use of indwelling intravenous catheters in the horse. *In Practice*, **25**, 264–271.

Ettlinger, J.J., Palmer, J.E., and Benson, C. (1992) Bacteria found on intravenous catheters removed from horses. *Veterinary Record*, **130**, 248–249.

Gardner, S.Y., Reef, V.B., and Spencer, P.A. (1991) Ultrasonographic evaluation of horses with thrombophlebitis of the jugular vein: 46 cases (1985–1988). *Journal of the American Veterinary Medical Association*, **199**, 370–373.

Geraghty, T.E., Love, S., Taylor, D.J., Mellor, D.J., and Hughes, K.K. (2009) Assessment of subclinical venous catheter-related diseases in horses and associated risk factors. *Veterinary Record*, **164** (8), 227–231.

Geraghty, T.E., Love, S., Taylor, D.J., Heller, J., Mellor, D.J., and Hughes, K.J. (2009) Assessing techniques for disinfecting sites for inserting intravenous catheters into the jugular veins of horses. *Veterinary Record*, **164** (2), 51–55.

Hay, C.W. (1992) Equine intravenous catheterization. *Equine Veterinary Education*, **4** (6), 319–323.

Kelmer, G., Catasus, C.T., Saxton, A.M., and Elliot, S.B. (2009) Evaluation of indwelling intravenous catheters for the regional perfusion of the limbs of horses. *Veterinary Record*, **165** (17), 496–501.

Lankyeld, D.P., Ensink, J.M., van Dijk, P., and Klein, W.R. (2001) Factors influencing the occurrence of thrombophlebitis after post-surgical long-term intravenous catheterization of colic horses: a study of 38 cases. *Journal of Veterinary Medicine A, Physiology, Pathology, Clinical Medicine*, **48**, 545–552.

Little, D., Keene, B.W., Bruton, C., Smith, L.J., Powell, S., and Jones, S.L. (2002) Percutaneous retrieval of a jugular catheter fragment from the pulmonary artery of a foal. *Journal of the American Veterinary Medical Association*, **220**, 212–214.

Scarrat, W.K., Pyle, R.L., Buechner-Maxwell, V., Karzenski, S., and Wallace, M.A. (1998) Transection of an intravenous catheter in six horses: effects and location of the catheter fragment. *Proceedings of the Annual Convention of the American Association of Equine Practitioners*, **44**, 294–295.

Spurlock, S.L., Spurlock, G.H., Parker, G., and Ward, M.V (1990) Long-term jugular vein catheterization in horses. *Journal of the American Veterinary Medical Association*, **196** (3), 425–430.

Traub-Dargatz, J.L. and Dargatz, D.A. (1994) A retrospective study of vein thrombosis in horses treated with intravenous fluids in a veterinary teaching hospital. *Journal of Veterinary Internal Medicine*, **8**, 264–266.

9

Chemical Restraint

Antonio José de Araujo Aguiar

9.1 Purpose

- To administer sedatives, tranquilizers and analgesics, or a combination of these drugs, to produce restraint or chemical immobilization, followed by sedation, anxiolysis, analgesia, and reduction of defensive behavior to external stimuli.
- To facilitate clinical examinations (including evaluate limbs, oral cavity, pinna and external auditory canal, perform ophthalmic examination and rectal palpation), perform diagnostic procedures (including bronchoscopy and gastroscopy, dentistry, ultrasonography and radiography, collection of cerebral-spinal fluid and trans-tracheal aspiration), or as anesthetic premedication.

9.2 Complications

- Cardiorespiratory depression
- Cardiac arrhythmias (e.g., alpha-2 agonists)
- Hypotension
- Marked ataxia
- Arousal and increased locomotion (e.g., opioids)
- Overdose
- Perivascular administration
- Adverse drug reaction (e.g., urticaria, anaphylactoid reaction)
- Accidental intra-arterial injection, leading to sudden recumbency and seizures.

Table 9.1 presents the concerns and facts to consider before sedation or tranquilization.

Table 9.1 Concerns and facts to consider before sedation or tranquilization

Factor	Facts to consider
Evaluation of the type of patient	Factors such as clinical condition, age, sex, breed and patient behavior are determinants in the selection of sedatives and tranquilizers, as well as the route and doses to be administered. Patient's state of excitement may affect quality and duration of sedation.
Clinical examination	Clinical evaluation of the cardiovascular and respiratory systems is required prior to administration of drugs that depress the central nervous system, especially alpha-2 agonists and opioids.
Weight measurement	Doses of sedatives and tranquilizers are established according to body weight in kilograms (kg). In order to avoid overdose and reduce the risks of adverse effects, it is very important to accurately measure or estimate the body weight of the animal. Body weight can be measured with use of scales for large animals, or estimated with the use of a weight tapes. Most weight tapes give an estimate of body weight based on the girth circumference (Figure 9.1). Others give an estimate based on girth circumference and body length. If body weight is measured in pounds (lb), it must be converted to kilograms (kg) by dividing by 2.2.

(continued)

Manual of Clinical Procedures in the Horse, First Edition. Edited by Lais R.R. Costa and Mary Rose Paradis.
© 2018 John Wiley & Sons, Inc. Published 2018 by John Wiley & Sons, Inc.

Factor	Facts to consider
Place where the chemical restraint is held	The environment must be calm and quiet because none of the sedative or tranquilizing agents will take adequate effect if the horse is stimulated before or immediately after drug administration. The administration should preferably be done at the place of the clinical procedure, avoiding unnecessary relocation of the animal, because of the ataxia and reluctance to walk induced by these drugs.
Venous access	Venous catheterization ensures reliable delivery of drugs by the IV route, avoiding the need for several punctures of the jugular vein, the risk of perivascular administrations of agents, and the risk of intra-arterial injection during the administration of supplementary doses. The placement of an IV catheter should be performed according to aseptic technique (see Chapter 8).
Interval between drug administration and the beginning of the clinical or diagnostic procedure	After administration of the sedatives or tranquilizers, it is very important to have an interval of time for the maximum effect to be observed before starting to handle the patient. This latency period is variable according to the route of administration (e.g., for the alpha-2 agonists, the latency period ranges from 2 to 5 minutes if the drug is given intravenously and from 20 to 30 minutes if given intramuscularly). Another fact is the chemical nature of the drug administered (e.g., the intramuscular absorption of acepromazine is slower than that of alpha-2 agonists).
Duration and intensity of drug effects in the central nervous system	The duration and intensity of sedation should be consistent with the length of time required to perform the clinical or diagnostic procedure, and the degree of stimuli that the horse will be subjected to. Sedatives and tranquilizers produce central nervous system depression to varying grades (from mild to intense) therefore horses under their effects are still able to produce sudden defense motor responses to external stimuli (noise, light, motion, palpation or touch at sensitive areas of body).
Availability of specific antagonists	In case of overdose of sedatives, depressive effects can be quickly stopped by the administration of specific antagonists, according to the pharmacological group. There are specific antagonists for alpha-2 agonists, opioids and benzodiazepines, but the effects of tranquilizing drugs can't be reversed (e.g., acepromazine).

9.3 Equipment Required

- Drugs:
  - sedatives: xylazine, detomidine, romifidine, medetomidine, dexmedetomidine
  - tranquilizers: acepromazine, diazepam, midazolam
  - opioids: butorphanol, morphine, methadone.
- Other materials:
  - sterile syringes: 1, 3, 5 or 10 ml
  - sterile needles: 18, 20 or 22 gauge, and 1″ or 1½″ in length
  - over-the-needle catheters: 14 or 16 gauge
  - three-way stopcock or injection port adaptor
  - cyanoacrylate glue or skin suture material
  - hair clipper
  - antiseptic solution (e.g., chlorhexidine and alcohol)
  - sterile gauze sponges
  - biohazard container.
- Halter and lead rope.
- "Twitch" (rope or chain).
- Stock for horses.

9.4 Restraint and Positioning

- The use of a halter and lead rope is essential for the proper positioning and control of the head of the animal during administration of medication.

- In case of restless, stressed or aggressive horses, it may be necessary to use a "twitch" or another physical restraint method.

- Depending on the procedure to be performed, it is preferable to place the horse into a stock for physical containment prior to administration of sedatives or tranquilizers.

9.5 Procedure: Selection of Drugs, Route of Administration and Calculation of Doses

Technical action	Rationale
Selection of drugs to be administered and route of administration (Table 9.2).	Based on the demeanor, characteristics, and clinical status of the patient, as well as the indications for the chemical restraint (e.g., loading and transporting the animal, type of clinical or diagnostic procedure to be performed, analgesia, premedication for local general anesthesia).
Calculation of the total volume of medication to be administered (ml). Use the formula: volume (ml) = (body weight (kg) × dose of drug (mg/kg or µg/kg))/concentration of the formulation (mg/ml or µg/ml)	Accurate calculation is a very important step in ensuring the administration of the correct dose to the patient, avoiding overdose and reducing the risks of adverse effects. If a scale is not available, body weight should be estimated using a weight tape (Figure 9.1). Care must be taken to double check the concentration of the drug being used, as some drugs come in different formulations of varying concentrations.
Preparation and administration of drugs by intravenous (IV) or intramuscular (IM) routes.	The techniques for IV and IM administration of sedatives, opioids, and tranquilizers follow those described in Chapter 6. When an IV catheter is to be placed, the reader is referred to Chapter 8.

Table 9.2 Drugs, doses, and route of administration

Drug group	Drug (brand name)	Concentration (mg/ml)	Dose (mg/kg)	Route
Phenothiazine	Acepromazine (*Promace*)	10	0.02–0.1	IV, IM
Alpha-2 agonists	Xylazine (*Rompun, Sedazine*)	100 or 20	0.5–1.0	IV, IM
	Detomidine (*Dormodesan*)	10	0.01–0.02	IV
			0.02–0.04	IM
	Romifidine (*Sedivet*)	10	0.05–0.12	IV, IM
	Medetomidine (*Domitor*)	1	0.0035–0.01	IV
	Dexmedetomidine (*Dexdomitor*)	0.5	0.003-0.005	IV
Alpha-2 antagonists	Atipamezol (*Antisedan*)	5	0.05–0.2	IV
	Yoimbine (*Antagonil, Yocon*)	5	0.04–0.15	IV

(continued)

Drug group	Drug (brand name)	Concentration (mg/ml)	Dose (mg/kg)	Route
	Tolazoline (*Tolazine*)	100	0.5–2	IV
Opioids	Butorphanol (*Torbugesic*)	10	0.02–0.04	IV, IM
	Morphine	50	0.05–0.1	IV, IM
	Methadone (*Dolophine, Methadose*)	10	0.05–0.2	IV
Benzodiazepines	Diazepam (*Valium*)	5	0.1–0.2	IV
	Midazolam (*Versed*)	5	0.1–0.2	IV

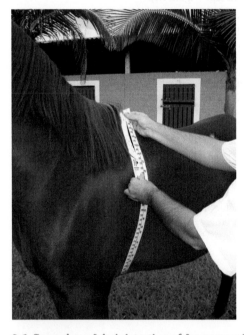

Figure 9.1 Estimation of the weight of a horse by the use of a weight tape, which is placed around the girth, can be achieved with reasonable accuracy. The accuracy of the weight estimation of young foals, very lean horses or donkeys using weight tape is poorer.

9.6 Procedure: Administration of Acepromazine

Technical action	Rationale
Based on the recommendations, determine if acepromazine is indicated. Note the dose range for acepromazine maleate: 0.02–0.1 mg/kg (IV or IM). Suggested dose: 0.02 to 0.05 mg/kg (IV or IM)	Recommended for: • horses with a calm demeanor that are quiet • stress control for loading into vehicles (Figure 9.2), during transportation or conditioning of the patient into a new environment, shoeing, sheath cleaning, and hair clipping • clinical or diagnostic procedures without production of noxious stimuli (minor procedures) • as anesthetic premedication.

Technical action	Rationale
Observe the patient closely. Note the expected effects and timing following the administration of acepromazine. Timing 15–20 minutes. Main effects: indifference to surroundings, reduced locomotion, mild ataxia, slight lowering of the head, ptosis of the eyelids and lips, flaccid protrusion of the penis. Repeated administration is not recommended because it will prolong the effect but not the level of tranquilization.	Expected effects: • time to peak effects 15–20 minutes (if given IV), 30–40 minutes (if given IM); duration is highly variable, often ranging from 4 to 6 hours. • mild to moderate tranquilization, anxiolysis • indifferent to the surrounding environment • reduction of locomotion • mild ataxia • slight lowering of the head, more evident in docile and calm horses (Figure 9.3a) • ptosis of eyelids and lips • drowsy expression • flaccid protrusion of the penis (long-lasting in some cases) (Figure 9.3b) • sudden motor reactions if stimulated.
Be aware of hypotension as a potential adverse effect associated with the administration of acepromazine.	Adverse effect: hypotension may be significant in hypovolemic horses, but clinically unimportant in normotensive animals.
Provide additional care if necessary.	Protection and support of the exposed penis with the use of non-compressive bandage (applied around the lumbar region).

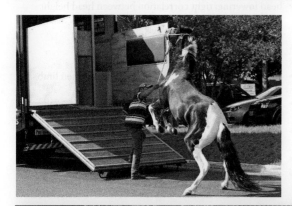

Figure 9.2 Administration of tranquilizers or sedatives prior to loading or transporting a horse is sometimes necessary. The calming and sedative effects make these procedures easier and safer for the animal and personnel.

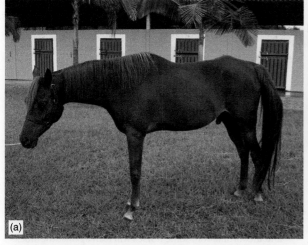
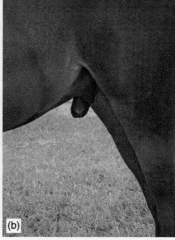

(a) (b)

Figure 9.3 Effects of acepromazine administration at 0.05 mg/kg IV to a horse. Note (a) the calm facial expression and mild lowering of head, and (b) penile relaxation.

9.7 Procedure: Administration of Alpha-2 Agonists

Technical action	Rationale
Based on the reported recommendations, determine if an alpha-2 agonist agent is indicated. Doses: • xylazine: 0.5–1.0 mg/kg (IV/IM) • detomidine: 0.01–0.02 mg/kg (IV); 0.01–0.04 mg/kg (IM) • romifidine: 0.05–0.12 mg/kg (IV/IM) • medetomidine: 0.0035–0.01 mg/kg (IV). • dexmedetomidine: 0.003-0.005 mg/kg (IV)	Recommended for: • fractious, unruly or stressed horses • control of stress during transportation • more complex clinical or diagnostic procedures requiring major manipulation (oral cavity, limbs, rectal palpation, radiographs, endoscopies, etc.) • control of visceral pain in colic patients, facilitating clinical examination and rectal palpation • sedation and immobilization techniques prior to local anesthetic procedures (minor surgical procedures) • as anesthetic premedication.

Observe the patient closely. Note the expected effects and timing following the administration of an alpha-2 agonist agent.
 	
Timing to peak effect varies depending on which alpha-2 agonist agent is used, ranging from 2 to 5 minutes if given IV.
 	
Main effects: indifference to surroundings, reluctance to move, mild to moderate ataxia, marked lowering of the head (dose-dependent), ptosis of the eyelids and lips, wide-based stance, relaxation of the penis.
 	
Starting dose varies depending on the desired level of sedation. The suggested starting dose is the lowest recommended dose:
 	
  – xylazine: 0.5 mg/kg IV
  – detomidine: 0.01 mg/kg IV
  – romifidine: 0.05 mg/kg IV
 	
Dosage should be titrated, such that administration is repeated as needed in order to achieve deeper level of sedation or increase the length of sedation.
	Expected effects:
	
	• time to peak effects is 2–5 minutes (IV) and 15–20 minutes (IM); duration of sedative effects varies greatly depending on the drug, the route of administration and the dose.
	• dose-dependent sedation (moderate to intense), visceral analgesia, and muscle relaxation
	• indifferent to the surrounding environment
	• dose-dependent ataxia and incoordination
	• reluctance to move
	• head lowering: tight correlation between head height and degree of sedation; the more intense the sedative effect, the lower the head (Figures 9.4 and 9.5)
	• marked drowsy expression (Figure 9.6).
	• ptosis of eyelids and lips (Figure 9.7)
	• wide-based stance = increased distance between limbs, most often the forelimbs (Figure 9.8)
	• resting a hindlimb by only the toe touching the ground (Figure 9.9); this may lead to loss of balance and stumbling
	• exteriorization/relaxation of penis (lasting according to the administered alpha-2 agonist agent) (Figure 9.10)
	• sweating
	• profuse urination 30–40 minutes after administration (hyperglycemic alpha-2 effect).

Be aware of potential adverse effects associated with the administration of an alpha-2 agonist agent. most notably bradycardia and bradyarrhythmias.	Side effects: • bradycardia • arrhythmias (atrioventricular blocks) • transient hypertension, followed by hypotension • mild respiratory depression • decreased gastrointestinal motility • tachypnea may occur in febrile animals (empirical observation).
Provide additional care if necessary: avoid walking and do not allow eating until fully recovered.	Avoid forcing the horse to walk after administration of alpha-2 agonists, especially when using higher doses of detomidine, because of the risk of accidents and injuries as a result of the severe ataxia and incoordination. When the sedated horse is standing in a stock, care must be taken with the neck position over the front bar, gate or rope because of the risk of tracheal obstruction, jugular vein occlusion, collapse, and fall. In case of intense ataxia and incoordination, some horses will lean against the stock side bars or the back gate. Place a muzzle if necessary, to prevent the horse from eating because of the risk of choke.

Technical action	Rationale
If indicated administer an alpha-2 antagonist: • atipamezol: 0.05–0.2 mg/kg (IV) • yohimbine: 0.04–0.15 mg/kg (IV).	Reversion is recommended in case of adverse effects, including: • overdose • marked cardiorespiratory depression • severe ataxia and incoordination (risk of recumbency).

9.8 Procedure: Administration of Opioids

Technical action	Rationale
Based on the reported recommendations, determine if an opioid is indicated. Drugs and doses: • butorphanol: 0.02–0.04 mg/kg (IV/IM) • morphine: 0.05–0.1 mg/kg (IV/IM) • methadone: 0.05–0.1 mg/kg (IV/IM). Starting dose varies depending on the desired level of analgesia and the associated drug. The suggested starting dose is the lowest recommended dose of the combination: butorphanol at 0.02 mg/kg IV associated with detomidine at 0.01 mg/kg IV Administration may be repeated as needed in order to achieve deeper level of analgesia or increase the length of analgesia.	Based on the desired effect: • analgesia: due to their analgesic properties, opioids are commonly used in horses with signs of pain and discomfort of various origins (e.g., trauma, fractures, osteoarticular lesions, visceral pain) • deep sedation: opioids in combination with acepromazine or alpha-2 agonists produce intense sedation; opioids exhibit only discrete sedative effects when administered alone, but they potentiate the sedation produced by other drugs • premedication for general anesthesia: in this case, opioids are often associated with acepromazine and alpha-2 agonists (e.g., orthopedic surgeries) • premedication for local or regional anesthesia prior to standing clinical or surgical procedures: in these cases, opioids are generally given in combinations with acepromazine or alpha-2 agonists.
Observe the patient closely. Note the expected effects following the administration of an opioid, especially when administered in combination with alpha-2 agonist agents.	Expected effects: • analgesia and reduction of discomfort caused by pain and distress • opioids associated with alpha-2 agonists (e.g., butorphanol and detomidine) result in: – moderate to intense sedation; – marked head lowering (lips close to the ground) – drowsiness, ptosis of eyelids and lips (Figure 9.11) – ataxia (moderate to intense).
Be aware of potential adverse effects associated with the administration of an opioid, most notably decreased gastrointestinal motility.	Side effects: • ataxia • increased locomotor activity • decreased gastrointestinal motility (more likely with higher doses and repeated administrations) • respiratory depression with higher doses of morphine or methadone.
Provide additional care as necessary: avoid walking and do not allow eating until fully recovered from sedation.	Avoid walking the horse after administration of opioids, especially if associated with alpha-2 agonists. Ataxia and severe incoordination increase the risk of accidents. Place a muzzle if necessary, to prevent the horse from eating because of the risk of choke.

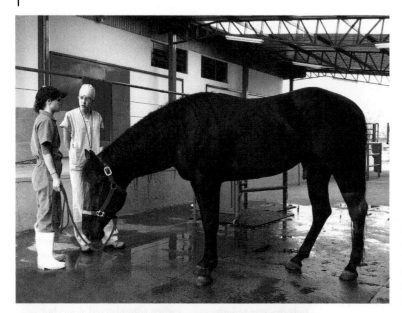

Figure 9.4 The sedative effect of xylazine at 0.5 mg/kg, 15 minutes after IV administration. Note the lowering of the head and penile relaxation.

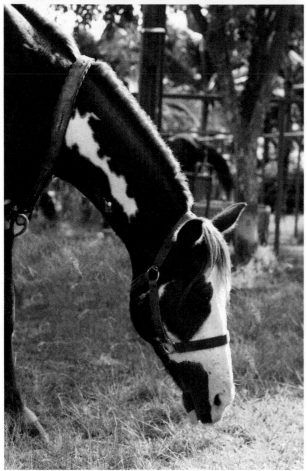

Figure 9.5 The "head lowering effect" produced by alpha-2 agonists is dose-dependent, correlating to the degree of sedation. The administration of a higher dose of xylazine (1.0 mg/kg, IV) results in lowering of the head almost to the ground.

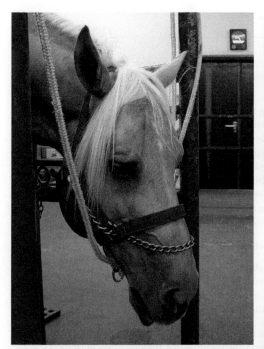

Figure 9.6 The sedative effect of detomidine at 0.01 mg/kg, 20 minutes after IV administration. Note the lowering of the head and drowsy expression.

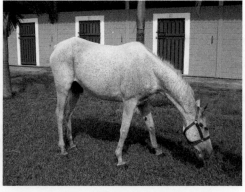

Figure 9.8 Wide-based stance of forelimbs and lowered head after IV administration of xylazine at 0.5 mg/kg.

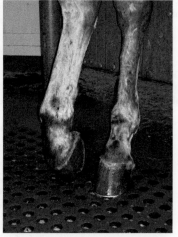

Figure 9.9 Horse resting a hindlimb by only the toe touching the ground after IV administration of detomidine at 0.01 mg/kg.

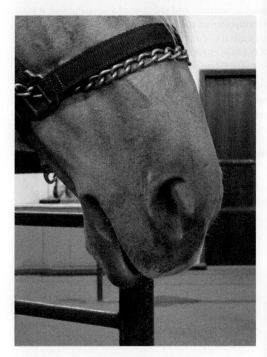

Figure 9.7 Ptosis of lips observed after IV administration of detomidine at 0.01 mg/kg.

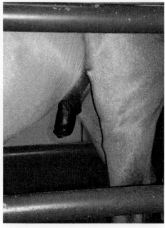

Figure 9.10 Relaxation of the penis following IV administration of detomidine at 0.01 mg/kg.

9.9 Procedure: Administration of Benzodiazepines

Technical action	Rationale
Based on the reported recommendations, determine if a benzodiazepine is indicated. Drugs and doses: • diazepam: 0.1–0.2 mg/kg (IV) • midazolam: 0.1–0.2 mg/kg (IV).	Recommended for: • sedation, chemical restraint, and anesthetic premedication of young foals • anesthetic induction of adult and young horses in combination with dissociative anesthetics (e.g., ketamine) and guaifenesin because the muscle relaxation effects produced by benzodiazepines counteract the hypertonia caused by dissociative agents. Specific considerations: benzodiazepines are not recommended as sole agents to sedate adult horses due to the intense ataxia and muscle relaxation.
Observe the patient closely. Note the expected effects following the administration of benzodiazepine, most notably ataxia and muscle relaxation.	Expected effects: • intense ataxia and incoordination • recumbency in foals • muscle relaxation • little cardiorespiratory depression.
Provide additional care to prevent injury due to severe ataxia. This is particularly important in foals given benzodiazepines.	After administration of benzodiazepines in foals there is intense ataxia and recumbency, therefore care must be taken to provide proper physical support and appropriate positioning of the patient in lateral or sternal recumbency on a pad or mat of adequate thickness for the animal's weight. Prior to chemical restraint and sedation of a neonatal foal, it is prudent to tranquilize or sedate the mare (using acepromazine or alpha-2 agonists) to control maternal stress caused by handling of the foal, ensuring the safety of the foal, the mare, and the personnel (Figure 9.12). The sedative effects of benzodiazepines can be long-lasting in foals. Physical support should be provided until there is complete recovery of the patient, preventing accidents and injuries.
If indicated administer a benzodiazepine antagonist. Drug and doses: • flumazenil: 0.01–0.05 mg/kg (IV).	Adverse effects of benzodiazepines and indication for reversal: • overdose • prolonged recumbency • ataxia and severe incoordination.

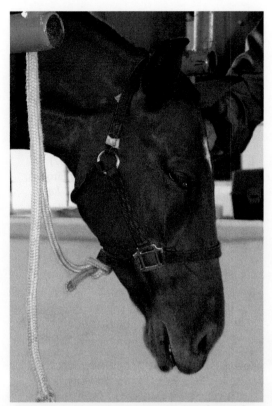

Figure 9.11 Effects of association of detomidine (0.01 mg/kg, IV) and butorphanol (0.02 mg/kg, IV) as premedication for minor surgery. The horse is heavily sedated, unaware of its surroundings, with the head lowered, ptosis of eyelids and lips.

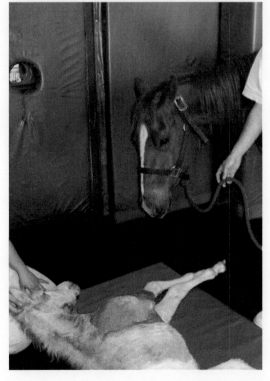

Figure 9.12 Mare sedated with xylazine (0.5 mg/kg, IV), shortly followed by premedication of her foal with diazepam (0.2 mg/kg, IV) prior to general anesthesia of the foal for orthopedic surgery.

Bibliography and Further Reading

Bettschart-Wolfensberger, R., Clarke, K.W., Vainio, O., Aliabadi, F.S., and Demuth, D.C. (1999) Pharmacokinetics of medetomidine in ponies and elaboration of a medetomidine infusion regime which provides a constant level of sedation. *Research in Veterinay Science*, **67** (1), 41–46.

Bryant, C.E., England, G.C.W., and Clarke, K.W. (1991) Comparison of the sedative effects of medetomidine and xylazine in horses. *Veterinary Record*, **129** (19), 421–423.

Clarke, K.W. and Paton, B.S. (1988) Combined use of detomidine with opiates in the horse. *Equine Veterinary Journal*, **20** (5), 331–334.

Clarke, K.W., England, G.C.W., and Goossens, L. (1991) Sedative and cardiovascular effects of romifidine, alone and in combination with butorphanol, in the horse. *Journal of Veterinary Anaesthesia*, **18** (1), 25–29.

Doherty, T. and Valverde, A. (2006) Management of sedation and anesthesia, in *Equine Anesthesia and Analgesia*, Blackwell Publishing, Oxford, pp. 206–259.

Elfenbein, J.R., Chris Sanchez, L., Robertson, S.A., Cole, C.A., and Sams, R. (2009) Effect of detomidine on visceral and somatic nociception and duodenal motility in conscious adult horses. *Veterinary Anaesthesia and Analgesia*, **36** (2), 162–172.

England, G.C.W. and Clarke, K.W. (1996) Alpha 2 adrenoceptor agonists in the horse – a review. *British Veterinary Journal*, **152** (6), 641–657.

Freeman, S.L. and England, G.C.W. (2000) Investigation of romifidine and detomidine for the clinical sedation of horses. *Veterinary Record*, **147** (18), 507–511.

Clarke, K.W., Trim, C.M., and Hall, L.W. (2014) Anaesthesia of the horse, in *Veterinary Anaesthesia*, Saunders-Elsevier, London, pp. 245–311.

Hofmeister, E.H., Mackey, E.B., and Trim, C.M. (2008) Effect of butorphanol on cardiovascular parameters in isoflurane-anesthetized horses – a retrospective clinical evaluation. *Veterinary Anaesthesia and Analgesia*, **35** (1), 38–44.

Lamont, L.A. and Mathews, K.A. (2007) Opioids, nonsteroidal anti-inflammatories, and analgesic adjuvants, in *Lumb & Jones' Veterinary Anesthesia and Analgesia*, Blackwell Publishing, Ames, pp. 241–271.

Lemke, K.A. (2007) Anticholinergics and sedatives, in *Lumb & Jones' Veterinary Anesthesia and Analgesia*, Blackwell Publishing, Ames, pp. 203–239.

Muir, W.W. (2009) Anxiolytics, nonopioid sedative-analgesics, and opiod analgesics, in *Equine Anesthesia: monitoring and emergency therapy*, Saunders Elsevier, St Louis, pp. 185-209.

Sellon, D.C., Monroe, V.L., Roberts, M.C., and Papich, M.G. (2001) Pharmacokinetics and adverse efects of butorphanol administered by single intravenous injection or continuous intravenous infusion in horses. *American Journal of Veterinay Research*, **62** (2), 183–189.

Taylor, P.M. and Clarke, K.W. (2007) Sedation and premedication, in *Handbook of Equine Anaesthesia*, Saunders Elsevier, Edinburgh, pp. 17–31.

Yamashita, K., Tsubakishita, S., Futaoka, S., Ueda, I., Hamaguchi, H., Seno, T., Katoh, S., Izumisawa, Y., Kotani, T., and Muir, W.W. (2000) Cardiovascular effects of medetomidine, detomidine and xylazine in horses. *Journal of Veterinary Medical Science*, **62** (10), 1025–1032.

10

Aseptic Technique

Colin Mitchell

10.1 Purpose

- To prevent or minimize the risk of infection following a surgical, diagnostic or therapeutic procedure because of contamination by pathogens (usually bacterial).
- To reduce the incidence of iatrogenic infections.

10.2 Complications

- Iatrogenic infection secondary to a procedure
- Iatrogenic infections increase patient morbidity, hospitalization time, and client expense.
- Iatrogenic infections can result in life- or career-threatening disease processes.

10.3 Equipment Required

- Hoof picks and stiff brush to clean feet.
- Brush and comb to remove loose hair, dander or larger debris from coat.
- Electric clippers with #40 blades
- Vacuum to remove clipped hair.

- Sterile gloves
- Sterile gauze sponges
- Scrub brushes
- Antiseptic scrub (usually chlorhexidene or povidone iodine-based products)
- Alcohol or sterile saline (to remove scrub)
- Sterile hand towels

10.4 Restraint and Positioning

- Restraint will depend on the type of procedure to be performed.
- If procedure is performed standing, a twitch may be applied to the horse's upper lip, sedation may be necessary depending upon the degree of invasiveness of the procedure, and/or local anesthetic techniques may be used to increase patient compliance.
- If the horse is anesthetized, it should be positioned appropriately before the area is prepared. If in an operating room, all personnel should be dressed accordingly with scrubs, surgical masks and caps.

10.5 Procedure: Aseptic Technique

Technical action	Rationale
The horse should be brushed off and have its feet picked out in an area separate from that where the procedure will be performed (Figure 10.1).	This will minimize contamination of the environment where the aseptic procedure will take place.
A wide area should be clipped using the #40 blade. Long-haired animals may need to be clipped twice, first with a #10 blade and then finished with a #40 blade (Figure 10.2).	Clipping the hair is less traumatic than using a razor and a wide area should be prepared so that if a more aggressive surgical incision has to be made, this area has already been aseptically prepared.

(continued)

Manual of Clinical Procedures in the Horse, First Edition. Edited by Lais R.R. Costa and Mary Rose Paradis.
© 2018 John Wiley & Sons, Inc. Published 2018 by John Wiley & Sons, Inc.

Technical action	Rationale
Clipped hair and debris should be removed, preferably by being vacuumed away from the surgery site.	This reduces the gross contamination of the site.
A rough prep should be performed first. The person performing this should wear sterile gloves. The antiseptic scrub is applied on gauze sponges. The sponge with the scrub should be applied in the center of the clipped region, then in concentric circles out towards the periphery. Once the edge is reached, a new sponge is used, starting at the center again. This continues until the site appears clean and no further debris/discoloration is observed on the sponge (Figure 10.3).	This rough prep removes the superficial debris and starts to kill any microorganisms on the site. By scrubbing from the center outwards, contaminants from the wound periphery will not be dragged into the center of the field.
	In some circumstances, an examination glove, rather than a sterile glove, may be used for the rough prep.
	As an alternative to sponge gauze, the site may be scrubbed with a surgical scrub sponge/brush. At least 5 minutes of contact time is recommended.
Alcohol or sterile saline is then used to remove the applied surgical scrub.	The antiseptic soap needs to be removed as it is usually cytotoxic when applied to open wounds or enters the skin following an incision or other penetration.
Another antiseptic scrub is performed with the person wearing a new pair of sterile gloves. The antiseptic scrubs require contact time to be effective, and 10 minutes of contact time is currently recommended in the horse. This can be removed with alcohol or sterile saline and left to air dry before the site is draped (if appropriate).	This scrub is performed on a cleaner surface than the initial area and helps the desired contact time be achieved to maximize the pathogen reduction.
The veterinarian and personnel performing the procedure should wash their hands and pick their nails out before performing a 5-minute scrub of the hands and arms with an antiseptic soap and scrub brush (Figure 10.4). The soap can be rinsed off before drying the hands on a sterile towel.	The hands often harbor large numbers of bacteria and other pathogens due to the degree and manner of patient contact.
If necessary, a gown can be put on before sterile gloving using a closed technique. Once sterile attire is applied, the site can be appropriately draped (Figure 10.5).	Gowning helps provide another aseptic barrier between the personnel performing aseptic procedures and the patient or drapes.

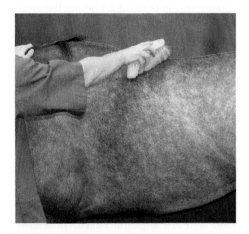

Figure 10.1 The horse is brushed off to remove any loose hair, shavings or dirt. This is performed outside the operating room to reduce the contamination of the room.

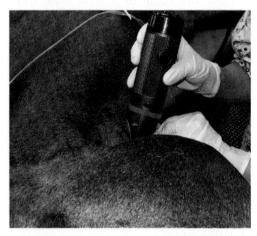

Figure 10.2 Once the horse is appropriately positioned, the surgical site can be clipped.

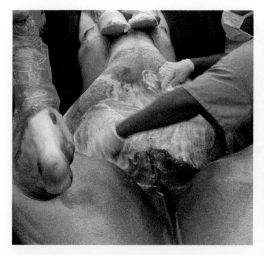

Figure 10.3 The initial, rough prep of the surgery site is performed.

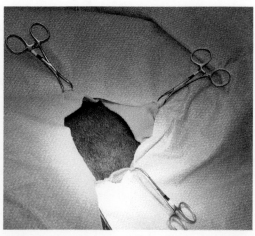

Figure 10.5 Once the sterile prep has been performed and the scrub solution has been removed using either alcohol or sterile water, the surgery site is draped.

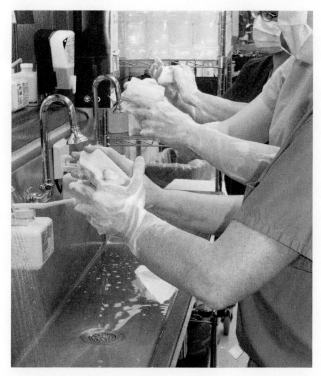

Figure 10.4 The personnel performing the sterile procedure or surgery must pick out their nails, and scrub hands and arms before applying sterile attire and sterile gloves for the procedure.

Bibliography and Further Reading

Auer, J.A. and Stick, J.A. (2006) *Equine Surgery*, 3rd edn, W.B. Saunders, Philadelphia.

Bassert, J.M. and McCurnin, D.M. (2010) *Clinical Textbook for Veterinary Technicians*, 7th edn, W.B. Saunders, Philadelphia.

Part II

Clinical Procedures by Body Systems: Digestive System

11

Oral and Dental Examination

Travis Henry and Molly Rice

11.1 Purpose

- To identify oral and dental abnormalities by conducting a thorough equine oral and dental examination comprising five components: extraoral, oral soft tissues, occlusion, periodontal status, and endodontic status.
- To develop a treatment plan based on the oral examination findings.

11.2 Complications

- Risks and complications associated with sedation (see Chapter 9).
- Oral trauma.

11.3 Equipment Required

- Sedation (see Chapter 9)
- Local anesthetic solution (2% lidocaine or mepivacaine) if regional perineural anesthesia is required (see Chapter 12).
- Full-mouth speculum (Figure 11.1a)
- Bright headlight (Figure 11.1b)
- Stainless steel bucket with antiseptic (0.05% chlorhexidine gluconate solution).
- Oral dosing syringe (Figure 11.1c)
- Dental mirror (Figure 11.1d)
- Periodontal depth probe (Figure 11.1e)
- Pulp horn explorer (Figure 11.1e)
- A dental examination form containing a dental chart (Figure 11.2).

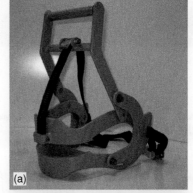
(a)

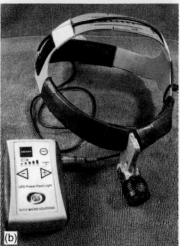
(b)

Figure 11.1 Essential equipment required for a complete oral and dental examination: (a) full-mouth speculum (pictured is the Aluma Spec), (b) bright head light (Rose Microsolutions), (c) oral dosing syringe, (d) dental mirror, and (e) dental scaler (top), pulp horn explorer (middle) and periodontal depth probe (bottom).

Manual of Clinical Procedures in the Horse, First Edition. Edited by Lais R.R. Costa and Mary Rose Paradis.
© 2018 John Wiley & Sons, Inc. Published 2018 by John Wiley & Sons, Inc.

Figure 11.1 (Continued)

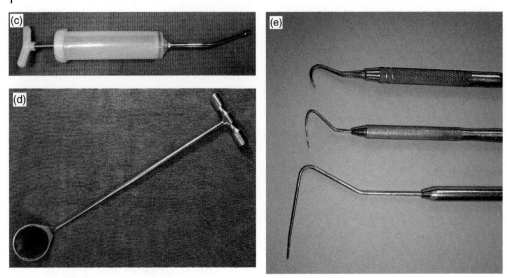

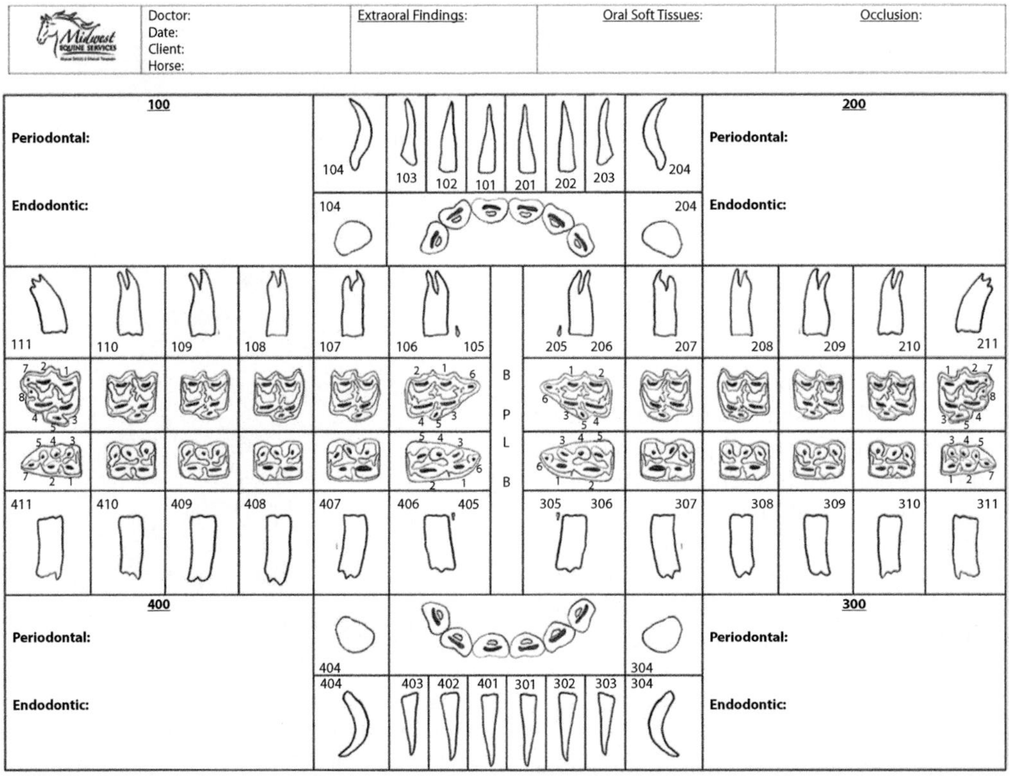

Figure 11.2 Dental chart to record findings.

11.4 Optional Equipment (Recommended but not Required)

- Dental scaler (Figure 11.1e)
- Alligator forceps (Figure 11.3a)
- Periodontal forceps (Figure 11.3b)
- Dental head stand (Figure 11.3c)
- Dental halter

11.5 Restraint and Positioning

- Use of stocks is preferred if available (Figure 11.4).
- Sedation is required for complete oral examination. Once the horse is sedated the preferable position for the head is resting on a headstand or supported in a dental halter.
- An assistant is required for restraining the head.

11.6 Procedure: Five-component Oral Examination

Technical action	Rationale
Obtain a complete medical and dental history. Identify problems and concerns that might be associated with oral and dental disorders, some of which affect the general health of the horse and lead to systemic manifestations.	Dental disease does not always correlate with a history of anorexia. Determine if the patient is a good candidate for sedation.
Evaluate the patient in an environment that is quiet and adequately illuminated, that is, well-lit for extraoral examination and with minimal backlighting for intraoral examination.	Proper environment for the examination minimizes the risk of missing abnormalities.
Each patient should have a five-component oral examination: 1) Extraoral 2) Oral soft tissues 3) Occlusion 4) Periodontal status 5) Endodontic status The findings should be recorded in the patient's medical record and dental chart (Figure 11.2).	Following a systematic approach to the oral examination minimizes the risk of missing minor pathologies. For review, a summary of equine dental nomenclature is presented in Table 11.1 and Figure 11.5. A dental eruption schedule is presented in Table 11.2 and Figure 11.6.

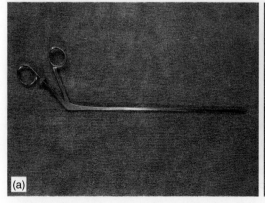
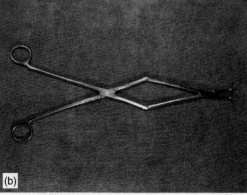

Figure 11.3 Additional equipment recommended to aid in the oral and dental examination: (a) alligator forceps, (b) periodontal forceps, and (c) dental head stand.

(continued)

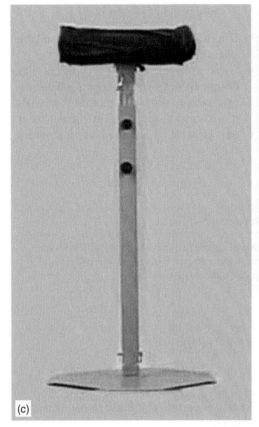

(c)

Figure 11.3 (continued)

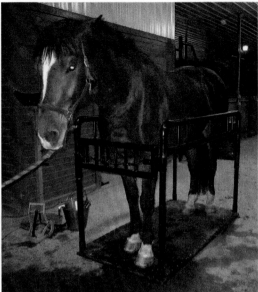

Figure 11.4 Horse restrained in portable stocks, which are often used in equine dentistry.

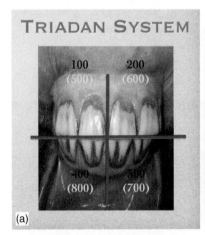

(a)

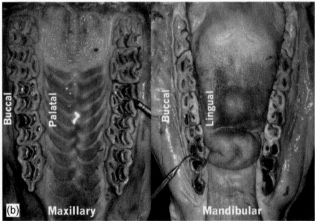

(b)

Figure 11.5 Terminology of equine dental examination. (a) Triadan system: the mouth is divided into four quadrants, permanent numbering in black, deciduous numbering in yellow: 100 (500) = upper right, 200 (600) = upper left, 300 (700) = lower left, 400 (800) = lower right. (b) Directional terminology: lingual, buccal, palatal. (c) Directional terminology: mesial, distal. (d) Normal occlusion angle of cheek teeth. (e) Incisors occlusal angle = 10–15 degrees. (f) Interocclusal space = 1–3 mm.

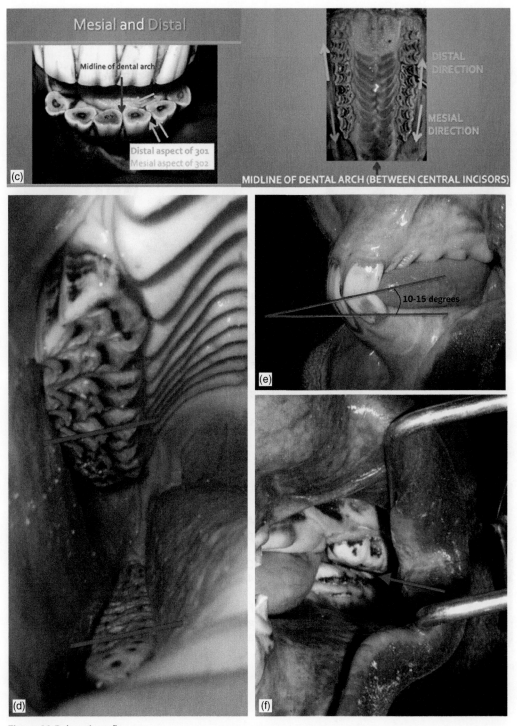

Figure 11.5 (continued)

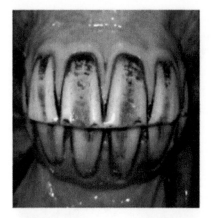

Dental Eruption Schedule: Incisors

Deciduous	Age	Permanent	Age
Central (01)	1 week	Central	2.5 yrs
Middle (02)	4-6 weeks	Middle	3.5 yrs
Corner (03)	6-9 months	Corner	4.5 yrs

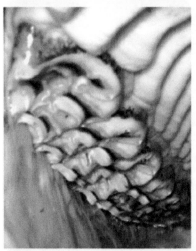

Premolars and Molars

Deciduous premolars (06-08's) are erupted at birth, or within the first week of life. Molars do not have deciduous precursors.

Premolars	Age	Molars	Age
06's	2 yrs, 8 mos	09's	1 year
07's	2 yrs, 10 mos	10's	2 years
08's	3 yrs, 8 mos	11's	3.5 years

Miscellaneous

- Adult cheek teeth erupt 2-3 mm per year

- Canines (04's) generally erupt by 4-6 years of age.

- First premolars (05's) or wolf teeth generally erupt by 6-12 months of age

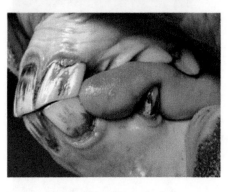

Figure 11.6 Dental eruption schedule.

Table 11.1 Equine triadan tooth numbering system

Nomenclature			Deciduous teeth				Permanent teeth			
			UR	UL	LL	LR	UR	UL	LL	LR
Incisors (I)	1st	Central	501	601	701	801	101	201	301	401
	2nd	Middle	502	602	702	802	102	202	302	402
	3rd	Lateral	503	603	703	803	103	203	303	403
Canine (C)			–	–	–	–	104	204	304	404
Pre-molar (PM)	1st	Wolf tooth	–	–	–	–	105	205	305	405
	2nd	1st cheek tooth	506	606	706	806	106	206	306	406
	3rd	2nd cheek tooth	507	607	707	807	107	207	307	407
	4th	3rd cheek tooth	508	608	708	808	108	208	308	408
Molar (M)	1st	4th cheek tooth	–	–	–	–	109	209	309	409
	2nd	5th cheek tooth	–	–	–	–	110	210	310	410
	3rd	6th cheek tooth	–	–	–	–	111	211	311	411

UR, upper right arcade; UL, upper left arcade; LR, lower right arcade; LL, lower left arcade.

Table 11.2 Summary of approximate equine teeth eruption age

Nomenclature		Deciduous teeth	Permanent teeth
Incisors (I)	1st I or central I	Birth to 1 week	2.5 years
	2nd I or middle I	3–6 months	3.5 years
	3rd I or lateral I	5–9 months	4.5 years
Canine (C)		Absent	4–5 years
Pre-molar (PM)	1st PM or wolf tooth	Absent	6 months to 3 years
	2nd PM or cheek tooth 1	Birth to 2 weeks	2.5 years
	3rd PM or cheek tooth 2	Birth to 2 weeks	3 years
	4th PM or cheek tooth 3	Birth to 2 weeks	4 years
Molar (M)	1st M or cheek tooth 4	Absent	9–12 months
	2nd M or cheek tooth 5	Absent	2 years
	3rd M or cheek tooth 6	Absent	3.5–4 years

Adapted from Hennig, G.E. and Steckel, R.R. (1995) Diseases of oral cavity and esophagus, in *The Horse: Diseases and clinical management* (eds C.N. Kobluk, T.R. Ames, and R.J. Geor), W.B. Saunders, Philadelphia, p. 290.

Technical action	Rationale
Extraoral Examination	
Extraoral examination should be performed before sedating the patient, if possible. For the extraoral examination, the examiner should stand in front of the patient.	Because sedation will affect head position, the appearance of the soft tissues/musculature of the head may be altered. Be cognizant of the risks of standing directly in front of an unsedated horse. Pay close attention to the horse's movements if the horse is not restrained in stocks.
Evaluate the following on extraoral examination: • the symmetry of the face and head • the presence of facial swelling • the presence of draining tracts • the presence and character of nasal discharge (bilateral or unilateral) • the presence of facial wounds • the presence (bilateral or unilateral) and character of ocular drainage • lymph node enlargement.	• Asymmetry of the face and head can involve muscle atrophy, and neurological and anatomical/developmental changes (Figure 11.7a,b). • Facial swelling can include bony or soft-tissue swelling. Location as it relates to the anatomy of the skull and teeth may be important. Careful examination to rule out fractures of the mandible or maxilla is important prior to opening the mouth with a full-mouth speculum (Figure 11.7c). • A correlation of the draining tract with an intraoral finding should be attempted. The location and nature of any drainage should be noted (Figure 11.7d). Radiographs of the affected area should be obtained for all draining tracts. Contrast media and/or metal probes combined with radiography can be utilized to determine the origin of the draining tract. • Nasal discharge may or may not be related to dental disease. In addition to oral examination, an endoscopic examination is recommended if purulent or sero-sanguinous nasal discharge is present (Figures 11.7d,e). • Facial wounds include cuts, scrapes and rubs resulting from trauma, and open lesions associated with swellings or draining tracts. • Ocular discharge may or may not be related to dental disease (Figure 11.7f). Ophthalmic examination should be performed to rule out injury or disease involving the eye(s). • The lymph nodes of the head and neck should be examined for enlargement.
Occlusion Evaluation	
Occlusion evaluation should be performed in the sedated patient. The assistant should restrain the horse's head such that the poll is level with the withers.	The sedated horse will be more cooperative and easier to evaluate. Positioning the poll level with the withers will avoid artificial rostro-caudal positioning of the jaw.
For occlusion evaluation the horse must first be evaluated without the full-mouth speculum and then with the speculum in place.	Visual assessment of the patient without the speculum allows evaluation of the incisor occlusion and relative relationship of the maxilla to the mandible.
Occlusion evaluation should identify skeletal or dental malocclusions, and examine lateral excursion of the mandible.	

Technical action	Rationale
Skeletal malocclusions are noted when there is maxillary–mandibular asymmetry, which can be seen in a rostro-caudal, side-to side, or dorso-ventral direction. Dental malocclusions are related to the teeth themselves, or an incorrect position of the tooth/teeth in their respective quadrant.	Assessment of the mouth with the speculum allows for evaluation of occlusion of the molar quadrants. The full-mouth speculum should only be placed once the horse is fully sedated.
Determine if there is a skeletal malocclusion. Skeletal malocclusions resulting from wearing of more than one specific tooth include: • wave mouth (Figure 11.8a) • incisor slants (Figure 11.8b) • dorsal or ventral curvature of the incisors • shear mouth (Figure 11.8c). Skeletal malocclusions resulting from skeletal deformations include: • asymmetrical conformation of the incisors (often caused by wry nose conformation of the skull) • relative maxillary prognathia (Figure 11.8d) • relative mandibular prognathia (Figure 11.8e).	Skeletal malocclusions involve several teeth in specific quadrants. They are the result of a discrepancy of size, shape, or position of the maxilla or mandible. Skeletal malocclusions can result in malocclusions of the premolars and molars such as mesial hooks (Figure 11.8f), when there is discrepancy between the mandible and the maxilla (relative maxillary prognathia).
Determine if there is a dental malocclusion. Dental malocclusions involve one specific tooth. Visual assessment of the patient without the speculum will allow evaluation of the incisors. Visual assessment of the patient with the full-mouth speculum will allow evaluation of the molar quadrants.	Dental malocclusions involve specific teeth, but skeletal relationship of the maxilla to the mandible is normal. When an overlong crown is observed, it is important to evaluate the opposing quadrant for pathology (Figure 11.8g). An overlong crown results from the complete or partial absence of opposing dentition (Figure 11.8h). A missing tooth or supernumerary teeth (Figure 11.8i) often contributes to dental malocclusions.
Evaluate lateral excursion and molar contact. The head should be held level with the withers. With the upper jaw held in a fixed position, the lower jaw is moved laterally. The point at which the incisors separate is the point of lateral excursion. Normal lateral excursion is roughly the width of 1–1½ incisors. As the jaw continues to move in a lateral direction, the incisors should separate approximately 2–6 mm.	Lateral excursion should be evaluated before and after floating the cheek teeth to determine if incisor reduction is indicated. This is especially important in geriatric patients that may have overlong incisors that are reducing or preventing normal molar occlusion.
Oral Soft Tissue Examination Oral soft tissues should be evaluated in the sedated patient with the full-mouth speculum in place. The assistant should restrain the horse's head on a head rest.	The horse must remain fully sedated while the full-mouth speculum is in place. The head position allows for a thorough examination.

(continued)

Technical action	Rationale
The oral soft tissues should be evaluated for the following:	Oral soft tissues include the tongue, lips, cheek, mucosa, gingiva, and hard and soft palate.
<ul><li>abrasions or ulcerations in the mouth (Figure 11.9a,b)</li><li>oral masses or swelling (Figure 11.9c)</li><li>draining tracts and fistulas (Figure 11.9d–f).</li></ul>	<ul><li>When abrasions or ulcerations are present it is important to evaluate the mouth for the underlying cause so that this can be addressed.</li><li>Differential diagnoses for oral masses or swelling include abscesses, tumors, polyps, and trauma. Biopsy is indicated to determine the definitive cause of most oral mass lesions.</li><li>Draining tracts or fistulas can be explored with probes (Figure 11.9e). Radiographs of the area should be obtained to thoroughly evaluate draining tracts and fistulas.</li></ul>

Periodontal Status Evaluation

Periodontal status should be evaluated on all teeth using the mirror and a bright light (Figure 11.10a):	Radiographs are necessary to stage the periodontal disease.
<ul><li>Periodontal pockets: the periodontal depth probe is utilized to explore the gingival sulcus and measure pocket depths.</li><li>Diastema (Figure 11.10b,c).</li><li>Gingival recession (Figure 11.10d).</li><li>The mobility of each tooth should be scored. Mobility scores range from 0 to 3 (see Chapter 12, Table 12.2).</li><li>Periodontal disease should be staged (see Chapter 12, Table 12.1).</li></ul>	<ul><li>The normal periodontal depth ranges from 3 to 5 mm. Note the depth and location of any periodontal pockets.</li><li>Diastema (pl. diastemata) should have all organic debris removed so that they can be evaluated for depth. Alligator forceps and/or periodontal forceps can assist in removal of debris.</li><li>The location and amount of gingival recession (in mm) should be noted. Tooth mobility should be evaluated.</li><li>Mobility scores (according to Klugh 2005): – 0 = no movement – 1 = first sign of movement – 2 = movement of up to 3 mm at the occlusal surface – 3 = movement of 3 mm or more at the occlusal surface</li></ul>

Endodontic Status Evaluation

Endodontic status should be evaluated for all teeth using the mirror and a bright light. It is important to thoroughly rinse the mouth prior to examination. Figure 11.11a,b depicts the nomenclature of tooth anatomy.	Areas where food is sticking to the surface of the teeth should be explored with a probe to determine if pathology is present.
<ul><li>The pulp horns/chamber should be visually evaluated on all teeth and the surface of the pulp horns should be probed using a pulp horn explorer (Figure 11.11c). Anatomical variations of the pulp horns/chambers should be noted (Figure 11.11d).</li><li>Infundibula should be visually evaluated on all maxillary cheek teeth with a bright light and mirror.</li><li>Dental caries should be staged (Stages 0–5) and recorded in the medical record and dental chart (see Chapter 12, Table 12.3).</li></ul>	<ul><li>Exposed pulp horns should be explored with the pulp horn explorer. Occlusal pulp exposure can occur in the equine patient in response to damage to the vital pulp. When pulp becomes non-vital, the odontoblasts cease to lay down the dentin that prevents exposure of the pulp horn/chamber at the occlusal surface due to attrition. Pulp exposure can lead to apical infection of the tooth in some cases. All patients with pulp horn/chamber exposure should have radiographs taken of the affected quadrant (Figure 11.11e).</li><li>Infundibula should be evaluated for abnormalities. Infundibula (singular infundibulum) are present in pairs in the maxillary cheek teeth, and as a single structure (cup) in the maxillary and mandibular incisors.</li></ul>

Technical action	Rationale
• Patent infundibulum is a condition most commonly found in young horses. Radiography is indicated in all cases.[4]	• It is important to be familiar with tooth anatomy to properly stage infundibular caries. All stage 5 caries and many stage 4 caries require extraction of the affected tooth (Figure 11.11f,g). Radiographs are indicated in cases of caries stage 2 and higher to evaluate the periapical structures and guide treatment planning. • Patent infundibulum is most often caused by premature loss of deciduous dentition as a result of trauma, iatrogenic removal, or anatomical failure of the deciduous tooth (Figure 11.11h). This results in disruption of normal development in the permanent tooth. This disruption often results in a patency through the infundibulum from the occlusal surface to the apex of the tooth. Radiography demonstrates patency of the infundibulum (Figure 11.11i,j) Clinical presentation is usually facial swelling associated with the affected tooth and/or nasal discharge. If cases are identified early enough, prompt endodontic treatments may save the permanent dentition. If significant periapical change is present on initial examination, extraction may be the only option.

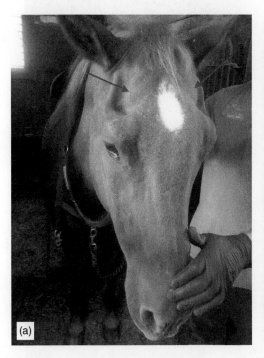
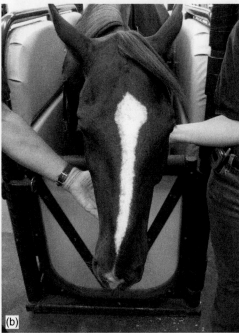

Figure 11.7 Extraoral examination is intended to identify external abnormalities. Examples of abnormalities noted during extraoral exam include (a) atrophy of the temporalis muscle, (b) laterally deviated maxilla (aka wry nose), (c) facial swelling, (d) draining tract, (e) nasal discharge, and (f) ocular discharge.

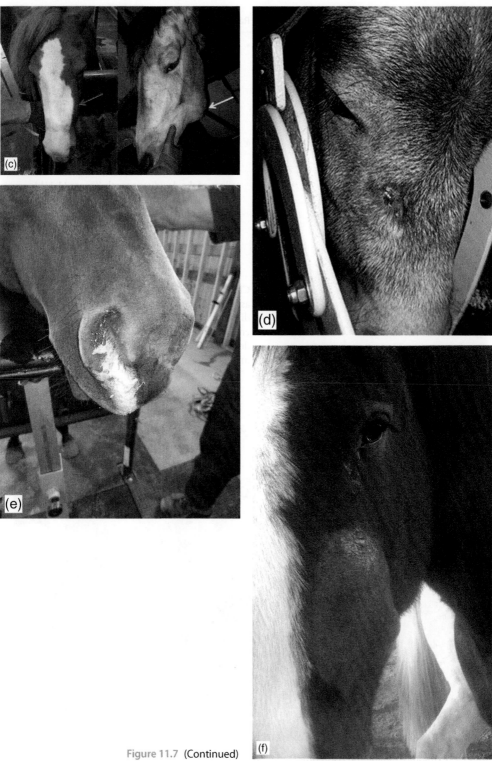

Figure 11.7 (Continued)

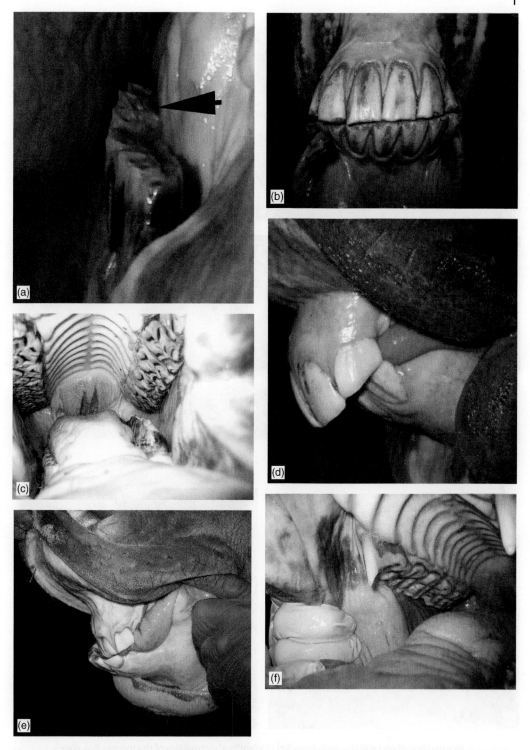

Figure 11.8 Examination of the occlusion is intended to identify skeletal and dental malocclusions: (a) wave mouth, (b) incisor slant, (c) shear mouth, (d) relative maxillary prognathia, (e) relative mandibular prognathia, (f) skeletal malocclusion leading to formation of mesial hooks on 106 and 206, (g) overlong crown on 109 leading to a step, (h) photograph and two radiographs of the 109 overlong crown associated with the loss of the opposing tooth (409), and (i) supernumerary tooth noted on examination and radiograph.

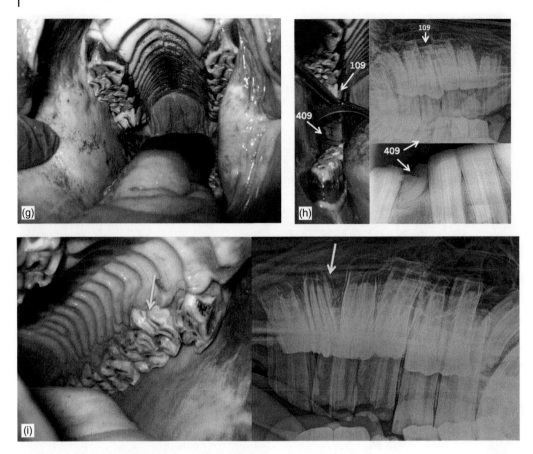

Figure 11.8 (Continued)

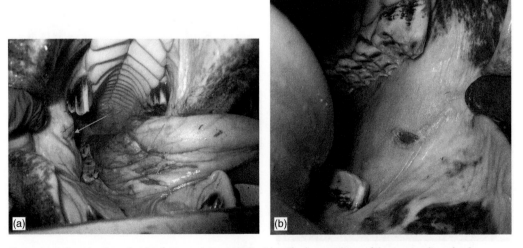

Figure 11.9 Examination of oral soft tissues is intended to identify abnormalities of the tongue, lips, cheek, mucosa, gingiva, and hard and soft palate: (a) oral abrasions in a geriatric horse, (b) oral ulceration associated with a hook, (c) oral mass that progressed over the course of 4 years, (d) draining tract associated with gingival recession on the palatal aspect of 108 and buccal aspect of 107, (e) draining tract associated with gingival recession on the palatal aspect of 108, and (f) draining tract associated with gingival recession on the buccal aspect of 207.

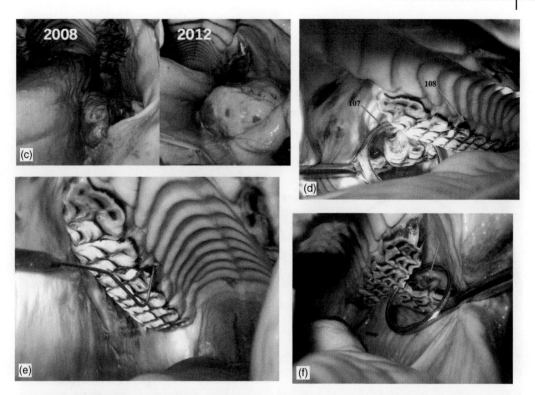

Figure 11.9 (Continued)

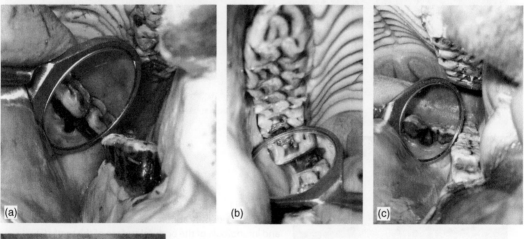

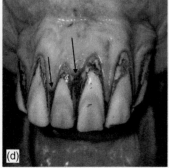

Figure 11.10 Examination of the periodontal status is intended to identify periodontal abnormalities: (a) periodontal pocket, (b) diastema after removal of the accumulated feed material, (c) valve diastema after removal of the accumulated feed material, (d) gingival recession on the maxillary incisors (101 to 201 and 101 to 102, as indicated by the arrows).

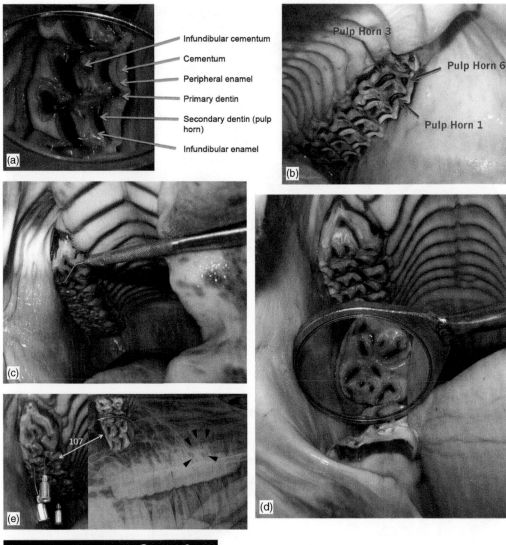

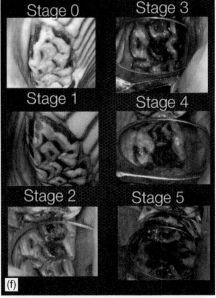

Figure 11.11 Examination of the endodontic status is intended to identify abnormalities of the dentin, enamel and infundibula of the occlusal surface of the teeth: (a) endodontic anatomy, (b) open pulp horn on 606, red arrows indicate the affected pulp horns, (c) open pulp horn in 106, (d) abnormal anatomical variations of the pulp horns/chambers, (e) multiple open pulp horns (two in 107 and one in 109), and a radiographic image demonstrating failure to narrow in the common pulp chamber and periapical lucency (black arrow heads), (f) stages of infundibular caries, (g) multiple open pulp horns indicating complete endodontic failure, (h) stage 2 caries mesial infundibulum in 209 (staging of infundibular caries is described in Chapter 13, Table 13.4), (i) patent mesial infundibulum in 208, and (j) radiograph of patent infundibula 107 Hedstrom endodontic files inserted in mesial and distal infundibulum. Note the large periapical lucency with external inflammatory root resorption.

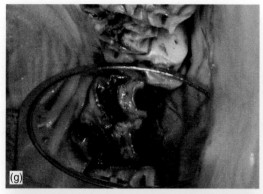

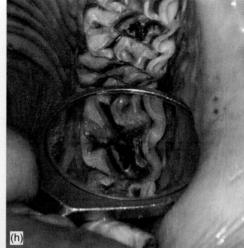

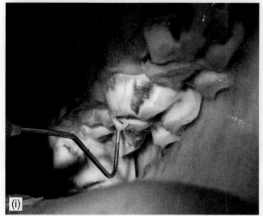

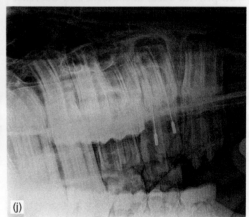

Figure 11.11 (Continued)

Bibliography and Further Reading

Baratt, R.M. (2010) How to recognize and clinically manage class 1 malocclusions in the horse. *Proceedings of the American Association of Equine Practitioners Convention*, **56**, 458–464.

Easley, K.J. (2004) Equine canine and first premolar (wolf) teeth. *Proceedings of the American Association of Equine Practitioners Convention*, **50**, 13–18.

Gieche, J.M. (2007) How to Assess Equine Oral Health. 53rd Annual Convention of the American Association of Equine Practitioners.

Johnson, T.J. (2003) Correction of common dental malocclusions with power instruments, in *Current Therapy in Equine Medicine 5* (ed. N.E.Robinson), W.B. Saunders, St Louis, pp. 81–87.

Klugh, D.O. (2005) Equine periodontal disease. *Clinical Techniques in Equine Practice*, **4**, 135–147.

Menzies, R.A., Lundstrom, T.S., Reiter, A.M., *et al.* (2012) Diagnostic imaging in veterinary dental practice. Incomplete formation of the apical infundibula of the permanent right maxillary second premolar tooth. *Journal of the American Veterinary Medical Association*, **240**, 949–951.

Rucker, B.A. (2002) Utilizing cheek teeth angle of occlusion to determine length of incisor shortening. *Proceedings of the American Association of Equine Practitioners Convention*, **48**, 448–452.

Staszyk, C, Bienert, A., Baümer, W., Feige, K., and Gasse, H. (2008) Simulation of local anaesthetic nerve block of the infraorbital nerve within the pterygopalatine fossa: Anatomical landmarks defined by computed tomography. *Research in Veterinary Science*, **85**, 399–406.

12

Perineural Anesthesia for Dental Procedures

Molly Rice and Travis Henry

12.1 Purpose

- To provide local anesthesia and decrease the discomfort associated with painful dental procedures.
- To decrease pain sensation and make the horse more tractable to dental procedures.

This chapter describes common perinerual anesthesia performed for dental procedures in the horse:

1. Infraorbital nerve block: provides anesthesia to the maxillary incisors and maxillary molar quadrants
2. Maxillary nerve block: provides anesthesia to the maxillary incisors and maxillary cheek teeth
3. Mental nerve block: provides anesthesia to the mandibular incisor quadrants
4. Inferior alveolar nerve block: provides anesthesia to the mandibular incisor and mandibular molar quadrants.

12.2 Complications

- Local irritation, inflammation.
- Hemorrhage or hematoma formation at the injection site.
- Self-trauma to the oral cavity.
- Abscess formation.

12.3 Complications Specific to Each Nerve Block

- *Infraorbital nerve block:*
  - postoperative neurogenic pain with self-mutilation
  - puncture of the infraorbital artery with hematoma formation
  - needle separation
  - inadvertent blockage of the facial nerve with alar collapse.
- *Maxillary nerve block:*
  - hemorrhage from inadvertent puncture of the infraorbital or palatine arteries
  - retrobulbar swelling or abscessation.
- *Mental nerve block:*
  - postoperative neurogenic pain with self-mutilation
  - hemorrhage from inadvertent puncture of the mental artery.
- *Inferior alveolar nerve block:*
  - numbness and paralysis of the tongue and self-inflicted lingual trauma
  - abscessation at the site of injection.

12.4 Equipment Required

- Surgical scrub and alcohol for prepping the injection site.
- Local anesthetic solution (2% lidocaine or mepivacaine) (Figure 12.1).
- Sterile needles and syringes of appropriate size for the nerve block (see Table 12.1).

Manual of Clinical Procedures in the Horse, First Edition. Edited by Lais R.R. Costa and Mary Rose Paradis.
© 2018 John Wiley & Sons, Inc. Published 2018 by John Wiley & Sons, Inc.

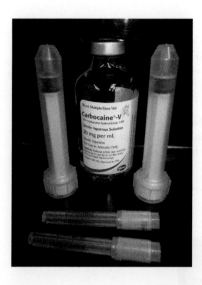

Figure 12.1 Local anesthetic 2% mepivacaine hydrochloride, Zoetis.

Table 12.1 Appropriate syringe and needle size for the dental nerve blocks

Nerve block	Infraorbital	Maxillary	Mental	Inferior alveolar
Needle size (gauge)	25	20	25	20
Needle length (″)	1 or 1½	1.5-3	1 or 5/8	5
Syringe size (ml)	3	12 or 20	3	12 or 20

12.5 Restraint and Positioning

- An assistant experienced in horse handling is required to restrain the head of the patient.
- The assistant should stand on the opposite side to the veterinarian.
- A twitch may be required.
- Sedation is necessary for the safety of the horse, the veterinarian, and the handler (see Chapter 9).

- Administration of perineural anesthesia of the infraorbital and mental nerve can be particularly noxious to some horses.
- It is important to never stand directly in front of the patient when performing a nerve block.

12.6 Procedure: Infraorbital Nerve Block

Technical action	Rationale
Restrain and sedate the patient appropriately.	Heavy sedation and capable restraint is recommended for this nerve block, since stimulation of the nerve can sometimes provoke a strong negative response from the patient, including rearing, striking, etc.
Locate the infraorbital foramen by placing the thumb at the nasoincisive notch and the little finger at the medial canthus of the eye. Halfway in between these points, the infraorbital foramen can be palpated (Figure 12.2).	The infraorbital nerve is blocked as it exits the infraorbital canal within the maxilla (Figure 12.3).

Technical action	Rationale
Stand to the side of the patient, place the fingers on the bridge of the nose, and elevate the levator nasolabialis muscle with the thumb. The thumb is placed just rostral to the infraorbital foramen.	Never stand in front of the horse, even if the horse is properly restrained and sedated.
Insert a 25-gauge 1½″ needle to infiltrate local anesthetic around the opening of the foramen (Figure 12.4a). Insert the needle into the infraorbital canal and deposit 3–5 ml of local anesthetic solution after aspiration is negative for hemorrhage (Figure 12.4b).	Insertion of the needle into the canal directly without first infiltrating the opening of the foramen will cause the horse to react violently.

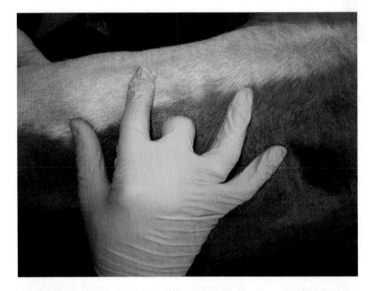

Figure 12.2 Landmarks for identifying the location of the infraorbital foramen.

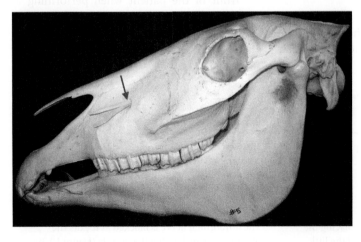

Figure 12.3 Skull showing the infraorbital nerve and the mental nerve, located in the infraorbital foramen (red arrow) and mental foramen (blue arrow), respectively.

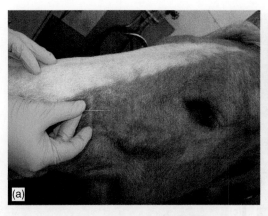

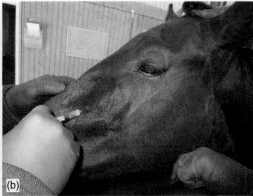

Figure 12.4 Infraorbital nerve block: (a) location of needle insertion for the infraorbital nerve block and (b) injecting local anesthetic solution into the infraorbital canal.

12.7 Procedure: Maxillary Nerve Block (by Extraperiorbital Fat Body Injection)

Technical action	Rationale
Restrain and sedate the patient appropriately.	Sedation is necessary for the safety of the horse and veterinarian/handler.
Locate the zygomatic arch near the posterior third of the eye, then insert the spinal needle perpendicular to the skin approximately 1–1.5 cm ventral to the zygomatic arch (Figure 12.5a).	The maxillary nerve is blocked as it enters the maxillary foramen below the eye.
Advance the needle until it makes contact with the caudal aspect of the maxillary bone (Figure 12.5b).	Staying close to the periosteum causes the anesthetic solution to be distributed more effectively to the surrounding the maxillary nerve (Figure 12.5c).
Inject 10–20 ml of anesthetic solution in this location after aspiration is negative for hemorrhage.	If hemorrhage is noted on aspiration, the needle should be repositioned prior to injecting the anesthetic solution.

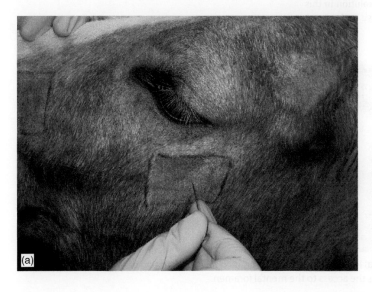

Figure 12.5 Maxillary nerve block: (a) location of needle insertion for the maxillary nerve block, (b) advancement of needle until it makes contact with the caudal aspect of maxillary bone, and (c) location of the maxillary foramen.

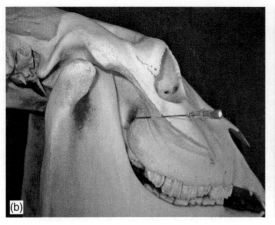
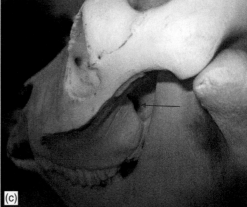

Figure 12.5 (Continued)

12.8 Procedure: Mental Nerve Block

Technical action	Rationale
Restrain and sedate the patient.	Heavy sedation and capable restraint is recommended for this nerve block, since stimulation of the mental nerve can provoke a negative response from the patient.
Locate the foramen on the lateral aspect of the mandible below the interdental space (Figure 12.6a).	The inferior alveolar nerve is blocked just prior to its exit from the mental foramen (Figure 12.3).
Stand to the side of the patient, place the thumb just rostral to the mental foramen, and elevate the depressor labii inferioris muscle dorsally (Figure 12.6b).	Never stand in front of the horse, even if the horse is properly restrained and sedated.
Insert a 25-gauge 1″ needle into the foramen and inject 2–3 ml of local anesthetic solution in this location after aspiration is negative for hemorrhage.	

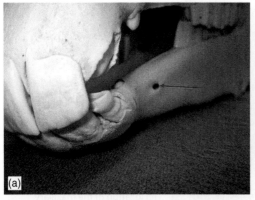
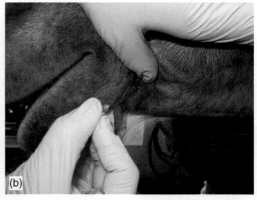

Figure 12.6 Mental nerve block: (a) location of the mental foramen and (b) elevation of the depressor labii inferioris muscle dorsally facilitates the access to the mental foramen.

12.9 Procedure: Inferior Alveolar Nerve Block

Technical action	Rationale
Restrain and sedate the patient appropriately.	Sedation is necessary for the safety of the horse and veterinarian/handler.
Locate the foramen by drawing a line along the occlusal surface of the mandibular cheek teeth, and another line perpendicular to the lateral canthus of the eye. The point of intersection of these two lines is the approximate location of the mandibular foramen, on the medial surface of the mandible (Figure 12.7a).	The inferior alveolar nerve is blocked as it enters the mandibular foramen on the medial surface of the mandible (Figure 12.7b).
The needle is inserted along the medial aspect of the mandible at the level of the rostral insertion of the masseter muscle (Figure 12.7c). The needle is advanced to an approximate depth of 3-3.5″ (Figure 12.7d).	It is important when performing this block to keep the needle directed in a lateral direction so that it does not stray from the medial surface of the mandible. This minimizes the risk of possible complications, such as paralysis of the tongue, leading to self-inflicted lingual trauma.
Inject 10–20 ml of anesthetic solution in this location after aspiration is negative for hemorrhage.	

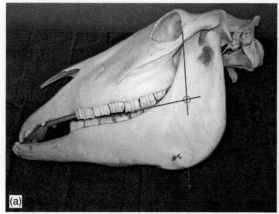
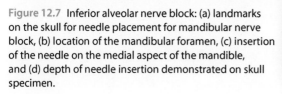
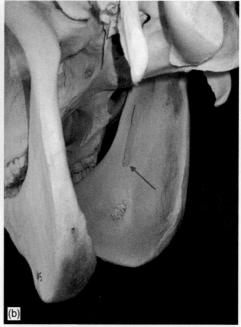

Figure 12.7 Inferior alveolar nerve block: (a) landmarks on the skull for needle placement for mandibular nerve block, (b) location of the mandibular foramen, (c) insertion of the needle on the medial aspect of the mandible, and (d) depth of needle insertion demonstrated on skull specimen.

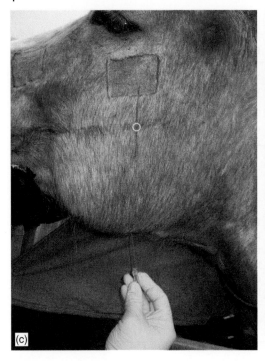

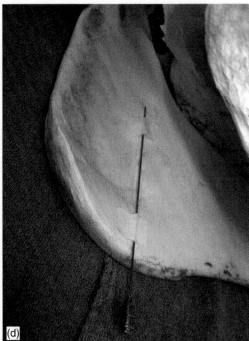

Figure 12.7 (Continued)

Bibliography and Further Reading

Fletcher, B.W. (2005) How to perform effective equine dental nerve blocks. *Horse Dentistry & Bitting*, **6**, 18–20.

Staszyk, C., Bienert, A., Baumer, W. *et al.* (2008) Simulation of local anaesthetic nerve block of the infraorbital nerve within the pterygopalatine fossa: anatomical landmark defined by computed tomography. *Research in Veterinary Science*, **85** (3), 399–406.

Tremaine, W.H. (2007) Local analgesic techniques for the equine head. *Equine Veterinary Education*, **19** (9), 495–503.

13

Common Dental Procedures

Molly Rice and Travis Henry

13.1 Purpose

- Treatment of routine dental abnormalities in the horse. The procedures described include occlusal adjustment, wolf tooth (P1) extraction, unerupted wolf tooth (P1) extraction, and deciduous tooth extraction.
- Diagnostic work-up and management of common dental abnormalities. The procedures described include fractured teeth, periodontal and endodontic disease, buccal luxation, and avulsion of incisors.

13.2 Complications

- Risks associated with sedation (see Chapter 9).
- Risks related to regional perineural anesthesia (see Chapter 11).

13.3 Equipment Required

- Sedation (see Chapter 9): local anesthetic (2% lidocaine or mepivacaine) may be required for regional perineural anesthesia (see Chapter 12).
- Oral examination instruments (see Chapter 11).
- Instruments for occlusal adjustment: hand instruments (floats) and/or motorized instruments.
- Instruments for extractions: luxators, elevators, dental spreaders, extraction forceps, scalpel handle with #15 or #12 blade, gauze and hemostats.

13.4 Restraint and Positioning

- Use of stocks is preferred if available.
- Sedation is required for most procedures. Once the horse is sedated the preferable position for the head is resting on a headstand or supported in a dental halter.
- The assistant should restrain the head, supported by the headstand or dental halter.

13.5 Procedure: Occlusal Adjustment

Technical action	Rationale
Occlusal adjustment includes: • the removal of sharp enamel points • reduction of overlong crowns resulting from abnormal physiological dental attrition, such as ramps, steps, waves • excessive transverse ridges.	Horses develop sharp enamel points due to attrition and the anisognathic anatomy of their oral cavity. Points normally develop on the buccal aspect of the maxillary cheek tooth quadrants and the lingual aspect of the mandibular cheek tooth quadrants. Depending on the type of feed materials and the anatomy of the patient, these can develop into severe focal malocclusions.

(continued)

Manual of Clinical Procedures in the Horse, First Edition. Edited by Lais R.R. Costa and Mary Rose Paradis.
© 2018 John Wiley & Sons, Inc. Published 2018 by John Wiley & Sons, Inc.

Technical action	Rationale
Select the instruments needed: full mouth speculum, dental headstand or dental halter, oral examination instruments (see Chapter 11), and instruments for occlusal adjustment.	Instrumentation for occlusal adjustment is largely based on personal preference and may include hand instruments (floats) and/or motorized instruments. Care must be taken to avoid thermal damage to the teeth if motorized instruments are used.
Perform complete oral and dental examination (see Chapter 11). Document all findings, ideally on a dental chart (see Chapter 11, Figure 11.2).	Corrections should only be done after complete oral and dental examinations have been performed and oral pathologies notated on a dental chart. Dental charting is part of a complete and accurate medical record.
Assess the lateral excursion and molar contact before the occlusal adjustment is made (see Chapter 11). Hold the head level with the withers. With the upper jaw held in a fixed position, move the lower jaw laterally. The point at which the incisors separate is the point of lateral excursion.	Normal lateral excursion is approximately the width of 1–1½ incisors. As the jaw continues to move in a lateral direction, the incisors should separate approximately 2–6 mm, as described by Rucker (2002).
Once charting is complete, prepare the instruments and position the horse to perform occlusal adjustments (Figure 13.1).	A systematic approach to occlusal adjustments (i.e., floating the mouth to remove sharp enamel points and correct malocclusions) will allow the veterinarian to be consistent and thorough (Figure 13.2).
Correct the distal hooks of incisors 103 and 203 (Figure 13.3) prior to placing the speculum.	Removal of hooks on incisors should be performed prior to placing the speculum for the comfort of the patient and to minimize risk of iatrogenic fracture.
Correct occlusion abnormalities as outlined in Figure 13.2. • Remove sharp enamel points as needed. • Perform crown reduction as needed. • Correct focal malocclusions as needed.	• Compare enamel points before and after floating (Figure 13.4). • Crown reduction should be performed in a sequential fashion (Figure 13.5). • Assess focal malocclusions before and after correction (Figure 13.6).
Reevaluate the occlusion by visual and digital assessment of the mouth.	Confirm that removal of sharp enamel points is complete and that malocclusions are corrected as best as possible.
Lateral excursion should be evaluated again after floating the cheek teeth to determine if incisor reduction is indicated.	This is especially important in geriatric patients that may have overlong incisors that are limiting or eliminating normal molar occlusion.

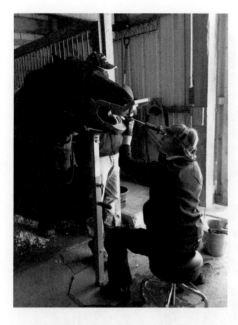

Figure 13.1 Position for occlusal adjustment.

OCCLUSAL ADJUSTMENT FLOWCHART

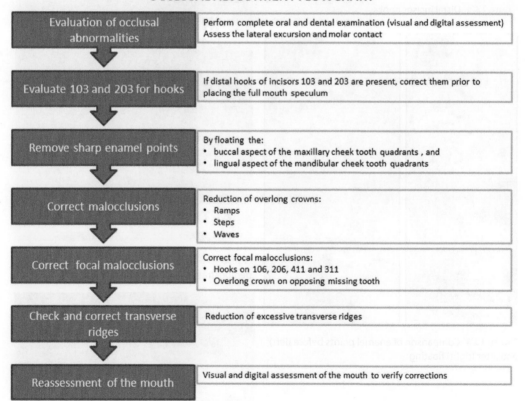

Evaluation of occlusal abnormalities	Perform complete oral and dental examination (visual and digital assessment) Assess the lateral excursion and molar contact
Evaluate 103 and 203 for hooks	If distal hooks of incisors 103 and 203 are present, correct them prior to placing the full mouth speculum
Remove sharp enamel points	By floating the: • buccal aspect of the maxillary cheek tooth quadrants , and • lingual aspect of the mandibular cheek tooth quadrants
Correct malocclusions	Reduction of overlong crowns: • Ramps • Steps • Waves
Correct focal malocclusions	Correct focal malocclusions: • Hooks on 106, 206, 411 and 311 • Overlong crown on opposing missing tooth
Check and correct transverse ridges	Reduction of excessive transverse ridges
Reassessment of the mouth	Visual and digital assessment of the mouth to verify corrections

Figure 13.2 Flowchart of occlusal adjustment.

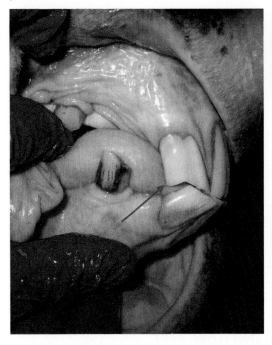

Figure 13.3 Distal incisor hooks.

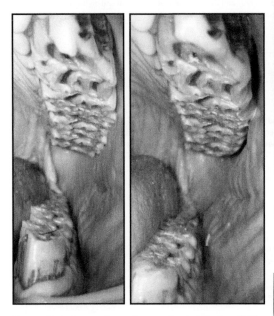

Figure 13.4 Comparison of enamel points before (left) and after (right) floating.

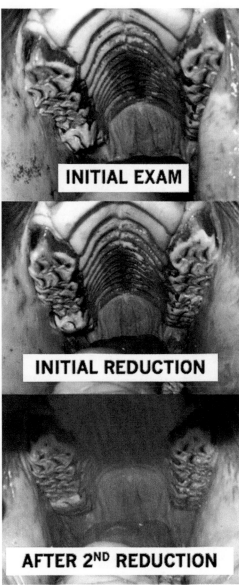

INITIAL EXAM

INITIAL REDUCTION

AFTER 2ND REDUCTION

Figure 13.5 Sequential crown reduction demonstrating the step for crown reduction.

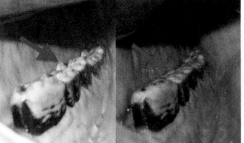

Figure 13.6 Correction of a focal malocclusion.

13.6 Procedure: Wolf Tooth/First Premolar Extraction

Technical action	Rationale
Wolf tooth extraction is the removal of the first premolar (P1) teeth: 105, 205, 305, and 405 (Figure 13.7).	First premolars most commonly erupt between the ages of 6 and 18 months. They are permanent teeth that do not come into occlusion with other teeth. First premolars are most commonly present in the maxillary quadrants (105, 205), but may occasionally be found in the mandibular quadrants (305, 405). Removal of these teeth is most commonly performed in young horses prior to commencement of training.
P1 extraction should only be performed after a complete oral examination has been performed.	Complete oral examination will allow for assessment of the anatomy and location of the first premolar in relation to the second premolar.\n\nIn horses that are 2–2½ years of age this is especially important if the second premolar is deciduous because of the close anatomical relationship of P1 to the unerupted permanent second premolar (Figure 13.8).
Consider postponing P1 extraction, in some cases until the deciduous second premolar has exfoliated and the permanent tooth has erupted.	Assertive extraction efforts in this area may potentially damage the unerupted permanent second premolar tooth. In some horses the P1 will be shed in the process of deciduous second premolar exfoliation.
Select the instruments needed: dental elevators, dental luxators, small dental extraction forceps, and full mouth speculum (Figure 13.9).	A variety of elevators or luxators may be required depending on the anatomy and location of the tooth in the mouth. Extraction is ideally performed with the aid of a full-mouth speculum. Specialized equine luxators have been developed with appropriate angles to facilitate working with the full-mouth speculum.
Infiltrate local anesthetic solution (2% lidocaine or mepivacaine) using a 3 ml luer lock syringe with a 20–22-gauge 1½″ needle (Figure 13.10).	Local anesthesia significantly improves patient compliance, which helps decrease the possibility of inadvertent palatine artery puncture.
Gingival margins are cut free using a sharp dental elevator or luxator.	Incising the gingival margin attachments allows for access to properly luxate and elevate the tooth.
Elevate and luxate the tooth along the length of the root. This frees the tooth from the alveolar attachments.	Care must be taken to avoid inadvertent puncture of the palatine artery, which is located in the palate running parallel to the maxillary molar quadrants.
Delivery of the tooth is performed with small dental forceps.	Dental forceps should not be applied until luxation is complete and the tooth is visualized moving in all planes. This will minimize the risk of separating a root tip. If delivery of the tooth is not progressing, radiography is indicated.

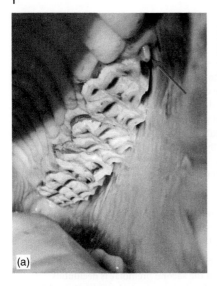

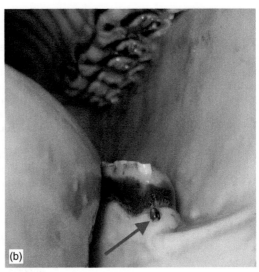

Figure 13.7 The first premolar (P1) teeth, also called wolf teeth, are 105, 205, 305, and 405: (a) maxillary wolf tooth (205) and (b) mandibular wolf tooth (305).

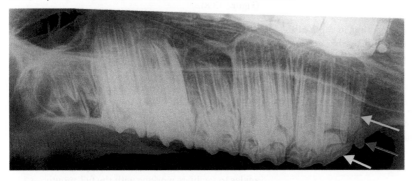

Figure 13.8 Intraoral radiograph of 2-year-old demonstrating close anatomical relationship of P1 to the unerupted permanent second premolar.

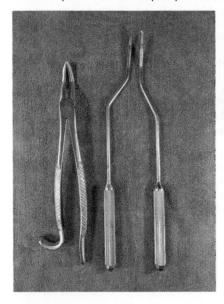

Figure 13.9 Instruments for wolf tooth extraction.

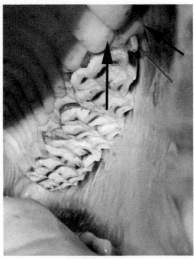

Figure 13.10 Local anesthetic placement for P1 extraction. Black arrows indicate injection sites and the red arrow indicates the wolf tooth.

13.7 Procedure: Blind Wolf Tooth/Unerupted Premolar 1 Extraction

Technical action	Rationale
Blind wolf tooth extraction is the removal of unerupted or retained first premolar teeth (105, 205, 305, 405).	Unerupted first premolar teeth can occur in any of the four dental quadrants.
Palpate the interdental space. The presence of a firm submucosal nodule rostral to the second premolar tooth (06) is suggestive of a retained first premolar. Differential diagnoses include: • exostosis of the mandible/maxilla • scar tissue from prior wolf tooth extraction • presence of a retained P1 tooth • presence of a separated P1 root tip.	Radiography is indicated to diagnose the presence of an unerupted P1 tooth and determine the orientation of the tooth prior to extraction (Figure 13.11).
Extraction of an unerupted or retained P1 tooth should only be performed after a complete oral examination has been performed.	Complete oral examination will allow for assessment of the anatomy and location of the first premolar in relation to the second premolar. In horses that are 2–2½ years of age this is especially important if the second premolar is deciduous because of the close anatomical relationship of P1 to the unerupted permanent second premolar.
Consider postponing extraction of an unerupted/retained P1 tooth until the deciduous second premolar has exfoliated and the permanent tooth has erupted.	Assertive extraction efforts in this area may potentially damage the unerupted permanent second premolar tooth.
Select the instruments needed: dental root elevators, dental luxators, small dental extraction forceps, dental speculum, #15 or #12 scalpel blade with handle, and gauze sponges.	Extraction should be performed with a full-mouth speculum to provide adequate visualization during the procedure.
Infiltrate the site with local anesthetic solution (2% lidocaine or mepivacaine) using a 3 ml syringe with a 20–22-gauge 1½″ needle.	Local anesthesia significantly improves patient compliance, which helps decrease the possibility of inadvertent palatine artery puncture.
Palpate the P1 tooth in the interdental space mesial to the second premolar and make an incision over the unerupted crown using the scalpel blade.	The incision should be made in a caudal-to-rostral direction to minimize risk of accidental puncture of the palatine artery.
Elevation and luxation of the tooth to expose the crown, and then along the length of its root promotes loosening of the periodontal attachments.	Radiography will help determine the orientation of the unerupted tooth, which will aid extraction and minimize risk of fracturing the tooth (Figure 13.12).
Deliver the tooth with small dental forceps.	Dental forceps should not be applied until luxation is complete and the tooth is visualized moving in all planes. This will minimize the risk of fracturing a root tip. If delivery of the tooth is not progressing, radiography is indicated.
The extraction site is left open to heal by second intention.	

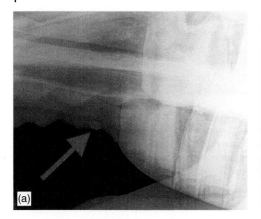 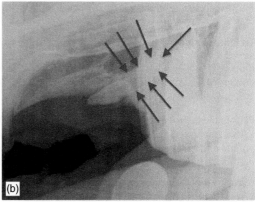

Figure 13.11 Radiography is indicated to diagnose the presence of an unerupted P1 (wolf) tooth: (a) radiograph of small blind wolf tooth (red arrow) and (b) radiograph of large blind wolf tooth (red arrows).

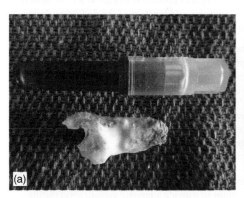 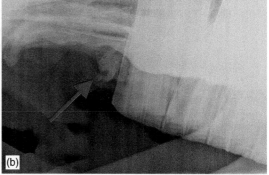

Figure 13.12 Large blind wolf tooth extraction: (a) extracted large wolf tooth and (b) radiograph showing location from where the large blind wolf tooth was extracted (red arrow).

13.8 Procedure: Deciduous Tooth Extraction

Technical action	Rationale
Extraction of deciduous teeth (aka, caps) is commonly performed in young horses (Figure 13.13). However, extraction of deciduous teeth solely based on the age of the horse is not recommended.	It is very important to know the normal eruption times for equine permanent teeth (see Chapter 11, Table 11.2). Premature removal of deciduous teeth can be detrimental to the development of the unerupted permanent teeth.
Criteria for removal of deciduous teeth: • the permanent tooth is visible in the mouth • mobility of the deciduous tooth is present • the deciduous tooth is fractured. At least one of these criteria should be present (Figures 13.14 and 13.15).	Eruption times can be variable in individual horses, and adhering to the criteria is important for avoiding complications. Possible complications of premature loss or extraction of deciduous teeth include patent infundibula (maxillary cheek teeth; Figures 13.16 and 13.17), tooth root abscess formation, eruption abnormalities, and failure to fully develop a permanent tooth.

Technical action	Rationale
If the patient appears to have persistent deciduous teeth that are not consistent with the age of the horse, radiographs should be obtained.	Radiography is recommended prior to extraction of persistent deciduous teeth.
Select the instruments needed: full-mouth speculum, dental elevators (spoon elevators), dental extractors, dental spreaders. For deciduous incisors: small dental forceps, milk tooth elevator, dental luxators.	Extraction of deciduous cheek teeth should be performed with the full-mouth speculum. Extraction of deciduous incisors should be performed without the speculum. Infiltration with local anesthetic solution and/or regional perineural anesthesia may be indicated in some patients to improve compliance and patient comfort.
Elevate the gingival margin if significant soft tissue attachment is present on the tooth. Deliver the tooth with extraction forceps.	Elevation of the gingiva minimizes soft tissue trauma when the tooth is extracted.
If delivery of the tooth is not progressing with extractors, dental spreaders can be utilized to aid extraction.	Deciduous cheek teeth are designed to withstand significant medial/lateral forces during mastication. Careful spreading along the distal margin of the tooth will place mesial force on the crown, causing the tooth to loosen its attachment and elevate the tooth in most cases.

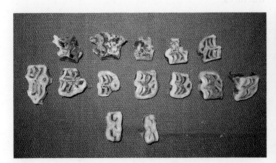

Figure 13.13 Deciduous teeth are also known as caps.

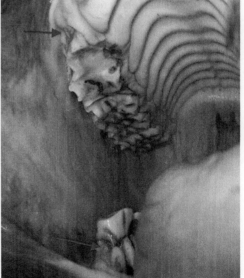

Figure 13.14 Retained caps are common in young horses. Note the erupting permanent teeth (red arrows) underneath the deciduous 506 and 806.

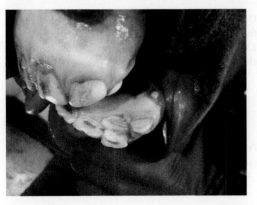

Figure 13.15 One of the criteria for removal of deciduous teeth is the permanent tooth visible in the mouth. Note the retained deciduous incisor (red arrow).

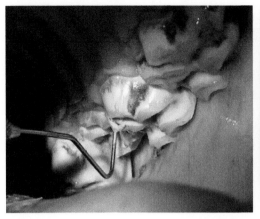

Figure 13.16 Pulp horn explorer used to demonstrate patent infundibulum on permanent tooth 208 following premature removal of deciduous tooth 608.

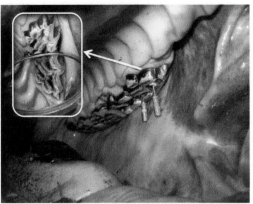

Figure 13.17 Permanent tooth 206 with patent infundibulum associated with premature deciduous tooth extraction.

13.9 Procedure: Management of Fractured Teeth

Technical action	Rationale/amplification
Fractured teeth identified on oral examination should be evaluated with a mirror to determine the structures of the tooth that are affected: • use the pulp horn explorer to detect pulp exposure (Figure 13.18) • use the periodontal depth probe to detect the extent of the fracture below the gingival margin and evaluate for possible draining tracts or loss of periodontal attachment • obtain radiographs to evaluate for apical pathology.	Proper knowledge of dental anatomy will allow the practitioner to accurately classify and diagnose tooth fractures. • Pulp exposure may indicate loss of vitality of the tooth. • Probing depth and location should be notated in the dental chart. • Apical pathology includes: – periapical lucency (Figure 13.19) – widening of the periodontal ligament space (Figure 13.20) – inflammatory root resorption (Figure 13.21) – hypercementosis, etc. In the case of maxillary P4 through M3, sinus involvement should also be evaluated.
Classify the type of tooth fracture based on visual inspection and radiologic interpretation into: 1. uncomplicated crown fracture (Figure 13.22) 2. complicated crown fracture (Figure 13.23) 3. uncomplicated crown root fracture (Figure 13.24) 4. complicated crown root fracture (Figure 13.25) 5. root fracture (Figure 13.26).	Use the classification of tooth fractures according to the American Veterinary Dental College. See Figure 13.27 and Table 13.1 for guidelines on tooth fracture classification.
If fractured teeth are found to be vital and demonstrate no apical pathology, management includes occlusal adjustment of the opposing quadrant.	Future dental examination should include radiographic evaluation.

Technical action	Rationale/amplification
If fractured teeth are found to be non-vital treatment consists of either extraction or endodontic treatment. Teeth that have significant apical pathology are usually recommended for extraction.	Radiography will determine if extraction is indicated. The presence of apical change and/or sinus involvement most often will result in extraction of the affected tooth.
In the case of uncomplicated crown or crown root fracture, extraction of any loose fragments of the fractured tooth is indicated: • excise the gingiva using spoon elevators • perform minor luxation to free the portion of the displaced crown	The fragments are removed to prevent further soft tissue irritation to the mucosa of the cheek or tongue, and prevent periodontal disease. Radiography is necessary to determine if the entire tooth should be recommended for extraction. In the cases where extraction is not recommended, follow up should include radiography and oral examination to evaluate for pulpar exposure and tooth vitality.
In cases of complicated crown root fracture involving both infundibula, the entire tooth must be extracted (Figure 13.28).	Extraction of fractured teeth in horses should only be performed by experienced practitioners due to the high technical ability and instrumentation required.

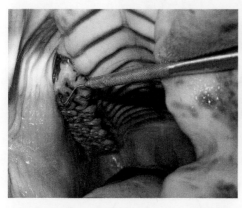

Figure 13.18 Use of the pulp horn explorer to detect pulp exposure.

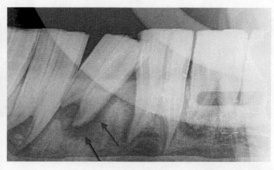

Figure 13.20 Periapical lucency and widening of the periodontal ligament. The red arrows indicate bone loss.

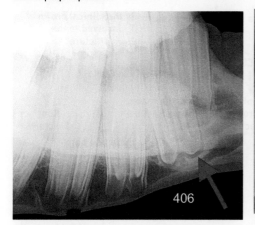

Figure 13.19 Periapical lucency (red arrow) on second premolar 406.

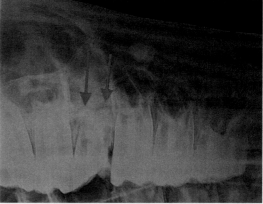

Figure 13.21 Inflammatory root resorption of 1st molar tooth (109). The red arrows indicate the affected tooth.

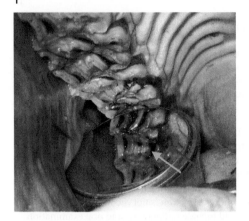

Figure 13.22 Uncomplicated crown fracture. The green arrow indicates the pulp horn 4 and the red arrow indicates the fracture.

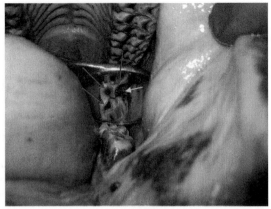

Figure 13.23 Complicated crown fracture. The yellow arrow indicates the fracture and the red arrow indicates the open pulp horns 1, 3, and 4 (counter-clockwise from right).

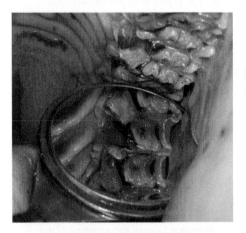

Figure 13.24 Uncomplicated crown root fracture.

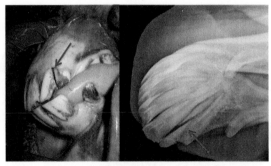

Figure 13.25 Complicated crown root fracture.

FRACTURED TOOTH

Is the fracture only above the gum line?

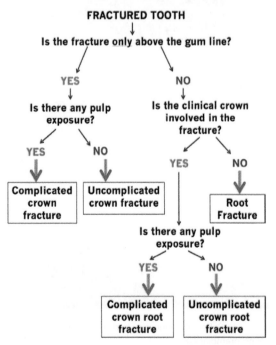

Figure 13.27 Flowchart demonstrating the decision tree concerning the classification of a fractured tooth.

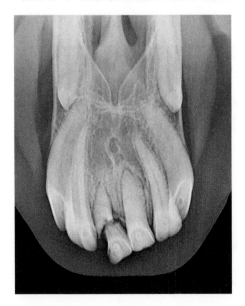

Figure 13.26 Root fracture.

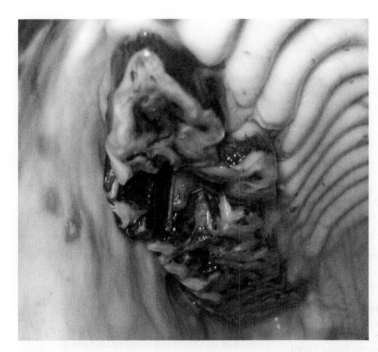

Figure 13.28 Saggital, complicated crown root fracture.

Table 13.1 Classification of tooth fracture (data from the American Veterinary Dental College)

Type of tooth fracture	Description and identification
Uncomplicated crown fracture (Figure 13.22)	The fracture of the tooth is only above the gingival margin and does not involve the pulp chamber or canal in such a way that a probe can be inserted. The tooth remains vital.
Complicated crown fracture (Figure 13.23)	The fracture of the tooth is above the gum line and there is exposure of the vital pulp horn or canal of the tooth where a probe can be inserted. The affected tooth structures are non-vital.
Uncomplicated crown root fracture (Figure 13.24)	The fracture of the tooth involves structures of the tooth above and below the gum line and does not involve the pulp chamber or canal in such a way that a probe can be inserted.
Complicated crown root fracture (Figure 13.25)	The fracture of the tooth involves structures of the tooth above and below the gum line, with exposure of the vital pulp horn or canal of the tooth where a probe can be inserted. The affected tooth is non-vital.
Root fracture (Figure 13.26)	The fracture of the tooth is only below the gum line, affecting the reserve crown or a root of the tooth.

13.10 Procedure: Management of Periodontal Disease

Technical action	Rationale
Thoroughly evaluate periodontal tissues to identify the presence and location of periodontal disease (PD). Periodontal examination is described in detail Chapter 11.	PD is considered a painful condition of the equine oral cavity. PD can be broken down into gingivitis and periodontitis: • gingivitis is the inflammatory process of the gingiva and gingival sulcus • periodontitis is the inflammatory process related to the alveolar bone and periodontal ligament.
PD should be staged. This will require radiography to evaluate for alveolar bone and attachment loss.	See Figure 13.29 and Table 13.2 for guidelines on PD staging. Loss of bone that occurs in advancing PD is thought to not be reversible.
Tooth mobility should be evaluated and scored.	See Table 13.3 for guidelines on scoring tooth mobility.
Establish a management plan for PD based on staging.	
Management of stage 0 PD (normal) • Occlusal adjustment.	*For stage 0 of PD* • Radiographs are generally not indicated unless there are other significant oral examination findings.
Management of stage 1 PD (gingivitis; Figure 13.30) • Occlusal adjustment. • Obtain radiographs.	*For stage 1 PD* • Radiographs are indicated to evaluate for attachment loss.
Management of stage 2 PD (early PD; Figure 13.31) • Diastemata, if present, should be evaluated for further treatment. • Occlusal adjustment should address imbalances that may be contributing to diastema formation and/or traumatic occlusion. • Obtain radiographs.	*For stage 2 PD* • Impacted feed material should be removed so that soft tissues can be properly evaluated. • Radiographs are required to properly evaluate attachment loss.
Management of stage 3 PD (moderate PD; Figure 13.32) • Similar to stage 2, but due to increased loss of attachment it is often not appropriate to manage these with occlusal adjustment alone. • Advanced treatments such as periodontal debridement with impression material application and antibiotic therapy are often indicated to prevent further advancement of PD.	*For stage 3 PD* • Proper follow-up care is important and owners should be aware that treatment of PD is an ongoing process. • Radiographs are required to evaluate attachment loss and any periapical change. Extraction may be indicated in some patients.
Management of stage 4 PD (advanced PD; Figure 13.33) • Similar to stage 3, it is not appropriate to manage these cases with occlusal adjustment alone. • Obtain radiographs. • Many teeth with mobility scores of 2, and all teeth with mobility scores of 3, should be recommended for extraction.	*For stage 4 PD* • Radiologic findings and mobility scores will help determine if extraction is indicated.

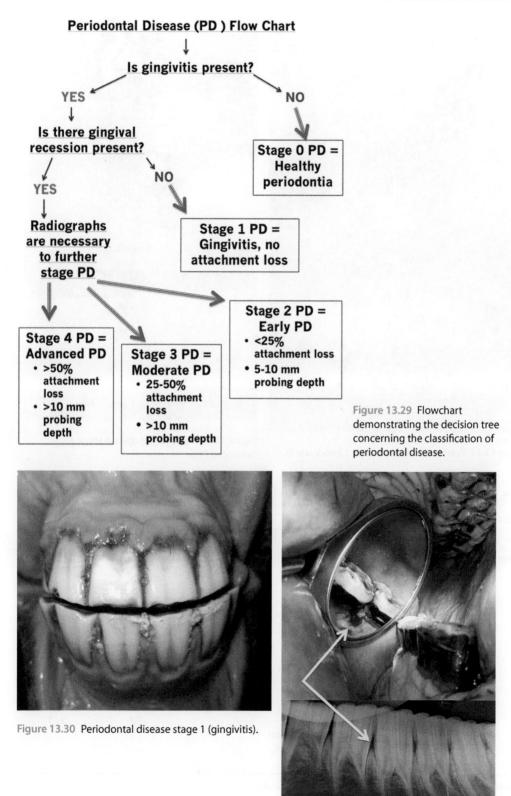

Periodontal Disease (PD) Flow Chart

Is gingivitis present?

YES → Is there gingival recession present?

NO → **Stage 0 PD = Healthy periodontia**

YES → Radiographs are necessary to further stage PD

NO → **Stage 1 PD = Gingivitis, no attachment loss**

Stage 4 PD = Advanced PD
- >50% attachment loss
- >10 mm probing depth

Stage 3 PD = Moderate PD
- 25-50% attachment loss
- >10 mm probing depth

Stage 2 PD = Early PD
- <25% attachment loss
- 5-10 mm probing depth

Figure 13.29 Flowchart demonstrating the decision tree concerning the classification of periodontal disease.

Figure 13.30 Periodontal disease stage 1 (gingivitis).

Figure 13.31 Periodontal disease stage 2 (early PD).

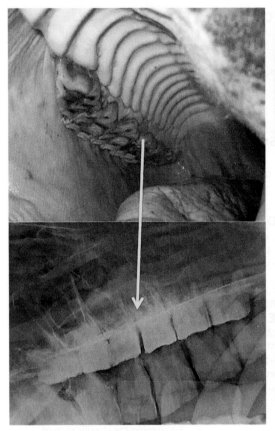

Figure 13.32 Periodontal disease stage 3 (moderate PD).

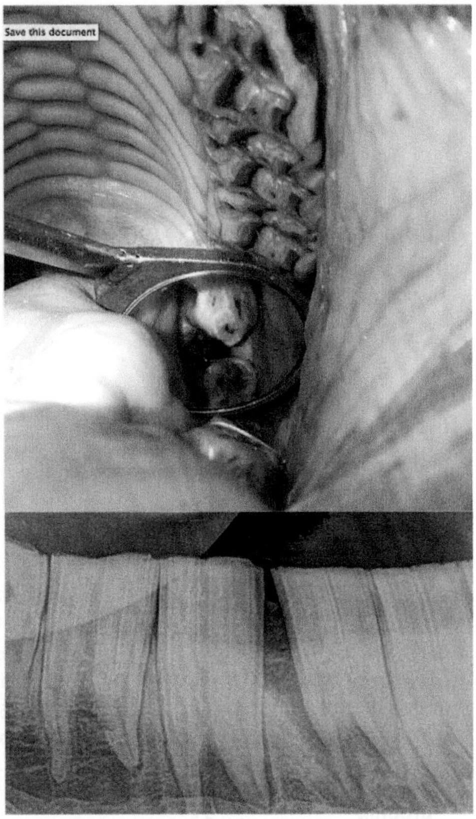

Figure 13.33 Periodontal disease stage 4 (advanced PD).

Table 13.2 Staging of periodontal disease: evaluation of gingiva and periodontal space (data from Klugh (2005))

Classification		Examination findings			
Stage	Description	Gingival appearance	Probing depth of gingival sulcus (mm)	Loss of attachment[a](%)	Tooth mobility
0	Normal	Normal gingiva	<5	None	None
1	Gingivitis	Inflamed gingiva	<5	None	None
2	Early PD	Gingivitis, gingival recession, feed impaction	5–10	<25	0–1
3	Moderate PD	Gingivitis, gingival recession, periodontal pocket, feed impaction	>10	25–50	1–2
4	Advanced PD	Oral examination findings may include gingivitis, gingival recession, periodontal pocket, feed impaction	>10	>50	2–3

[a]Alveolar bone attachment loss is determined radiographically.

Table 13.3 Scoring tooth mobility: evaluation of tooth mobility (data from Klugh (2005))

Score	Stage of tooth mobility	Description
0	Normal	No tooth mobility
1	Mild	Represents the first distinguishable sign of movement greater than normal
2	Moderate	Movement of up to approximately 3 mm at the occlusal surface
3	Severe	Movement >3 mm in any direction and/or tooth can be depressed into the alveolus

13.11 Procedure: Management of Endodontic Disease

Technical action	Rationale
Evaluate all teeth visually and probe the surface of the pulp horns and infundibula using a pulp horn explorer. Endodontal evaluation is described in detail in Chapter 11. See Table 13.4.	Thoroughly evaluate endodontal structures to identify the presence and location of endodontal disease. Radiographs should be obtained of any teeth that have an endodontic finding. Draining tracts and fistulas can often be noted from non-vital teeth.
Obtain radiographs of any teeth with abnormal findings.	Diagnostics are aimed at determining whether the affected tooth is vital or non-vital.
Teeth affected with endodontal disease are treated by extraction or endodontic treatment.	Treatment of endodontic disease in the horse often requires specialized instrumentation. Referral for treatment may be warranted.

Table 13.4 Classification of stages of infundibular caries

Stage	Classification	Description
0	Normal	
1	Caries involving the cementum	Food impaction in the enlarged vascular remnant of the infundibulum , with caries involving infundibular cementum
2	Caries involving the cementum and enamel	Caries of the infundibulum involves the cementum and infundibular enamel
3	Caries involve the cementum, enamel and surrounding pulp horn dentin	The carious process has breached the infundibular enamel and is affecting the surrounding pulp horn dentin
4	Caries have lead to tooth fracture	The tooth has lost integrity and has fractured and potentially missing crown
5	Tooth is fractured through both infundibula	Mesial to distal fracture through the infundibula with one fragment displaced buccal and the other lingual Tooth is non-vital

13.12 Procedure: Buccal Luxation and Tooth Avulsion of Incisors

Technical action	Rationale/amplification
Determine if there is a buccal luxation or tooth avulsion. Buccal luxation is the displacement of a tooth in a buccal direction from the alveolus. The tooth still remains attached to the buccal periodontia. This often affects incisor teeth. Tooth avulsion is the traumatic removal of a tooth from the alveolus. The tooth is free of periodontal attachment. This often affects incisor teeth.	Radiographs are indicated for any luxation or avulsion cases. Buccal luxation is usually caused by a traumatic event; it occurs most often in juvenile horses. Tooth avulsion is usually caused by a traumatic event.
If the tooth is not fractured and it is a recent luxation or avulsion (Figure 13.34), the tooth can be re-implanted and splinted with orthopedic wire and composite to the surrounding normal teeth (Figure 13.35). Endodontic treatment of the affected tooth may be indicated once the periodontia has healed. This is due to the vascular supply of the avulsed or luxated tooth being compromised and the tooth becoming non-vital. Treatments would include radiographs and root canal treatment.	Tooth resorption can be a result of luxation or avulsion. Radiographs must be obtained at regular intervals to determine if tooth resorption is present and if the tooth remains vital. Endodontic treatment must be recommended for any teeth that are splinted or reimplanted. This is done in 2–4 weeks, after the periodontia has healed. Radiographs are indicated at 3 months post endodontic procedure to confirm the success of the endodontic procedure.
If the root of the luxated/avulsed tooth is fractured in a juvenile horse and/or a large amount of time has passed: • the free portion of the of tooth should be extracted • the fractured portion of the deciduous root should be left • warn the client that the horse may not develop a permanent tooth in that location.	The permanent tooth develops from germinal cells that are located near the apex of the deciduous tooth. Attempting to extract a separated root of a deciduous tooth may cause disruption of the germinal cells and failure of a permanent tooth to develop. Failure to develop a permanent tooth may occur in any case of luxation or avulsion of a deciduous tooth.
If the root of the luxated/avulsed tooth is fractured in an adult horse: The separated root must be extracted along with the tooth. Loose bone fragments are debrided and the mucosa is sutured with 2-0 Monocryl on a reverse cutting needle in a simple interrupted pattern.	The extraction process is similar to that previously described incisor extractions.

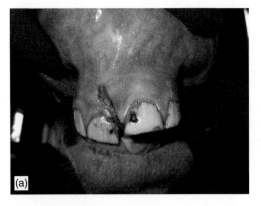 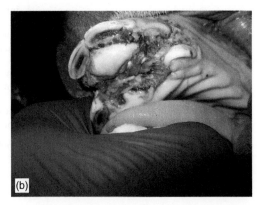

Figure 13.34 Buccal luxation of incisors in a 2-year-old colt: (a) frontal view of buccal luxation of incisors and (b) ventral view of buccal luxation of incisors.

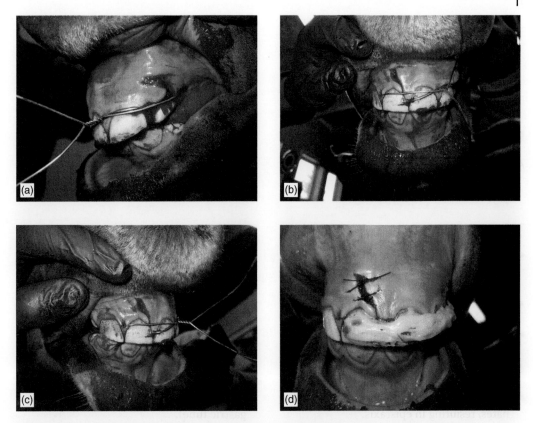

Figure 13.35 Repair of buccal luxation with orthopedic wire in the 2-year-old colt in Figure 13.31: (a) application of the wire, left side view, (b) application of the wire, frontal view, (c) application of the wire, right side view, and (d) after suture of the gingiva and application of composite.

Bibliography and Further Reading

Dixon, P.M., Barakzai, S., Collins, N., and Yates, J. (2008) Treatment of equine cheek teeth by mechanical widening of diastemata in 60 horses (2000–2006). *Equine Veterinary Journal*, **40** (1), 22–28.

Easley, R.J. (2004) Equine canine and first premolar (wolf) teeth, in *Proceedings of the American Association of Equine Practitioners Convention*, Vol. 50, American Association of Equine Practitioners, Lexington, KY, pp 13-18.

Klugh, D. (2005) Equine periodontal disease, in *Clinical Techniques in Equine Practice*, Elsevier Saunders, pp. 135–147.

Rucker, B.A. (2002) Utilizing cheek teeth angle of occlusion to determine length of incisor shortening. *American Association of Equine Practice Proceedings*, **48**, 448–452.

Staszyka, C., Bienertb, A., Kreutzerc, R., Wohlseinc, P., and Simhoferd, H. (2008) Equine odontoclastic tooth resorption and hypercementosis. *Veterinary Journal*, **178** (3), 372–379.

Tremaine, W.H. and Schumacher, J. (2010) Exodontia, in *Equine Dentistry*, 3rd edn (eds J. Easley, P.M. Dixon, and J. Schumacher), Saunders Elsevier, pp. 319–344.

14

Nasogastric Intubation

Alfredo Sanchez Londoño

14.1 Purpose

- Gastric decompression to relieve excess gas, fluid (such as enteral reflux) or gastric impaction.
- Administration of fluids, medications, nutritional gruel or supplements.
- To relieve esophageal obstructions.

14.2 Complications

- Trauma to the nasal mucosa and turbinates, resulting in epistaxis.
- Rhinitis from long-term placement of the nasogastric tube.
- Necrosis of the nasal mucosa when a large bore tube is kept indwelling for extended period of time.
- Pharyngitis/laryngitis resulting from trauma following attempts to have the horse swallow the nasogastric tube or from long-term placement of the nasogastric tube.
- Aspiration pneumonia from inadvertently administering liquid through tube passed into the trachea instead of the esophagus.
- Esophagitis or esophageal rupture following excessive force applied when trying to relieve an esophageal obstruction.

14.3 Equipment Required

- Sedation, optional (see Chapter 9).
- Twitch, optional (see Chapter 2).
- Nasogastric tube:

  – Choose the appropriate length and size for the animal.
  – Mark the tube with an indelible marker to record the approximate distance from the nostril to the pharynx. This can be estimated by measuring the distance from the nostril to the lateral canthus of the eye (Figure 14.1).
- Lubrication (lidocaine gel, water-soluble gel or any other lubricant at tip of nasogastric tube).
- Stomach pump or funnel that adapts to end of the tube.
- Two buckets: one empty, one with a premeasured amount of warm water.
- Liquid (e.g. water, electrolyte solution, fluids, mineral oil), medication or nutritional support to be administered.
- Additional supplies if the nasogastric tube is to be maintained as indwelling tube:
  – roll of 1″ white tape
  – a syringe or syringe case that fits snugly into the free end of the nasogastric tube
  – a muzzle

14.4 Restraint and Positioning

- Sedation and/or application of a twitch may be necessary.
- For the best personal protection the clinician should stand on the same side of the horse as the person who is providing the restraint.

Manual of Clinical Procedures in the Horse, First Edition. Edited by Lais R.R. Costa and Mary Rose Paradis.
© 2018 John Wiley & Sons, Inc. Published 2018 by John Wiley & Sons, Inc.

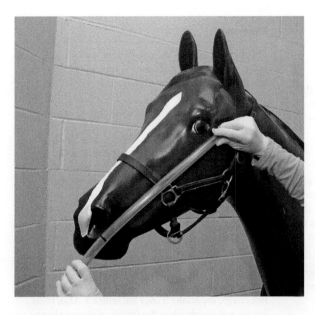

Figure 14.1 The distance from the nostril to the pharynx can be approximated by measuring the distance from the nostril to the lateral canthus of the eye. The tube can then be marked to indicate its location after insertion into the nose.

14.5 Procedure: Nasogastric Intubation

Technical action	Rationale
Gather all the materials prior to beginning the nasogastric intubation (Figure 14.2).	Make sure to get the appropriate size nasogastric tube that fits the horse's nasal passages properly. Also make sure the end of the tube fits snugly on the pump nozzle or the funnel. If using a pump, make sure the pump is working properly (not leaking at the top).
Lubricate several inches of the outside of the tube (Figure 14.3).	This will decrease the friction of the tube on the nasal mucosa.
Preferably, stand on the left side of the horse's head. Have the handler stand just behind you.	Standing on the left side allows the clinician to visualize the neck and observe the tube sliding down the neck as it passes through the cervical esophagus. Some clinicians opt to stand on the right side of the horse.
Choose which nasal passage is to be used (see below for the two options). Lubricate the nasal passage, preferably with lubricant containing lidocaine since the horse reacts most strongly to the first 6″ of the tube insertion.	The insertion of the initial 6″ of tube is best done as gently but as quickly as possible. Care should be taken when advancing the tube. The ethmoids may be encountered, which will feel like a hard structure. If this occurs the tube will need to be slightly pulled back and redirected more ventrally.
Option 1: Same side tube insertion Place the right hand over the bridge of the horse's nose and insert the right thumb into the external nares, slightly elevating the alar fold. With the left hand, the lubricated nasogastric tube is advanced into the ventral meatus using the thumb in the nostril to guide it ventromedially (Figure 14.4).	Most clinicians/operators are most comfortable with this option. Make sure to not occlude the opposite nostril when putting your hand over the bridge of the horse's nose.

(continued)

Technical action	Rationale
Option 2: Opposite side tube insertion Place the right hand over the bridge of the horse's nose and insert the middle finger and the ring finger into the nostril of the opposite side. Use these fingers to press the tube ventromedial as you pass the tube (Figure 14.5).	This technique gives the clinician/operator a little more control of the head during tube passage. It is less likely to occlude the nostril.
Once the tube reaches the pharyngeal area, judged by distance, swallowing is required to advance the tube into the esophagus. Flexion of the horse's head promotes swallowing of the tube (Figure 14.6). Be prepared to quickly advance the tube down the esophagus several inches when the horse swallows by positioning the left hand on the tube several inches from the nares.	It is helpful to have the mark on the tube indicating the length to the pharynx. Swallowing may occur spontaneously or may be stimulated by sliding the tube in and out, by rotating the tube, or by inserting a finger in the interdental space.
Correct positioning of the tube in the esophagus must be assessed before any liquid is placed into the tube. This can be done by: • detecting negative pressure on the tube when applying suction • visualizating or palpating the tube on the left side of the neck as it passes down the esophagus (Figure 14.7) • noting the increased resistance to passage of the tube into the esophagus as compared to that of the trachea • detecting a rattle of the tube against the trachea wall when shaking the trachea from side to side if the tube is placed into the trachea instead of the esophagus.	Do not rely on the horse coughing to tell you that the tube is in the trachea because some horses will not cough, especially if they are sedated. Also, some horses will cough when the tube is in the esophagus due to irritation of the tube passing over the larynx. In some horses, the esophagus may be anatomically located more to the right than the left side, in this case the tube may not be visualized from the left as it slides down the cervical esophagus.
Positioning of the nasogastric tube incorrectly into the trachea can be fatal if anything is administered into the tube. Make sure to check, especially for the lack of negative pressure when suctioning the tube.	Fatal aspiration pneumonia can occur if the tube is inadvertently placed in the trachea and fluid is pumped into the lungs.
Once in the esophageal lumen, advance the tube to the stomach. Judging by the length of tube passed, one can estimate that the stomach has been reached. Mild resistance may be encountered at the cardia. If gentle pressure or blowing into the tube does not allow passage into the stomach, instillation of 10 ml of lidocaine in 50 ml of water into the tube may cause relaxation of the cardia.	Presence of spontaneous reflux is abnormal, so any fluid obtained spontaneously should be measured to determine the amount present. If no spontaneous reflux is present, an effort to initiate reflux by creating a siphon should be attempted before administering any kind of medication through the tube.
To recover gastric fluid via a siphon effect, the tube is filled with water via either pump or gravity flow (using a funnel), and then allowed to drain by quickly lowering the external end of the tube to start a siphon effect. If no reflux is obtained initially, this procedure should be repeated multiple times until it is confirmed that there is no evidence of excessive gastric contents. The amount of fluid recovered in a normal situation is the same or slightly less than what was pumped in.	Any excess amount of fluid should be considered gastric reflux. The true amount of reflux should be determined by subtracting the original volume of water used to create a siphon from the final amount of reflux. This is referred to as the net reflux. The characteristics of the reflux should be noted. The pH will be acid if gastric in origin or basic if refluxing from the small intestine. The pH of the content should be tested with pH test strips (if these are not available, urine dipsticks can be used instead).

Technical action	Rationale
If the purpose of the nasogastric intubation is administration of fluid, mineral oil or any kind of medication or supplement, the appropriate amount of liquid, medication or gruel should be administered, followed by an amount of water sufficient to push all the medication out of the tube and into the stomach.	If net reflux is obtained, the administration of any liquid such as mineral oil, medications, gruel or supplements is not recommended.
If the nasogastric tube is to be maintained as an indwelling tube for continuous or intermittent reflux of gastric contents, or administration of liquids, the end should be taped to the horse's halter.	It may be necessary to keep a muzzle, to prevent the horse from eating the bedding and from rubbing the nose and removing the tape securing the tube to the halter.
To remove the tube, obstruct the lumen of the tube by placing a thumb in the end of the tube or folding it over to prevent contamination of the pharynx with gastric contents. The horse's head should be lowered as you pull the tube out with one continuous motion.	Maintain downward pressure on the tube by the other hand in the nostril to prevent the tube from flipping on exit and traumatizing the ethmoids, resulting in epistaxis.

Epistaxis may appear dramatic, but is generally of little significance unless a coagulopathy is present. |

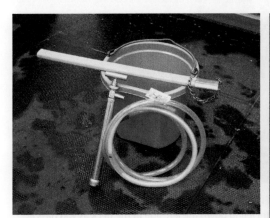

Figure 14.2 Supplies needed for the procedure: an appropriate size nasogastric tube, lubricant for the tube, a pump or funnel (that fit snuggly on the end of the nasogastric tube), and an empty bucket. Additional supplies not in this figure include a bucket with water to be administered for syphoning gastric contents, and, if that is the case, the fluid to be administered (e.g., mineral oil). If the tube is to be kept indwelling, additional materials include a roll of 1″ white tape, a syringe or syringe case that fits snuggly into the free end of the nasogastric tube, and a muzzle.

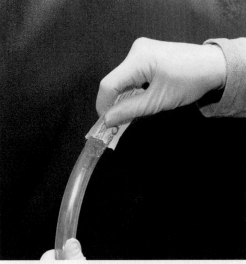

Figure 14.3 For ease of passage the end of the nasogastric tube should be lubricated.

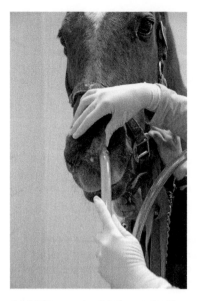

Figure 14.4 The nasogastric tube can be inserted in the nostril on the same side that you are standing on by placing your thumb in the nostril and passing the tube ventral medially up the nostril.

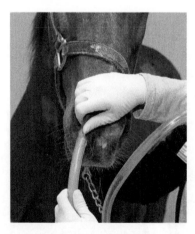

Figure 14.5 The nasogastric tube can be inserted in the nostril on the opposite side that you are standing on by placing your hand on the bridge of the nose and using your middle and ring finger to direct the tube ventromedial.

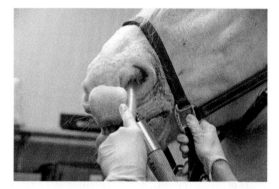

Figure 14.6 Swallowing the tube can be encouraged by flexing the neck and moving the tube back and forth in the pharynx.

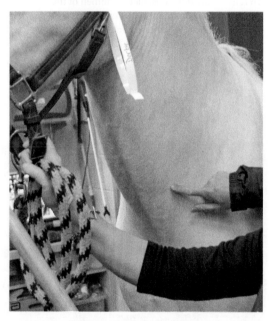

Figure 14.7 In most horses you can visualize the tube traveling down the left side of the neck as you pass it.

Bibliography and Further Reading

Dallap, B.S. (2008) Gastrointestinal system diagnostic and therapeutic procedures, in *Equine Emergencies: Treatment and Procedures*, 3rd edn (eds J.A.Orsini and T.J.Divers), W.B. Saunders, Philadelphia.

Hardy, J. (1998) Critical care, in *Equine Internal Medicine*, 2nd edn (eds S.Reed and W.Bayly), W.B. Saunders, Philadelphia.

Wilfong, D.A. and Waldridge, B. (2009) Technical procedures, in *AAEVT's Equine Manual for Veterinary Technicians*, Wiley-Blackwell, Ames.

Wimer, C.L. (2012) Nasogastric intubation, in *Clinical Veterinary Advisor: The Horse* (ed. D.A.Wilson), Elsevier Saunders, St Louis.

15

Abdominocentesis

Alfredo Sanchez Londoño

15.1 Purpose

- To obtain a sample of peritoneal fluid aseptically to diagnose or evaluate abdominal disease, including colic, complications associated with post abdominal surgery, peritoneal effusion, weight loss, chronic diarrhea, weight loss, and cases of fever of unknown origin.

15.2 Complications

- Enterocentesis: If the instrument used for peritoneal collection penetrates the bowel, ingesta will be recovered. The sample will show plant material, bacteria, possibly protozoa and debris, but no evidence of inflammatory cells. It is important to differentiate between intestinal rupture and enterocentesis. In a case of intestinal rupture, cytology will most likely show neutrophils, extracellular bacteria and phagocytized bacteria within the neutrophils. Differentiation between enterocentesis and intestinal rupture can be difficult, especially in the acute phase of a rupture, when inflammatory infiltrate may not have taken place. Antimicrobials should be administered in cases of enterocentesis. Intestinal rupture carries a grave prognosis.
- Splenic puncture or laceration: The position of the spleen is variable and it may be displaced medially or to the right of the midline. Puncture of the spleen results in hemorrhage into the abdominal cavity, which interferes with interpretation of abdominal fluid analysis. Splenic rupture is usually characterized by the presence of platelets, whereas intraabdominal hemorrhage of 12 hours duration may not have platelets and erythophagocytosis may be present. The packed cell volume (PCV) of splenic blood is often greater that peripheral PCV.
- Inadvertent prolapse of omentum can occur when abdominocentesis is performed with a teat cannula in foals.

15.3 Equipment Required

- Clippers.
- Antiseptics (alcohol and another antiseptic scrub).
- 2–3 ml of 2% lidocaine with 25-gauge ¾″ and 22-gauge 1½″ needles for local anesthesia.
- 18-gauge 1½″ or 18-gauge 3″ needle, teat cannula or bitch catheter (Figure 15.1).
- Sterile syringes.
- Sterile gloves.
- Sterile gauze.
- #15 scalpel blade.
- EDTA and no additives evacuated tubes.
- Ultrasound (if available).

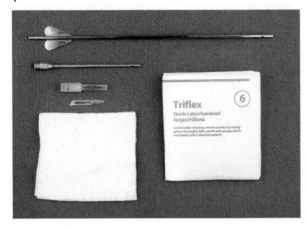

Figure 15.1 Material for performing an abdominocentesis in horse: (top to bottom) a bitch catheter, a teat cannula, an 18-gauge 1½″ needle, scalpel blade #15, 4 x 4 sterile gauze and sterile gloves.

15.4 Restraint and Positioning

- Positioning the horse in stocks provides a more secure environment for the person performing the procedure.
- The operator should be positioned near the forelimb of the patient, to the side, out of the range of the arc of the hind limb.
- Adequate sedation should be used.
- A nose twitch can be applied during the procedure.

15.5 Procedure

Technical action	Rationale
Locate the appropriate site. Ideally the location should be slightly to the right of the ventral midline caudal to the xiphoid (Figure 15.2).	This location may prevent accidental puncture of the spleen. Ultrasonography of the ventral midline will help identify the location of the spleen and any visible fluid (Figure 15.3). The sternal flexure of the large colon may lie on the lowest point of the abdomen.
The area should be clipped and aseptically prepared (Figure 15.4). An injection of 2–3 ml of 2% lidocaine is given subcutaneously and into the abdominal musculature (Figure 15.5). The area should be rescrubbed aseptically (Figure 15.6).	The subcutaneous bleb should be visible. Detailed description of aseptic technique is given in Chapter 10.
Option 1: While wearing sterile gloves, palpate the site. The needle is inserted through the skin and gently advanced (through the muscle layers, if off the midline) into the abdomen. Release the needle once it is in the abdomen. The hub of the needle will rotate slightly as the bowel moves around the shaft of the needle. A second needle can be inserted next to the first one to obtain some fluid.	Needle size will vary depending on the size of the horse. An 18-gauge 1½″ needle should be enough for a small or thin horse, but an 18-gauge 3″ needle may be needed for an obese or very large horse. The needle technique has a high risk of enterocentesis or blood contamination.
Option 2: If using a teat cannula or a bitch catheter, a small stab skin incision should be made with the #15 blade over the locally anesthetized area (Figure 15.7). To prevent blood contamination from the skin vessels, the cannula or the bitch catheter should be placed through a sterile 4 × 4 gauze (Figure 15.8).	The bitch catheter is preferred when obtaining abdominal fluid from a very large horse (i.e., draft breeds) or from obese animals. Caution must be exercised when using the teat cannula technique in foals. Inadvertent prolapse of the omentum through the abdominocentesis site can occur as the cannula

Technical action	Rationale
The cannula is then inserted into the small incision that was made in the skin and gently advanced through the muscle layers and into the abdominal cavity (Figure 15.9). A distinct "pop" can be felt as the teat cannula goes through the peritoneum.	is removed. If this happens then the exposed omentum should be removed and the remaining omentum tucked into the abdomen with another sterile teat cannula and a belly bandage applied.
If no fluid is obtained after penetrating the abdominal cavity, the needle or cannula can be rotated, slowly advanced, removed or redirected. If still no fluid is obtained the needle or cannula should be removed and a bitch catheter inserted deeper into the abdominal cavity.	In horses that are extremely dehydrated it may be very difficult to obtain peritoneal fluid as it is reabsorbed by the body.
The fluid that is obtained should be collected in a plain tube (red-top tube) for culture and sensitivity, and in an EDTA-containing tube (lavender-top tube) for fluid and cytologic analysis.	If blood contamination occurs in the process of fluid collection, analysis will be affected.
After fluid collection is complete, the needle, cannula or bitch catheter is removed and the area is cleaned with an alcohol wipe.	There is no need to place any sutures at the site of the incision.

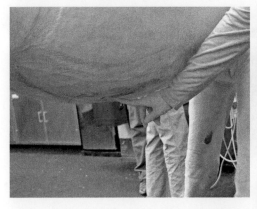

Figure 15.2 If done without the use of ultrasound, the site is located to the right of the ventral midline of the horse at the most ventral part of the abdomen in an attempt to avoid a splenic puncture.

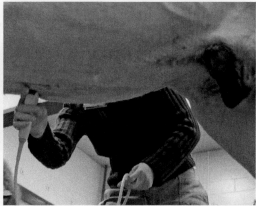

Figure 15.3 If ultrasound is used then a site may be chosen where there is a visible hypoecchoic area indicating a "pocket" of fluid.

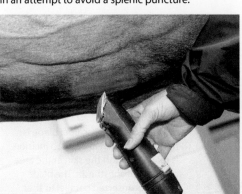

Figure 15.4 A square area (10 × 10 cm) is clipped and scrubbed with surgical scrub and alcohol.

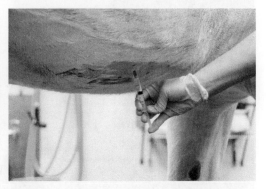

Figure 15.5 Local anesthetic (2–3 ml of 2% lidocaine) is injected both subcutaneously and deeper into the muscle layer of the abdominal wall.

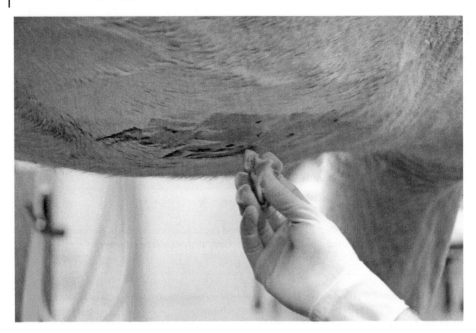

Figure 15.6 A final surgical preparation is performed with sterile gloves and surgical scrub and alcohol after local anesthesia.

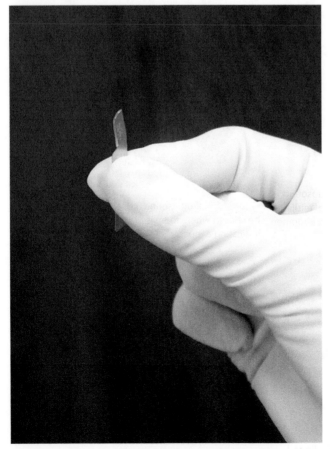

Figure 15.7 A #15 scalpel blade is held at the notch and a stab incision is made through the skin at the area of the local anesthesia. The blade should be inserted parallel to the linea alba.

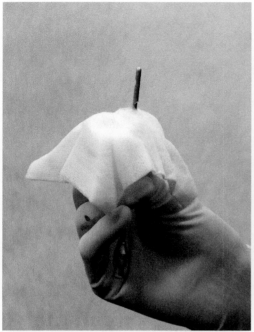

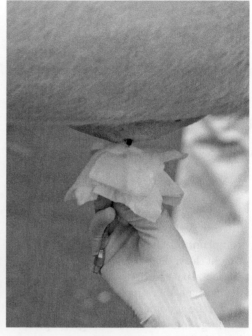

Figure 15.8 To avoid contaminating the sample of peritoneal fluid with blood from the stab incision, the teat cannula should be inserted through a 4 × 4 gauze.

Figure 15.9 The teat cannula is introduced through the incision in the skin, through the muscle layers and into the abdominal cavity. A distinct "pop" may be felt as the teat cannula goes through the peritoneum.

Bibliography and Further Reading

Freeman, D. (2010) How to do and evaluate abdominal paracentesis, in *Proceedings of the Annual Meeting of the Italian Association of Equine Veterinarians*, Carrara, Italy, pp. 194–197.

Hardy, J. (1998) Critical care, in *Equine Internal Medicine*, 2nd edn (eds S.Reed and W. Bayly), W.B. Saunders, Philadelphia.

Jones, S.L. and Blikslager, A.T. (1998) Disorders of the gastrointestinal system, in *Equine Internal Medicine*, 2nd edn (eds S.Reed and W. Bayly), W.B. Saunders, Philadelphia.

Jones, S.L. and Smith, B.P. (2009) Diseases of the alimentary tract, in *Large Animal Internal Medicine*, 4th edn (ed. B.Smith), Mosby, St Louis.

Kaneps, A.J. (2012) Abdominocentesis, in *Clinical Veterinary Advisor: The Horse* (ed. D.A.Wilson), Elsevier Saunders, St Louis.

16

Rectal Examination

Alfredo Sanchez Londoño

16.1 Purpose

- To thoroughly evaluate a horse with a complaint of abdominal discomfort or weight loss. Rectal palpation is a fundamental part of this routine examination.
- To evaluate the structures in the caudal half of the abdomen, including portions of the large intestine, caudal edge of spleen, left kidney, aorta, mesenteric root, peritoneal surface, reproductive tract of mares, and inguinal rings in stallions.
- To determine any changes in the size, shape, distension or positioning of structures within the caudal portion of the abdomen.
- To determine the reproductive status of a mare, evaluate the fetus in case of pregnancy,

and evaluate the post-parturient mare (see Chapters 36, 39, and 41, respectively).

16.2 Complications

- Rectal tears (see Table 16.1).
- Injury to the person performing the rectal examination.

16.3 Equipment Required

- Stocks (if available) or stall doorway or hay bales.
- Sedation.
- Twitch.
- Rectal sleeve and glove.
- Lubricant gel.
- Shirt guard (optional) (Figure 16.1).

Table 16.1 Classification and management of rectal tears: rectal tears require immediate attention

Grades	Severity	Management
Grade I	Mucosa and submucosa only are involved	Reduce straining to prevent progression: sedation, epidural, administration of parasympatolytic such as scopolammonium (Buscopan®), and stool softners; careful removal of feces from rectum and tear; administration of broad spectrum antibiotics, anti-inflammatories, tetanus prophylaxis.
Grade II	Muscle layer involved, while mucosa and submucosa remain intact	
Grade III	All layers except the serosa are torn	All above recommendations and immediate referral to a surgical facility for repair and further evaluation. Pack the rectum with a cotton-filled stockinette prior to shipping. Guarded prognosis.
Grade IV	Complete perforation	Immediate referral to a surgical facility. Poor prognosis because of fecal contamination of the peritoneal cavity.

Manual of Clinical Procedures in the Horse, First Edition. Edited by Lais R.R. Costa and Mary Rose Paradis.
© 2018 John Wiley & Sons, Inc. Published 2018 by John Wiley & Sons, Inc.

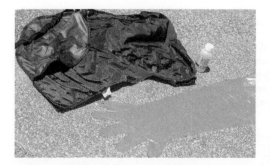

Figure 16.1 Rectal sleeve and shirt guard.

16.4 Restraint

- If possible, the horse should be placed in stocks (Figure 16.2). If it is not possible to place the horse in stocks, a safe location for the handler and performer (veterinarian) must be used, including utilizing a stall doorway or stack of bales of hay as barrier.
- The handler should have complete control of the horse and be paying attention to the

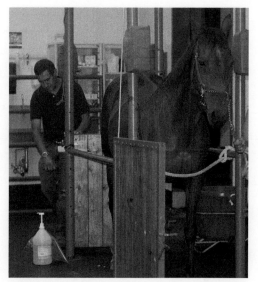

Figure 16.2 Horse in stocks.

instructions and indications that the veterinarian is giving.

16.5 Procedure

Technical action	Rationale
Administration of sedatives and application of a nose twitch may be required in uncooperative horses (see Chapter 2 for restraint and Chapter 9 for sedation)	This examination can be dangerous for both the horse and the veterinarian. Adequate restraint is important in preventing catastrophic injury. A horse handler should be in control of the horse as the veterinarian performs the examination.
The tail can be wrapped with brown gauze (Figure 16.3a), a neoprene tail wrap (Figure 16.3b) or placed in a plastic bag to prevent it from getting dirty.	If the tail is to be tied, it must be tied to the horse itself (Figure 16.4). The tail should never be tied to stocks or other objects. When the tail is tied around the horse's neck, a forelimb should be included to avoid blocking the jugular veins.
Place rectal sleeve and glove over arm that will be performing the examination.	A thin rectal sleeve with no creases should be placed over the palpating arm. The fingertips of the sleeve can be removed and a surgical glove placed over it to improve sensitivity (Figure 16.5).
Apply a generous amount of lubricating gel on the palm of the glove and also on the dorsal surface extending towards the elbow (Figure 16.6).	Because the anus will tighten around the hand, causing the applied lubricant to be removed, one can directly place lubricant into the rectum using a 60 ml catheter tip syringe.

(continued)

Technical action	Rationale
The sleeved and gloved hand should approach the rectum with the fingers extended. To enter the rectum, the fingers should gently dilate the anal sphincter (Figure 16.7). If the anal sphincter tightens, place one finger at a time, so that the hand is gradually advanced. Fecal material should be evacuated from the rectum to allow for adequate evaluation (Figure 16.8).	If the horse is straining or intestinal contractions occurs, the hand should be removed to prevent rectal tears. As the rectum relaxes, the hand and arm are gently advanced deeper to palpate the different structures.
Perform rectal examination to identify all the palpable structures within the caudal abdomen (see Table 16.2).	Carefully localize and evaluate all palpable structures (Figures 16.9 through 16.15).
Removal of arm and hand from rectum: The gloved hand should be gently removed from the rectum. It is important to remember to remove the fingers in a closed and tight position to prevent the possibility of lacerating the rectal wall.	Upon exiting, the sleeve and glove should be checked for the presence of blood. Any presence of blood should be investigated further to determine the source. This can be done with a bare hand and arm to feel for any tears in the rectum.
If a rectal tear is suspected, it should be confirmed carefully. Management of rectal tears requires immediate attention.	See Table 16.1 for grading rectal tears and management guidelines.

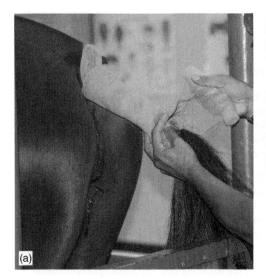

(a)

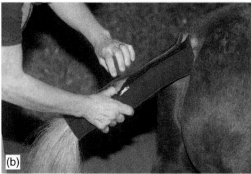

(b)

Figure 16.3 The tail can be wrapped with (a) brown gauze or (b) neoprene tail wrap. (Courtesy of Dr. Lais R.R. Costa).

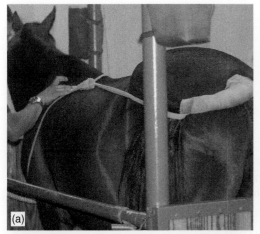

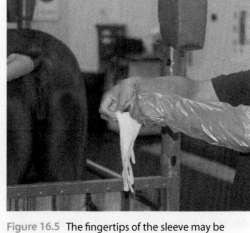

Figure 16.5 The fingertips of the sleeve may be removed and an examination or surgical glove placed over it to improve sensitivity.

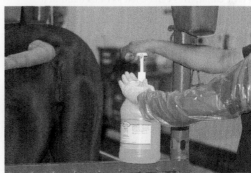

Figure 16.6 A generous amount of lubricating gel is applied on the palm of the glove and also on the dorsal surface extending towards the elbow.

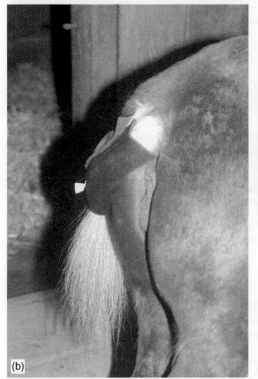

Figure 16.4 Tail can be tied around the horse's neck: (a) brown gauze or (b) neoprene tail wrap. (Courtesy of Dr. Lais R.R. Costa). The tail should be never tied to an object (e.g., stocks, stall gate, etc.).

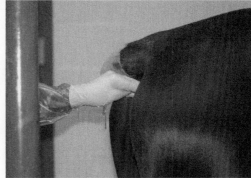

Figure 16.7 To introduce the hand into the rectum, the fingers should gently dilate the anal sphincter.

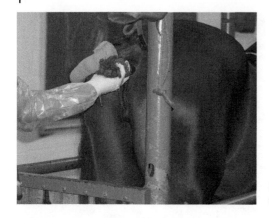

Figure 16.8 Fecal material should be evacuated from the rectum to allow for adequate evaluation.

Table 16.2 Localization of some palpable structures during rectal examination

Localization of palpable structures	Interpretation of findings
Pelvic canal: This can be felt as one's hand first enters the rectum.	The pelvic canal should be symmetrical with no abnormal masses present.
Bladder: The bladder is located cranially and ventrally over the brim of the pelvis.	The bladder may not be palpable when it is empty.
Uterus: The uterus in the mare can be found dorsal to the bladder by extending the arm over the brim of the pelvis, curling the fingers down and gently retracting the hand.	In a pregnant mare the uterus and the fetus can also be palpable. Depending on the stage of pregnancy, the uterus will hang over the brim of the pelvis.
Ovaries: After the uterus is located, one can follow each horn up to each of the ovaries.	Palpation of a mare's ovaries allows the clinician to determine the stage of her estrus cycle.
Inguinal rings: Located on the caudal ventral aspect (floor) of the abdominal wall (at 5 and 7 o'clock), the normal inguinal rings will be palpated as a fold of tissue. In intact stallions the spermatic cord can be felt entering the ring.	The inguinal rings are of major importance in stallions with suspected inguinal hernias.
Aorta: Dorsally and on the midline, the aorta can be felt pulsing. The aorta will serve as a landmark for identification of the mesenteric root located cranially (Figure 16.9).	The aorta can be followed caudally to the bifurcation to iliac arteries. It is important to determine if the pulses are equal on the left and right iliac arteries.
Small colon: The small colon is located in the caudal middle of the abdomen and is identified by the presence of two taenia or bands and the presence of fecal balls within and sacculations.	The small colon should be the most obvious and identifiable structure.
Left kidney: The caudal pole of the left kidney is found by directing the hand towards the left dorsal abdominal wall, just lateral to the aorta. It will be felt as a firm structure (Figure 16.10).	Only the caudal pole of the left kidney is palpable. The right kidney is located beyond the clinician's reach.
Spleen: The caudal edge of the spleen can usually be found by advancing the hand cranially along the left body wall (Figure 16.11).	Gently waving your hand laterally from the left body wall will often allow you to feel the sharp edge of the spleen.

Localization of palpable structures	Interpretation of findings
Nephrosplenic ligament (space): Located between the left kidney and the dorsal edge of the spleen.	The nephrosplenic space can be palpated in some of horses. This is an area where the large colon can become displaced and cause signs of colic.
Pelvic flexure: The pelvic flexure of the colon should be palpable as a soft and relaxed structure just cranial to the pelvic brim, either on midline or slightly to the left. It generally feels smooth with no palpable taenia (the one taenia is located on the mesocolon) (Figure 16.12).	Impaction of the pelvic flexure can be readily palpated on rectal examination. It feels like a smooth firm structure approximately 10–12 cm in diameter. If larger it may extend across the midline or back into the pelvic canal.
Cecum: The cecum can be palpated on the right side of the abdominal cavity. The cecum has four taenia or bands, but only the ventral and medial bands are palpable on the caudal aspect of the cecal base (Figure 16.13).	In the normal horse the cecum may be difficult to discern. In cases of cecal impaction, the cecum will become more prominent and when tugging on the ventral taenia of the cecum one will have the impression that the cecum is heavy. In cecal tympany one will feel a gas-filled structure on the right side of the abdomen that may actually be palpable in the mid abdomen (Figure 16.14).
Small intestine: In a normal healthy horse it should not be possible to identify small intestinal loops in the caudal portion of the abdomen.	When the small intestine is dilated it can be felt in the central portion of the abdomen by gently sweeping your hand up and down (Figure 16.15). The bowel is smooth and can vary in diameter from 3 to 6 cm.
Peritoneal surface: The peritoneal surfaces should also be palpated and they should feel smooth and not be painful.	In a horse with a ruptured bowel the peritoneal surfaces may have a "gritty" feel to them.

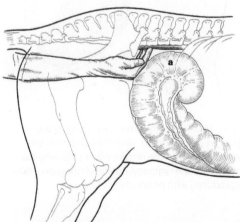

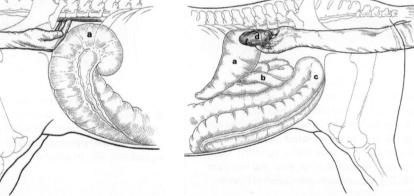

Figure 16.9 Identification of the aorta during rectal palpation. Note the position of the examiner's arm in the rectum. The aorta lies in the midline attached to the dorsal body wall. A pulse should be felt. The base of the cecum is shown (a). Rose and Hodgson (2000). Reproduced with permission of Elsevier.

Figure 16.10 Identification of the left kidney during rectal palpation. Note the position of the examiner's arm in the rectum when palpating the left kidney (d). The kidney is dorsal and medial to the spleen (a), and it is attached to the body wall. b, small intestine; c, pelvic flexure. Rose and Hodgson (2000). Reproduced with permission of Elsevier.

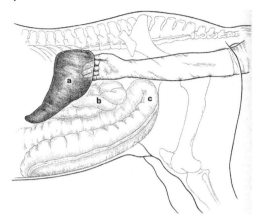

Figure 16.11 Identification of the spleen during rectal palpation. Note the position of the examiner's arm in the rectum when palpating the spleen (a). The spleen normally lies in the dorsal part of the abdomen on the left-hand side adjacent to the body wall. b, small intestine; c, pelvic flexure. Rose and Hodgson (2000). Reproduced with permission of Elsevier.

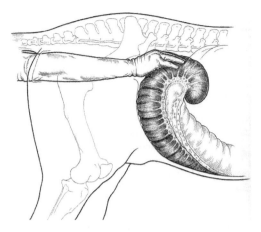

Figure 16.13 Identification of the cecum during rectal palpation. Note the position of the examiner's arm in the rectum when palpating the cecum. Rose and Hodgson (2000). Reproduced with permission of Elsevier.

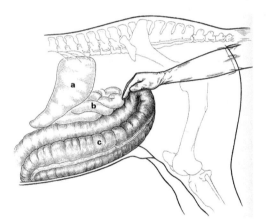

Figure 16.12 Identification of the pelvic flexure during rectal palpation. Note the position of the examiner's arm in the rectum when palpating the pelvic flexure (c) of the large colon. It lies just over the pelvic brim on the left-hand side of the midline on the ventral abdominal wall. a, spleen; b, small intestine; c, left ventral colon. Rose and Hodgson (2000). Reproduced with permission of Elsevier.

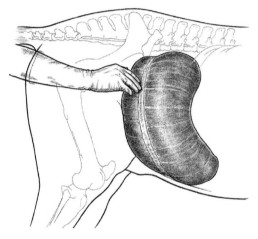

Figure 16.14 Identification of cecum tympany during rectal palpation. Note the position of the examiner's arm in the rectum when palpating the cecum with the tympany. Rose and Hodgson (2000). Reproduced with permission of Elsevier.

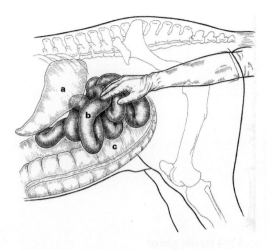

Figure 16.15 Identification of distended small intestine during rectal palpation. Note the position of the examiner's arm in the rectum when palpating the distended small intestine loops (b). Taut loops of gas- and fluid-filled small intestine are often palpable. a, spleen; c, left ventral colon. Rose and Hodgson (2000). Reproduced with permission of Elsevier.

Bibliography and Further Reading

Adams, S.B. and Fessler, J.F. (2000) Management of rectal tears, in *Atlas of Equine Surgery*, W.B. Saunders, pp. 121–127.

Ethell, M.T., Dart, A.J., Hodgson, D.R., and Rose, R.J. (2000) Alimentary System, in *Manual of Equine Practice*, 2nd edn (eds R.J.Rose and D.R.Hodgson), W.B. Saunders, Philadelphia.

Hunt, J. (1987) Rectal examination of the equine gastrointestinal tract. *In Practice*, **9**, 171–177.

Jones, S.L. and Blikslager, A.T. (1998) Disorders of the gastrointestinal system, in *Equine Internal Medicine*, 2nd edn (eds S.M. Reed and W. Bayly), W.B. Saunders, Philadelphia, pp. 769–780.

Jones, S.L. and Smith, B.P. (2009) Diseases of the alimentary tract, in *Large Animal Internal Medicine*, 4th edn, Mosby, pp. 667–668.

Rose, R.J. and Hodgson, D.R. (2000) *Manual of Equine Practice*, 2nd edn, W.B. Saunders, Philadelphia.

Sherlock, C. (2012) Rectal tear, in *Clinical Veterinary Advisor: The Horse* (ed. D.A.Wilson), Elsevier Saunders, St Louis.

The Glass Horse Equine Colic, DVD, V. 1.1. University of Georgia Research Foundation, Athens, GA, 2007.

White, N.A. (1998) Rectal examination for the acute abdomen, in *Current Techniques in Equine Surgery and Lameness*, 2nd edn, W.B. Saunders, Philadelphia, pp. 262–270.

17

Percutaneous Cecal Trocharization

Mustajab H. Mirza and Lais R.R. Costa

17.1 Purpose

- To relieve cecum or large colon tympany when the severe gaseous distension of the cecum and large colon results in unrelenting pain and surgery is not an option.
- To relieve cecum or large colon tympany when the severe gaseous distension compresses the veins draining the abdomen, resulting in poor venous return and compromised cardiovascular status of the patient, and surgery is not an option.
- To reduce cecum or large colon gas distension associated with large colon displacement in cases when conservative medical treatment, instead of surgical treatment, is pursued.

17.2 Complications

- Septic peritonitis secondary to leakage of intestinal content into the abdomen.
- Visceral laceration.
- Puncture of diaphragm.
- Puncture of kidney.
- Hematoma formation.
- Abscess formation in the body wall due to seeding of bacteria from withdrawal of trocar.
- Hemoperitoneum

17.3 Equipment Required

- 14-gauge 5″ catheter (such as Angiocath 5¼″)
- #15 surgical scalpel blade

- 4 × 4 sterile gauze
- Sterile gloves
- Aseptic scrub supplies
- 2% lidocaine or 1.5% or 2% carbocaine
- 22-gauge 1″ needle and 5 ml syringe
- 20″ luer slip extension set
- Specimen cup filled with sterile saline or sterile water
- Optional: gentamicin (total of 200 mg) diluted in physiologic saline, total volume of 10 ml
- Sterile saline and sterile 10 ml syringe

17.4 Restraint and Positioning

- Positioning the horse in stocks provides a more secure environment for the person performing the procedure. However, as the horse might be very uncomfortable and unable to stand safely in the stocks, the procedure might have to be performed in a stall.
- The operator should be positioned on the right side of the patient, next to the thorax, out of the range of the arc of the hind limb.
- The handler should be positioned on the same side of the horse.
- Adequate sedation should be used.
- A nose twitch can be applied during the procedure if deemed necessary.

Manual of Clinical Procedures in the Horse, First Edition. Edited by Lais R.R. Costa and Mary Rose Paradis.
© 2018 John Wiley & Sons, Inc. Published 2018 by John Wiley & Sons, Inc.

17.5 Procedure: Percutaneous Cecal Trocharization

Technical action	Rationale
The indication for cecal trocarization must be determined during detailed physical examination and a rectal palpation.	Cecal trocarization is a palliative procedure and the condition is likely to recur if the cause of the tympany is not addressed.
	In general, cecal trocarization is performed in cases of severe abdominal distension when surgery is not an option. Relief of gas distension is helpful in the medical management of large colon impactions.
The site location for the cecal trocarization is the right flank, lateral to epaxial musculature, caudal to the last floating rib, and cranial to the great trochanter. The site is in the middle of the upper flank region (Figures 17.1 and 17.2).	The base of the cecum is in the upper right flank. This is where gas will accumulate in cecal tympany. It is important to determine whether the abdominal distention is cecal in origin because the procedure is contraindicated in gas accumulation in the small intestine. Rectal palpation is crucial to confirm cecal tympany and rule out gas accumulation in the small intestine or colon torsion.
Perform percussion of the upper right flank to locate a gas cap (or "ping") to confirm that cecal tympany is indeed present (Figure 17.3).	Place a stethoscope in the right flank and percuss the surrounding area by flicking the middle finger between the thumb and the body wall, which will produce an audible resonant sound if there is gas in the cecum.
Prepare all materials for the procedure (Figure 17.4).	
Clip hair over a large area (10 × 10 cm) using a #40 clipper blade (Figure 17.5).	Remove the hair to decrease the possibility that organic debris and bacteria lead to local infection.
Wearing examination gloves, aseptically prepare the site and the surrounding area (Figure 17.6).	Use at least 5-7 minutes of antiseptic contact time to reduce bacterial skin contamination (see Chapter 10).
Inject 3 ml of lidocaine into the subcutaneous tissue and external abdominal oblique muscle (Figure 17.7). Repeat the aseptic scrub while wearing sterile gloves.	Local anesthetic may reduce patient movement during insertion of the catheter.
Perform a stab incision in the center of the lidocaine block with a #15 scalpel blade (Figure 17.8).	The stab incision decreases the drag of the catheter through the skin.
Insert a 14-gauge 5″ or 5 1/4″ catheter through the stab incision and advance into the abdomen as the tip points towards the xiphoid (Figure 17.9).	This angled position will decrease the chance of puncturing the right kidney.
Insert approximately three-quarters of the catheter and monitor for exit of gas. Inability to evacuate gas may occur because of occlusion of the catheter by cecal contents.	If the catheter is appropriately placed in the lumen of the gas-distended cecum, gas will escape and noise and cecal aroma of methane will be evident. If gas is not escaping, adjust the catheter placement.
Once the catheter is properly placed, remove the stylet. Hold the hub of the catheter gently (Figure 17.10a). You will notice the catheter being tugged as the cecum moves.	The stylet should be removed to avoid lacerating the intestinal wall.

(continued)

Technical action	Rationale
Note the gas being evacuated from the cecum by the smell and attach an extension set to the hub of the catheter (Figure 17.10b).	This will prevent gut contents that might exit the catheter from contaminating the insertion site and allows continuous monitoring of gas evacuation.
The free end of the extension set is submerged into sterile water or saline in a sterile specimen cup (as depicted in Figure 17.2) to monitor the gas exit.	The position of the catheter might need to be adjusted during evacuation of the gas.
Continue to monitor the evacuation of gas because after decompression the viscus might pull away from the body wall, dislodging the catheter from the lumen.	If the catheter becomes free in the abdominal cavity, it will contaminate the peritoneal cavity.
If gas is no longer escaping, but satisfactory evacuation of gas has not been achieved, flush the catheter with sterile saline and recheck for gas.	Sometimes the catheter will be plugged with intestinal content. Flushing may restart the gas flow. Often gas will continue to escape for 10–15 minutes.
Once it has been determined that there is no more gas flow, flush the catheter with sterile saline once more and inject gentamicin as the catheter is withdrawn.	During withdraw of the catheter diluted gentamicin may offer some protection to the body wall from contamination.
If there is concern about contamination, monitor the horse for any signs of peritonitis or abscess formation.	When contamination of the peritoneal cavity is suspected, prompt treatment with systemic antibiotic therapy is recommended.

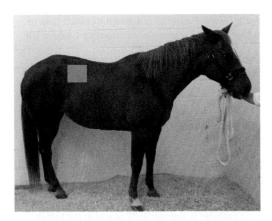

Figure 17.1 The site for the cecal trocarization is the middle of the upper right flank region, lateral to epaxial musculature, caudal to the last floating rib and cranial to the great trochanter.

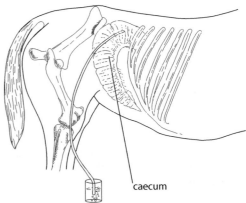

Figure 17.2 The positioning of the catheter during evacuation of the gas from the cecum. Rowe (2008). Reproduced with permission of John Wiley & Sons, Inc.

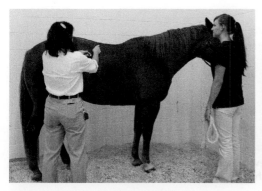

Figure 17.3 Percussion of the right flank area to identify the area of resonant sound.

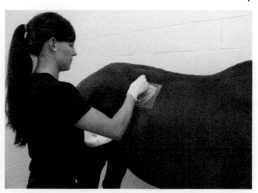

Figure 17.6 Aseptic scrubbing of the skin in preparation for percutaneous trocharization.

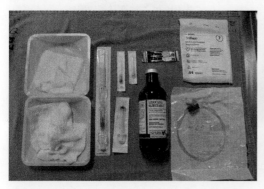

Figure 17.4 Materials needed for cecal trocarization include 14-gauge 5" catheter (such as the Angiocath 5¼), #15 surgical scalpel blade, 4 × 4 sterile gauze, sterile gloves, aseptic scrub supplies, local anesthetic (2% lidocaine or 2% carbocaine), 22-gauge 1" needle and 5 ml syringe, 20" luer slip extension set.

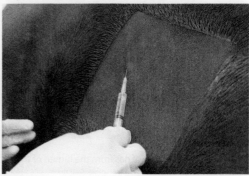

Figure 17.7 Injection of local anesthetic at the site of the stab incision.

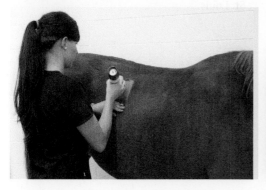

Figure 17.5 In preparation for percutaneous trocharization, a 10 × 10 cm area of hair is clipped.

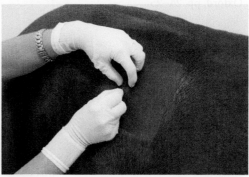

Figure 17.8 Performing the stab incision using a #15 blade.

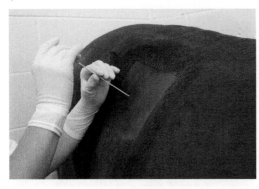

Figure 17.9 Insertion of the 14-gauge catheter for evacuation of gas from cecum and advancement into the abdomen as the tip points towards the xiphoid.

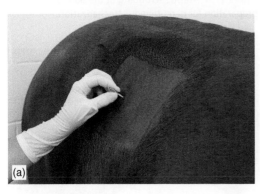

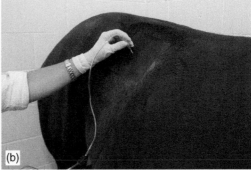

Figure 17.10 Evacuation of gas from the lumen of the cecum (a) prior and (b) after attachment of an extension set.

Bibliography and Further Reading

Rowe, E. (2008) Percutaneous trocarisation, in *The Equine Hospital Manual* (eds K.Corley and J. Stephen), Blackwell, Oxford, pp. 24–25.

Wimer, C.L. (2012) Cecal trocarisation, in *Clinical Veterinary Advisor: The Horse* (ed. D.A.Wilson), Elsevier Saunders, St. Louis.

18

Gastroscopy and Esophagoscopy

Patrick Loftin, Joshua A. Cartmill, and Frank M. Andrews

18.1 Purpose

- To visualize the esophagus (esophagoscopy), stomach (gastroscopy), and proximal duodenum (duodenoscopy) to inspect and assess mucosal defects such as erosion, ulceration, thickening and discoloration (hyperkeratosis or hyperemia), desquamation (peeling off of the mucosa), and raised areas (tumors or polyps) using an endoscope.
- To identify abnormalities such as stricture, diverticulae, and/or impaction of the esophagus, stomach, and proximal duodenum in horses showing clinical signs of colic, regurgitation, and/or dysphagia.

18.2 Complications

- Abrasion, irritation, and hyperemia of the nasal and nasopharyngeal mucosa.
- Epistaxis.
- Abrasion, irritation, and hyperemia of the esophageal, gastric, and duodenal mucosa.
- Abdominal pain (colic) due to over-distension of the stomach and/or duodenum with air.
- Esophageal or gastric rupture.

18.3 Equipment Required

- 2.5–3 m fiberoptic or video endoscope (Figure 18.1) with:
  - 9–13 mm outer diameter
  - air/water feed and suction buttons (Figure 18.2)
  - biopsy/water flush channel
  - 90–120° deflection in all directions.
- Video monitor (Figure 18.3).
- Video processor.
- Light source: 150–300* halogen light.
- Air compressor (Figure 18.4) attached to a video processor or separate*.
- Suction device: bottle (glass or plastic) for collection of gastric fluid (Figure 18.5).
- Water source: 60 ml syringe or external pump to flush debris from the stomach mucosa.
- Optional-mouth gag or a large bore, short nasoesophageal guide tube to minimize the risk of damaging the scope in case it is misdirected into the oral cavity.

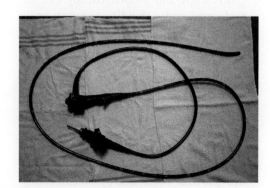

Figure 18.1 A 3 m endoscope.

Manual of Clinical Procedures in the Horse, First Edition. Edited by Lais R.R. Costa and Mary Rose Paradis.
© 2018 John Wiley & Sons, Inc. Published 2018 by John Wiley & Sons, Inc.

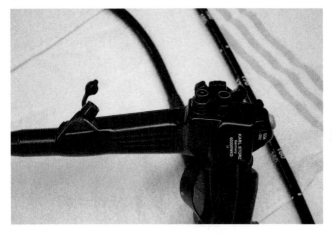

Figure 18.2 Endoscope with air/water feed (blue), suction buttons (red), and biopsy channel (black with cap).

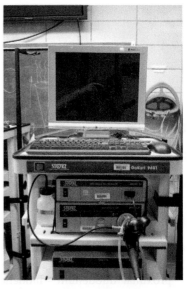

Figure 18.3 Video monitor, processor, and light source for an endoscope.

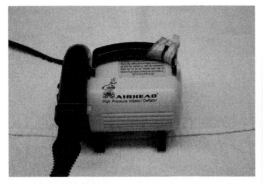

Figure 18.4 A small air compressor can be attached to the biopsy channel to facilitate insufflation of the stomach.

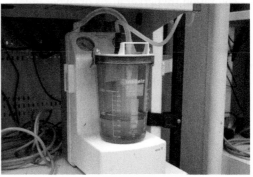

Figure 18.5 Suction bottle to collect gastric juice.

18.4 Restraint and Positioning

- Gastroscopy and esophagoscopy can be performed under standing sedation or in a horse that is under general anesthesia.

18.4.1 Standing Esophagoscopy and Gastroscopy

- Three people are needed to perform a thorough standing endoscopic examination in a horse: one restrains the horse, one passes the endoscope, and one drives the endoscope.
- The horse can be placed in stocks or a stall with the head controlled by a technician.

- Sedation with xylazine (0.5 mg/kg, IV) or detomidine (0.01-0.02 mg/kg, IV) is administered and the horse is left undisturbed until it appears sedated and drops its head.
- A twitch may be applied to the horse's muzzle on the opposite side from which the endoscope will be passed.
- Flexion of the neck aids in passing the endoscope into the esophagus.

18.4.2 General Anesthesia Esophagoscopy and Gastroscopy

- To perform endoscopy under general anesthesia it is best to place the horse in right lateral recumbency so that the stomach is up.

- Care must be taken not to over-insufflate the stomach as this could result in air escaping into the small and large intestine, resulting in bloating and abdominal pain during recovery.

18.5 Procedure: Gastroscopy and Esophagoscopy

Technical action	Rationale/amplification
Feed should be withheld for 12–14 hours and water for 4 hours, and the horse properly restrained and sedated. The tip of the endoscope is coated with sterile water-soluble lubricant and passed into the nostril. The lubricant should not be placed over the lens as it may obscure the view.	Withholding feed and water decreases the amount of feed and fluid present in the stomach so that the mucosa can be better visualized. Lubrication of the endoscope aids in reducing irritation to the nasal mucosa and facilitates passage of the endoscope.
Using the index finger placed dorsally on the endoscope, the endoscope is directed into the ventral portion of the middle meatus of the nasal cavity and directed caudally approximately 20 cm to view the nasopharynx. The orientation can be confirmed by viewing the dorsal pharyngeal recess at the 12 o'clock position, the two guttural pouch openings at 10 and 2 o'clock, and the tongue-shaped epiglottis at 6 o'clock (Figure 18.6).	If necessary, the scope should be rotated clockwise or counterclockwise to the correct orientation.
The endoscope is directed dorsally to the arytenoids cartilages. Once the endoscope reaches the rima glottis, air and water can be released from the end of the scope to stimulate swallowing. Once the horse swallows, the endoscope is directed into esophagus. Every effort must be made to determine that the endoscope is in the esophagus and not in the oral cavity.	If the endoscope enters the oral cavity it may be damaged. The use of a mouth gag will prevent the horse from chewing the endoscope, if it accidentally ends up in the oral cavity.
To ensure entry and smooth passage into the esophagus, air can be injected to distended the esophagus and facilitate advancing the endoscope (Figure 18.7).	
On accidental entry into the trachea, the tracheal rings will be observed and the structure will maintain its lumen without the need for distention. In this instance reverse the endoscope back into the nasopharynx and repeat the procedure above.	Entry into the trachea may cause coughing and distress the animal. Improper passage of the endoscope may also result in retroflexion of the tip of the endoscope into the oral cavity. In this case the endoscope should be withdrawn immediately as damage to the endoscope may occur.
Alternative option: A guide tube can be inserted into the nares as one would pass a nasogastric tube and pass it into the proximal esophagus. The gastroscope can then be inserted through the guide tube into the esophagus. The gastroscope should be well lubricated to assist in the passage.	The guide tube is used to ensure the safety of the endoscope. Because the long flexible scope is less stiff, it can bend in an S shape and become positioned under the soft palate, in the oral cavity. If not recognized, severe damaged is likely to occur as the horse bites the scope. The guide is also useful when used to relieve an esophageal obstruction because the scope can be passed through the guide tube multiple times without the concern of having the horse swallow repetitively. This improves patient cooperation.

(continued)

Technical action	Rationale/amplification
Once entry into the esophagus has been confirmed, the esophagus can be dilated by depressing the air feed button on the endoscope handle to facilitate passing the endoscope quickly. At approximately 180 cm, resistance due to the lower esophageal sphincter will be encountered.	By distending the esophagus, the endoscope is passed more easily and quickly. Evaluation of the esophagus mucosa is better done while exiting the esophagus, after the gastroscopy has been completed.
Gentle manipulation of the endoscope will allow entrance into the stomach. Once in the stomach, a small air compressor can be attached to the biopsy channel to insufflate the stomach for better visualization. Proper distension is achieved when the ruggae have disappeared.	Air insufflation expands the stomach and flattens out the folds and ruggae, allowing a better examination of the mucosal surfaces.
A water pump or 60 ml syringe can be attached to the biopsy channel and water can be flushed to remove adherent food and mucus from the mucosal surfaces (Figure 18.8). Initially, the saccus cecus (proventricular region) and greater curvature can be viewed from one position just inside the lower esophageal sphincter. The saccus cecus rarely contains gastric ulcers but should be viewed to determine the orientation of the endoscope.	Withholding feed from the horse for 12–14 hours prior to the endoscopy procedure ensures an empty stomach, but adherent food material, mucus, and debris may be on the mucosal surface of the stomach, which may obscure ulcers or other lesions.
The greater curvature (Figure 18.9) is viewed just ventrally to the saccus cecus and contains white nonglandular mucosa dorsally and pink glandular mucosa ventrally, separated by a cuticular ridge or margo plicatus.	The margo plicatus area should be closely inspected, as this region typically contains gastric ulcers (Figure 18.10).
Once the greater curvature has been examined the endoscope may be passed along the margo plicatus until it is retroflexed and can be viewed entering the stomach from the esophagus. The lesser curvature can then be examined (Figure 18.11).	The lesser curvature region should be viewed closely as gastric ulcers are frequently seen in this area (Figure 18.12).
Once the lesser curvature has been viewed the endoscope can be advanced ventral to the lesser curvature, into the pyloric antrum. Here the pylorus can be visualized (Figure 18.13).	The pyloric antrum is positioned ventral to the lesser curvature, such that retroflexion of the endoscope is required to visualize this structure as well as the lesser curvature between them.
The endoscope can be guided through the pyloric opening and the proximal duodenum viewed for duodenal ulcers.	
Prior to removing the endoscope, a suction pump attached to the endoscope biopsy channel can be used to remove air from the stomach.	Leaving the stomach distended may cause discomfort and result in post-gastroscopy abdominal pain or colic.
On exiting the stomach, the endoscope should be removed slowly so that the esophageal mucosa can be examined for hyperemia and ulceration.	The esophagus is most easily assessed for ulceration or other damage as the endoscope is being removed. In the case of esophageal obstruction, this would be encountered on introduction and passage of the endoscope into the esophagus.

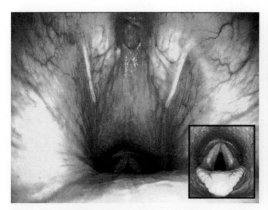

Figure 18.6 View of the nasopharynx showing the tongue-shaped epiglottis, arytenoids cartilages, and the openings to the guttural pouches.

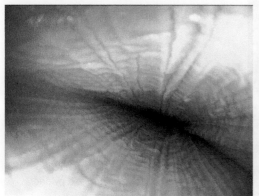

Figure 18.7 The esophagus is distended with air during passage of the endoscope.

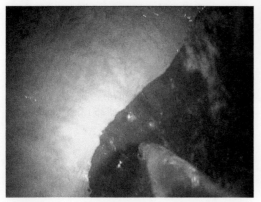

Figure 18.8 Water being flushed through the biopsy channel to wash off excess debris.

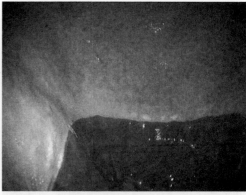

Figure 18.9 The tip of the endoscope is just inside the lower esophageal opening and the greater curvature is in view. The smooth white mucosa is the non-glandular, or squamous, portion of the stomach, and the pink mucosa ventrally is the glandular region of the stomach. The delineation between the two is the cuticular ridge or margo plicatus.

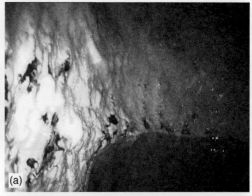

(a)

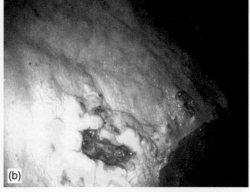

(b)

Figure 18.10 The area where gastric ulcers are commonly seen. (a) Multiple ulcerations of the squamous mucosa along the greater curvature at the level of the margo plicatus. (b) A closer view of a large ulceration of the squamous mucosa along the greater curvature at the level of the margo plicatus.

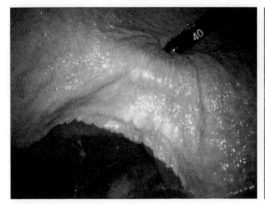

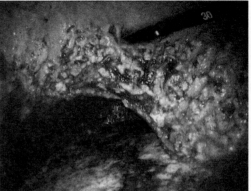

Figure 18.11 Lesser curvature of the stomach. Note the endoscope entering the stomach at the 12 o'clock position.

Figure 18.12 Multifocal severe gastric ulceration on the nonglandular mucosa at the margo plicatus on the lesser curvature of the stomach.

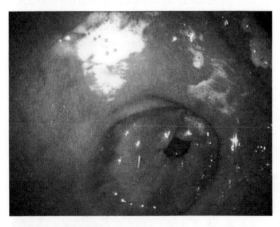

Figure 18.13 The pyloric antrum and pyloric opening.

Bibliography and Further Reading

Bell, R.J.W., Mogg, T.D., and Kingston, J.K. (2007) Equine gastric ulcer syndrome in adult horses: a review. *New Zealand Veterinary Journal*, **55** (1), 1–12.

Davis, J.L. and Jones, S.L. (2004) Examination for disorders of the gastrointestinal tract, in *Equine Internal Medicine*, 2nd edn (eds S.M.Reed, W.M.Bayly, and D.C.Sellon),Saunders Elsevier, St Louis, pp. 769–780.

Sanchez, L.C.(2004) Diseases of the stomach, in *Equine Internal Medicine*, 2nd edn (eds S.M. Reed, W.M. Bayly, and D.C.Sellon), Saunders Elsevier, St Louis, pp. 863–873.

Videla, R. and Andrews, F.M. (2009) New perspectives in equine gastric ulcer syndrome. *Veterinary Clinics of North America Equine Practice*, **25** (2), 283–301.

Part III
Clinical Procedures by Body Systems: Respiratory System

19

Percutaneous Sinocentesis

Mustajab H. Mirza, Jill R. Johnson, and Lais R.R. Costa

19.1 Purpose

- As a diagnostic procedure to collect fluid from the paranasal sinus for cytologic evaluation, culture, and sensitivity.
- As a therapeutic procedure to perform lavage of the paranasal sinus.
- The most common indications for performing paranasal sinocentesis include primary sinusitis, secondary sinusitis associated with periapical infections, and sinus cysts.
- To access the maxillary and conchofrontal sinuses percutaneously (Figures 19.1– 19.4 and Table 19.1)

19.2 Complications

- Epistaxis and hemorrhage
- Wound infection/cellulitis
- Subcutaneous emphysema
- Periapical infections secondary to damage to the apices of the premolar and molar teeth
- Pneumocephalus (very rare potential complication)

19.3 Equipment Required

- Clippers with #40 blade.
- Surgical scrub (gauze soaked in antiseptic solution and gauze soaked in 70% alcohol).
- Local anesthetic (e.g., 2% lidocaine or 2% mepivacaine).
- 25-gauge hypodermic needle.
- 6–12 ml sterile syringe.

- Sterile gloves of appropriate size
- Jacobs chuck
- Steinmann pins and pin guard
- #10 or #15 scalpel blade

For aspiration

- 18-gauge 1″ hypodermic needle
- 20, 35 or 60 ml luer slip sterile syringe

For lavage

- 16- or 14-gauge short (2-3″) intravenous catheter, for example:
  - Angiocath™ 16-gauge, 2 or 3″ (gray)
  - Angiocath™ 14-gauge, 2 or 3″ (orange)
- 20 Fr Foley catheter and 2-0 nylon suture
- Sterile fluid solution for lavage (e.g., 0.9% saline solution) warmed to body temperature
- Fluid administration set or 60 ml syringes
- Three-way stopcock valves (optional)

19.4 Restraint and Positioning

- Sinocentesis is performed with the animal in a standing position, preferably restrained in stocks.
- The veterinarian and handlers should try to position themselves to the side of the animal, not directly in front of the animal.
- Chemical restraint should be administered; a combination of alpha-2 agonist (e.g., xylazine or detomidine) and an opioid agonist-antagonist (e.g., butorphanol) is recommended. See Chapter 9.

Manual of Clinical Procedures in the Horse, First Edition. Edited by Lais R.R. Costa and Mary Rose Paradis.
© 2018 John Wiley & Sons, Inc. Published 2018 by John Wiley & Sons, Inc.

Table 19.1 Relevant features of the seven pairs of paranal sinuses

Accessibility	Sinuses	Features	Anatomical location
Direct percutaneous sinocentesis	Caudal maxillary	In horses under 6 years of age, the crown of the maxillary cheek teeth fill a significant portion of the maxillary sinuses	Landmarks for the maxillary sinus are depicted in Figure 19.1.
	Rostral maxillary	The bony septum separating the caudal maxillary sinus from the rostral maxillary sinus may vary in location	
	Frontal	The frontal sinus communicates with the caudal maxillary sinus	Landmarks for the conchofrontal sinus are depicted in Figure 19.2.
Indirect access through the frontal sinus	Dorsal conchal	The frontal sinus and the dorsal conchal sinus communicate, forming the conchofrontal sinus	
Indirect access through the rostral maxillary sinus	Ventral conchal	Communicates with the rostral maxillary sinus through the conchomaxillary aperture	
No percutaneous access	Sphenopalatine	Communicates with the caudal maxillary sinus	

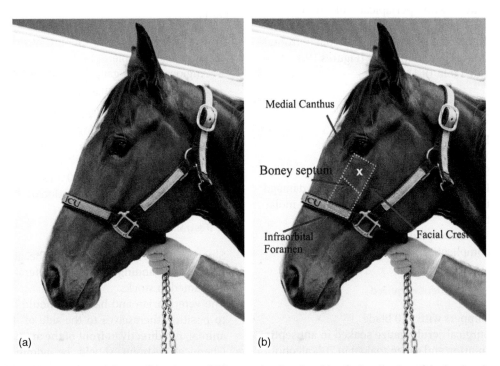

(a) (b)

Figure 19.1 Location of the maxillary sinuses. (a) Appropriate head position for localization of the landmarks. (b) Draw a box extending from the medial canthus of the eye to the infraorbital foramen (digitally palpable) ventrally to the facial crest and then caudally along the facial crest, then dorsally at the level of the medial canthus of the eye. The irregular boney septum is located approximately midway in the sinus (dotted line dividing the box). The X marks the site of entry into the caudal compartment of the maxillary sinus.

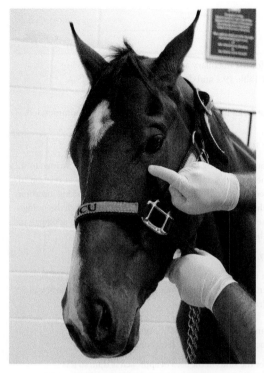

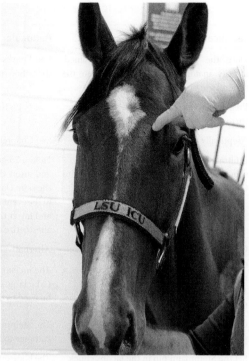

Figure 19.2 Point for sinocentesis of the caudal compartment of the maxillary sinus.

Figure 19.4 Point for sinocentesis of the conchofrontal sinus.

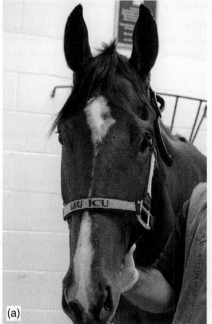

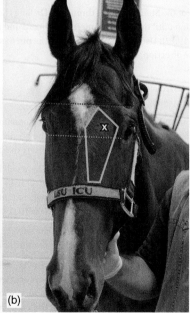

(a)

(b)

Figure 19.3 Location of conchofrontal sinuses. (a) Appropriate head position for localization of the landmarks. (b) Draw a box starting near the midline at level of the middle of the zygomatic arches extending to a point just above the medial canthus of the eye, then down to a rostral line drawn between the midline to the infraorbital foramen (digitally palpable as a nasomaxillary notch), and back up over the midline.

19.5 Procedure: Sinocentesis of the Maxillary and Frontal Sinuses

Technical action	Rationale
Once the patient is properly restrained, identify anatomical landmarks to locate the surgical site by palpating the facial crest.	Landmarks for the maxillary and conchofrontal sinuses are described in Table 19.1 and depicted in Figures 19.1–19.4.
Prepare the site by clipping an area 6 × 6 cm surrounding the chosen site (Figure 19.5).	Although the facial hair is often thin, clipping is still recommended.
Aseptically prepare the site (Figure 19.6).	See Chapter 10.
Infiltrate 3–5 ml of local anesthetic subcutaneously centered on the chosen site (Figure 19.7).	Hold a 25-gauge needle by the hub without attaching the syringe to it, and insert the needle at approximately a 30-degree angle in relation to the skin. Direct the tip of the needle away from the eye during insertion in the event the horse moves in response to the needle. Attach the syringe and inject the local anesthetic. Subcutaneous anesthesia is adequate to anesthetize the skin and periostium.
Confirm that the local anesthesia has taken effect by pricking the skin with a sterile needle. Using a #15 scalpel blade (Figure 19.8) make a stab incision through the skin to the depth of the bone (Figure 19.9).	Alternatively, a #10 blade might be used. The incision needs to be the full thickness of the skin and it needs to be large enough to accommodate the Steinmann pin, which will be used to drill through the bone.
Choose the appropriate size of Steinmann pin (Figure 19.10).	The Steinmann pin must be slightly larger than the needle or catheter to be used to penetrate the sinus.
Set the Steinmann pin in the Jacobs chuck with ½″ (1.5 cm) exposed (Figure 19.11a).	The bone over the sinus in the area of approach is thin, so it is unnecessary to leave more than ½″ (1.5 cm) of the pin exposed. Limiting the pin exposure will prevent damage to deeper structures once the sinus is entered. If the pin extends out the back of chuck, install a pin guard to avoid stabbing yourself (Figure 19.11b).
Insert the tip of the Steinmann pin through the stab incision until the tip encounters bone (Figure 19.12). Using firm rotating motion in one direction, drill through bone into the sinus.	Drilling the pin will feel like drilling the pin into a thin wooden board and requires moderate force. Once through the bone, expect the pin to suddenly fall into the sinus up to the hub of the chuck.
Once in the sinus, rotate the pin several times to establish the opening in the bone.	
Remove the pin and insert a hypodermic needle or catheter into the sinus, following the path created by the pin.	The opening in the bone may be surprisingly difficult to locate with the needle or catheter. Try to recreate the angle that was used to insert the pin.
Attach the syringe and aspirate a sample of sinus contents, if appropriate.	There will be no fluid in a normal sinus cavity. If retrieval of fluid is difficult, 20–30 ml of warmed sterile physiologic solution can be injected into the cavity and then aspirated to yield sample collection (Figure 19.13).
If a lavage is to be performed, attach the fluid administration set or 60 ml syringe to the catheter or needle and instill warmed sterile physiologic solution into sinus. The fluid from the sinus will drain into the nasal cavity and be voided from the nares.	Intuitively, pre-warming the fluid used for lavage will be more comfortable for the patient. If an indwelling catheter is to be placed for serial lavages, insert the 20 Fr Foley catheter through the opening. You may need to use a small forceps at the end of the Foley catheter to push it into the opening. The cuff of the catheter needs to be inflated with 5 ml of sterile water or saline. The conchofrontal sinus may take at least a volume of 120 ml of fluid before the fluid exits from the nares. The caudal maxillary sinus requires a minimal of 50 ml of fluid before the fluid exits from nares. The rostral maxillary sinus requires a minimal of 35 ml volume to recover fluid from nares.

Technical action	Rationale
Remove the needle or catheter from the sinus after completing the sample collection or lavage.	If subsequent lavages are indicated, the indwelling Foley catheter should be sutured using the nylon suture in a purse-string and chinese finger trap technique (Figure 19.14). The end portion of the Foley catheter needs to be attached to the horse; this can be done by taping the Foley to the forelock, or placing a duct tape butterfly to the distal third of the Foley catheter and suturing it to the forehead. The end of the Foley catheter can be plugged with a syringe plunger or covered with a glove finger to prevent contamination.
Placing a skin suture after removal of the catheter is optional.	The size of the incision determines whether a suture is necessary.

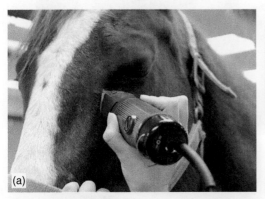

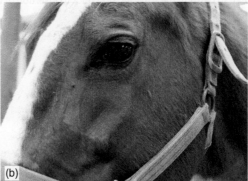

Figure 19.5 Preparation of the site. (a) Clipping the hair on the chosen site. (b) 6 × 6 cm clipped area.

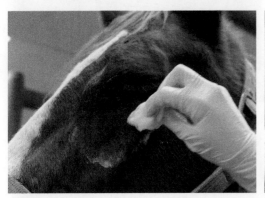

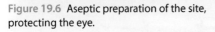

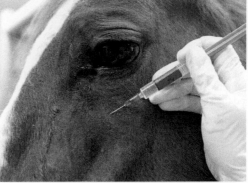

Figure 19.6 Aseptic preparation of the site, protecting the eye.

Figure 19.7 Infiltration of 3–5 ml of local anesthetic subcutaneously at the chosen site. Introduce needle pointing away from the eye. May introduce the needle by itself first, then attach the syringe.

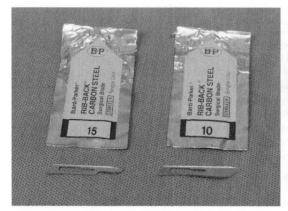

Figure 19.8 The two sizes of scalpel blades that can be used to perform the small incision prior to insertion of the Steinmann pin.

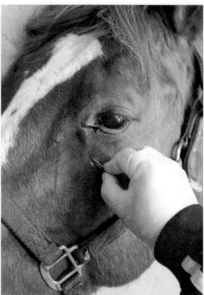

Figure 19.9 Make the stab incision large enough to allow insertion of the Steinmann pin.

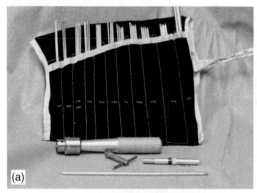

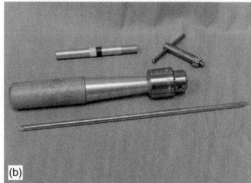

Figure 19.10 Jacobs chuck and a set of Steinmann pins of various sizes, ranging from 0.035" to 0.25" in diameter. (b) Materials required for this procedure: Jacobs chuck, Steinmann pin of appropriate size, pin guard and the key to tighten the Jacobs chuck.

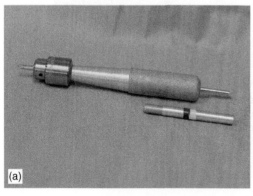

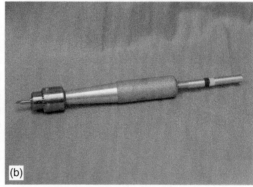

Figure 19.11 Steinmann pin inserted into the Jacobs chuck. (a) ½" of the pin is exposed. (b) A pin guard installed to protect the exposed end of the pin.

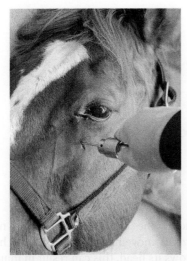

Figure 19.12 Positioning the Steinmann pin through the stab incision.

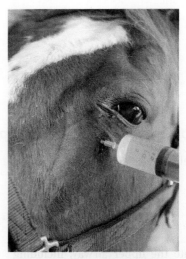

Figure 19.13 Injection of warmed sterile physiologic solution to flush the sinus cavity to obtain a sample for evaluation.

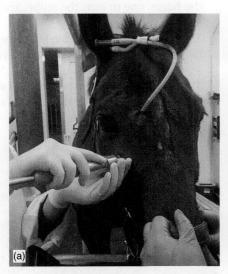

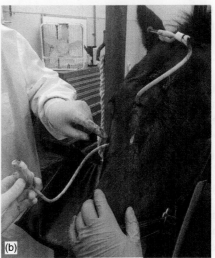

Figure 19.14 Indwelling catheter placement into the sinus for serial lavages: (a) A Foley catheter (20 Fr) is placed into the right conchofrontal sinus (note the chinese finger trap suture holding the Foley catheter in place, the end of the Foley catheter is plugged with a syringe plunger, and the catheter is attached to the horse's forelock), while a Jacobs chuck is used to drive a Steinmann pin into the right maxillary sinus. (b) A 20 Fr Foley catheter is inserted through the opening into the maxillary sinus, subsequently the cuff of the Foley catheter will need to be inflated with 5 ml of sterile water.

Bibliography and Further Reading

Barakzai, S. (2008) Standing sinus surgery in the horse: Indications, techniques and complications. *In Practice*, **30** (5), 252–262.

Mair, T. (2010) Examination of the paranasal sinuses, in *Diagnostic Techniques in Equine Medicine* (eds F.G.Taylor, T.J.Brazil, and M.H.Hillyer), Saunders Elsevier, Edinburgh, pp. 222–228.

Schumacher, J. and Moll, H.D. (2006) Sinocentesis, in *Manual of Equine Diagnostic Procedures*, Teton New Media, Jackson, pp. 51–56.

Stephen, J. (2008) Sinocentesis, in *The Equine Hospital Manual* (eds K.Corley and J.Stephen), Blackwell, Oxford, pp. 77–78.

20

Endoscopic Examination of the Upper Respiratory Tract

Colin Mitchell

20.1 Purpose

- To evaluate the upper airway, including nasal passages, nasal septum, ethmoturbinates, nasomaxillary opening, pharynx, guttural pouches (aka auditory tube diverticulum), larynx, and palate, for structural and functional abnormalities.

20.2 Complications

- Epistaxis (usually self-limiting).
- Failure to visualize all structures due to patient's lack of compliance or the presence of lesion obstructing or impairing complete examination.

20.3 Equipment Required

- Flexible endoscope (1 m) with biopsy channel.
- Water-soluble lubricant to aid passing the scope through the nasal passages.
- Light source (usually halogen source).
- Video monitor or eyepiece for viewing images.
- Biopsy or grasping instruments.
- Chambers mare catheter.
- Specialized catheters for aspirating, injections or providing constant drainage.

20.4 Restraint and Positioning

- As a minimum, a twitch should be applied to the horse's upper lip (Figure 20.1).
- Sedation is contraindicated until laryngeal and palatal function has been evaluated.

- Placing the horse in stocks will minimize its movement, although if the horse throws its head, this can result in injury.
- A minimum of three people is necessary to perform this procedure: one to handle the horse, one to pass the scope, and one to drive the scope.
- The handler should hold the lead rope and twitch on the side of the horse that the endoscope is not being passed up (Figure 20.1).
- The person passing the scope should stand slightly off to the side of the horse to avoid being injured if the horse strikes.

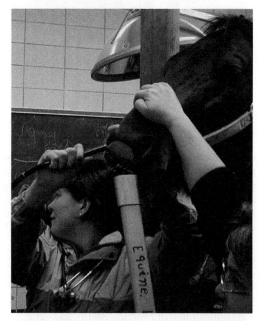

Figure 20.1 Horse restrained using a twitch applied to its nose for endoscopy. The scope is being passed up the right nasal passage and the handler has the lead rope and twitch on the left side.

Manual of Clinical Procedures in the Horse, First Edition. Edited by Lais R.R. Costa and Mary Rose Paradis.
© 2018 John Wiley & Sons, Inc. Published 2018 by John Wiley & Sons, Inc.

20.5 Procedure: Rhinolaryngoscopy

Technical action	Rationale
The endoscope should be held correctly, with the handpiece balanced between the thumb and first finger of the left hand. This leaves the other fingers of the left hand free to use the suction and air/flush valves. The right hand is used to control the angulation knobs and direct the scope (Figure 20.2).	Sedation should not be administered prior to evaluation of laryngeal and palatal function. Using the endoscope appropriately will allow diagnostic examinations to be consistently performed.
When placing the endoscope, the passer must elevate the nasal cartilage and direct the scope towards the nasal septum and ventral meatus. The non-dominant hand is placed over the muzzle and the thumb is used to keep the scope medial and ventral, while the dominant hand advances the scope (Figure 20.3).	The ventral meatus is wide and the scope can usually be passed up without traumatizing the nasal passageways (Figure 20.4). Care should be taken to direct the scope below and away from the ethmoturbinates.
The scope should be advanced into the nasopharynx, ensuring that it passes ventrally to the ethmoturbinates. During the passage of the endoscope into the nasopharynx, the nasal passages and the ethmoids may be evaluated (Figure 20.5). When the scope reaches the nasopharynx, all the structures should be identified (Figure 20.6) and anatomical abnormalities should be recorded (Figure 20.7).	Knowledge of the normal anatomy of the nasopharynx is critical during endoscopic evaluation of the upper respiratory tract.

(continued)

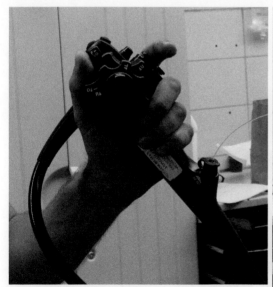

Figure 20.2 The endoscope is held firmly in the left hand in such a way that the index or middle finger can be used to activate the flush or suction buttons on the endoscope. The right hand can be used to direct the scope or advance the laser fiber placed through the biopsy channel.

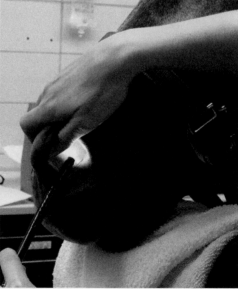

Figure 20.3 The nasal cartilage is elevated with one hand and the scope is introduced into the ventral meatus. If necessary, the thumb of the right hand (as depicted in this picture) can be used as a guide to direct the scope towards the ventral meatus.

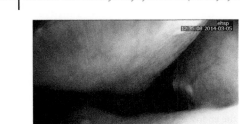

Figure 20.4 Endoscopic view of the ventral meatus during passage of the endoscope into the nasal passages.

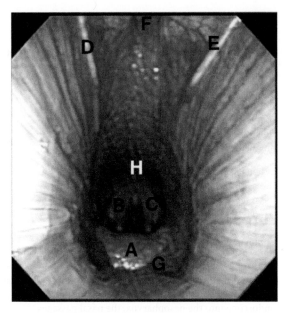

Figure 20.6 Once the endoscope reaches the nasopharynx, the structures of the larynx and pharynx should be identified: A, epiglottis (which should rest over the soft palate; B and C, corniculate processes of the arytenoid cartilages; D and E, the openings of the guttural pouches; F, dorsal pharyngeal recess; G, soft palate; H, palatopharyngeal arch.

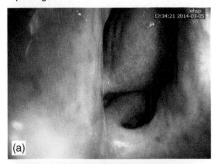

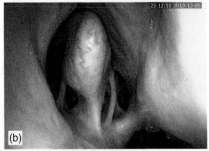

Figure 20.5 Endoscopic view of the ethmoids during passage of the endoscope: (a) normal ethmoidturbinates and (b) view of the ethmoid crypt.

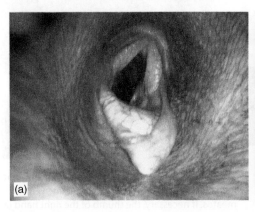

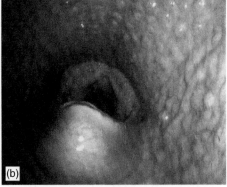

Figure 20.7 Endoscopic evaluation of the nasopharynx should first identify abnormalities of the structures of the larynx and pharynx: (a) epiglottic entrapment, (b) large epiglottic entrapment (note the pharyngeal lymphoid hyperplasia), (c) epiglottis not visible because of dorsal displacement of the soft palate, and (d) paralysis of the right arytenoid in a case of fourth brachial arch defect.

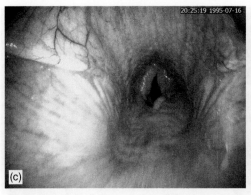
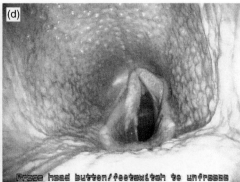

Figure 20.7 *(Continued)*

Technical action	Rationale
The laryngeal and palatal function should be evaluated, and all abnormalities should be recorded:	Knowledge of the normal laryngeal and palatal functions is very important.
• Evaluation of laryngeal function - after occlusion of the nostrils and after flushing water through the endoscope, which induces swallowing: – evaluate the laryngeal abductor and adductor movement - the first breath should display full abduction of both arytenoid cartilages (Figure 20.8a–c; Table 20.1)	Table 20.1 depicts the grading for laryngeal function. Once laryngeal and palatal functions have been evaluated, the remainder of the upper airway can be examined, using sedation if necessary.
• Evaluation of palatal function – the epiglottis may temporarily "disappear" as the soft palate is displaced dorsally (Figure 20.8d). The soft palate and epiglottis should be replaced to their normal position after swallowing.	Evaluate lymphoid tissue and note if lymphoid hyperplasia is present (Figure 20.7b).

Table 20.1 Grading system for laryngeal function

Grade	Description
1	Synchronous full abduction and adduction of the left and right arytenoid cartilages, which can be provoked by occlusion of the nostrils. Full abduction occurs during exercise.
2	Asynchronous movement (hesitation, flutter, abductor weakness) of the left arytenoid cartilage. Full abduction left arytenoid cartilage can be provoked by occlusion of the nostrils. Full abduction occurs during exercise.
3	Asynchronous movement (hesitation, flutter, abductor weakness) of the left arytenoid cartilage during any phase of breathing. Full abduction cannot be provoked with occlusion of the nostrils. During exercise full abduction of the arytenoid cartilages may occur, but these horses might undergo dynamic collapse of the arytenoid cartilage.
4	Marked asymmetry of the larynx at rest without significant movement of the left arytenoid cartilage during any phase of breathing. Full abduction cannot be provoked with occlusion of the nostrils. During exercise, these horses undergo dynamic collapse of the arytenoid cartilage.

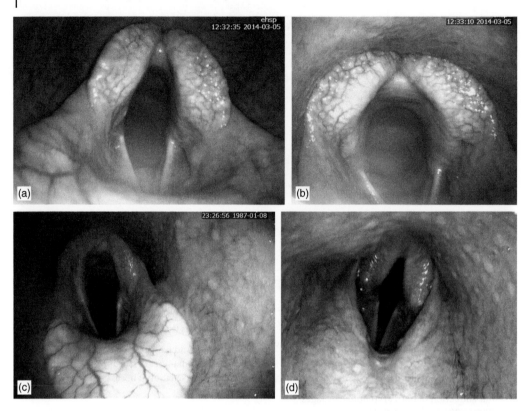

Figure 20.8 With the endoscope in the nasopharynx, the laryngeal and pharyngeal functions should be evaluated: (a) arytenoid cartilages are resting (aka relaxed position of the arytenoids), (b) on occlusion of the nostrils both arytenoid cartilages are abducted (note the symmetry of the right and left arytenoids), (c) on occlusion of the nostrils, only the right arytenoid cartilage is fully abducted, whereas the left arytenoid cartilage remains "relaxed" (case of idiopathic laryngeal hemiplegia), and (d) on occlusion of the nostrils, the epiglottis is no longer resting on the soft palate in a case of dorsal displacement of the soft palate.

Technical action	Rationale
Accessing the guttural pouches requires opening of the pharyngeal orifice prior to scope placement. This can be achieved using a biopsy instrument through the endoscope biopsy channel or a Chambers mare catheter placed up the contralateral nasal passageway (Figure 20.9; see Chapter 24).	If a biopsy instrument is used, it is vital that it remains closed, as there are vital structures within the guttural pouch that it could potentially damage as it is inserted blindly into the pouch to act as a guide for the scope to be advanced over. The Chambers mare catheter is safer as it is used to open the orifice to allow the scope to be advanced into the pouch, but its placement in the contralateral nasal passageway is often poorly tolerated.
Once the endoscope has entered the guttural pouch, the biopsy instrument is retracted and the pouch is evaluated in its entirety (see Chapter 24).	Evaluation of the contralateral guttural pouch may require the scope to be passed into the opposite nasal passage.
The ethmoturbinates, nasal maxillary opening, nasal septum, conchae, and meati can be evaluated as the scope is being withdrawn. It is important to evaluate the contralateral nasal passageway as unilateral abnormalities are common.	Advancing the scope outside of the ventral meatus can result in iatrogenic trauma, which can be mistaken for real pathology. The other structures can be evaluated by directing the scope as it is withdrawn without creating significant trauma.

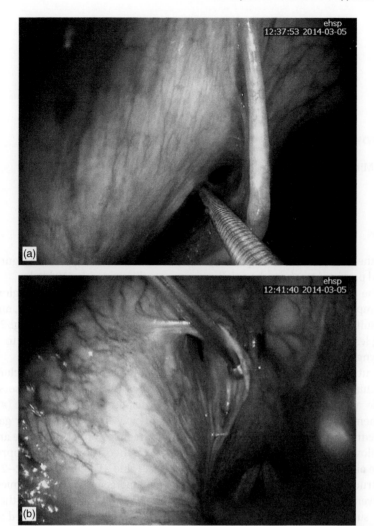

Figure 20.9 Access to the guttural pouches is gained by opening of the pharyngeal orifice prior to scope placement (a) by using a biopsy instrument through the endoscope biopsy channel or (b) by placing a Chambers mare catheter up the contralateral nasal passageway.

Bibliography and Further Reading

Freeman, D.E. and Hardy, J. (2007) Guttural pouch, in *Equine Infectious Diseases* (eds D.C.Sellon and M.T.Long), Saunders Elsevier, St. Louis, pp. 13–20.

Hardy, J. and Léveillé, R. (2003) Diseases of the guttural pouches. *Veterinary Clinics of North America Equine*, **19**, 123–158.

McGorum, B.C., Dixon, P.M., Robinson, N.E., and Schumacher, J. (2007) *Equine Respiratory Medicine and Surgery*, W.B. Saunders, Philadelphia.

McKenzie, H. (2008) Endoscopy of the guttural pouch, in *The Equine Hospital Manual* (eds K.Corley and J.Stephen), Blackwell Publishing, pp. 66–68.

Slovis, N.M. (2004) *Atlas of Equine Endoscopy*, Mosby, St Louis.

Rose, R.J. and Hodgson, D.R. (2000) Respiratory system, in *Manual of Equine Practice*, 2nd edn, W.B. Saunders, Philadelphia.

Stephen, J. (2008) Endoscopy of the respiratory tract, in *The Equine Hospital Manual* (eds K.Corley and J.Stephen), Blackwell Publishing, pp. 65–66.

21

Tracheostomy

Mustajab H. Mirza, Jill R. Johnson, and Lais R.R. Costa

21.1 Purpose

- To bypass the nasal passages, nasopharynx, larynx, and proximal trachea when airflow through the upper airway is partially or almost completely impaired due to conditions resulting in obstruction or space-occupying lesions (e.g., nasal obstruction, retropharyngeal lymphoadenopathy and cellulitis, guttural pouch empyema), congenital occlusion (e.g., choanal atresia).
- To provide airflow in an emergency situation when an immediate, potentially life-threatening impairment of the upper airway airflow is present.
- To provide airflow in an elective situation when obstruction is anticipated after surgical intervention (e.g., post nasal septum resection surgery or pharyngeal mass removal) or to bypass oral and nasal cavities in order to perform oral, mandibular or maxillary surgery.

21.2 Complications

- Local wound infection
- Subcutaneous emphysema
- Tracheal strictures
- Mediastinitis
- Pneumonia
- Necrosis of the tracheal mucosa due to compression by the inflated cuff.

21.3 Equipment Required

- Elective tracheostomies (Figure 21.1):
  - clippers with #40 blade
  - examination and sterile gloves
  - antiseptic scrub, alcohol, and gauze
  - local anesthetic agents (e.g., 2% lidocaine)
  - needles and syringes to administer local anesthetic
  - minor surgical pack, including scalpel for #10 or #20 blade, scissors, hemostats
  - disposable surgical blade (#10 or #20)
  - heavy suture material or gauze to affix tracheostomy tube to the animal
  - tracheostomy tube of appropriate size (Table 21.1, Figures 21.2–21.4).
- In emergency tracheostomies speed is imperative to save the life of the patient and minimal equipment is needed to establish a patent airway. Clipping the hair and infusing local anesthetic agent may not be an option in an effort to save the life of the patient. Essential materials required include:
  - minor surgical pack, including scalpel handle for blade sizes #10 and #20, scissors, hemostats
  - disposable surgical blades (#10 and #20)
  - heavy suture material, umbilical tape or gauze to affix tracheostomy tube to the animal (if not using a self-retaining tracheostomy tube)
  - tracheostomy tube of appropriate size

Manual of Clinical Procedures in the Horse, First Edition. Edited by Lais R.R. Costa and Mary Rose Paradis.
© 2018 John Wiley & Sons, Inc. Published 2018 by John Wiley & Sons, Inc.

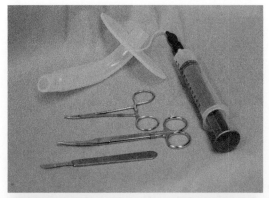

Figure 21.1 Essential supplies for tracheostomy: scalpel with #10 or #20 blade, scissors, hemostats, tracheostomy tube.

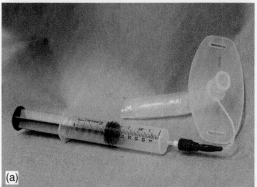

(a)

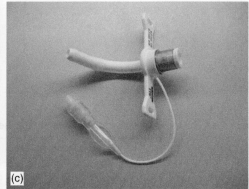

(c)

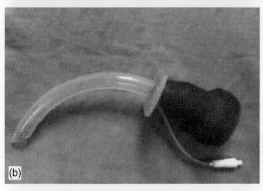

(b)

Figure 21.2 J-type cuffed, silicone tracheostomy tubes: (a) Bivona™ 16 mm ID (no longer commercially available) for use in adult horses, (b) Jorgensen Lab™ 15, 20 or 25 mm ID with funnel adapter, for use in adult horses, and (c) Surgivet™ 5–10 mm ID, for use in miniature horses or foals.

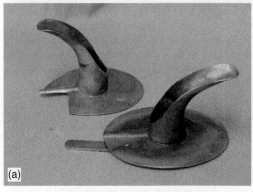

(a)

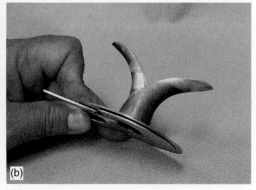

(b)

Figure 21.3 Self-retaining metal tracheostomy tube: (a) the outer part, which has the latch, and the inner part displayed separately, (b) the inner part inserted into the outer part, and (c) the two parts latched together.

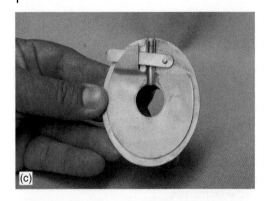

Figure 21.3 (*Continued*)

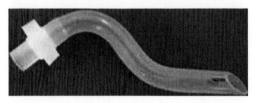

Figure 21.4 Cuffless, fenestrated silicone tracheostomy tubes used in adult horses, Jorgensen Lab™ 12 mm ID.

Table 21.1 Types of tracheostomy tubes commonly used in horses

Name	Description	Placement
J-type	Silicone, with cuff, beveled tip, fenestrated For adult horses, sizes 12–25 mm ID (Figure 21.2a,b)	Easy insertion (Figure 21.9) Secured by umbilical tape from the holes of the tube flange (neck plate) to loop stay sutures in the skin or tethered around the neck with kling gauze tied to the holes on each side of the tube flange
J-type	Silicone, with cuff, unfenestrated, with obturator for placement For foals and miniature horses, sizes 5–10 mm ID (Figure 21.2c)	Easy insertion Obturator is used while the tube is inserted and then removed The tube is secured by tethering around the neck with kling gauze tied to the holes on each side of the tube flange
Metal J-type	Stainless steel, uncuffed, beveled tip, flattened dorsoventrally, fenestrated or unfenestrated	Easy insertion Secured by umbilical tape from the holes on the tube flange to loop stay sutures in the skin or tethering around the neck with kling gauze tied to the holes on each side of the tube flange
Metal self-retaining	Self-retaining or metal interlocking cannulas (Figure 21.3)	Insertion is more cumbersome The outer part with the latch is inserted with its tip pointing toward the lungs, then the inner part is inserted with its tip pointing toward the head After positioning, the latch is closed (Figure 21.10)

Name	Description	Placement
Other, for adult horses	Silicone, cuffless, beveled tip, fenestrated (Figure 21.4)	Somewhat easy insertion and removal Tube is tethered around the neck with kling gauze tied to the holes on each side of the tube flange
Human J-type, disposable	Cuffed or cuffless, fenestrated or unfenestrated with outer and inner cannulas and obturator for placement	May be used in miniature horses and foals Easy insertion and removal Tube is tethered around the neck with kling gauze tied to the holes on each side of the tube flange

21.4   Restraint and Positioning

- Most elective tracheostomies are performed with the animal in a standing position, preferably restrained in stocks.
- The surgeon and handlers should position themselves to the side of the animal, not in front.
- Sedation with an alpha-2 agonist (e.g., xylazine at a dose of 0.5 mg/kg) and an opiod agonist-antagonist (e.g., butorphanol at a dose of 0.04 mg/kg) is recommended. Care should be taken to avoid heavy sedation. For detail, see Chapter 9.
- In life-threatening emergencies, it may not be possible or advisable to sedate the animal and restraint may rely on a handler who holds the head using a halter and lead rope. With the safety of the handler and the surgeon in mind, it is advisable to approach the tracheotomy surgical site from the side of the horse and not from the front, especially if the horse is agitated and unmanageable.

21.5   Procedure: Tracheostomy

Technical action	Rationale
Identify anatomical structures: midline musculature (sternothyrohyoideus muscles) and the tracheal rings. Locate the site by palpating the tracheal rings, where the trachea is most superficial (Figure 21.5).	The tracheostomy is performed to bypass the nasal passages, nasopharynx, larynx, and proximal trachea, therefore the tracheostomy is performed at the junction of the upper and middle third of the neck, just above the junction of the sternothyrohyoideus muscles.
Prepare the site by clipping a 10 × 10 cm area on the ventral side of the neck, in the proximal third of the neck (Figure 21.6).	In a life-threatening emergency one may proceed immediately without clipping the hair.
Wearing examination gloves, aseptically prepare the tracheostomy site.	In a life-threatening emergency, one may proceed immediately without aseptic preparation.
Infiltrate local anesthetic subcutaneously on a line approximately 8 cm in length on the ventral midline over the tracheal rings to be approached.	In a life-threatening emergency when the patient is in respiratory distress speed is essential, so one may proceed immediately without local anesthesia.
Make a midline incision of the skin, subcutaneous tissue, and cutaneous muscles about 8 cm in length with a #10 or #20 scalpel blade (Figure 21.7a). Bluntly dissect the incised area, retracting the sternothyrohyoideus muscles and exposing the tracheal cartilages (Figure 21.7b).	If the procedure is performed in the lower half of the cervical trachea, the trachea will be covered by the sternocephalicus muscles, making it much more difficult to expose the tracheal rings. Figure 21.8 is a schematic representation of the procedure.

(continued)

Technical action	Rationale
Incise the annular ligament between two cartilaginous tracheal rings with a #10 scalpel blade entering the lumen of the trachea (Figure 21.7). The incision is extended laterally to include a quarter to a third of the luminal diameter.	Penetration of the tracheal lumen will result in a gush of air through the incision. The size of the incision in the annular ligament will be dictated by the size of the tracheostomy tube to be used. Generally, the incision should not exceed one-third of the luminal diameter. Remember that the carotid artery is located on either side of the trachea and should be avoided when incising the tracheal ring.
Insert a tube into the tracheal incision, assuring patency of the stoma created by the tracheostomy (Figures 21.9 and 21.10), and check the airflow through the tube.	The placement of the tracheostomy tube will vary with the type of tube used (Table 21.1). Easy-to-insert tubes such as a silicone or metal J-type tubes (silicone or metal) are preferable in emergency situations (Figure 21.9).
Secure the tracheostomy tube in position. This will depend on the type of tube.	The appropriate method of securing the tracheostomy tube will vary with the type of tube used (see Table 21.1). J-type tubes are secured with umbilical tape or heavy suture to loop-sutures placed in the skin on each side of the tracheostomy site. Alternatively, the tube can be secured with gauze run through the flanges on the tube and tied around the neck (Figure 21.11). Self-retaining tubes do not need any additional method for securing them.
When using a cuffed tracheostomy tube, decide if inflation of the cuff is necessary. If the cuff is to be inflated, make sure to use the proper amount of air to avoid over-inflation of the cuff and compression of the tracheal mucosa.	Inflation of the cuff is generally unnecessary, except during volatile general anesthesia or if the animal is to be ventilated. An over-inflated cuff increases the risk of necrosis of the tracheal mucosa.
The tracheostomy tube must be checked for patency regularly and the lumen of tube must be cleaned as often as is necessary, at least twice daily. Manage the surgical site as an open wound. Apply a small amount of petroleum jelly ventral to the incision to decrease skin scaling associated with exudate drainage.	Proper cleaning usually requires removal of the tube from the stoma, except if the tube has an inner cannula (in which case the outer cannula is left in place, keeping the stoma open). Take the tube or inner cannula, clean it thoroughly, and replace it. If the animal immediately becomes dyspneic when the tracheostomy tube is removed and the stoma is left without a tube, a second tube should be available for immediate replacement when the first tube is removed for cleaning.
Remove the tracheostomy tube when normal airflow through the upper airway has been restored.	Evaluation of airflow can be performed by temporary manual occlusion of the tracheostomy site. Following removal of the tube, the animal must be closely monitored and a tube should be left available in case the animal becomes dyspneic and the tube needs to be replaced.
The trachea and skin incision should be allowed to heal by second intention. The wound should be cleaned twice a day.	Exuberant or polypoid masses of granulation tissue may form. They often resolve without treatment.

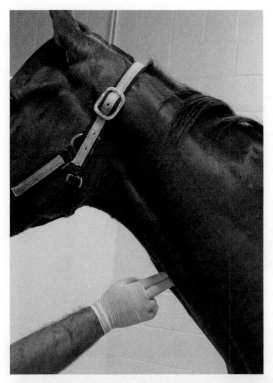

Figure 21.5 Palpating site for tracheostomy.

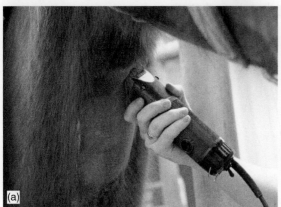

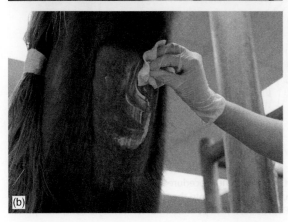

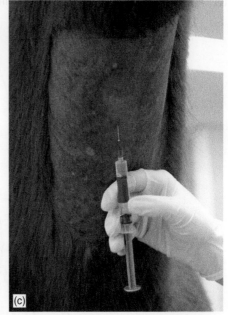

Figure 21.6 Preparing the site for tracheostomy: (a) clipping the hair, (b) performing aseptic surgical scrub, and (c) injecting local anesthetic.

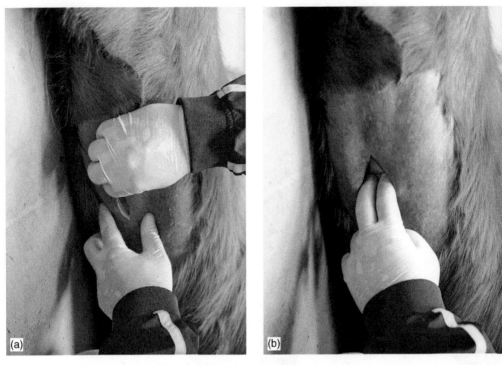

Figure 21.7 Surgical approach: (a) incision of the skin, subcutaneous tissue, and cutaneous colli muscles, and (b) blunt dissection of the sternothyrohyoideus muscles to locate the trachea.

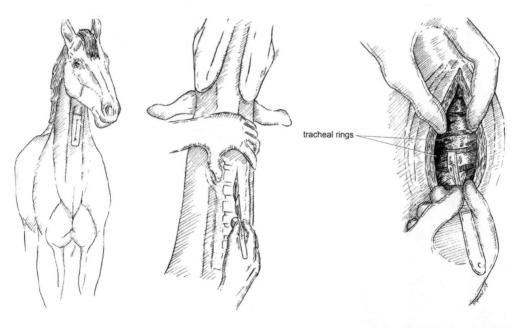

Figure 21.8 Tracheostomy procedure. Schematic of the site for the procedure at the junction of the proximal and mid third of the ventral neck, the incision of the skin, and the incision into the tracheal annular ligament between two tracheal cartilages. Corley and Stephen (2008). Reproduced with permission of John Wiley & Sons, Inc.

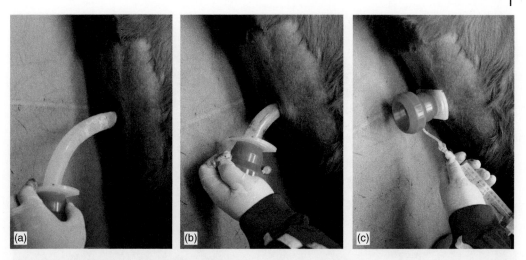

Figure 21.9 (a) Insertion of the J-type silicone tracheostomy tube through the skin, (b) placement of the tube all the way into the trachea, and (c) inflation of the cuff (optional).

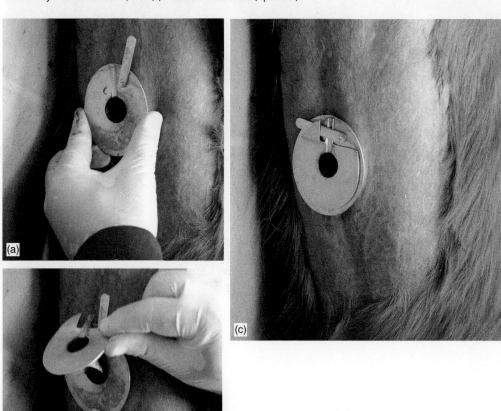

Figure 21.10 Placement of the self-retaining metal tracheostomy tube: (a) insertion of the outer part, which has the latch, pointing the tip of the tube toward the lungs, (b) insertion of the inner part with the tip pointing toward the head, and (c) locking the latch.

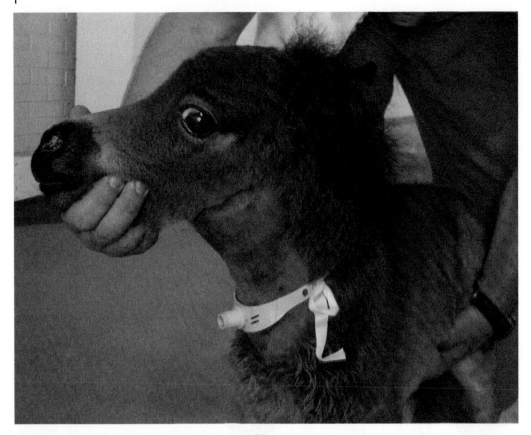

Figure 21.11 Miniature foal wearing a Jorgensen Lab™ silicone tracheostomy tube 6 mm, secured with kling gauze around the neck.

Bibliography and Further Reading

Freeman, D.E. (1991) Trachea, in *Equine Respiratory Disorders* (ed. J. Beech), Lea & Febiger, Philadelphia, pp. 395.

Hardy, J. *Equine emergency procedures in the respiratory tract.* http://www.vet.ohio-state.edu/assets/courses/vm70016/respemergency.pdf.

Stephen, J. (2008) Emergency tracheostomy, in *The Equine Hospital Manual* (eds K. Corley and J. Stephen), Blackwell Publishing, Oxford, pp. 60.

22

Nasopharyngeal Sampling

Lais R.R. Costa and Ashley G. Boyle

22.1 Purpose

- To obtain a swab or wash sample from nasopharyngeal secretions for the purposes of virus isolation, bacterial culture, and/or molecular diagnostics (e.g., immunoassay, nucleic acid detection by PCR) of potential pathogens.
- Nasopharyngeal swabs are often used in horses for detection of equine viral pathogens such as influenza virus, rhinovirus, herpes virus 1 and 4, equine viral arteritis, and adenovirus. Swabs can be used for the retrieval of bacterial pathogens such as *Streptococcus equi* subspecies *equi*.
- Nasopharyngeal lavage in horses is most often used for retrieval of bacterial pathogens such as *S. equi* subspecies *equi*. Lavage covers a large area of the nasopharynx, thus increasing the chance of recovery of the organism, if present. Lavage sample can also be submitted for detection of viral pathogens such as influenza virus, rhinovirus, herpes virus 1 and 4, equine viral arteritis, and adenovirus.
- Sampling of nasopharyngeal secretions is a diagnostic procedure indicated in cases of nasal discharge, cough, and fever, as well as outbreaks of contagious respiratory disease.

22.2 Complications

- Epistaxis (unusual).
- Failure to obtain a sample due to the patient's lack of compliance or the presence of a lesion obstructing or impairing completion of the procedure.

22.3 Equipment Required

- Appropriate protective clothing (including examination gloves, disposable plastic boots, and disposable coveralls).
- For collecting nasopharyngeal swab:
  - gauze
  - examination gloves
  - sterile culture swab (for PCR testing, calcium alginate swabs should be avoided):
    - long shaft: standard cotton or polyester swab (e.g., 8″ or 16″[1]), or protected equine uterine culture swab (e.g., guarded or double guarded culture swab, ranging from 27″ to 33″ in length; if necessary these can be cut to appropriate size)[2], or guarded pharyngeal swab (tube within a tube) kit[3].
  - For performing nasopharyngeal lavage:
    - gauze
    - examination gloves
    - rectal sleeve (not necessary to be sterile)
    - long cannula:
      - sterile uterine pipette or
      - sterile polypropylene catheter (8–10 Fr)
    - 60 ml syringe, filled with 50 ml of sterile isotonic (0.9%) saline.

Manual of Clinical Procedures in the Horse, First Edition. Edited by Lais R.R. Costa and Mary Rose Paradis.
© 2018 John Wiley & Sons, Inc. Published 2018 by John Wiley & Sons, Inc.

– For sample preparation:
  ○ aerobic transport media for bacterial culture: BBL™ CultureSwab™ Collection and Transport System
  ○ viral transport medium: Universal Viral Transport Medium;[4] maybe obtained from diagnostic laboratories upon request.
  ○ three sterile evacuated tubes without additives (red-top vacutainer tubes):
    ○ one with 0.5 ml of sterile saline to keep swab moist, not wet
    ○ one plain to add the wash sample
    ○ one plain for PCR-based diagnostics
  ○ small evacuated tubes with EDTA (purple-top vacutainer tubes, 3 ml, for cytology)
  ○ cold packs and a styrofoam container.

22.4 Restraint and Positioning

- Although the degree of restraint varies depending on the age, demeanor, and training of the horse, in general sampling of the nasopharynx requires moderate sedation.
- In most cases, sedation with an alpha-2 agonist (e.g., xylazine, detomidine, etc.) is effective; combination with butorphanol might be indicated (see Chapter 9).
- Ensure all personnel wear the appropriate protective clothing as generally nasopharyngeal sampling is performed in horses suspected of shedding/harboring highly contagious infectious agents.

22.5 Procedure: Nasopharyngeal Swab

Technical action	Rationale
Following sedation, clean the nostril with gauze.	This will eliminate the chance of gross contamination of the swab.
Remove guard from swab if it exists (Figure 22.1). Measure the distance between the nostril and the eye of the horse to estimate the length of the swab necessary to reach the horse's nasopharynx (Figure 22.2). Make a small mark on the swab handle if desired.	This will help orient how far the swab should be advanced.
Immobilize the head by wrapping the arm under the horse's jaw and placing it over the bridge of the nose. Open the nostril by lifting the false nostril to allow introduction of the swab (Figure 22.3a).	This will give control of the head and allow introduction of the swab into the nostril even if the horse moves. Alternatively, have an assistant immobilize the head to facilitate the introduction of the swab into the nostril (Figure 22.3b).
Introduce the swab into the ventral meatus of the chosen (right or left) nostril.	Advancement into the ventral meatus avoids contact with the ethmoid turbinates.

Technical action	Rationale
Advance the swab into the pharynx, then carefully advance it until there is resistance. Gently rotate the swab in the nasopharynx.	Make sure to allow time for the pharyngeal secretions to soak into the swab.
Remove the swab swiftly, avoiding touching any surfaces.	Place the swab immediately into the appropriate container (see below). Collection of two or more swabs may be necessary.
Prepare the swabs for submission. Check the requirements of the specific laboratory and test prior to collection. Insert the swab into the appropriate tube and break the swab shaft (Figure 22.4): 1. For bacterial culture and molecular detection, place the swab into a bacterial transport medium such as a BBL™ Culture Swab tube. 2. For virus isolation place the swab into an appropriate virus transport medium. 3. For viral detection by molecular detection, immunoassay, etc. place the swab in a red-top tube with or without 0.5 ml of 0.9% sterile saline to keep tip wet immediately after collection (Figure 22.5).	1. Bacterial culture and molecular detection assays are intended to isolate *S. equi* subspecies *equi*. 2. If virus transport medium is not available, the material should be placed in a red-top tube containing 0.5 ml of sterile saline and chilled or rapidly frozen. (Some laboratories will accept dry samples.)
Keep the culture medium at room temperature. Keep remaining samples on ice until ready to ship. Samples should be shipped refrigerated (cold packs) to the appropriate diagnostic laboratory in a styrofoam container as soon as possible.	If it will take longer than 24 hours for the samples to arrive, check with the diagnostic laboratory if they are still acceptable.

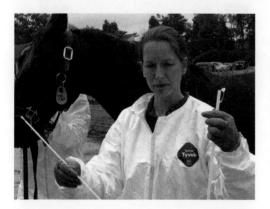

Figure 22.1 Remove guard from swab if it exists.

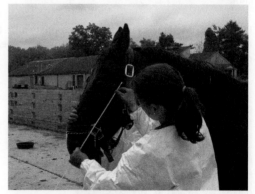

Figure 22.2 Estimate the length of (a) the swab or (b) the catheter necessary to reach the horse's nasopharynx by measuring the distance from the nostril to the eye.

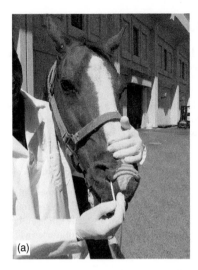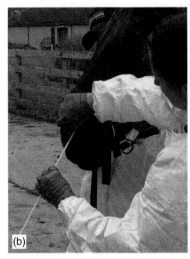

Figure 22.3 Immobilize the head and open nostril to introduce the swab into the ventral meatus of the chosen (right or left) nostril. (a) Place the hand under the jaw and over the bridge of the nose and lift the false nostril. Pusterla et al. (2006). Reproduced with permission of Elsevier. (b) Have an assistant immobilize the head, place a hand over the bridge of the nose, and lift the false nostril to open the nares.

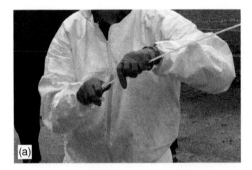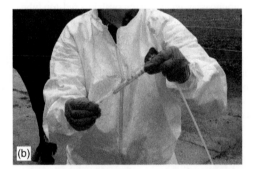

Figure 22.4 Insert the swab into the appropriate tube. (a) Break the swab shaft. (b) If using a tube for bacterial transport medium such as a BBL™ Culture Swab™ tube, squeeze the bottom of the tube to break into the medium compartment.

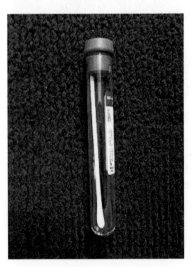

Figure 22.5 Proper sample preparation for viral detection by molecular detection, immunoassay, etc. Place the swab into a red-top tube with or without 0.5 ml of 0.9% sterile saline immediately after collection.

22.6 Procedure: Nasopharyngeal Lavage

Technical action	Rationale
Following sedation, clean the nostril with gauze.	This will eliminate the chance of gross contamination of the sample.
Estimate the length of the catheter or pipette necessary to reach the horse's nasopharynx by measuring the distance between the nostril and the eye of the horse (Figure 22.6a). Make a small mark if desired.	This will guide how far the polypropylene catheter or pipette should be advanced.
Pass the sterile polypropylene catheter (8–10 Fr) or pipette through from the outside to the inside of a rectal palpation sleeve approximately 5″ from the opening of the sleeve (Figure 22.6b).	
Immobilize the head by wrapping the arm under the horse's jaw and placing it over the bridge of the nose. Open the nostril by lifting the false nostril to allow introduction of the pipette, as shown for swabbing.	This will give control of the head and allow introduction of the pipette into the nostril even if the horse moves. Alternatively, have an assistant immobilize the head to facilitate the introduction of the pipette into the nostril as shown for swabbing (Figure 22.3b).
Pass the pipette up the ventral nasal meatus (Figure 22.7).	This and the next two steps should be performed in quick succession to minimize the amount of time the sleeve is over the nose.
Place the opening of the rectal palpation sleeve over the horse's nose (Figure 22.8).	A small breathing hole can be made in advance if necessary but could allow leakage of the sample.
Advance the catheter or pipette into the pharynx at the marked spot. Flush 50 ml of sterile saline through the pipette/catheter (Figure 22.9).	
Catch reflux fluid that drains from the nostrils into the rectal palpation sleeve (Figure 22.10a).	The rectal sleeve fits well around the horse's muzzle, improving the retrieval of the lavage fluid. There is no need to use a sterile sleeve. Alternatively, a wide-mouth container is used for collection of the fluid.
Collect the retrieved lavage fluid from the fingers of the sleeve by aspirating it with your pipette and original saline syringe (Figure 22.10b).	
Prepare the sample for submission to the appropriate laboratory: 1. For bacterial culture and molecular detection, place the sample in a plain (red top) vacutainer tube (Figure 22.11). If desired, a separate aliquot can be placed in container with bacterial culture media. 2. For cytologic evaluation, place the sample into a small evacuated tube with EDTA (purple-top vacutainer tubes, 3 ml)	Bacterial culture and molecular detection assays are generally aimed to isolate *S. equi* subspecies *equi*. Check with the diagnostic laboratory which tube is best for specific tests.

Technical action	Rationale
Refrigerate samples except BBL™ Culture Swab™ culture media.	Do not freeze samples.
If washes are being performed on multiple horses, exercise caution to avoid cross-contamination of the samples.	

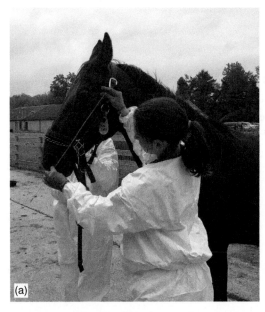

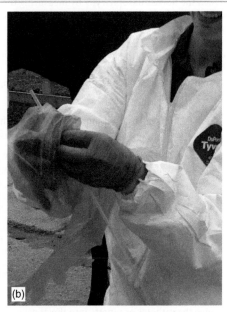

Figure 22.6 In preparation for collection of nasopharyngeal lavage sample, pass a sterile pipette or polypropylene catheter (8–10 Fr) through the outside to the inside of a rectal palpation sleeve approximately 5″ (12.5 cm) from the opening of the sleeve.

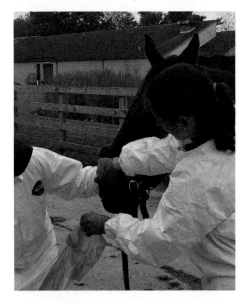

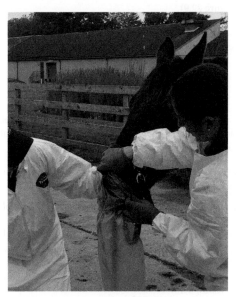

Figure 22.7 With the pipette or catheter inserted through the rectal sleeve, pass the pipette or catheter up the ventral nasal meatus and into the nasal passage.

Figure 22.8 Place the opening of the rectal palpation sleeve over the horse's nose.

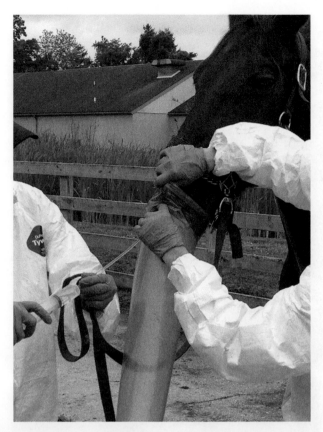

Figure 22.9 Flush 50 ml of sterile saline through the pipette/catheter.

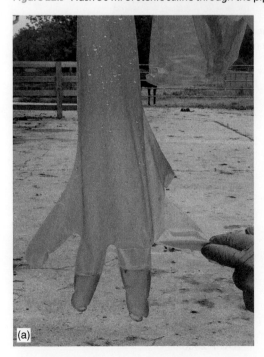

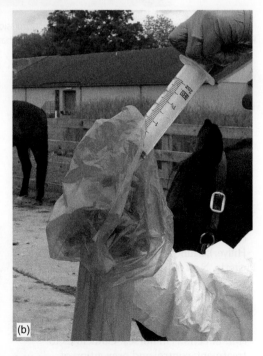

Figure 22.10 Collection of the lavage fluid. (a) Catch reflux fluid that drains from the nostrils into the rectal palpation sleeve. (b) Collect the retrieved lavage fluid from the fingers of the sleeve by aspirating it with a pipette.

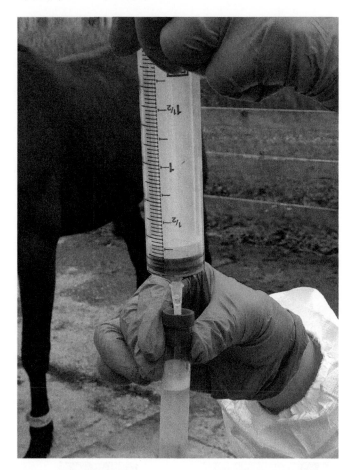

Figure 22.11 Preparation of the wash sample for submission for bacterial culture and bacterial molecular detection. Place an aliquot of the retrieved lavage fluid into a tube that has no additives (e.g., an evacuated red-top tube).

Bibliography and Further Reading

Boyle, A.G. (2011) *Streptococcus equi* subspecies *equi* infection (Strangles) in horses. *Compendium: Continuing Education for Veterinarians*, Vetlearn.com. https://s3.amazonaws.com/assets.prod.vetlearn.com/ca/9442c0b24011e08712005056 8d3693/file/PV0311_Boyle_CE.pdf.

Mair, T.S. (2010) Respiratory disease, in *Diagnostic Techniques in Equine Medicine*, 2nd edn (eds F.G.R. Taylor, T.J. Brazil, and M.H. Hillyer), Saunders Elsevier, Edinburgh, pp. 242.

Pusterla, N. *et al.* (2006) Diagnostic approach to infectious respiratory disorders. *Clinical Techniques in Equine Practice*, **5**, 174–186.

Sweeney, C.R., Timoney, J.F., Newton, J.R., and Hines, M.T. (2005) *Streptococcus equi* infections in horses: Guidelines for treatment, control and prevention of strangles. *Journal of Veterinary Internal Medicine*, **19**, 123–134.

Notes

1. Manufacturers of swabs 8″ and 16″ in length include Fox Converting Inc.
2. Manufacturers of swabs ranging from 27″ to 33″ in length include Jorgensen Laboratories, Inc., VetOne, MAI Animal Health, and Kalayjian Industries, Inc.
3. Manufactured by MILA International, Inc.
4. Manufacturers of viral transport medium include BD™ and Copan™.

Nasopharyngeal wash: see the following links to AAEP guidelines. http://www.aaep.org/custdocs/Respiratory Guidelines.pdf and http://www.aaep.org/custdocs/Streptococcus equi var.pdf; © Copyright AAEP 2006.

23

Nasotracheal Intubation

Mustajab H. Mirza, Jill R. Johnson, and Lais R.R. Costa

23.1 Purpose

- To maintain a patent airway and administer supplemental oxygen during recovery from general anesthesia.
- To maintain a patent airway in patients with edema of the nasal passages (e.g., snake bite, bee sting, thrombi and obstruction of the jugular vein bilaterally).
- To allow administration of volatile anesthetic agent for induction of general anesthesia in foals or adult horses undergoing general anesthesia when orotracheal intubation is not possible (e.g., for oral surgery).
- To perform assisted ventilation, as an alternative to assisted ventilation via orotracheal intubation.

- To prevent increased abdominal pressure during fetal reposition in dystocia.

23.2 Complications

- Coughing due to tracheal irritation.
- Trauma to the nasal meatus, nasal mucosa, ethmoid turbinates, pharyngeal mucosa, dorsal pharyngeal recess, arytenoid cartilages, and tracheal mucosa.
- Arytenoid chondritis.

23.3 Equipment Required

- Nasotracheal tube of appropriate size for the animal, cuffed or non-cuffed (cuffed tubes are often preferred) (Table 23.1 and Figure 23.1).

Table 23.1 Equine nasotracheal tube sizes recommended according to the approximated weight of the animal.

Size of the Animal (kg)		ID (mm)	OD (mm)	Length (cm)
Adult horses	>450	18–22	22–30	75–90
	250–450	14–16	18–22	55–70
	<250	12–14	16–19	55
Foals	(30–60)	7–10	10–14.3	55
Adult miniature horses	75–95	7–8	10–11	34–55
Miniature foals	(5–10)	5–6	7.3–8.7	20–28

ID, inner diameter; OD, outer diameter. The diameter of the ventral meatus will determine the adequate size of the tube that can be used for nasotracheal intubation. Endotracheal tube sizes are generally given based on the inner diameter (ID). The outer diameter is variable according to manufacturer.

The required length of the tube is determined by the distance between the nostril to the proximal third of the trachea (6 to 10 cm pass the larynx).

Manual of Clinical Procedures in the Horse, First Edition. Edited by Lais R.R. Costa and Mary Rose Paradis.
© 2018 John Wiley & Sons, Inc. Published 2018 by John Wiley & Sons, Inc.

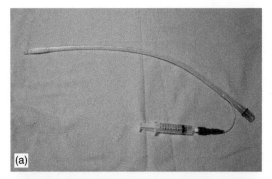

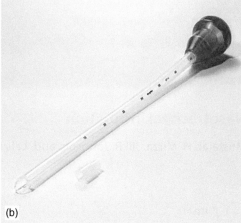

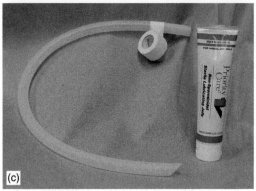

Figure 23.1 Supplies for nasotracheal tube placement: (a) silicone cuffed nasotracheal tube (8 mm ID, 11 mm OD, 55 cm length), (b) silicone non-cuffed nasotracheal tube (14 mm ID, 19 mm OD, 40 cm in length) with funnel adaptor that prevents the tube from being inserted all the way into the horse (courtesy of Lisa Kor), and (c) silicone non-cuffed nasotracheal tube, 1″ white tape, sterile lubricant.

- White tape, 1″
- 60 ml syringe
- Sterile water-soluble lubricant
- Oxygen supply, with a small-diameter long tube to be inserted into the nasotracheal tube.

23.4 Restraint and Positioning

- Nasotracheal intubation is most often performed in anesthetized horses, while they are in lateral or dorsal recumbency.

- Nasotracheal intubation of the animal in a standing position may require sedation with an alpha-2 agonist (e.g., xylazine at a dose of 0.5 mg/kg) in conjunction with an opioid agonist-antagonist (e.g., butorphanol at a dose of 0.04 mg/kg) (see Chapter 9). Avoid excessive sedation.
- Helpers passing the tube or restraining the horse should stand to the side of the horse, and not directly in front of the horse.

23.5 Procedure

Technical action	Rationale
Clean any debris from the external nares.	This will reduce amount of contamination of the trachea.
Apply water-soluble, sterile lubricant to the distal few inches of the end of the nasotracheal tube that will be inserted into the nares.	Lubricating jelly will facilitate passage of the tube through the nasal turbinates.

Technical action	Rationale
Lubricate the nostril with sterile lubricant as well.	If the animal to be intubated is awake, use lubricant gel containing a topical anesthetic. Topical anesthetic is not necessary if the animal is anesthetized (when the purpose of nasotracheal intubation is administration of oxygen during recovery).
Direct the tube into the ventral nasal meatus by digitally pressing the tip of the tube ventrally and medially in either nostril (Figure 23.2). Make sure the horse's head and neck are extended. Advance the tube until positioned at the opening to the larynx. Wait until the horse inhales then quickly advance the tube into the trachea.	Extension of the head and neck facilitate placement of the tube into the trachea. If the horse swallows during advancement of the tube, the tube may be displaced into the esophagus instead of being advanced into the trachea.

If the tube advances into the trachea, minimal resistance will be encountered to advancement, whereas if the tube enters the esophagus more resistance is encountered. Once into the trachea, a flow of air through the tube should be detectable. |
| Once positioned in the trachea, secure the tube to prevent inhalation of the tube or extubation.

Place a few wraps of white tape around the tube where it exits from the external nares then continue to wrap the tape around the horse's muzzle to secure the tube in place (Figures 23.3–23.5).

Other alternative for securing the nasotracheal tube is inflating the cuff, if using a cuffed nasotracheal tube (Figure 23.1a). | Securing the tube to the horse with tape prevents accidental dislodgement of the tube.

For cuffed tubes, it is important to check the integrity of the cuff and the appropriate amount of air for inflation of the cuff. The volume of air to inflate the cuff will depend on the size of the tube. Typically 20-30 ml are used in tube sizes 16 to 22 mm ID. It is best to verify the volume necessary for the particular tube, prior to intubating the horse. Do not over-inflate the cuff; it is better to under-inflate the cuff.

Some tubes have a funnel adaptor attached, which is designed to prevent the nasotracheal tube from being aspirated (Figure 23.1b). |
To administer oxygen, insert a smaller diameter oxygen supplementation tube into the nasotracheal tube's lumen.	Oxygen can be administered while preserving the flow of air around the tube, leaving the system open for expiration of carbon dioxide.
Administer oxygen flow at a rate appropriate for patient needs.	Oxygen may be delivered from a mobile tank or house oxygen system. The oxygen flow rate for an adult horse is typically set around 15 liters/minute; for foals the oxygen flow is set around at 3–4 liters/minute.
To extubate, remove the tape securing the tube to the muzzle and pull the tube out through the nostril.	If using a cuffed nasotracheal tube, make sure to deflate the cuff before extubation.

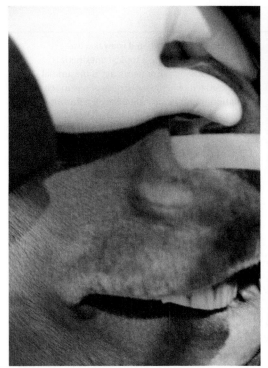

Figure 23.2 Passing the nasotracheal tube via ventral nasal meatus into the trachea.

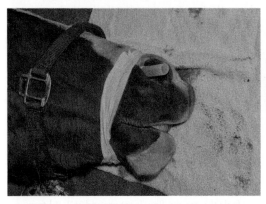

Figure 23.4 Nasotracheal tube in place and taped to the muzzle.

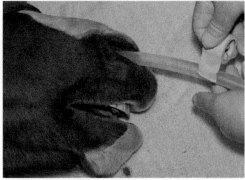

Figure 23.3 Passing white tape around the free end of the nasotracheal tube after it has been placed into the trachea.

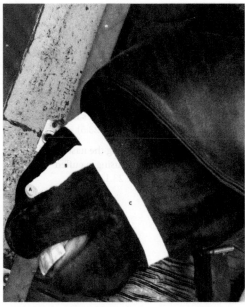

Figure 23.5 Placement of white tape around the muzzle: A, the opening of the nasotracheal tube; B, free end of the nasotracheal tube to which the white tape has been wrapped around; C, white tape wrapped around the muzzle.

Bibliography and Further Reading

Corley, K. (2008) Nasotracheal and orotracheal intubation, in *The Equine Hospital Manual* (eds K. Corley and J. Stephen), Blackwell Publishing, Oxford, pp. 120.

Holland, M., Snyder, J.R., Steffey, E.P., and Heath, R.B. (1986) Laryngotracheal injury associated with nasotracheal intubation in the horse. *Journal of the American Veterinary Medical Association*, **189** (11), 1447–1450.

Schaer, B.D. and Orsini, J.A. (2008) Nasotracheal and orotracheal tube placement, in *Equine Emergencies*, 3rd edn (eds J.A. Orsini and T.J. Divers), Saunders, pp. 435.

24

Endoscopy and Catheterization of the Guttural Pouch for Sampling and Lavage*

Lais R.R. Costa and Jill R. Johnson

24.1 Purpose

- To evaluate the guttural pouches via naso-pharyngeal endoscopy and determine the presence of abnormalities such as guttural pouch empyema, guttural pouch mycosis, and temporohyoid ostearthropathy.
- To obtain a wash sample from guttural pouches for the purposes of cytologic evaluation, microbiological culture, and molecular diagnostics (e.g., immunoassay, nucleic acid detection by polymerase chain reaction) of potential pathogens. Sampling of guttural pouches is the best diagnostic procedure for the detection of *Streptococcus equi* subspecies *equi*, particularly identification of chronic infection and carriers of *S. equi* subspecies *equi*.
- To perform drainage and lavage of, or to administer local treatment to, the guttural pouches in the management of guttural pouch infections such as guttural pouch empyema and guttural pouch mycosis.
- To place an indwelling catheter in the guttural pouch(es) to provide constant drainage and a means for repeated lavage or treatment. Guttural pouch catheterization is best performed with the aid of an endoscope.

24.2 Complications

- Epistaxis
- Failure to enter the guttural pouches due to the patient's lack of compliance or the

presence of a lesion obstructing or impairing completion of the procedure.
- Damage to vascular or neural structures within the guttural pouch (Table 24.1).

24.3 Equipment Required

- Appropriate protective clothing if contagious pathogen is suspected (see Chapter 22, Figure 22.1).
- For evaluation and sampling of guttural pouches:
  - gauze
  - examination gloves
  - water-soluble lubricant to aid passing the scope through the nasal passages
  - small-diameter (best if 10 mm OD or less), 1 m endoscope with biopsy channel
  - biopsy instrument appropriate for the endoscope
  - light source (usually halogen)
  - video monitor or eyepiece for viewing
  - aspiration catheter appropriate for the endoscope*
  - Chambers mare catheter (56 cm, 8 gauge) or a uterine infusion pipette with a 20° bend approximately 3.75 cm at one end
  - two 60 ml syringes, each filled with 50 ml of sterile isotonic (0.9%) saline
  - aerobic transport media for bacterial culture (Amies Bacterial Transport Medium)
  - two sterile evacuated tubes without additives (red-top vacutainer tubes, 7–10 ml volume)

---

*Manufacturers of aspiration catheters to be introduced through the endoscope channel include MILA International Inc. and Olympus.

Manual of Clinical Procedures in the Horse, First Edition. Edited by Lais R.R. Costa and Mary Rose Paradis.
© 2018 John Wiley & Sons, Inc. Published 2018 by John Wiley & Sons, Inc.

Table 24.1 Structures within the guttural pouch structure

Location	Structure		Comments
Separation between the two compartments	Bones and muscles	Stylohyoid bone	Articulates with the petrous temporal bone dorsally
			Vestibulocochlear (CN VII) in close proximity to the lateral aspect of the temporostylo-hyoid joint
		Stylopharyngeal muscle	Runs along the stylohyoid bone
Medial compartment	Vascular structures	Internal carotid artery	
The largest (two-thirds) overlies the retropharyngeal lymph nodes	Neural structures	Glossopharyngeal (CN IX)	Nerves are visible traveling in a fold of mucosa next to the internal carotid artery
		Vagus (CN X)	
		Accessory (CN XI)	
		Hypoglossal (CN XII)	
		Recurrent laryngeal nerve (branch of CN X)	
		Sympathetic nerves	
		Cranial cervical ganglion	
		Pharyngeal branches of CN IX and CN X	Nerves travel in a rostroventral direction along the lateral and medial walls of the medial compartment
Lateral compartment	Vascular structures	External carotid artery	Branches into the maxillary and linguofacial artery
The smaller one (one-third) overlies the parotid and mandibular glands			Courses along the separation of the lateral and medial compartments
		Maxillary artery	The maxillary artery gives off the temporal and the auricular arteries
		Auricular artery	
		Temporal artery	
		Maxillary-facial vein	
	Neural structures	Facial nerve (CN VII)	Exits the skull via the stylomastoid foramen

- two small evacuated tubes with EDTA (purple-top vacutainer tubes, 3 ml, for cytology and PCR-based diagnostics).
- For placement of an indwelling catheter in the guttural pouch to provide constant drainage and a means for repeated lavage or treatment administration:

  - Option 1: Foley catheter of adequate length for the patient. For an average size, light breed horse a 26 Fr Foley catheter, 16″ (40 cm) in length is adequate, with a balloon that when inflated prevents the catheter from sliding out of the guttural pouch, and a Chambers mare catheter (56 cm, 8 gauge).

- Option 2: A long catheter with a coil at one end and an introducer (e.g., Indwelling guttural pouch coiled catheter kit**, which includes a 12-gauge polyurethane catheter, 135 cm in length, with a coiled end, a bendable introducer, and an attachable luer lock adapter).

24.4 Restraint and Positioning

- Endoscopy and placement of a catheter for sampling or lavage of the guttural pouch requires moderate sedation.
- In most cases, sedation with an alpha-2 agonist (e.g., xylazine, detomidine, etc.) is effective. Combination with butorphanol might be indicated (see Chapter 9).
- These procedures generally require at least three people: a handler, one person to pass the scope, and one person to drive the scope. Additional assistants would be helpful.
- Ensure all personnel wear the appropriate protective clothing if infection with *S. equi* subspecies *equi* is suspected.
- The handler and the person passing the scope should stand slightly off to the side of the horse to avoid being injured if the horse strikes.

24.5 Procedure: Collection of Guttural Pouch Lavage Samples using an Endoscope

Technical action	Rationale
Following sedation, clean the nostril with gauze and apply topical lidocaine gel to the mucosa along the ventral meatus on both nostrils.	Making the nasal mucosa numb might reduce the reaction of the animal to the stimulation of the mucosa while passing the endoscope and catheter.
Have the handler immobilize the head of the horse to allow the introduction of the endoscope into the chosen nostril.	Introduce the endoscope into the ipsilateral nostril (on the same side of the guttural pouch to be catheterized).
Introduce the endoscope into the ventral meatus of the chosen (right or left) nostril, and advance it until both openings of the guttural pouches can be seen (Figure 24.1). Make an assessment of the pharynx for symmetry, presence of discharge, lymphoid hyperplasia, and any other abnormalities.	See Chapter 20 for endoscopic evaluation of the upper respiratory tract (URT). Note the presence and character of drainage from the guttural pouches openings: • mucoid secretion (Figure 24.2a) • purulent discharge (Figure 24.2b) • blood or blood clot (Figure 24.2c). Note if there is a fistula between the guttural pouch and the pharynx (generally at the pharyngeal recess).
Advance the endoscope, directing it against the lateral pharyngeal wall just ventral to the openings of the chosen guttural pouch. Introduce the biopsy instrument into the channel until the tip of the biopsy instrument is visible.	Most endoscopes have the biopsy channel exiting in an eccentric point at the tip of the scope. The endoscope has to be rotated such that the biopsy channel is closest to the guttural pouch opening.
Advance the biopsy instrument such that it enters the opening of the chosen guttural pouch (Figure 24.3). As soon as the horse swallows and the guttural pouch opening flaps open, advance the endoscope into the pouch.	The biopsy instrument acts as a guide for the scope to be advanced over it. The biopsy instrument must remain closed at all times to avoid damage to structures within the guttural pouch.

**An indwelling guttural pouch catheter kit is available from MILA International Inc.

Technical action	Rationale
Alternatively, introduce the Chambers catheter into the contralateral nasal passage and advance it to the nasopharynx. Use the tip of the catheter to pry open the fibrocartilagenous flap of the guttural pouch opening. Once the guttural pouch flap is open, the endoscope is advanced into the pouch (Figure 24.5).	Estimate the length of the Chambers catheter necessary to reach the guttural pouch (Figure 24.4). The Chambers catheter is safe because of it has a round, non-traumatic tip.
Once inside the guttural pouch, retract the biopsy instrument promptly. Observe all structures in both medial and lateral compartments.	Locate the vascular and neural structures that are normally visible inside the guttural pouch (Table 24.1 and Figure 24.6).
Identify any abnormalities in the guttural pouch.	See Figure 24.7.
Remove the biopsy instrument from the endoscope channel and replace it with the aspiration catheter. Advance the catheter through the channel until it is visible.	The long through-the-channel aspiration catheter can be single or multiple lumen. If a catheter is not available, the lavage may be performed using the biopsy channel itself.
Flush 50 ml of sterile (ideally warmed) saline through the catheter and aspirate the lavage fluid, directing the endoscope tip such that the tip of the catheter is submerged into the fluid.	Try to collect all the lavage fluid draining from the nostrils into a bucket to decrease environmental contamination of potentially contagious pathogens. Alternatively, the lavage fluid draining from the nostrils may be collected in a rectal sleeve (See Chapter 22, Figure 22.8).
In most cases both guttural pouches must be examined and sampled. Once the wash sample of one guttural pouch has been obtained, proceed to collect the sample from the other guttural pouch. Remove the endoscope from the first nostril.	
Introduce the endoscope into the other nostril to access the other guttural pouch. Repeat the lavage procedure as described above.	Typically the endoscope is placed into one nostril and the ipsilateral guttural pouch is sampled. It is possible to sample both the ipsilateral and the contralateral guttural pouches without replacing the endoscope, but this requires more skill and experience.
Prepare the lavage sample for submission to the appropriate laboratory: • for bacterial culture, place an aliquot of the lavage fluid in a sterile container or vial immediately after collection • for molecular detection, place an aliquot of the lavage fluid in an evacuated EDTA tube • for cytologic evaluation, place the sample in a small evacuated tube with EDTA. Refrigerate samples.	Bacterial culture and molecular detection assays are generally aimed to isolate *S. equi* subspecies *equi*. An evacuated tube without additive is ideal to send a sample of lavage fluid for culture. Do not freeze the sample. Check with the diagnostic laboratory which tube is best for specific tests. Typically either an EDTA evacuated tube or and evacuated tube without additives are adequate for molecular diagnostic tests and cytologic evaluation. Do not freeze samples.
Keep samples on ice until ready to ship. Samples should be shipped refrigerated (cold packs) to the appropriate diagnostic laboratory in a styrofoam container as soon as possible.	
The endoscope should be cleaned and cold sterilized. Follow manufacturer's guidelines.	Make sure that the protective clothing of all personnel is changed, and disinfection of any restraint device such as twitch, lip chain, etc. is performed.

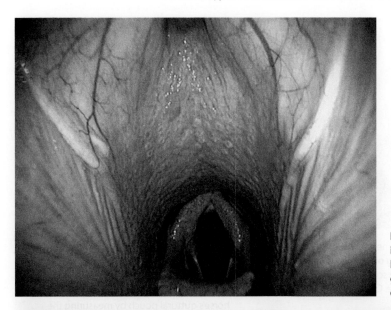

Figure 24.1 Once the scope is in the pharynx, observe both openings of the guttural pouches. Courtesy of Dr. Daniel Burba.

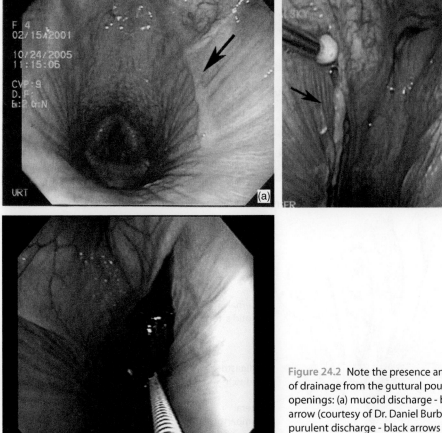

Figure 24.2 Note the presence and character of drainage from the guttural pouches openings: (a) mucoid discharge - black arrow (courtesy of Dr. Daniel Burba), (b) purulent discharge - black arrows (courtesy of Dr. Daniel Burba), and (c) blood clot protruding from the guttural pouch opening (courtesy of Dr. Maria Masri).

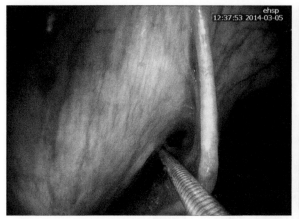

Figure 24.3 Once the scope is next to the pharyngeal wall near the fibrocartilagenous opening of the guttural pouch, advance the biopsy instrument into the scope's channel until the tip of the biopsy instrument is visible. Courtesy of Dr. Colin Mitchell.

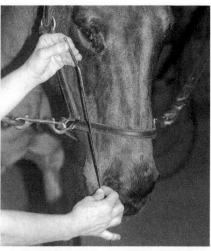

Figure 24.4 Estimate the length of the Chambers catheter necessary to reach the horse's guttural pouch by measuring the distance from the nostril to the lateral canthus.

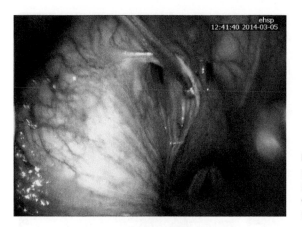

Figure 24.5 The Chambers catheter is used to pry the fibrocartilagenous flap of the guttural pouch open. Once the guttural pouch flap is open, the endoscope can be advanced into the pouch. Courtesy of Dr. C. Mitchell.

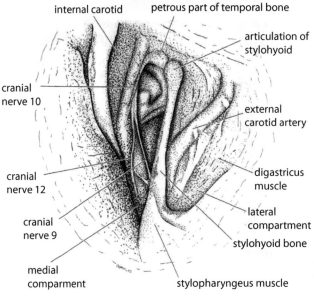

Figure 24.6 The vascular and neural structures normally visible on endoscopy of the guttural pouches. Corley and Stephen (2008). Reproduced with permission of John Wiley & Sons, Inc.

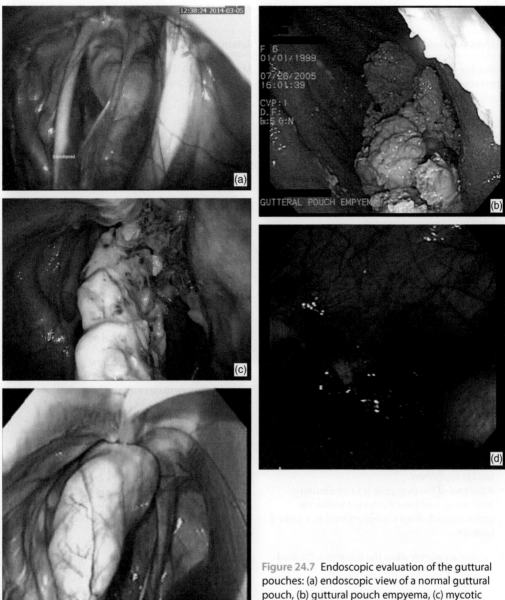

Figure 24.7 Endoscopic evaluation of the guttural pouches: (a) endoscopic view of a normal guttural pouch, (b) guttural pouch empyema, (c) mycotic plaque in guttural pouch mycosis, (d) bleeding in guttural pouch mycosis, and (e) thickening of the stylohyoid bone. Courtesy of Dr. D. Burba.

24.6 Procedure: Catheterization of the Guttural Pouch without the Endoscope

Technical action	Rationale
Following sedation, clean the nostril with gauze and apply topical lidocaine gel to the mucosa along the ventral meatus on both nostrils.	Making the nasal mucosa numb might reduce the reaction of the animal to the stimulation of the mucosa while passing the catheter.
Measure the distance from the middle of the ipsilateral nostril and the medial canthus of the eye (Figure 24.4).	If possible, make a mark on the catheter or pipette. This will guide you when it is time to turn the catheter in order to enter the guttural pouch.
Have the handler immobilize the head of the horse. Introduce the Chambers catheter into the ventral meatus of the ipsilateral nostril.	Alternatively, a uterine pipette with a 60° bend at one end can be used. The Chambers catheter is safer because of it has a round, non-traumatic tip.
When the catheter reaches the marked point, rotate it laterally about 150°, moving the catheter into a more dorsal and lateral position over the alar fold. As soon as the horse swallows (causing the guttural pouch openings to flap open) advance the catheter into the pouch.	Rotating the catheter about 150° laterally places the catheter tip in contact with the pharyngeal wall and lifts the guttural pouch flap. If you are unable to insert the catheter further, the catheter has not entered the guttural pouch. Insertion is only possible if the tip of the catheter is correctly placed into the guttural pouch
Once in place, administer the fluid for lavage or medication for infusion.	Blind catheterization of the guttural pouch is recommended as a once-only procedure. If the procedure needs to be performed repeatedly, an indwelling tube should be placed.
Position the horse's head appropriately: • if the goal of the catheterization is to lavage and drain the guttural pouch, make sure the horse's head is kept down • if the goal of the treatment is to administer a medication, and have it retained within the guttural pouch, keep the horse's head in a neutral position.	Lowering the head will facilitate drainage of the lavage fluid into the nasopharynx and exit through the nostrils. If lavage is being performed in a horse with suspected or confirmed *S. equi* subspecies *equi* infection, try to collect the drainage into a bucket lined with a garbage bag in order to decrease environmental contamination.
Remove the catheter when the infusion is finished.	

24.7 Procedure: Placement of an Indwelling Tube into the Guttural Pouch with the Aid of an Endoscope

Technical action	Rationale
Following sedation, clean the nostril with gauze and apply topical lidocaine gel to the mucosa along the ventral meatus on both nostrils.	Making the nasal mucosa numb might reduce the reaction of the animal to the stimulation of the mucosa while passing the endoscope.
Estimate the length of the Foley catheter and Chambers catheter necessary to reach the horse's guttural pouch by measuring the distance between the nostril and the lateral canthus of the eye (Figure 24.8).	Make a small mark on the catheter. If using the indwelling guttural pouch catheter kit make the mark on the introducer. This will help estimate how far the catheter should be advanced.
Have the handler immobilize the head of the horse because the procedure will require the introduction of the catheter into the ventral meatus of the ipsilateral nostril and the endoscope into the contralateral nostril.	The catheter is introduced into the side of the guttural pouch to be catheterized and the endoscope is introduced into the other nostril.
Insert the tip of the Chambers catheter through the side hole of the Foley catheter and push it to the tip.	Check that the cuff of the Foley catheter does not have any leaks.
Introduce the catheter into the ventral meatus of the ipsilateral nostril with the tip pointed down, and advance it up to 3–5 cm from the mark. Introduce the endoscope into the contralateral nostril. Advance the endoscope and the Chambers/Foley catheter combo until the tip of the Foley catheter can be seen. While keeping the endoscope in place, rotate the Chambers catheter about 150° laterally, pointing the tip against the pharyngeal wall. As soon as the guttural pouch opening flaps open, advance the catheter into the pouch.	If using the indwelling guttural pouch coiled catheter**, insert the introducer into ventral meatus and follow the manufacturer's instructions for endoscopic-guided insertion of the coiled polyurethane catheter.
Once into the guttural pouch, inflate the cuff of the Foley catheter with the appropriate amount of sterile water. Carefully remove the Chambers catheter, leaving the Foley catheter in place.	Observe the guttural pouch opening while and after removing the Chambers catheter to make sure that the Foley catheter stays in place. Do not over-inflate the cuff.
The Foley (or coiled) catheter can be used for lavage or administration of treatment to the guttural pouch. Attach a fluid line that is connected to an isotonic fluid bag and lavage the pouch or administer non-irritating medication properly diluted.	Use only non-irritating solution in the guttural pouches to ensure that no damage is caused to the nervous and vascular structures within the pouch (see Table 24.1). For lavage, make sure the horse's head is low to the ground (best achieved by sedation with alpha-2 agonists). If administering medication the head might be kept in a neutral position to retain the medication in the pouch.
When the infusion is finished, detach the administration set from the catheter. Do not remove the catheter.	The catheter can be left in place for as long as necessary, but be cognizant that the indwelling catheter might induce considerable irritation to the mucosa of the guttural pouch.

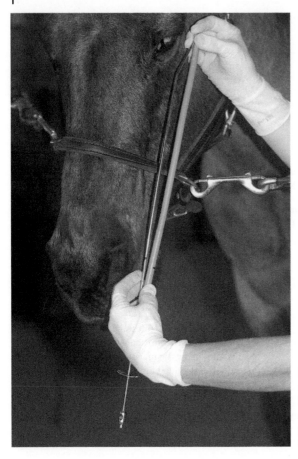

Figure 24.8 For placement of an indwelling catheter in the guttural pouch, estimate the length of the Chambers catheter and the Foley catheter necessary to reach the horse's guttural pouch by measuring the distance from the nostril to the lateral canthus.

Bibliography and Further Reading

Boyle, A.G. (2011) *Streptococcus equi subspecies equi infection (Strangles) in horses.* Compendium: Continuing Education for Veterinarians, Vet learn.com. https://s3.amazonaws.com/assets.prod.vetlearn.com/ca/9442c0b24011e08712005056 8d3693/file/PV0311_Boyle_CE.pdf.

Greet, T.R. (1987) Outcome of treatment in 35 cases of guttural pouch mycosis. *Equine Veterinary Journal,* **19** (5), 483–487.

Guttural Pouch Sampling. See links to AAEP guidelines: http://www.aaep.org/custdocs/Respiratory Guidelines.pdf

http://www.aaep.org/pdfs/control_guidelines/Streptococcusequivar.pdf.

Hardy, J. and Léveillé, R. (2003) Diseases of the guttural pouches, in (ed. E.J. Parente) *Veterinary Clinics of North America, Equine,* **19** (1), 123–158.

Judy, C.E., Chaffin, M.K., and Cohen, N.D. (1999) Empyema of the guttural pouch (auditory tube diverticulum) in horses: 91 cases (1977–1997). *Journal of the American Veterinary Medical Association,* **215** (11), 1666-1670.

Mair, T.S. (2010) Respiratory disease, in *Diagnostic Techniques in Equine Medicine,* 2nd edn (eds F.G.R. Taylor, T.J. Brazil, and M.H. Hillyer), Saunders Elsevier, Edinburgh, pp. 242.

Pusterla, N., Watson, J.L., and Wilson, W.D. (2006) Diagnostic approach to infectious respiratory disorders. *Clinical Techniques in Equine Practice,* **5**, 174–186.

Rose, R.J. and Hodgson, D.R. (2000) Respiratory system, in *Manual of Equine Practice,* 2nd edn, W.B. Saunders, Philadelphia.

McKenzie, H. (2008) Endoscopy of the guttural pouches, in *The Equine Hospital Manual* (eds K. Corley and J. Stephen), Blackwell Publishing, Oxford, pp. 66.

25

Bronchoalveolar Lavage of Adults and Foals

Brett Sponseller and Beatrice Sponseller

25.1 Purpose

- To obtain a sample from the lower airways for cytologic characterization, particularly when a non-infectious cause of lower airway disease is suspected.
- As part of the diagnostic workup for horses with a cough without fever, epistaxis, poor performance or dyspnea.
- To evaluate the airway anatomic structures such as the larynx, trachea, and larger bronchi and collect sample via bronchoscopy of a specific area of the tracheobronchial tree where more inflammation or discharge is noted. The endoscope can be guided to that specific location.

BAL can be performed via a BAL catheter/tube or via endoscopy.

25.2 Complications

- Bronchopleural fistula
- Bronchopneumonia

25.3 Equipment Required

25.3.1 Bronchoalveolar Lavage via a Bronchoalveolar Lavage Catheter

- BAL catheter, typically 2.4 or 3 m in length, with 10 or 11 mm outer diameter (OD). (Equine bronchoalveolar lavage catheters are available from Bivona (3 m length, 11 mm OD), Equivet (240 cm length, 10 mm OD), Cook (240 cm length, 10 cm

OD or 300 cm length, 10 cm OD), and Mila (240 cm length, 10 cm OD or 300 cm length, 10 cm OD)

- 6 ml syringe to inflate BAL catheter cuff
- 10–20 ml of local anesthetic (2% lidocaine hydrochloride without epinephrine) for the nasal passages
- 30 to 40 ml of undiluted pre-warmed local anesthetic (2% lidocaine hydrochloride without epinephrine) or 60 ml of 0.4% w/v diluted pre-warmed lidocaine solution to instill into the airways.
- Sterile gloves
- Four 60 ml syringes, each filled with isotonic (0.9%) pre-warmed sterile saline (to avoid osmotic lysis of cells).
- Two evacuated tubes containing EDTA (lavender top). The small (3 ml) tube should suffice for each cytology and PCR-based diagnostics.

25.3.2 Bronchoalveolar Lavage via Endoscopy

- 3 m endoscope for adult horses or a pediatric endoscope for foals
- 50 ml local anesthetic (2% lidocaine hydrochloride or mepivicaine) or 60 ml of 0.4%w/v dilute pre-warmed lidocaine solution without epinephrine
- Sterile gloves
- Four 60 ml syringes, each filled with pre-warmed, isotonic (0.9%) sterile saline (to avoid osmotic lysis of cells).
- Two evacuated tubes containing EDTA (lavender top). 3 ml would suffice for each cytology and PCR-based diagnostics.

Manual of Clinical Procedures in the Horse, First Edition. Edited by Lais R.R. Costa and Mary Rose Paradis.
© 2018 John Wiley & Sons, Inc. Published 2018 by John Wiley & Sons, Inc.

25.4 Restraint

25.4.1 Bronchoalveolar Lavage via a Catheter

- The degree of restraint will depend on the age, training and disposition of the horse.
- In general, moderate sedation with an alpha-2 agonist (xylazine, detomidine, etc.) in combination with butorphanol is effective.
- A twitch is often indicated, depending on the horse's demeanor and response to the twitch.

25.4.2 Bronchoalveolar Lavage via Endoscopy

- The degree of physical and chemical restraint will depend on the age, training, and disposition of the horse.

- In general, moderate sedation with an alpha-2 agonist (xylazine, detomidine, etc.) in combination with butorphanol, and the use of a twitch are often indicated.
- Restraint in stocks to protect the endoscopic equipment and for the safety of the horse is advised.
- Foals are often restrained in sternal recumbency under heavy sedation on a foal table with the thoracic limbs over the leading edge of the table, facing the endoscopist.

25.5 Procedure: Bronchoalveolar Lavage via a Catheter

Technical action	Rationale
Sedate the horse. Typically a combination of alpha-2 agonist (xylazine, detomidine, etc.) and butorphanol is recommended.	Moderate sedation will facilitate the procedure and decrease coughing. Allow sufficient time prior to beginning the procedure itself for the sedation to take full effect.
Take the BAL catheter from the sterile package and keep it coiled within a sterile field (Figure 25.1).	The technique is not sterile, but using a sterile BAL catheter/tube can mitigate the introduction of infectious agents to the patient.
Check the BAL tube cuff by insufflating 5 ml of air then deflate completely (Figure 25.2).	A functioning cuff is helpful in retaining the fluid in the lung segment being lavaged.
Clean the nostril and instill 10-20 ml of lidocaine along the nasal meatus (Figure 25.3).	Cleaning the nostril mitigates dragging debris into the pharynx and upper airway. Topical lidocaine is an inexpensive aid in decreasing the patient's response to trigeminal nerve stimulation.
Put on (sterile) latex gloves.	The technique is not sterile, so sterile gloves are not required. Gloves can mitigate introduction of infectious agents to the patient during passage of the BAL tube.
Apply a small amount of sterile lubricant to the tip of the BAL tube (Figure 25.4).	Lubricant will facilitate passage of the tube.
Apply a twitch if necessary. Be mindful of the need to access the nostril easily when applying the twitch.	Control of the nose is greatly facilitated with application of a twitch, but the demeanor and response of the horse to the twitch need to be weighed against not using it.

Technical action	Rationale
Elevate the head and extend the neck (Figure 25.5).	This position facilitates eventual passage of the BAL tube into the trachea. A flexed neck facilitates undesired passage into the esophagus.
Advance the BAL tube ventrally and medially through the nasal passage, through the glottis by angling the tip ventrally, and expediently through the trachea past the carina.	Ventromedial positioning through the nasal passages avoids bumping the ethmoid with resultant epistaxis. Angling the curved tip ventrally through the glottis helps avoid induction of swallowing and passage of the BAL tube into the esophagus.
The horse may experience coughing when the tube is in contact with the larynx or the carina of the trachea. Instillation of 20–30 ml of diluted 0.4% lidocaine without epinephrine at these two locations will help to decrease the coughing.	Alternatively, 5–10 ml of undiluted lidocaine might be infused followed by 20 ml of air. Most horses have cough receptors at the larynx and the tracheal bifurcation (carina). Sometimes the cough is quite violent. Use of the lidocaine will desensitize these areas and allow the procedure to continue with less distress to the horse.
Once resistance to the passage of the BAL tube is detected, inflate the cuff with about 5 ml of air.	The resistance that you feel is the tube wedging in a fourth- or fifth-generation segmental bronchus. The inflated cuff helps to retain the infused saline within the segment of lung being lavaged.
Attach each 60 ml syringe and infuse the entire 240 ml volume of saline (Figure 25.6).	
Immediately aspirate with the same syringe (Figure 25.7).	The BAL tube will contain approximately 20 ml of dead space, so actual lung lavage sample will not be obtained until more than 20 ml is aspirated.
Continue aspirating gently with each syringe consecutively. Alternatively, infuse and aspirate the content of each syringe at a time until 30–50 ml of sample is obtained.	Given the diameter of the BAL tube, the lung segment where the tube is placed can generally accommodate >240 ml of saline. Repeated infusion/aspiration of saline up to this amount will safely allow for lavage of the lung segment. The use of large volumes with rapid aspiration may cause barotrauma to the airway. In order to avoid causing barotrauma, it is recommended to infuse and aspirate 60 ml at a time.
Once an adequate sample volume has been retrieved, deflate the cuff of the BAL tube, carefully withdraw it and, remove the twitch (Figure 25.8).	Care during withdrawal of the tube is necessary to avoid bumping the ethmoid and causing epitaxis.
Gently mix the contents of all the syringes and fill two EDTA tubes (Figure 25.9).	EDTA preserves the cells for cytology and improves fluid analysis. The quality of the cells decreases with time. If submission to the laboratory is likely to take more than 8 hours, prepare two slides.

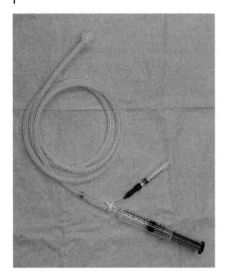

Figure 25.1 BAL catheter is kept coiled within a sterile field.

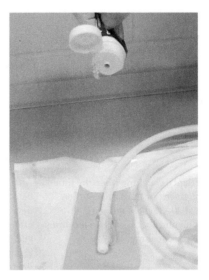

Figure 25.4 Coat the end of the BAL tube with sterile lubricant to facilitate passage through the nostril.

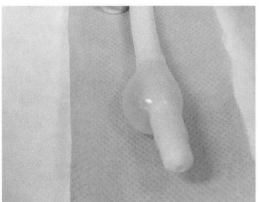

Figure 25.2 Test the inflation of the cuff on the BAL tube before beginning the procedure.

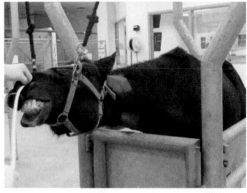

Figure 25.5 The head of the horse should be lifted and the neck straightened to facilitate the passage of the tube into the trachea instead of the esophagus.

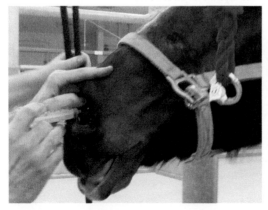

Figure 25.3 Clean the nostril and instill 20 ml of 2% lidocaine to improve the comfort of the horse.

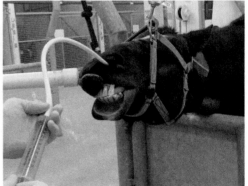

Figure 25.6 Inject one 60 ml syringe of 0.9% saline through the BAL tube.

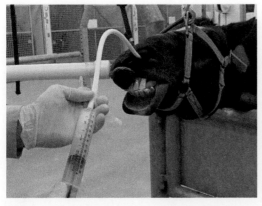

Figure 25.7 Immediately aspirate with the same syringe.

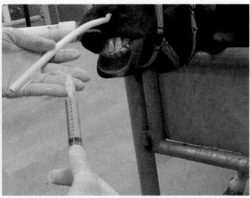

Figure 25.8 Be sure to deflate the cuff of the BAL catheter after lavage is completed and before withdrawing from the bronchi.

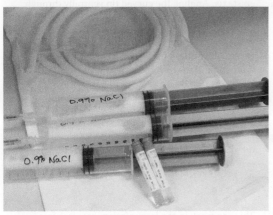

Figure 25.9 Thoroughly mix the sample and place an aliquot into two EDTA collection tubes.

25.6 Procedure: Bronchoalveolar Lavage via Endoscopy

Technical action	Rationale/amplification
Restrain and sedate the horse. A combination of alpha-2 agonist (xylazine, detomidine, etc.) and butorphanol is recommended.	Moderate sedation will facilitate the procedure and decrease coughing. Allow some time prior to beginning the procedure itself for the sedation to take full effect.
Assemble the endoscope.	
Clean nostril and instill 10–20 ml of lidocaine along nasal meatus.	Cleaning the nostril mitigates dragging debris into the pharynx and upper airway. Topical lidocaine is an inexpensive aid in decreasing the patient's response to trigeminal nerve stimulation.
Put on (sterile) latex gloves.	The technique is not sterile, so sterile gloves are not required. Gloves can mitigate introduction of infectious agents to the patient during passage of the endoscope.
Apply a small amount of sterile lubricant to the tip of the endoscope and turn on the light source.	Lubricant will facilitate passage.

(continued)

Technical action	Rationale/amplification
Apply a twitch if necessary. Be mindful of the need to access the nostril easily when applying the twitch.	Control of the nose is greatly facilitated with application of a twitch, but the demeanor and response of the horse to the twitch need to be weighed against not using it.
Elevate the head and extend the neck.	This position facilitates eventual passage of the endoscope into the trachea. A flexed neck facilitates undesired passage into the esophagus.
It is prudent to observe closely the route of the endoscope through the nasal passage and pharynx to avoid flexure of the endoscope and accidental passage into the oral cavity.	Avoid passage of the endoscope into the oral cavity, where the teeth can damage the scope.
Advance the endoscope ventrally and medially through the nasal passage, through the glottis by angling the tip ventrally, and expediently through the trachea, and towards the carina.	Ventromedial positioning through the nasal passages avoids bumping the ethmoid with resultant epistaxis. Angling the curved tip ventrally through the glottis helps avoid induction of swallowing and passage of the endoscope into the esophagus.
The lavage via bronchoscope allows for evaluation of the tracheobronchial tree.	Images illustrating findings during endoscopic evaluation of the lower airways are depicted in Figure 25.10.
Once in the trachea, instill mepivicaine (or lidocaine), making sure to cover points of airway bifurcation, including the carina. Continue instilling the local anesthetic drug while advancing the endoscope. The horse may experience coughing when the tube is in contact with the larynx or the carina of the trachea.	Airway mechanoreceptors are concentrated at airway bifurcations. Sometimes the cough is quite violent. Use of topical anesthetic will desensitize these areas and lessen coughing, making the procedure less traumatic to the lung and safer for the patient.
Advance the endoscope, selecting airways closest to the median plane and angling dorsally.	This approach in the large airways requires few turns, less pressure of the scope against airway bifurcations, and incites less coughing. Angling dorsally may allow for a better sample recovery.
Advance the endoscope until resistance to the passage of the endoscope is detected, then gently retract the endoscope enough to reduce pressure on the airway and prepare to instill sterile (preferably warm) saline.	Firm wedging of the scope is unnecessary as the process of instilling saline will enable pooling of the sample to be aspirated beyond the tip of the endoscope.
Administer the sterile solution and suction the lavage fluid using the biopsy channel *For a full size horse (450 kg, 1000 lb)*: Attach the first 60 ml syringe and infuse the entire 60 ml volume. *For a foal (45 kg, 100 lb*: Attach one 35 ml syringe and infuse approximately 25 ml.	The volume to be infused is determined by the volume of the segment of lung beyond the endoscope and, in part, by the diameter of the tip of the endoscope, with narrower scopes advancing further into the bronchial tree.
Observe the saline as it is instilled. Once the bronchial segment is being filled with saline, small bubbles should be observed emanating distal to the endoscope.	There should be little resistance to infusion of the saline. Resistance could signal that the endoscope is firmly wedged in the bronchial segment and that the segment is fully filled.

Technical action	Rationale/amplification
Gently aspirate the instilled saline into the same syringe immediately.	The endoscope will contain approximately 10–20 ml of dead space, so actual lung lavage sample will not be obtained until the volume in the dead space is completely aspirated.
Continue with additional 60 ml syringes of saline, infusing and aspirating until 30–50 ml of sample is obtained.	Serial addition and aspiration of aliquots of saline helps ensure that a excessive amount of saline is not instilled, resulting in barotrauma to the lung segment. The alternative technique is to infuse larger volumes 120 or 240 ml at once and then aspirate it. The problem with the larger volume, particularly with the narrow diameter endoscopes commonly used (the 3 m, which are about 9 mm in diameter) is that the narrow endoscope can get further into the airway than the BAL tube/catheter. And especially if the endoscopist follows the "dorsal/mid-line" approach, the volume of saline infused might overwhelm the lung segment, leading to barotrauma.
Once adequate sample volume has been retrieved, carefully withdraw the endoscope and remove the twitch.	Care during withdrawal of the endoscope is necessary to avoid bumping the ethmoid and causing epitaxis.
Gently mix the contents of the syringe and fill two EDTA tubes.	EDTA preserves the cells for cytology and improves fluid analysis. The quality of the cells decreases with time. If submission to the laboratory is likely to take more than 8 hours, prepare two slides.

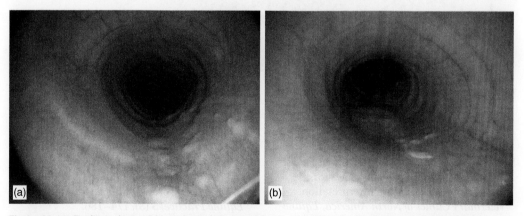

Figure 25.10 Findings during BAL via bronchoscope: (a) accumulation of a small amount mucopurulent secretion on the walls of the trachea, (b) accumulation of a moderate amount of mucopurulent secretion in the floor of the horizontal portion of the trachea, (c) accumulation of a large amount of mucopurulent secretion in the floor of the horizontal portion of the trachea, (d) normal appearance of the mucosa at the carina, and (e) hyperemic mucosa at the carina. Courtesy of Lais Costa and Jackie Bowser.

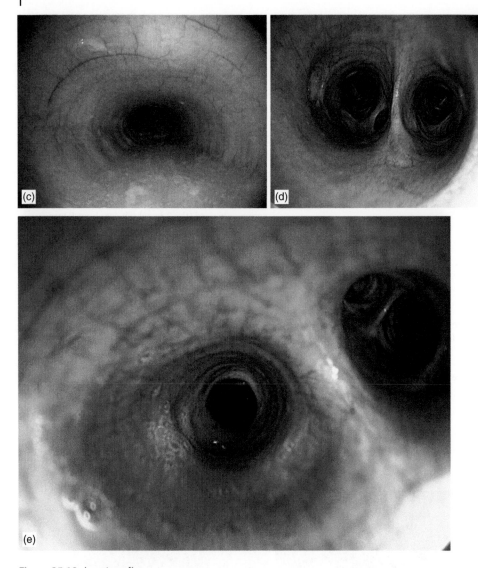

Figure 25.10 (continued)

Bibliography and Further Reading

Hoffman, A.M. (2008) Bronchoalveolar lavage: sampling technique and guidelines for cytologic preparation and interpretation. *Veterinary Clinics of North America, Equine Practice*, **2**, 423–435.

Mansmann, R.A. and King, C. (1998) How to perform bronchalveolar lavage in practice. *Proceedings of the Annual Convention of the AAEP*, **44**, 186–188.

McKenzie, H. (2008) Broncholaveolar lavage, in *The Equine Hospital Manual* (eds K. Corley and J. Stephen), Blackwell, Oxford, pp. 70–71.

Pusterla, N., Watson, J.L., and Wilson, W.D. (2006) Diagnostic approach to infectious respiratory disorders. *Clinical Techniques in Equine Practice*, **5** (3), 174–186.

Viel, L. and Hewson, J. (2003) Bronchoalveolar lavage, in *Current Therapy in Equine Medicine*, 5th edn (ed. N.E. Robinson), W.B. Saunders, Philadephia, pp. 407–411.

26

Transtracheal Aspiration of Adults and Foals

Brett Sponseller and Beatrice Sponseller

26.1 Purpose

- To obtain an uncontaminated wash sample from pulmonary secretions for the purposes of bacterial culture and/or virus isolation, detection of nucleic acid of potential pathogens, and cytologic characterization.
- Transtracheal aspiration is a diagnostic procedure indicated in cases of cough with fever, a productive cough, evidence of pleural irregularities and fluid with thoracic ultrasound examination, and/or evidence of pulmonary consolidation and/or pleural fluid with thoracic radiography.

26.2 Complications

- Laceration of jugular vein or common carotid artery
- Subcutaneous emphysema
- Pneumomediastinum
- Iatrogenic infection

26.3 Equipment Required

- 15-gauge cannula with 16-gauge intraluminal needle (approximate sizes), about 8 cm long (the cannula and catheter can be obtained individually or as a kit).
- Semi-rigid catheter, approximately 60 cm long (the cannula and catheter can be obtained individually or as a kit).
- Bladed clippers with a #40 blade.

- 4 × 4 gauze sponges soaked with 2% chlorhexidine scrub and 70% alcohol.
- Local anesthetic (2% lidocaine hydrochloride).
- #15 scalpel blade (in order to pierce the skin to reduce drag of cannula/needle).
- Sterile gloves
- Two 60 ml syringes, each filled with 20–40 ml of isotonic (0.9%) sterile saline to avoid osmotic lysis of equine and bacterial cells.
- One small syringe (3–12 ml volume).
- Three sterile evacuated tubes without additives (red-top vacutainer tubes, 7–10 ml volume, for sample transfer to the laboratory).
- Two small evacuated tubes with EDTA (purple-top vacutainer tubes, 3 ml, for cytology and PCR-based diagnostics).
- Antibiotic ointment
- Elastikon, 3″ (or similar)
- Sterile 4 × 4 gauze sponges

26.4 Restraint and Positioning

- The degree of restraint will depend on the age, training, and disposition of the horse.
- In general, moderate sedation with an alpha-2 agonist (xylazine, detomidine, etc.) in combination with butorphanol is effective (see Chapter 9).
- A twitch is often indicated, depending on the horse's demeanor and response to the twitch.

Manual of Clinical Procedures in the Horse, First Edition. Edited by Lais R.R. Costa and Mary Rose Paradis.
© 2018 John Wiley & Sons, Inc. Published 2018 by John Wiley & Sons, Inc.

26.5 Procedure: Transtracheal Aspiration

Technical action	Rationale
Following sedation, elevate the head and extend the neck. Identify where the trachea is most easily palpated in the mid-cervical region (at the junction of the upper and the middle third of the neck).	This position facilitates palpation of the trachea and lateralizes the cervical strap muscles, increasing exposure of the trachea.
Clip the hair in a square approximately 10 × 10 cm and scrub the skin surface.	An aseptic field large enough to permit stabilization of the trachea is necessary.
Identify the tracheal rings. In between two tracheal rings, on the center of the aseptically prepared site, inject a 2–5 ml lidocaine bleb subcutaneously (Figure 26.1).	Tracheal puncture occurs in between the tracheal rings, on the midline. Lidocaine should not be injected into the tracheal wall or lumen.
Perform a final scrub of the clipped area.	The site may be contaminated during the previous step if palpation is required to identify site for lidocaine injection.
Open sterile gloves. Use the sterile field afforded for opening a #15 blade, cannula/needle, and long, semi-rigid catheter. Loop the long catheter so it retains itself (Figure 26.2).	This approach allows the clinician to perform the procedure with minimal assistance, as might be necessary in a field situation.
Put on sterile gloves following aseptic technique.	The gloves will help maintain sterility during the procedure and enable direct contact with the long catheter.
Make a small stab incision in the skin with the #15 blade in the blocked area, on midline, overlying the space between the tracheal rings (Figure 26.3).	This step may be omitted, but it is recommended because it reduces drag on the large cannula/needle during tracheal puncture.
With one hand, stabilize the trachea. With the other, insert the cannula/needle at the point of the stab incision (Figure 26.4).	The trachea needs to be well stabilized. Considerable pressure is required to advance the cannula/needle through the trachea. Usually a noticeable "pop" will be felt when entering into the trachea. Should the cannula/needle deviate from the trachea, laceration of the jugular vein or common carotid artery is possible.
Advance the cannula/needle to the hub, within and down the trachea.	It is possible to puncture the deep (dorsal) aspect of the trachea with perpendicular advancement of the cannula/needle.
Remove the needle from the stylet and either note air movement or aspirate with a small syringe (Figure 26.5).	There should be no negative pressure on aspiration if the cannula is within the trachea.
Thread the semi-rigid catheter approximately two-thirds of the way through the cannula in the foal, and further in the adult (Figure 26.6).	This depth should place the catheter tip approximately where the trachea parallels the ground.
Inject 20–40 ml of sterile saline through the semi-rigid catheter into the trachea. Begin aspirating immediately, advancing or withdrawing the semi-rigid catheter if no fluid is aspirated. Be sure the cannula does not back out. Usually >20 ml can be recovered per 50 ml injected (Figures 26.7 and 26.8). The horse is likely to cough at this time. It is important to keep the catheter pointing down so that the force of the cough does not bend the catheter up into the pharynx.	The tip of the semi-rigid catheter will need to be in the pool of injected fluid for sample collection. Maintaining the cannula parallel to the trachea and allowing the horse's neck to be almost parallel (not below) to the ground surface will facilitate fluid collection. Maintain the cannula in this position so that the potentially contaminated semi-rigid catheter does not introduce bacteria, etc. that could result in peri-tracheal infection, possibly extending to the mediastinum.

Technical action	Rationale
If recovery of fluid is unsuccessful, instill another 20-40 ml of sterile saline and aspirate immediately.	Neck position, catheter depth, and coughing all influence the recovery efficiency of the instilled fluid.
Remove the semi-rigid catheter through the cannula.	The cannula protects tissue planes from infection on withdrawal of the semi-rigid catheter, a rare but significant complication.
Remove the cannula (Figure 26.9).	
Antibiotic ointment and a sterile gauze can be applied to the puncture site and the site can be wrapped loosely with Elastikon®.	Local cellulitis and emphysema at the puncture site are rare, but antibiotic ointment and bandaging may mitigate these complications.
Prepare the sample for delivery to the appropriate laboratories. The tests requested should take into account other relevant clinical findings (Figure 26.10). Typically a sample of the fluid is placed in: (a) an evacuated tube with EDTA (i.e., purple-top vacutainer tube) for cytology (b) an evacuated tube with no additives (i.e., a red-top vacutainer tube) for microbial culture Preparation of additional tubes or slides may be indicated.	Samples of the fluid are: (a) placed in a purple-top vacutainer tube (evacuated tube with EDTA) and chilled to allow preservation of cell morphology for cytologic evaluation (b) placed in a red-top vacutainer tube and chilled to allow preservation of microorganisms for microbial culture (c) placed in a purple-top vacutainer tube for PCR-based diagnostic testing (d) placed in a red-top vacutainer tube (evacuated tube with no additives) and chilled for virus isolation (e) added to two slides and allowed to air dry for cytologic evaluation it will take more than 8 hours for the sample to be submitted to the laboratory.

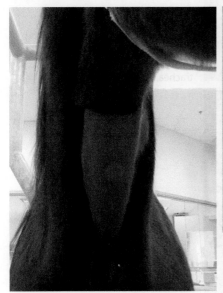

Figure 26.1 An area of the ventral mid-cervical region is clipped and surgically prepared. Subcutaneous lidocaine is injected on the midline just over the palpable trachea.

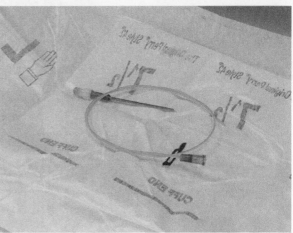

Figure 26.2 The glove wrapping can act as a sterile field for the cannula, rigid catheter, and blade. The catheter should be looped together to prevent inadvertent contamination.

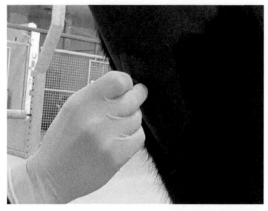

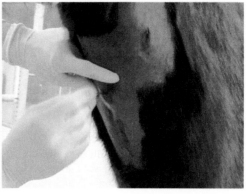

Figure 26.3 A vertical stab incision is made through the skin and subcutaneous tissue at the lidocaine bleb site.

Figure 26.4 The cannula is inserted through the stab incision. The tip of the cannula can be used to feel for the indent between the tracheal rings. The trachea is stabilized with the other hand by tensing the skin over the trachea.

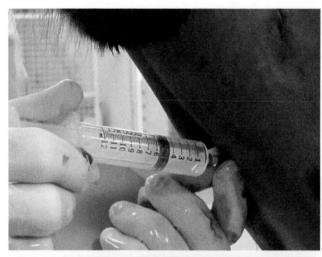

Figure 26.5 After the stylet of the cannula is removed, a syringe can be attached. Aspiration of air will confirm the placement of the cannula in the trachea.

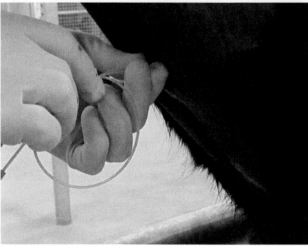

Figure 26.6 The rigid catheter is threaded through the cannula, keeping the cannula pointed down the trachea. This is important because if the horse coughs it may flip the catheter upward into the pharyngeal region.

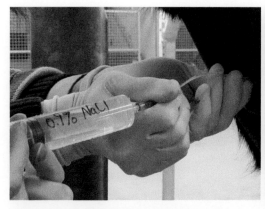

Figure 26.7 Up to 50 ml of sterile isotonic saline is quickly instilled through the catheter. The horse is likely to cough at this time.

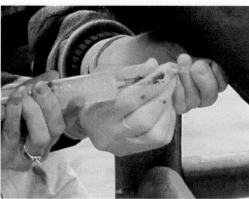

Figure 26.8 The sample should be aspirated using the same syringe immediately after the fluid has been instilled.

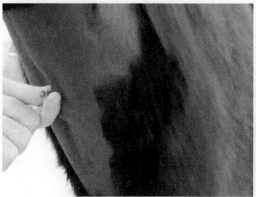

Figure 26.9 Once a sufficient sample has been obtained, the catheter can be removed followed by removal of the cannula.

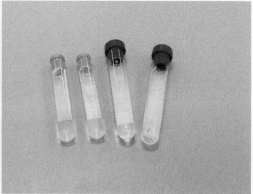

Figure 26.10 After thoroughly mixing the sample, it should be placed in the appropriate tubes for analysis and culture.

Bibliography and Further Reading

Hodgson, J.L. and Hodgson, D.R. (2003) Tracheal aspirates: indications, techniques and interpretation, in *Current Therapy in Equine Medicine*, 5th edn (ed. N.E. Robinson), W.B. Saunders, Philadelphia, pp 401–406.

McKenzie, H. (2008) Tracheal aspiration, in *The Equine Hospital Manual* (eds K. Corley and J. Stephen), Blackwell, Oxford, pp. 68–70.

Part IV

Clinical Procedures by Body Systems: Locomotor System

27

Lameness Examination

Daniel J. Burba

27.1 Purpose

- To determine the cause of musculoskeletal unsoundness (lameness) in the horse by pinpointing where the source of lameness is occurring and using additional diagnostic imaging to specify the etiology.
- To perform and record a subjective evaluation of the horse's lameness, using the universally accepted grading scale for lameness established by the American Association of Equine Practitioners to classify the degree of lameness (Table 27.1).

27.2 Complications

None.

27.3 Equipment Required

- Form to record findings
- Hoof testers
- Hoof pick
- Lunge rope and whip
- Firm, flat working surface
- Local anesthetic, syringes, and hypodermic needles, supplies for aseptic scrub (see Chapters 28 and 29).
- Imaging capabilities, such as an X-ray unit, ultrasound unit with tendon probe, etc., are needed to confirm lameness examination findings.

27.4 Restraint and Positioning

- It is important to have an assistant with good horse-handling and restraint skills when performing lameness examination.
- Horses often object to injections in the lower limbs.
- Use of a nose or shoulder twitch may be necessary during the injections.

Table 27.1 American Association of Equine Practitioners grading scheme for lamenesses in horses

Grade 1	Difficult to observe; not consistently apparent regardless of circumstances, i.e. weight carrying, circling, inclines, hard surfaces, etc.
Grade 2	Difficult to observe at a walk or a trot in a straight line; consistently apparent under certain circumstances, i.e. weight carrying, circling, inclines, hard surfaces, etc.
Grade 3	Consistently observable at a trot under all circumstances
Grade 4	Obvious lameness; marked nodding, hitching, or shortened stride, reluctance to move
Grade 5	Minimal weight bearing in motion and/or at rest; inability to move

Manual of Clinical Procedures in the Horse, First Edition. Edited by Lais R.R. Costa and Mary Rose Paradis.
© 2018 John Wiley & Sons, Inc. Published 2018 by John Wiley & Sons, Inc.

27.5 Procedure: Lameness Examination

Technical action	Rationale
Obtain a history. How did the owner notice the unsoundness? Did it occur after a specific event? How long has the horse been lame? What is the use of the horse?	Getting an accurate history can facilitate the localization and etiology of the pain.
Evaluate the horse's conformation. Start by looking at the horse from the front, then the sides and rear. Compare one side to the other for asymmetry or swelling.	The relationship between conformation and lameness is well established, such that poor conformation can predispose a horse to certain types of lameness.
Palpate the horse's back (Figure 27.1). Start by palpating along the thoracic and lumbar vertebrae by placing your thumbs on one side of the dorsal spine and fingers on the contralateral side and gently, yet firmly, pressing along the epaxial muscles.	Back soreness can be a cause of locomotor disorders or the result of compensation for lameness. A horse with muscle soreness that is sensitive to touch will flinch.
Palpation of the forelimb starts at the shoulder and moves distally. Firmly push on the horse at the point of the shoulder. Grasp the biceps insertion just distal to the point of the shoulder (Figure 27.2).	If a painful response is elicited, it indicates bicipital tendonitis or bursitis.
Next, palpate the dorsum of carpal joints and palpate the palmar pouches of the metacarpophalangeal (fetlock) joints (Figure 27.3).	If the joint feels distended, this indicates joint effusion.
Palpate the flexor tendons and suspensory ligament by running the thumb on one side and the fingers on the contralateral side (Figure 27.4).	Identify any abnormalities of the superficial and deep digital flexor tendons and the suspensory ligament by palpating individually.
Work down the entire structure, feeling for thickening, swelling, edema, heat, or pain.	If a painful response is identified, it indicates tendonitis or desmitis.
Pick up each forelimb and flex the carpus and fetlock separately to assess the range of motion and any pain response to flexion.	If pain is elicited or there is reduced range of motion, then this may be an indication of capsulitis.
While the limb is picked up, apply thumb pressure at the insertion of the suspensory, at the palmar aspect of the proximal metacarpus (Figure 27.5).	If pain reflex is elicited it indicates proximal suspensory desmitis.
Pick the forelimb up and grasp the foot and pull the leg forward (Figure 27.6).	If the horse objects to this by trying to pull away this may be an indication of scapulohumeral joint or triceps pain.
Palpation of the hindlimb starts at the croup and moves distally. First, apply pressure over the croup, tuber coxae, tuber ischia, and greater trochanter (point of hip) with your fingers (Figure 27.7).	Pain response to pressure may be an indication of trochanteric bursitis.

Technical action	Rationale
Palpate the front of the stifle area, just above the tibial crest (Figure 27.8).	If effusion is present this may indicate gonitis (inflammation of the femoropatellar joint).
Palpate the front of the hock (i.e., the tarsocrural joint) (Figure 27.9).	If effusion is present this may indicate bog spavin.
Palpate the fetlock joint.	Refer to palpation of the forelimb fetlock.
Palpate the flexor tendons and suspensory apparatus with thumb and forefingers.	Refer to palpation of the forelimb flexor tendons.
Inspection of the foot. Clean each hoof out with a hoof pick (Figure 27.10).	This is important for the assessment of the integrity of the sole and frog, and for white line disorders.
Apply hoof testers to each foot (Figures 27.11 and 27.12). Use farrier's stance when applying the hoof testers to a hoof. For the forelimb, the limb is flexed and the examiner stands next to the forelimb, facing the rear of the horse, and places the forelimb between their legs and grasps the horse's limb at the pastern with their knees (Figure 27.11). For the hindlimbs, the examiner faces the rear of the horse, picks up the limb, takes two steps behind the horse, and rests the limb on the thigh (Figure 27.12).	This frees up the hands to perform the examination. Hoof testers are routinely not applied to the rear feet unless there is complaint or suspicion of hindlimb lameness. An eight-point pressure technique is applied around the hoof wall to determine if there is response to pressure applied to the hoof (see Chapter 32). Generally a pain response by a horse is a withdrawal reflex of the limb. It has to be repeatable before it is considered it a true pain response.
Observation of the horse in motion. Examine the horse going away, coming towards, and passing by you (Figure 27.13). Perform this first at a walk then at a trot with someone on a lead line. Pay particular attention to the up and down movement of the head, rise and fall of the croups, length of the stride of the fore- and hindlimbs, and the amount of drop of the fetlocks.	A rise in the head when the horse is landing on a forelimb indicates lameness in that leg. This is best seen from the side as the horse is moving at a trot on a lead. If the lameness is emanating from a hindlimb, the hip will rise on the lame limb. This is best seen from the side and rear with the horse moving at a trot on a lead. Look at the stride of the limbs, particularly the hindlimbs in relation to the forelimbs. If the lameness is in a hindlimb the distance of the placement of the foot in relation to the front foot will be a longer distance compared to the contralateral limb.
Have the horse lunged in a 20 m circle to the left and right (Figure 27.14).	This often will exacerbate the lameness when the affected limb is to the inside of the circle.
Perform flexion tests. Each flexion test is performed for 60 seconds. After 60 seconds, the limb is quickly but quietly placed on the ground and the horse is immediately trotted off to see if lameness is induced or a pre-flexion lameness is exacerbated. Each flexion test is performed on the contralateral limb before moving on to the next joint flexion.	Flexion tests add stress to the horse's joints, thus intensifying the lameness and helping to localize the source of the unsoundness.
Distal forelimb flexion. Pick up the limb, move to the front of the horse, and place an arm on either side of the limb (medial and lateral), clasping your hands around the hoof (Figure 27.15). Push the carpus toward your chest, slightly extending the carpus but focusing on flexing the distal limb. Perform the same examination on the contralateral limb.	This flexion helps to isolate the source of the lameness to the metacarpal phalangeal or interphalangeal joints of the forelimb. Care must be taken to not flex the carpal joint during this test.

(continued)

Technical action	Rationale
Carpal flexion. Pick up the limb, face toward the side of the horse, place a hand on the medial and lateral aspect of the limb, cradle the metacarpus with your hands, and pull it up against the back of the antebrachium so that the carpus is pointing toward the front of the horse (Figure 27.16).	Generally the timed flexion tests are not performed proximal to the carpus as they are often difficult to interpret. However, the radiohumeral joint and the scapulohumeral joints can be manipulated to try to elicit pain by picking up the limb and flexing and extending each joint.
Distal rearlimb flexion. Flex the distal limb by picking up the limb, moving a couple steps behind the horse, placing a hand on each side of the limb, and clasping the hoof with your hands (Figure 27.17). Slightly extend the limb backward while the flexion is focused on the distal limb.	This flexion helps to isolate lameness to the metatarsophalangeal and phalangeal joints.
Spavin flexion. Flex the tarsus by standing beside the hindlimb, picking up the limb by grabbing the metatarsus with a hand placed medially and laterally, straightening your back, and pulling up on the limb until the metatarsus is horizontal to the ground (Figure 27.18).	This flexion will also flex the stifle due to the reciprocal apparatus.
Perineural/intraarticular anesthesia. Once the lameness has been localized to a limb(s), perineural or intraarticular anesthesia may be necessary to localize the lameness to a specific site (see Chapter 28).	
Diagnostic imaging. Once the source of the lameness has been identified, diagnostic imaging is used to characterize the lesion. Imaging modalities often used to further evaluate lameness in horses include: (a) ultrasonography (b) radiography (c) computed tomography (d) magnetic resonance imaging (MRI) (e) nuclear medicine (aka bone scan) The choice of the modality will depend on the structures suspected to be the source of the lameness.	Ultrasonography is excellent for imaging tendons, ligaments, bursi (biceptial and trochanteric) or skeletal muscle. It is also helpful in certain joints, such as the coxafemoral and femorotibial joints. Radiography and computed tomography are excellent for visualizing skeletal lesions of the distal limb. Magnetic resonance imaging (MRI) provides detailed images of soft tissue lesions of the distal limb. Nuclear scintigraphy (bone scan) helps localize non-specific causes of lameness.

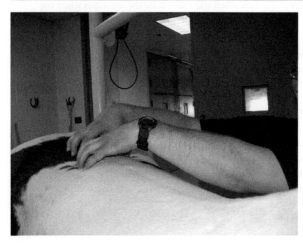

Figure 27.1 To assess back soreness, thumbs are placed on one side of the dorsal spine and fingers on the contralateral side, and pressure is gently, yet firmly, placed along the epaxial muscles.

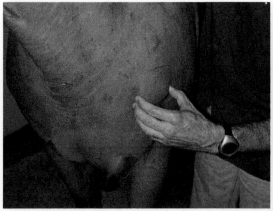

Figure 27.2 To assess bicipital tendonitis or bursitis, the biceps tendon is grasped just distal to the point of the shoulder.

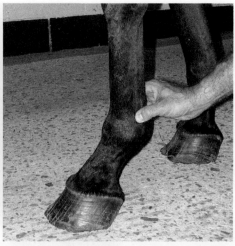

Figure 27.3 Palpation of the palmar pouch of the metacarpophalangeal joint for effusion.

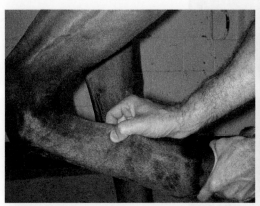

Figure 27.4 Palpation of the forelimb flexor tendons. The tendon is grasped between the thumb and forefingers.

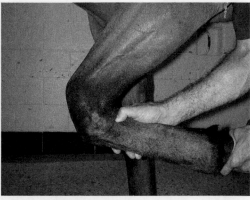

Figure 27.5 Palpation of the proximal forelimb suspensory. Thumb pressure is applied to the insertion of the suspensory, at the palmar aspect of the proximal metacarpus.

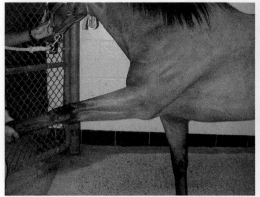

Figure 27.6 Evaluation for scapulohumoral joint or triceps pain. The forelimb is picked up by the foot and the limb is pulled forward.

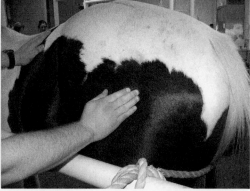

Figure 27.7 To assess trochanteric bursal pain, pressure is applied to the point of the hip (greater trochanter).

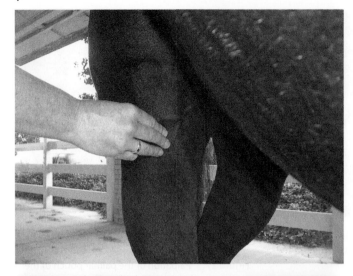

Figure 27.8 The front of the stifle area is palpated, just above the tibial crest, to assess for femorpatellar effusion.

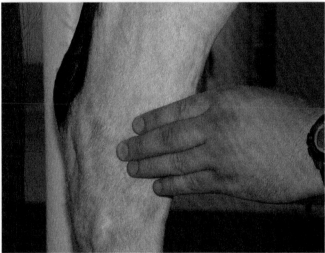

Figure 27.9 Palpation of the tarsocrural joint for effusion.

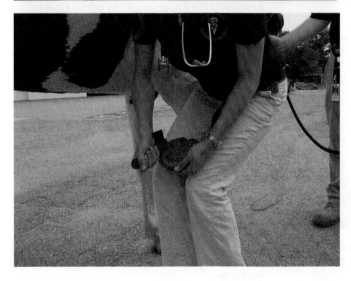

Figure 27.10 The foot is cleaned out with a hoof pick to assess the integrity of the sole and frog, and for white line disorders. This should be performed prior to applying hoof testers to the hoof.

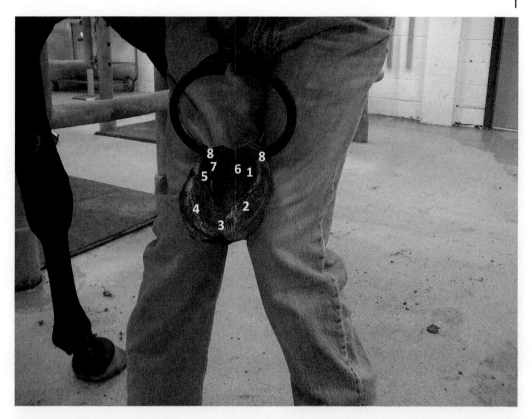

Figure 27.11 The proper position for applying hoof testers to the forelimb hoof. The eight-point application of hoof testers: (1) lateral heel, (2) lateral quarter, (3) toe, (4) medial quarter, (5) medial heel, (6) lateral sulcus, (7) medial sulcus, (8) across the heels. One jaw of the hoof testers is placed on the outer wall with the other placed on the sole at the various points.

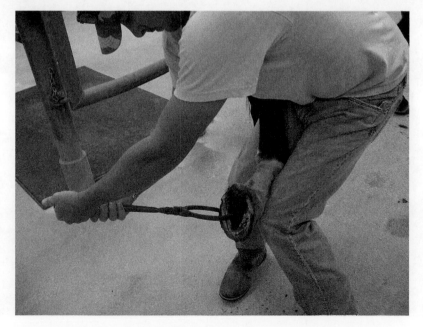

Figure 27.12 Proper position for holding the distal limb to apply hoof testers to the hind feet.

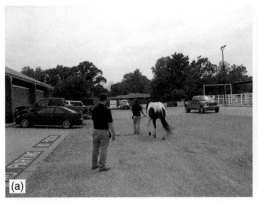

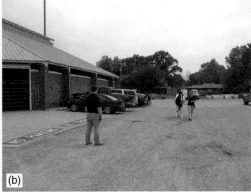

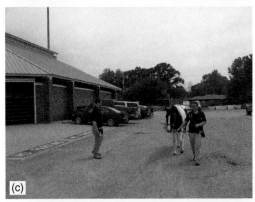

Figure 27.13 Evaluation of a horse for lameness. The horse should be observed (a) moving away from the evaluator, (b) moving toward the evaluator, and (c) from the side.

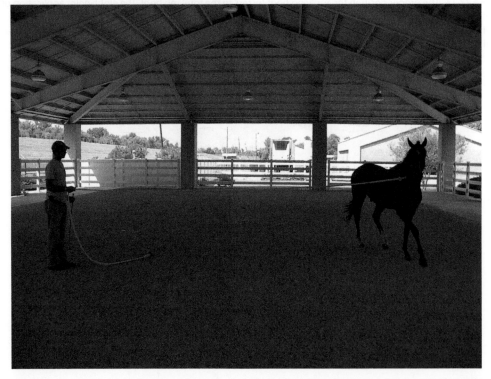

Figure 27.14 As part of a lameness examination the horse is observed on a lunge line moving in both directions.

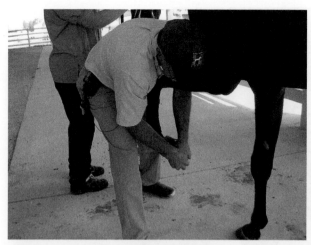

Figure 27.15 Flexion of the distal forelimb.

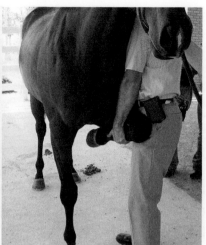

Figure 27.16 Flexion of the carpus.

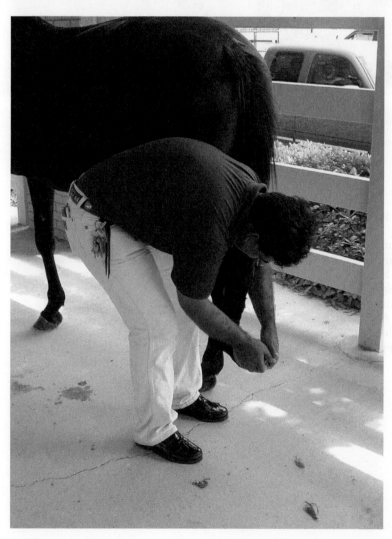

Figure 27.17 Flexion of the distal hindlimb.

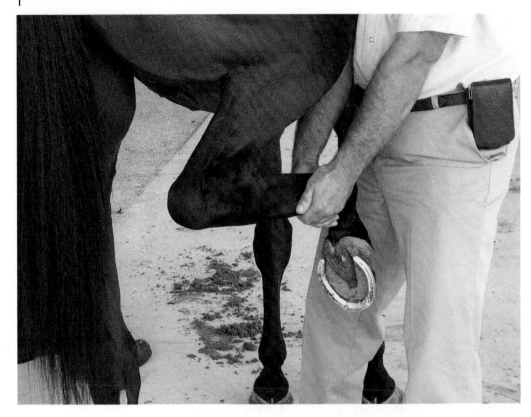

Figure 27.18 Flexion of the hock/stifle (spavin test).

Bibiography and Further Reading

Ross, M.W. (2003) The lameness examination, in *Diagnosis and Management of Lameness in the Horse* (eds M.W. Ross and S.J. Dyson), W.B. Saunders, Philadelphia.

Stashak, T.S. (2002) Examination for lameness, in *Adam's Lameness in Horses*, 5th edn (ed. T.S. Stashak), Lippincott Williams & Wilkins, Philadelphia, pp. 113–183.

Lameness exams: Evaluating the lame horse (2005). AAEP, https://aaep.org/horsehealth/lameness-exams-evaluating-lame-horse

28

Perineural Anesthesia of the Limbs

Daniel J. Burba

28.1 Purpose

- To confirm or identify the site (or sites) of pain that is (are) causing lameness.
- To localize the source of pain. Perineural anesthesia therefore must be performed in a systematic manner, starting with the distal extremity and progressing upward.

- To further localize the lameness of the forelimb or hindlimb that was not specifically identified on baseline observation of the horse.
- Table 28.1 summarizes the nerve blocks discussed in this chapter.

Table 28.1 Description of the nerve blocks and the corresponding areas and structures desensitized

Name of the nerve block	Nerves and locations	Area anesthetized	Significant structures desensitized
Palmar/plantar digital	Palmar/plantar digital nerves (lateral and medial) just above the heels	The heel region of the foot.	Navicular bone, navicular bursa, distal insertion of the DDFT and digital cushion, corium of the frog, palmar/plantar third of the lamellar corium, corium of the sole, palmar/ plantar third of the distal phalanx.
Abaxial sesamoid	Palmar/plantar digital nerves (lateral and medial) along the abaxial surface proximal sesamoidal bones.	The entire foot.	All three phalanges, proximal and distal interphalangeal joints, lamellar corium and corium of the sole, dosral branches of the suspensory ligament, distal insertions of the digital extensor and flexor tendons, distal sesamoidean ligaments.
Low four-point	Palmar/plantar nerve (lateral and medial) and palmar/plantar metacarpal/metatarsal nerves at the level of distal end of the second and fourth metacarpal/ metatarsal bones.	The limb distal to the fetlock.	Same structures as above and metacarpo/tarsophalangeal joint, flexor tendon sheath, branches of the suspensory ligament.

(continued)

Manual of Clinical Procedures in the Horse, First Edition. Edited by Lais R.R. Costa and Mary Rose Paradis.
© 2018 John Wiley & Sons, Inc. Published 2018 by John Wiley & Sons, Inc.

Name of the nerve block	Nerves and locations	Area anesthetized	Significant structures desensitized
High four-point	Palmar/plantar digital nerve (lateral and medial) and palmar/plantar metacarpal/metatarsal nerves at the level of the proximal metacarpus/metatarsus.	Palmar/plantar region of the metacarpus/metatarsus.	Suspensory ligament, SDFT, DDFT and the limb distally, except the third metacarpal or metatarsal bone.
Ulnar	Ulnar nerve about 10 cm above the accessory carpal bone on the caudal aspect of the forearm.	Distal forearm and distally to the fetlock.	The carpal canal, portion of the accessory carpal bone, proximal suspensory ligament, and proximal flexor tendons.
Median	Median nerve at the caudal aspect of the radius, cranial to the origin of the flexor carpi radialis muscle.	Part of the carpus and antebrachium area.	Alone it will desensitize the suspensory ligament, SDFT, DDFT, and the limb distally, except the third metacarpal or metatarsal bone. When used in conjunction with the ulnar nerve block, it will block out most of the distal limb.
Tibial	Tibial nerve about 10 cm above the point of the hock on the medial aspect of the limb, between the Achilles tendon and the deep flexor tendon.	Plantar tarsus In conjunction with the blocking of the deep and superficial peroneal nerves, will desensitize the hock and distal structures.	Plantar metatarsus, Achilles tendon, and calcaneus
Superficial and deep peroneal	Superficial and deep peroneal (fibular) nerves about 10 cm above the point of the hock on the lateral aspect of the limb.	Tarsus and distally	Tarsal structures, suspensory ligament, DDFT and SDFT.

DDFT, Deep digital flexor tendon; SDFT, superficial digital flexor tendon.

28.2 Complications

- Post-injection edema.
- Post-injection infection (rare).

28.3 Equipment Required

- 4 × 4 gauze soaked in disinfectant scrub
- 4 × 4 gauze soaked in alcohol
- Examination gloves
- 22-gauge × 1.5″ and 25-gauge hypodermic needles
- Syringes: 3, 6, and 10 ml
- Nose twitch
- Bottle of local anesthetic drug (carbocaine or lidocaine)

28.4 Restraint and Positioning

- It is important to have an assistant with good horse-handling skills and restraint when performing perineural anesthesia.
- Horses often object to injections in the lower limbs.
- Use of a nose or shoulder twitch may be necessary.
- Sedation is not ideal because the animal will need to be examined in motion 5–10 minutes after the injection of local anesthetic drug.

28.5 Procedure: General

Technical action	Rationale
Hair over injection site(s) generally does not need to be clipped.	If hair over the site is extremely long, clip the hair.
Prep the skin with disinfectant scrub, alternating with alcohol (Figure 28.1).	It is best to use three scrub cycles.
Use 3 ml syringes and draw up the anesthetic.	
Insert a 25-gauge needle subcutaneously at the injection site, then connect the loaded syringe and inject the anesthetic. The volume of anesthetic varies for each block (see specific blocks).	It is important to have a thorough working knowledge of the neurovascular anatomy of the equine limbs.
Allow 5–10 minutes to lapse, text the area for desensitization then jog the patient on a lead.	The patient is observed to determine if the lameness has improved.

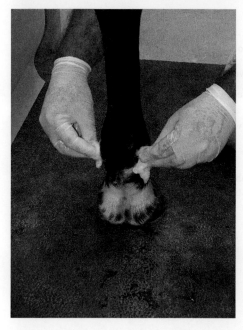

Figure 28.1 Preparation of the skin with disinfectant alternating with alcohol for a perineural injection of anesthetic.

28.6 Procedure: Injection of Specific Perineural Sites

Palmar/Plantar Digital

This block is used to anesthetize the heel region of the foot.

Technical action	Rationale
Prep the site: the medial and lateral abaxial surface of the deep flexor tendon just above the heel bulbs.	
Insert a 25-gauge needle alongside the flexor tendon (medial and lateral) over the palmar digital neurovascular bundle just above the heel bulb (Figure 28.2). Inject 2 ml of anesthetic into each site.	Try to leave the horse standing on the limb. In some horses it may be less challenging to pick up the foot to perform the injection.

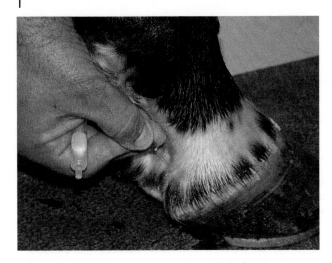

Figure 28.2 Placement of needle for a palmar digital nerve block. Inject 2 ml of anesthetic into each site.

Abaxial Sesamoid

This block is used to anesthetize the entire the foot.

Technical action	Rationale
Prep the site: the medial and lateral abaxial surface of the metacarpophalangeal joint over the sesamoid bones.	Nerves blocked: • medial and lateral palmar/plantar nerves.
Palpate the neurovascular bundle along the abaxial surface of the sesamoids (medial and lateral).	You will be able to roll it under your finger.
Insert the needle alongside the neurovascular bundle on each side (medial and lateral) (Figure 28.3). Inject 2 ml of anesthetic into each site.	A subcutaneous bleb should be seen as the anesthetic is injected.

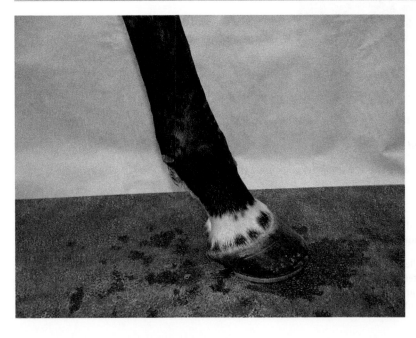

Figure 28.3 Needle placed at the site for an abaxial nerve block. Inject 2 ml of anesthetic into each site.

Low Four-point

This block is used to anesthetize the limb from the fetlock distally.

Technical action	Rationale
Prep the site: medial and lateral surface of the distal metacarpus/metatarsus from the button of splints to just above the fetlock.	Nerves blocked: • medial and lateral metacarpal/metatarsal nerves • medial and lateral palmar/plantar nerves.
Insert a 25-gauge needle just palmar/plantar to the suspensory ligament alongside the abaxial edge of deep digital flexor tendon on the medial (block 1) and lateral (block 2) side (A in Figure 28.4). Inject 3 ml of anesthetic into each site.	This will block the medial and lateral palmar nerves.
Insert a 25-gauge needle at the distal tip of the button of the medial (block 3) and lateral (block 4) splint bones (B in Figure 28.4). Inject 3 ml of anesthetic into each site.	This will block the medial and lateral metacarpal/metatarsal nerves. The needles are inserted at the level as the buttons of the splint bones. Each block is performed individually.

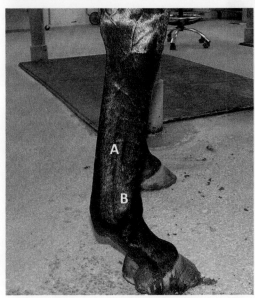

Figure 28.4 Low four-point nerve block: A, needle inserted at the site for palmar nerve block (medial and lateral); B, needle positioned at the site for a metacarpal nerve block (medial and lateral). Inject 3 ml of anesthetic into each of the 4 sites.

High Four-point

This block is used to anesthetize the suspensory, flexor tendons, and the limb distally, not including the metacarpal or metatarsal bone.

Technical action	Rationale
Prep the site: palmar/plantar on the proximal region of the medial and lateral metacarpus/metatarsus distal to the carpus/tarsus.	Nerves blocked: • medial and lateral metacarpal/metatarsal nerves • medial and lateral palmar/plantar nerves.
Insert a 22-gauge needle in a horizontal fashion in the groove between the suspensory ligament and the deep digital flexor tendon on the medial and lateral side of the limb (A in Figure 28.5). Inject 3 ml of anesthetic into each site.	This will block the proximal medial and lateral palmar/plantar nerves. You should feel the needle pop through heavy fascia.

(continued)

Technical action	Rationale
Insert a 22-gauge needle horizontally in the space between the splint bone (B in Figure 28.5) and the suspensory ligament, on the medial and lateral side of the limb. Inject 3 ml of anesthetic into each site.	This will block the medial and lateral proximal metacarpal/metatarsal nerves. The needle is slid off the back edge of the splint bone and directed toward the axial surface of the splint bone to a depth of approximately ¾″.

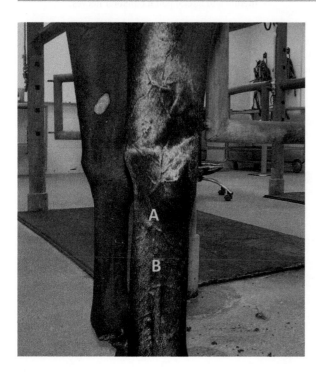

Figure 28.5 High four-point nerve block: A, needle inserted at the site for palmar nerve block (medial and lateral); B, needle positioned at the site for a metacarpal nerve block (medial and lateral). Inject 3 ml of anesthetic into each of the 4 sites.

Ulnar Nerve

This block is used to anesthetize the carpal canal and proximal suspensory.

Technical action	Rationale
Prep the site: 4 × 4 cm area centered 10 cm proximal to the accessory carpal bone on the caudal surface of the distal antebrachium (Figure 28.6a).	
Palpate the groove between the flexor carpi ulnaris and ulnaris lateralis muscles. Insert a 22-gauge needle horizontally in this groove to a depth of approximately 1.5 cm below the skin surface and inject 5-10 ml of local anesthetic (Figure 28.6b).	The depth of the nerve is variable. The use of 10 ml of local anesthetic increases the change of blocking both deeply and superficially.

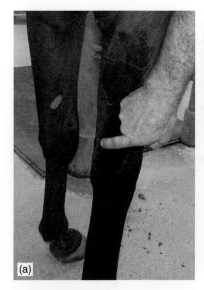

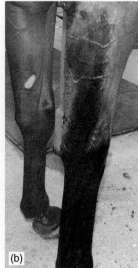

Figure 28.6 Ulnar nerve block. (a) Site for an ulnar nerve block. (b) Needle inserted at the site for an ulnar nerve block. Inject 5 ml of anesthetic into this site.

Median Nerve

This block is used to anesthetize part of the carpus and antebrachium, and when used in conjunction with the ulnar nerve block it will block out any pain distal to the block.

Technical action	Rationale
Prep the site: 5 × 5 cm area centered over the mid-diaphysis of the radius, on the medial side of the antebrachium.	
Palpate the radius where it lies directly underneath the skin distal to the pectorals (Figure 28.7a).	The nerve lies subcutaneously and directly on the caudal surface of the radius.
Insert a 22-gauge needle horizontally along the caudal cortex and inject 6 ml of anesthetic (Figure 28.7b).	

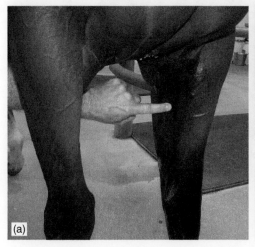

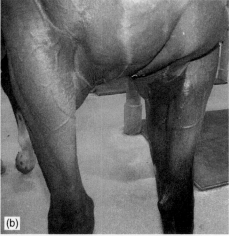

Figure 28.7 Median nerve block. (a) Site for a median nerve block. (b) Needle inserted at the site for a median nerve block. Inject 6 ml of anesthetic into this site.

Tibial Nerve

In conjunction with the blocking of the deep and superficial peroneal nerves, this block will desensitize the hock and distal structures.

Technical action	Rationale
Prep the site: 5 × 5 cm area centered approximately 10 cm above the point of the hock on the medial region of the gaskin.	Local injection of the skin with 1 ml of local anesthetic may make it easier to place the large needle.
Insert a 22-gauge, 1.5″ needle horizontally between the Achilles and deep flexor tendons (Figure 28.8).	The leg can be flexed to facilitate palpation of the nerve.
Inject 10 ml of anesthetic, deep and superficially.	Performing this block alone will block the proximal suspensory.

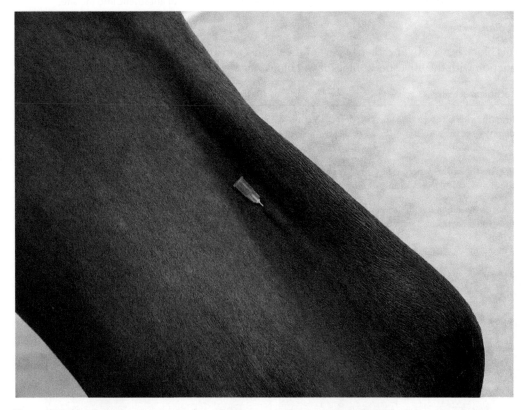

Figure 28.8 Needle inserted at the site for a tibial nerve block. Inject 10 ml of anesthetic into this site.

Superficial and Deep Peroneal Nerves

This block is used to complete the anesthesia of the hock.

Technical action	Rationale
Prep the site: 5 × 5 cm area centered approximately 10 cm above the point of the hock on the lateral region of the gaskin.	Local injection of the skin with 1 ml of local anesthetic may make it easier to place the large needle.
Insert a 22-gauge 1.5″ needle horizontally in a groove formed between the muscle bellies of the lateral digital extensor and long digital extensor muscles (Figure 28.9).	
Insert the needle deep (to the hub) and inject 10 ml. Retract the needle and in doing so inject another 10 ml to get the superficial peroneal nerve.	A total volume to be injected is 20 ml for adequately block the peroneal nerves. Loss of skin sensation over the plantar region of the pastern and heels will occur.

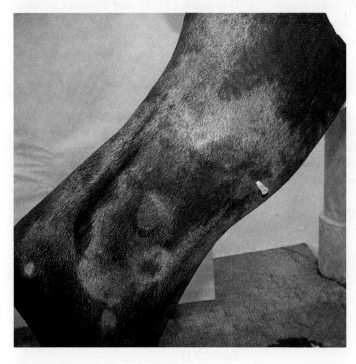

Figure 28.9 Needle inserted at the site for a deep and superficial peroneal nerve block. Inject 10 ml of anesthetic into the deep site, and another 10 ml superficially as you retract the needle.

Bibliography and Further Reading

Bassage, L.H. and Ross, M.W. (2011) Diagnostic analgesia, in *Diagnosis and Management of Lameness in the Horse* (eds M.W. Ross and S.J. Dyson), W.B. Saunders, Philadelphia.

Moyer, W., Schumacher, J., and Schumacher, J. (2007) *A Guide to Equine Joint Injection*, 4th edn (eds W. Moyer, J. Schumacher, and J. Schumacher), Veterinary Learning Systems, Yardley.

Stashak, T.S. (2002) Procedures for examination, in *Adams' Lameness in Horses*, 5th edn (ed. T.S. Stashak), Lippincott Williams & Wilkins, Philadelphia, pp. 160–167.

29

Arthrocentesis and Intraarticular Analgesia/Anesthesia

Daniel J. Burba

Arthrocentesis must be performed under strict aseptic conditions. Moreover, the appropriate technique requires a thorough working knowledge of joint anatomy. Some joints can be injected by more than one approach, but for simplicity only one approach will be described for each joint.

29.1 Purpose

- To obtain a sample of synovial fluid for analysis. This is important in assessing if a joint is septic, especially in foals.
- To inject an anesthetic into an articular space to assess if the joint is the source of lameness.
- To inject a therapeutic agent into the joint.

29.2 Complications

- Iatrogenic septic arthritis

29.3 Equipment Required

- Electric hair clippers
- 4 × 4 gauze soaked in disinfectant scrub
- 4 × 4 gauze soaked in alcohol
- Examination gloves
- Sterile surgical gloves
- Disposable 18-, 20- and 22-gauge needles (Table 29.1):
  - for most joint injections a 20-gauge 1½″ needle is recommended, except for the femoropatellar joint
  - an 18- or 19-gauge 3½″ spinal needle is recommended for injection of the femoropatellar joint.
- Disposable sterile syringes (Table 29.1): 12, 20, 35, and 50 ml (if injecting an anesthetic).
- Sterile evacuated tube containing EDTA (lavender top), if a sample of synovial fluid is to be collected for fluid analysis.
- Sterile evacuated tube without additives (red top), if sample of synovial fluid is to be collected for bacterial culture/sensitivity.
- Nose twitch
- Sedation (optional)
- New unused bottle(s) of carbocaine or lidocaine (the volume of anesthetic drug appropriate for each joint is listed in Table 29.1).

Table 29.1 Supplies for injection of anesthetics into specific synovial structures. Length of the needles should be 1 ½″, except for those indicated by *, which should be spinal needles 3 ½″ with stylet.

Synovial Structure	Syringe size (ml)	Needle size (gauge)	Drug volume (ml)
Distal interphalangeal joint	12	20	6
Navicular bursa	12	18, 19*	5
Proximal interphalangeal joint	12	20	6
Metacarpophalangeal/metatarsophalangeal joint	12	20	10
Middle carpal and radiocarpal joints	12	20	10
Tarsocrural joint	20	20	15
Distal intertarsal joint	6	22	3
Tarsometatarsal joint	6	20	3
Femoropatellar joint	60	18, 19*	50
Lateral femorotibial joint	20	20	20
Medial femorotibial joint	20	20	20

Table 29.2 Approach for specific joints

Joint	Area to be prepared	Approach
Distal interphalangeal	Distal dorsal region of the pastern just above and including the coronary band	Point of needle insertion: on the midline, 1 cm dorsal to the coronary band, perpendicular with the dorsal surface of the hoof wall.
Navicular bursa	Heel bulbs (especially the sulci between the heel bulbs)	Palmar/plantar approach: with the distal limb flexed.
	Make a mark on the lateral hoof wall at a point ½″ distal to the coronary and halfway between the palmar and dorsal aspects of the coronary band.	Point of needle insertion: immediately above the coronary band, aiming toward the mark on the lateral hoof wall at a point ½″ distal to the coronary and halfway between the palmar and dorsal aspects of the coronary band, staying mid-sagittal.
Proximal interphalangeal	Palmaro/plantarolateral pastern region	With the limb flexed
		Point of needle insertion: from a lateral to medial direction with the needle point pointing distally toward the midline, just above the palmar/plantar border of the lateral eminence of P2.

(continued)

Joint	Area to be prepared	Approach
Metacarpophalangeal and metatarsophalangeal	Dorsal surface of joint	Dorsolateral approach
		Point of needle insertion: from lateral to medial just above the palpated dorsolateral eminence of P1, directing the needle slightly caudally and slightly angled distally toward the midline.
Middle carpal and radiocarpal	Dorsal surface of joints	Dorsolateral approach: with the carpus flexed and correctly positioned, identify the joint spaces located just abaxial to the extensor carpi radialis tendon.
		Point of needle insertion: from dorsal to caudal, directing it slightly axially.
Tarsocrural	Dorsomedial surface of joint pouch; medial to the saphenous vein	Point of needle insertion: dorsomedially, directing axially and plantarolaterally.
Distal intertarsal	Medial surface of tarsus between medial malleolus and proximal splint	Point of needle insertion: over the top edge of the cunean tendon at the intersection of a line between the medial malleolus and the top of the medial splint.
Tarsometatarsal	Plantarolateral surface of the tarsus and just above the proximal protuberance of the lateral splint	Point of needle insertion: in a depression just proximal to the top of the lateral splint.
		The needle is directed distally and 45 degrees to the vertical, aiming from plantar to medial toward the midline.
Femoropatellar	4″ × 4″ area between the medial and middle patellar ligaments just above the tibial crest	Point of needle insertion: 2 cm proximal to the top edge of the tibial crest between the medial and lateral patellar ligaments, and aiming from distal to proximal directing axially.
Lateral femorotibial joint	4″ × 4″ over the lateral patellar ligament	Point of needle insertion: just caudal to the palpable lateral patellar ligament.
		The needle is positioned horizontally and inserted directly lateral to medial.
Medial femorotibial joint	4″ × 4″ over the medial patellar ligament	Point of needle insertion: just caudal to the palpable medial patellar ligament.
		The needle is positioned horizontally and inserted directly medial to lateral.

29.4 Restraint

- Proper restraint is critical when performing arthrocentesis because movement may result in damage to the joint capsule or underlying cartilage.
- Application of a nose twitch is often adequate for most anesthetic joint injections.

- Restraint must be balanced with the need to have the horse fully awake if one is attempting to block out lameness. Once a joint is injected with an anesthetic, 20 minutes should be allowed to pass before jogging the horse.
- If septic arthritis is suspected, heavy sedation or possibly general anesthesia is required to obtain the sample of synovial fluid, flush the joint, and inject antibiotics.

29.5 Procedure: General preparations

Technical action	Rationale
If required, the horse is sedated.	Light sedation or twitch only if joint is being blocked for lameness diagnostic purposes (see Chapter 9).
Clip hair over the injection site(s) if the hair over the joint(s) to be injected is excessively long.	Clipping improves the ability to disinfect the skin more thoroughly.
Prepare skin with antiseptic scrub alternating with alcohol. Aseptic technique is imperative.	See Chapter 9 on aseptic preparation. It is best to use at least five scrub cycles. Leave the last scrub application on the skin until ready to inject. At that time an assistant can wipe it off with alcohol.
Put on surgical gloves.	Use the sterile paper liner that the gloves are wrapped in as a sterile working surface (Figure 29.1).
Have an assistant carefully open a syringe case and dump the syringe into the palm of your hand (Figure 29.1).	This will reduce the chances of contaminating the syringe.
Have an assistant open a needle case (usually an 18-gauge needle) and carefully place the syringe tip into the needle hub and remove the needle from the casing.	This will reduce the chances of contaminating the needle. This needle will be used to draw the medication or anesthetic drug.
Draw up the medication or anesthetic drug into the syringe. Place it on the sterile field.	Be careful not to contaminate the tip of loaded syringe. Do not use the same needle to draw the medication and to inject the joint. After drawing the medication or anesthetic drug, discard the needle.
Obtain a new needle from an assistant. A 20-gauge 1½″ needle is used for most joints. An 18-gauge 3½″ spinal needle is used for the femoropatellar, joint.	Changing needles between drawing up medication and placing a needle into the joint decreases the chance of joint contamination.
Have another assistant apply the nose twitch to the horse and ensure the horse is properly restrained.	Restraint is necessary to prevent the horse from moving when the needle enters the joint. Movement may result in joint trauma or loss of the needle onto the ground.
Have an assistant wipe the injection site with one last alcohol sponge with a single swipe, staying within the scrubbed area.	This removes the disinfectant scrub from the entry site.

(continued)

Technical action	Rationale
With the needle in one hand and an empty (dry) syringe in the other, insert the needle into the joint pouch with a quick and deliberate move.	Having a thorough working knowledge of joint anatomy is important when performing an arthrocentesis.
Once the needle is positioned correctly, the dry syringe is connected and aspiration of the synovial fluid is attempted. If the synovial fluid is to be analyzed, place a sample into an EDTA tube. A sample can also be placed in a sterile tube or culturette if a culture is needed.	Inability to obtain fluid does not mean the needle is not in the joint. Collection of fluid is not performed if a sample of synovial fluid is not needed. Placing a synovial fluid sample in blood culture media broth and incubating for 24 hours will enhance bacterial culture.
Disconnect the dry syringe, connect the syringe containing the medication or anesthetic, and proceed with the injection.	Medications can be antibiotics or anti-inflammatory drugs. Sterile physiologic solutions are used to flush the joint, if septic.
Remove the needle and wipe the injection site with alcohol.	This is performed to clean any blood from the injection site.
If anesthetic has been injected, 20 minutes is allowed to lapse.	The horse is walked on a lead during this time. This delay is necessary to allow the anesthetic to take full effect.
The patient is then jogged to determine if the anesthetic has localized the painful joint.	See Chapter 27 on lameness examination.

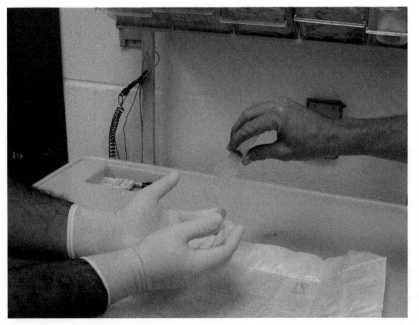

Figure 29.1 An assistant has carefully opened a syringe case and is dumping the sterile syringe into the palm of gloved hands. Notice the use of the sterile paper liner that the gloves were wrapped in as a sterile working surface.

29.6 Procedure: Injection of Anesthetics in Specific Synovial Structures

Technical action	Rationale/amplification
Table 29.2 summarizes the area to be prepared and the approach for each synovial structure described below.	
Distal interphalangeal joint	Generally, 6 ml of anesthetic is used to block this joint.
• Prepare the distal dorsal area of the pastern, including the coronary band. • Insert the needle on the midline, 1 cm dorsal to the coronary band. Place the needle perpendicular with the dorsal surface of the hoof wall (Figure 29.2). • Advance the needle until P2 is encountered and then retract it approximately 2 mm. • Inject the anesthetic.	
Navicular bursa	Generally, 5 ml of anesthetic is used to block this synovial structure.
• Prepare heel bulbs, paying particular attention to the sulci between the heel bulbs. • Using a marker pen, make a spot on the lateral hoof wall at a point ½″ distal to the coronary and halfway between the palmar and dorsal aspects of the coronary band. Using a palmar/plantar approach flex the distal limb. Rest the foot on a Hickman block or have someone hold it. • Insert a 3.5″ spinal needle immediately above the coronary band, aiming toward the spot marked on the hoof wall, staying mid-sagittal (Figures 29.3 and 29.4). • Advance the needle until you feel resistance to further advancement, which should be approximately 1.5–2″. • Inject the anesthetic.	
Proximal interphalangeal joint	Generally, 6 ml of anesthetic is used to block this joint.
• Prepare the palmaro/plantarolateral pastern region. • Flexing the limb, palpate the palmar/plantar border of the lateral eminence of P2 (Figure 29.5). Insert a 20-gaige needle from a lateral to medial direction just above the lateral eminence to a depth of approximately 2.5 cm (Figure 29.6). • Direct the needle along the edge of the flexor tendon. • Inject the anesthetic.	
Metacarpo/metatarsophalangeal joint	Keep the limb in weight-bearing mode when injecting this joint.
• Prepare the dorsal surface of the joint. • Using the dorsolateral approach, palpate the dorsolateral eminence of P1 to determine the place of needle insertion. • Insert a 20-gauge needle from lateral to medial just above the palpated dorsolateral eminence (Figure 29.7). • Direct the needle caudally and slightly angled distally. • Inject the anesthetic.	Generally, 10 ml of anesthetic is used to block this joint.

(continued)

Technical action	Rationale/amplification
Middle carpal and radiocarpal joints • Prepare the dorsal surface of the joints. • Using a dorsolateral approach, have an assistant place the limb between your knees with the carpus flexed to insert the needle (Figure 29.8). • Palpate the joint spaces located just abaxial to the extensor carpi radialis tendon. • Insert a 20-gauge needle from dorsal to caudal, directing it slightly axially (Figure 29.9). • Inject the anesthetic.	In a non-distended joint, a "dimple" or depression can be felt between the carpal bones. This is where the needle should be inserted. Generally, 10 ml of anesthetic is used to block each joint.
Tarsocrural joint • Prepare an area on the dorsomedial surface of joint pouch, medial to the saphenous vein. • Insert a 20-gauge needle dorsomedially, directed axially and plantarolaterally (Figure 29.10). • Inject the anesthetic.	Generally, 15 ml of anesthetic is used to block this joint.
Distal intertarsal joint • Prepare the medial surface of the tarsus between the medial malleolus and the proximal splint. • Insert a 22-gauge needle on a line drawn between the medial malleolus and the top of the medial splint and at the junction where this line crosses over the top edge of the cunean tendon (Figure 29.11). • Inject the anesthetic.	Deep palpation at the top edge of the cunean tendon with a gloved fingernail often reveals the indentable joint space. If the needle does not drop into the joint, walk the needle off the bone until does. Generally, 3 ml of anesthetic is used to block this joint.
Tarsometatarsal joint • Prepare the plantarolateral surface of the tarsus around the proximal protuberance of the lateral splint. • Palpate a depression just proximal to the top of the lateral splint. • Insert a 20-gauge needle at this depression, just proximal to the top of the lateral splint (Figure 29.12). • Direct the needle dorso-medially and distally at a 45-degree angle. • Inject the anesthetic.	Generally, 3 ml of anesthetic is used to block this joint.
Femoropatellar joint • Prepare a 4″ × 4″ area between the medial and middle patellar ligaments just above the tibial crest (Figure 29.13). • Insert a 3″ spinal needle 2 cm proximal to the top edge of the tibial crest between the medial and lateral patellar ligaments (Figure 29.14). • Direct the needle axially. • Inject the anesthetic.	Generally, 50 ml of anesthetic is used to block this joint.

Technical action	Rationale/amplification
Lateral femorotibial joint • Prepare a 4″ × 4″ area over the lateral patellar ligament. • Insert a 20-gauge needle horizontally into the palpable depression just caudal to the palpable lateral patellar ligament (Figure 29.15). • Inject the anesthetic.	Generally, 20 ml of anesthetic is used to block this joint.
Medial femorotibial joint • Prepare a 4″ × 4″ area over the medial patellar ligament. • Insert a 20-gauge needle horizontally into the palpable depression just caudal to the palpable medial patellar ligament (Figure 29.16). • Inject the anesthetic.	Generally, 20 ml of anesthetic is used to block this joint.

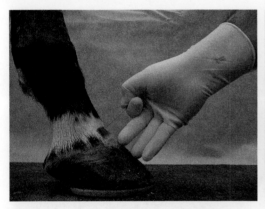

Figure 29.2 Injection of the distal interphalangeal joint. The needle is inserted into the joint perpendicular to the dorsal surface of the hoof wall approximately ½″ (1.25 cm) above the coronay band. Notice that the hair over the injection site has been clipped.

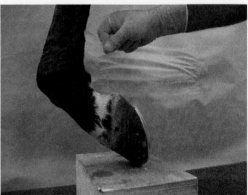

Figure 29.3 Injection of the navicular bursa. Using a marker pen, a spot (black) is made on the lateral hoof wall at a point ½″ (1–1.5 cm) distal to the coronary and halfway between the palmar and dorsal aspects of the coronary band. A Hickman block can be used to rest the tip of the foot on or someone can hold the foot with the distal limb flexed.

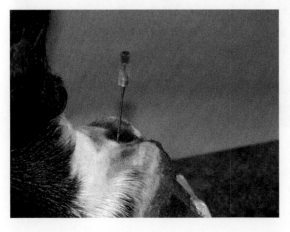

Figure 29.4 Injection of the navicular bursa. The needle is inserted immediately above the coronary band, aiming toward the spot marked on the hoof wall, staying mid-sagittal.

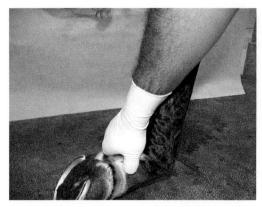

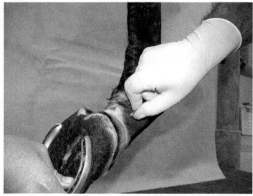

Figure 29.5 Injection of the proximal interphalangeal joint. The distal limb is flexed. The lateral eminence is palpated on palmaro/plantarolateral region of proximal of P2.

Figure 29.6 Injection of the proximal interphalangeal joint. The needle is inserted from a lateral to a medial direction just above the lateral eminence of P2 along the flexor tendon to a depth of approximately 2.5 cm.

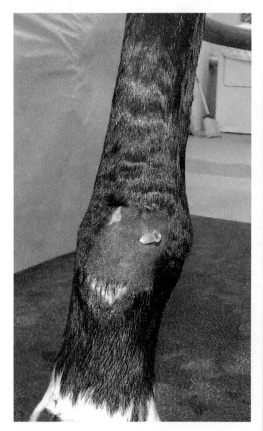

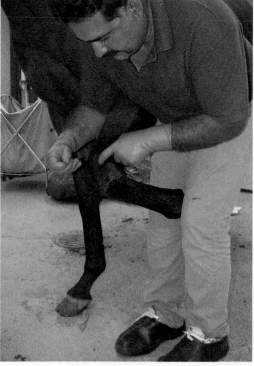

Figure 29.7 Injection of the metacarpophalangeal joint. A dorsolateral approach is taken. The dorsolateral eminence of P1 is palpated and the needle is inserted from lateral to medial just above the dorsolateral eminence. The needle is directed slightly caudally and angled slightly distally.

Figure 29.8 Injection of the radiocarpal and middle carpal joints. An assistant places the limb between the knees of the injector with the carpus flexed. The joint spaces are palpated just abaxial to the extensor carpi radialis tendon.

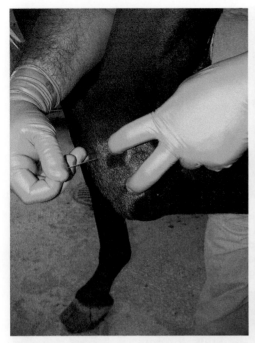

Figure 29.9 Injection of the radiocarpal and middle carpal joints. The needle is inserted dorsolaterally from dorsal to caudal, directing it slightly axially.

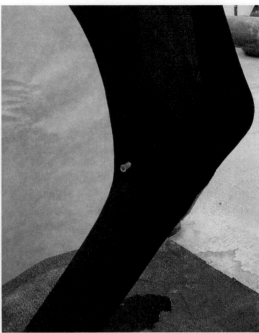

Figure 29.10 Injection of the tarsocrural joint. The needle is inserted dorsomedially and medial to the saphenous vein and directed axially and plantarolaterally.

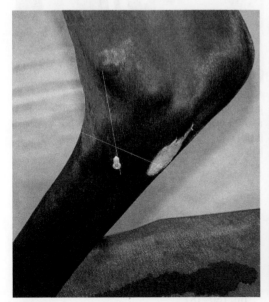

Figure 29.11 Injection of the distal intertarsal joint. The needle is inserted medially at a site determined by a line drawn between the medial malleolus and the top of the medial splint and at the junction where this line crosses over the top edge of the cunean tendon.

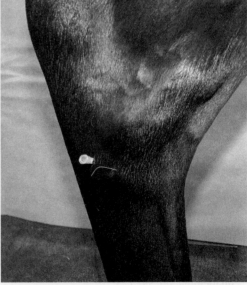

Figure 29.12 Injection of the tarsometatarsal joint. The needle is inserted just proximal to the top of the lateral splint in a depression felt by deep palpation with a gloved fingernail. The needle is directed dorsomedially and distally at 45 degrees. The curved line depicts the top of the fourth metacarpus.

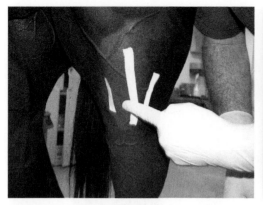

Figure 29.13 Site for injection of the femoropatellar joint. This is located between the middle and medial patellar ligaments, just above the tibial crest. The patellar ligaments are depicted by the strips of tape.

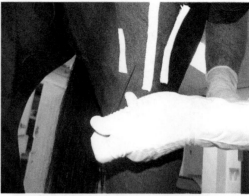

Figure 29.14 Injection of the femoropatellar joint. A spinal needle is inserted 2 cm proximal to the top edge of the tibial crest between the medial and lateral patellar ligaments and directed axially. The patellar ligaments are depicted by the strips of tape.

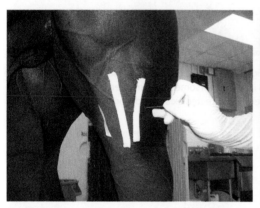

Figure 29.15 Injection of the lateral femorotibial joint. The needle is inserted horizontally just caudal to the palpable lateral patellar ligament. The needle is placed into the palpable depression. The patellar ligaments are depicted by the strips of tape.

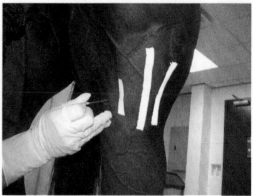

Figure 29.16 Injection of the medial femorotibial joint. The needle is inserted horizontally just caudal to the palpable medial patellar ligament. The needle is placed in the palpable depression. The patellar ligaments are depicted by the strips of tape.

Bibliography and Further Reading

Bassage, L.H. and Ross, M.W. (2011) Diagnostic analgesia, in *Diagnosis and Management of Lameness in the Horse* (eds M.W. Ross and S.J. Dyson), W.B. Saunders, Philadelphia, pp. 99–123.

Moyer, W., Schumacher, J., and Schumacher, J. (2007) *A Guide to Equine Joint Injection*, 4th edn, Veterinary Learning Systems, Yardley.

Stashak, T.S. (2002) Procedures for examination, in *Adams' Lameness in Horses*, 5th edn (ed. T.S. Stashak), Lippincott Williams & Wilkins, Philadelphia, pp. 160–181.

30

Intravenous Regional Limb Perfusion in Adult Horses

Mustajab H. Mirza, Jill R. Johnson, and Lais R.R. Costa

30.1 Purpose

- The principle of intravenous regional limb perfusion (IVRLP) is to occlude venous drainage from the limb then, under pressure, retro fill the vascular space distal to the tourniquet with antimicrobial solutions, which are temporarily retained in the vascular space by tourniquet and allowed to diffuse into the surrounding tissues of the isolated region.
- To achieve high levels of antimicrobials in target tissues of the distal limb of the horse, specifically below the stifle and elbow, by delivering a high concentration of antibiotics intravenously in the region.
- To provide adjunctive treatment for septic conditions of the distal limb of the horse, including iatrogenic septic arthritis subsequent to intra-articular injection of the carpus, tarsus, metacarpo-phalangeal, metatarsal-phalangeal, and distal inter-phalangeal joints, osteomyelitis, and soft tissue infections of the distal limb refractory to topical and systemic antimicrobial treatment alone.
- Regional limb perfusion in neonatal foals is discussed in Chapter 59.

30.2 Complications

- Perivascular leakage of antimicrobial drugs
- Venous thrombosis
- Hematoma
- Cutaneous necrosis
- Cellulitis

- Distal limb ischemia and sloughing of tissue.
- In the presence of cellulitis, there is a chance that regional perfusion under pressure will facilitate the spread of the infection, therefore, the use of IVRLP in horses with primary cellulitis should be avoided.

30.3 Restraint and Positioning

- IVRLP can be performed in anesthetized horses while they are in lateral or dorsal recumbency (see Chapter 76) or on standing horses. When IVRLP is performed on the animal in the standing position, it requires heavy sedation with a alpha-2 agonist (e.g., xylazine at a dose of 0.5 mg/kg) in combination with an opioid agonist-antagonist (e.g., butorphanol at a dose of 0.04 mg/kg). See Chapter 9 for detailed discussion of sedation.

30.4 Equipment Required

- Clippers
- Supplies for aseptic preparation of injection site (see Chapter 10).
- Esmarch compression bandage (6″ wide is preferred) to drain blood from the distal limb.
- Wide tourniquet, either:
  - pneumatic tourniquet and E-type CO_2 tank (Figure 30.1); or
  - wide Esmarch rubber compression bandage (6″ wide is preferred).

Manual of Clinical Procedures in the Horse, First Edition. Edited by Lais R.R. Costa and Mary Rose Paradis.
© 2018 John Wiley & Sons, Inc. Published 2018 by John Wiley & Sons, Inc.

- Two rolls of brown gauze
- Sterile gloves
- 21-gauge ¾″ butterfly needle or a 20-gauge over-the-wire catheter with an injection cap
- Heparinized saline
- 60 ml syringe
- Sterile 0.9% saline (volume up to 60 ml)
- Antibiotic solution (preferably selected based on an antibiogram). Commonly used antibiotics include amikacin, gentamicin, penicillin, and ceftiofur sodium (Table 30.1).
- 1″ white tape
- 4″ × 4″ gauze
- Topical anti-inflammatory cream (optional)
- Bandage material to apply a sterile bandage to immobilize the area surrounding the site.

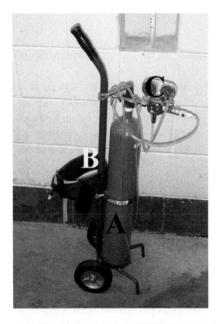

Figure 30.1 Components of the pneumatic tourniquet: A, CO_2 cylinder; B, pneumatic cuff; C, pressure gauges.

Table 30.1 List of commonly used antimicrobial drugs in intravenous regional limb perfusion (the doses listed are for an average size adult horse, see Table 30.2 for more information on the total volume to be administered)

Antibiotic drug (concentration)	Dose of antimicrobial (volume)	Volume (ml) of saline for dilution to achieve a total volume of 60 ml
Amikacin	1 gram	56
(250 mg/ml)	(4 ml)	
Ceftiofur	1 gram	50
(100 mg/ml)	(10 ml)	
K penicillin	3,000,000 IU	54
(500,000 IU/ml)	(6 ml)	
Gentamycin	1 gram	50
(100 mg/ml or 50 mg/ml)	(10 ml or 20 ml)	
Cefazolin	1 gram	50
(100 mg/ml)	(10 ml)	

The volume of antimicrobial will change if the horse weighs less than 500 kg. The dose of antimicrobial should not exceed one-third of the calculated systemic dose of the antimicrobial. Some antimicrobials (e.g., gentamicin) if given at doses greater than 1 g are reported to cause soft tissue sloughing.

30.5 Procedure: IVRLP of the Distal Limb of an Adult Horse

Technical action	Rationale
Select the antimicrobial to be administered via IVRLP: • based on an antibiogram of the organism isolated from the infected site (ideal) • empirical.	There are several factors that are relevant when deciding what antimicrobial drug to use for IVRLP, such as the choice between a concentration-dependent antibiotic (e.g., aminoglycoside) and a time-dependent antibiotic (e.g., K penicillin, ceftiofur sodium). Guidelines for the selection of antimicrobials are beyond the scope of this chapter.
Choose the total volume of perfusate adequate for the case. (See Table 30.1 and Table 30.2). Consider the size of the patient and the vessel to be injected.	In general, for an average size adult horse (450–500 kg): • 60 ml administered to the cephalic or saphenous vein • 40 ml administered to the palmar or plantar digital vein. For IVRLP in neonatal foals, see Chapter 59.
Dilute the antibiotic with a compatible sterile isotonic fluid solution.	Antibiotics must be diluted appropriately to avoid vasculitis and necrosis of the perfused area.
Administer medication for heavy sedation or short general anesthesia, depending on whether the procedure is to be performed with the horse in standing or recumbent positions, respectively.	The procedure requires more about 45 minutes to allow adequate time for performance of the procedure and 30 minutes post injection for perfusion into the tissues to take place.
Clip the hair and prepare the site of injection aseptically. If an intravenous catheter is to be placed, place it prior to application of the compression bandage and the tourniquet. Place the catheter in a distad direction.	See Chapters 8 and 10. Directing the catheter distally is thought to favor perfusion into surrounding tissue. Protect the catheter to prevent dislodgement during placement of the compression bandage and tourniquet.
Apply an Esmarch compressive bandage to the distal limb starting at the hoof and ascending to the level below where the venous approach is to be made. Each turn of the compressive bandage should overlap by about half of its width.	Draining the blood of the distal limb with elastic compression bandage prior to injection is recommended but not absolutely necessary.
Place a roll of gauze over the vein proximal to the site of injection, such that the gauze compresses the vein once the tourniquet is placed. Apply a tourniquet at level proximal to the injection site.	The roll of gauze over the vein will ensure occlusion of the vein. If a catheter was not placed, additional aseptic prep might be necessary after placement of the tourniquet prior to insertion of the butterfly needle.
If using a pneumatic tourniquet, pressurize the tourniquet to 150 mmHg.	The tourniquet should provide pressures of about 50 mmHg above the patient's systolic pressure. Even if using a rubber compressive bandage, as a tourniquet the venous pressures achieved during perfusion will equal the effective tourniquet pressures.
If using a butterfly needle, insert the needle in a distad direction into the lumen of the vein draining the region distal to the tourniquet.	Directing the injection distally is thought to favor perfusion into surrounding tissue.

(continued)

Technical action	Rationale
Inject the diluted antibiotic as a bolus into the vein over 1–3 minutes (Figures 30.2–30.4).	The volume of drug to be administered depends on the size of the patient and how distal the vessel is, but the time should remain the same.
Apply pressure over the injection site with a gauze and white tape wrapped around circumferentially.	This is to prevent backflow of the drug from the injection site.
Allow the tourniquet to remain in position for 30 minutes then release the pressure to allow resumption of blood flow to the area.	A minimal of 20 minute, ideally 30 minutes, is recommended for the drug to perfuse into the surrounding tissues.
Apply a support bandage to the area.	If an indwelling catheter has been used and will be left in place, apply a protective bandage over the insertion site.
The IVRLP procedure is generally repeated, and the frequency and length of treatment varies.	IVRLP of time-dependent antibiotics should be performed daily whereas IVRLP of concentration-dependent antibiotics may be performed at intervals of 24–36 hours to avoid developing phlebitis at the injection site.

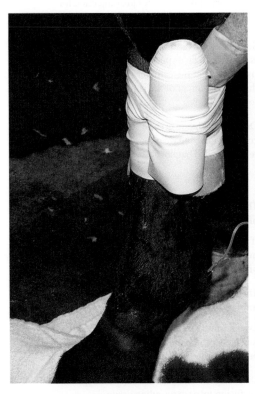

Figure 30.2 Administration of IVRLP of a digital vessel in a standing horse. The tourniquet is placed at the level of the proximal metacarpal bone and the IVRLP is administered to the lateral digital vein.

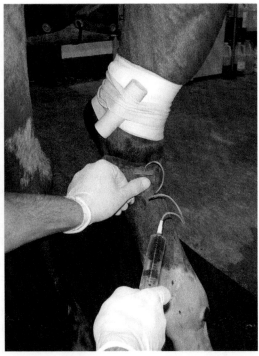

Figure 30.3 Administration of IVRLP to a metatarsal vessel in a standing horse. The tourniquet is placed at the level of the distal tibia and the IVRLP is administered to the dorsal common digital vein.

Table 30.2 Guidelines for performing intravenous regional limb perfusion in an average size adult horse.

	Tourniquet placement	Vessel used for injection	Total volume of infusate (ml)
Front limb	Mid-radius	Cephalic vein	60
	Mid-metacarpal	Palmar digital vein	40
Hind limb	Mid-tibia	Saphenous vein	60
	Mid-metatarsal	Plantar digital vein	40

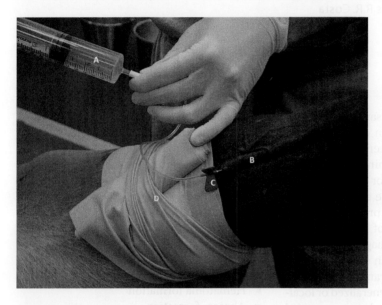

Figure 30.4 Performing IVRLP to the medial saphenous vein. The horse is anesthetized and placed in lateral recumbency over the side of the affected limb, the tourniquet is placed at the level of the distal tibia, and the IVRLP is administered to the medial saphenous vein: A, antibiotic diluted in saline; B, medial saphenous vein; C, butterfly needle; D, Eshmarch bandage.

Bibliography and Further Reading

Levine, D.G. (2014) Regional perfusion, intraosseous, and resuscitation infusion techniques, in *Equine Emergencies*, 4th edn (eds J.A. Orsini and T.J. Divers), W.B. Saunders, Philadelphia, pp. 16–18.

Lugo, J. (2009) Regional limb perfusion with antimicrobials, in *Current Therapy in Equine Medicine 6*, 6th edn (eds N.E. Robinson and K.A. Sprayberry), Saunders Elsevier, St. Louis, pp. 529–531.

Palmer, S. and Hogan, P.M. (1999) How to perform a regional limb perfusion in the standing horse. *Proceedings of the 45th Annual Convention of the AAEP*, Albuquerque, December 5-8, pp. 124–127.

Schaer, B.D. and Orsini, J.A. (2008) Regional limb perfusion, in *Equine Emergencies*, 3rd edn (eds J.A. Orsini and T.J. Divers), W.B. Saunders, Philadelphia, pp. 17–18.

Scheuch, B.C., Van Hoogmoed, L.M., Wilson, W.D. *et al.* (2002) Comparison of intraosseous or intravenous infusions for delivery of amikacin sulphate to the tibiotarsal joint of horses. *American Journal of Veterinary Research*, **63**, 374–380.

Stashak, T.S. and Theoret, C.L. (2007) Local antimicrobial therapy, in *Equine Emergencies*, 3rd edn (eds J.A. Orsini and T.J. Divers), W.B. Saunders, Philadelphia, pp. 206–208.

Stashak, T.S. and Theoret, C.L. (2014) Local antimicrobial therapy, in *Equine Emergencies*, 4th edn (eds J.A. Orsini and T.J. Divers), W.B. Saunders, Philadelphia, pp. 251–253.

Stephen, J. (2008) Application of a tourniquet and regional limb perfusion, in *The Equine Hospital Manual* (eds K. Corley and J. Stephen), Blackwell Publishing, Oxford, pp. 108–110.

Southwood, L. (2008) Regional limb perfusion in *The Equine Hospital Manual* (eds K. Corley and J. Stephen), Blackwell Publishing, Oxford, pp. 602–604.

31

Collection of Muscle Biopsy in Horses

Mustajab H. Mirza and Lais R.R. Costa

31.1 Purpose

- To obtain a diagnostic sample of a muscle biopsy for evaluation of morphologic and biochemical characteristics of skeletal muscle tissue to determine the diagnosis of suspected muscular or neuromuscular disorders, and formulate a plan for management and long-term prognosis.
- Histologic evaluation of muscle biopsy specimen is part of the diagnostic work-up of horses presenting with exercise intolerance, muscle stiffness, cramping, pain, fasciculation, or atrophy (generalized or localized). These signs might be accompanied by increased activity of muscle-specific isoenzymes, for example creatine kinase (CK), and aspartate aminotransferase (AST).
- This chapter describes two techniques for obtaining a muscle biopsy specimen: incisional and needle muscle biopsy. Obtaining a needle muscle biopsy is the least invasive of the two techniques, but incisional biopsy harvests more tissue. The advantage of the needle biopsy is that it does not require layup time after biopsy collection. The disadvantages are: (1) it requires a specialized instrument, (2) it requires experience to obtain an adequate size sample, and (3) it does not ship as well as the larger surgical biopsy.
- Muscles frequently sampled include semimembranosus, semitendinosus, sacrocaudalis dorsalis medialis, dorsal compartment of the gluteus medius, and longissimus lumborum (Table 31.1). Prior to collecting muscle biopsy samples, review the specimen handling instructions from the laboratory where the samples are to be submitted.

31.2 Complications

- Seroma formation
- Hematoma formation
- Abscess formation
- Suture dehiscence and open wound formation

31.3 Restraint and Positioning

- The procedure is generally performed in a sedated, standing horse.
- Restraining the horse in stocks provides a safer environment for the person performing the procedure.
- Sedation with a combination of alpha-2 agonist (such as xylazine or detomidine) and opioid agonist-antagonist (such as butorphanol) is usually adequate (see Chapter 9).
- A nose twitch can be applied during the performance of the procedure (see Chapter 2).

Manual of Clinical Procedures in the Horse, First Edition. Edited by Lais R.R. Costa and Mary Rose Paradis.
© 2018 John Wiley & Sons, Inc. Published 2018 by John Wiley & Sons, Inc.

Table 31.1 Location of muscle to be sampled

Muscle to be sampled	Anatomical location	Major rule-out
Semimembranosus	Centrally located in the body of the muscle about 10 cm below the tuber ischii (Figure 31.1)	Polysaccharide storage myopathy Exertional myopathies/rhabdomyolysis
Gluteus medius	One-third of the distance between the tuber coxae and the tail head (Figure 31.2)	Exertional myopathies/rhabdomyolysis Compartmental/pressure necrosis myopathy
Sacrocaudalis dorsalis medialis	Above the tail head on either side of the dorsal spinous processes of the sacrocoxygeal vertebra (Figure 31.3)	Equine motor neuron disease
Longissimus lumborum	Lumbar area, 5–7 cm off the midline (Figure 31.4)	Polysaccharide storage myopathy Exertional myopathies/rhabdomyolysis
Sample affected muscle that is suspected to be atrophied by gross, ultrasonographic or EMG examination	Often gluteal or epaxial muscles are affected	Localized muscle atrophy Immuno-mediated myositis

EMG, electromyogram.

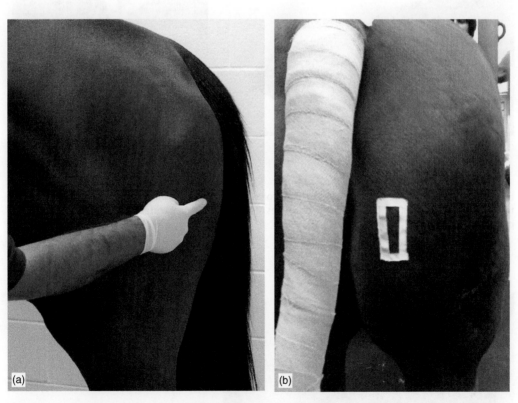

(a)   (b)

Figure 31.1 Location of the sampling site for the semimembranosus muscle. Sample the central portion in the body of the muscle about 10 cm below the tuber ischia: (a) lateral view and (b) posterior view.

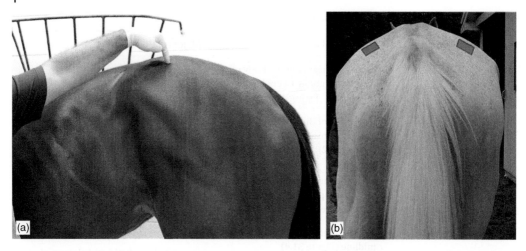

Figure 31.2 Location of the sampling site for the middle gluteal muscle. Sample at the site one-third of the distance between the tuber coxae and the tail head: (a) lateral view and (b) posterior view.

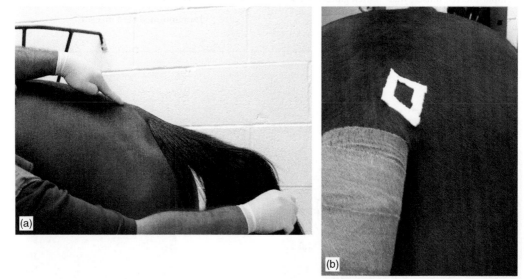

Figure 31.3 Location of the sampling site for the sacrocaudalis dorsalis medialis muscle. Sample above the tail head on either side of the dorsal spinous processes of the sacrocoxygeal vertebra: (a) lateral view and (b) posterior view.

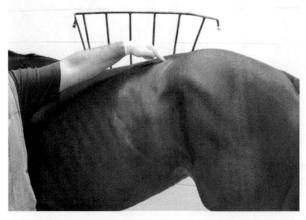

Figure 31.4 Location of the sampling site for the longissimus lumborum muscle. Sample a site at the lumbar area, 5–7 cm off the midline.

31.4 Equipment Required

- Chemical and/or physical restraint.
- Brown gauze or neoprene tail wrap
- Clippers
- 4″ × 4″ gauze soaked in disinfectant scrub
- 4″ × 4″ gauze soaked in alcohol
- Examination gloves
- 22-gauge 1" or 25-gauge 5/8" hypodermic needles
- Syringes: 3 and 6 ml
- Local anesthetic (carbocaine or lidocaine or mepivicaine)
- Sterile gloves
- 4″ × 4″ gauze damped with saline
- 10% buffered formalin (optional)

- Specimen container
- Non-absorbable suture material or skin staples
- Specific supplies for incisional muscle biopsy:
  - scalpel blade #10 and handle
  - scissors (Metzenbaum)
  - thumb forceps
  - Gelpi retractors
  - tongue depressor
  - absorbable suture material.
- Specific supplies for needle muscle biopsy:
  - scalpel blade #15 on a #3 BP handle
  - muscle core biopsy needle (Bergström needle).

31.5 Procedure: Incisional Muscle Biopsy

Technical action	Rationale
Locate the appropriate site to obtain the muscle specimen (Table 31.1, Figures 31.1–31.4).	Knowledge of the anatomy is important.
Apply a tail wrap.	For details see Chapter 60.
Clip the hair in the area of the biopsy.	Removal of hair is necessary for appropriate aseptic technique.
Aseptically prepare the site.	A detailed description of aseptic technique is given in Chapter 10.
Anesthetize the area using an inverted U or an inverted L regional block with 2% lidocaine or other local anesthetic agent.	Avoid injecting anesthetic agent directly into the muscle tissue to be sampled to avoid distortion of the tissue. The injected skin may appear slightly raised where the lidocaine is injected (Figure 31.5a).
Incise skin over the muscle to be sampled. Make a 4–6 cm incision (Figure 31.5b).	A shorter incision in the muscle than in skin allows closure with less dead space.
If available, apply Gelpi retractors to retract the skin.	The use of Gelpi retractors ensures good surgical exposure because they are self-retaining.
Bluntly dissect two parallel separations to muscle fibers about 3–5 cm in length, approximately 1–1.5 cm apart.	Avoid crushing muscle tissue with instruments during manipulation to prevent morphological artifacts. Handle only one corner of the tissue.
Transect the segment of muscle tissue proximally and distally, taking care not to crush the tissue.	The piece of tissue will be approximately the size of a cube of 1.5 cm.

(continued)

Technical action	Rationale
Prepare the sample for submission: All or the majority of the tissue should be wrapped in slightly damped (with saline) gauze and refrigerated (do not freeze).	A fresh sample allows for performance of different tests.
	Aligning the muscle sample on a piece of tongue depressor will preserve the linearity of the muscle fibers during fixation.
	Biochemical tests are performed on fresh muscle sample. Although some techniques are performed in frozen tissue samples, special processing is required before freezing, therefore the sample is sent refrigerated to the laboratory.
	Optional: One small segment of the sample may be fixed in buffered formalin.
Close the muscular fascia and the subcutaneous tissue with absorbable suture material.	Suture the fascia (perimysium) which surrounds the muscle belly rather than the muscular tissue itself. In addition, the subcutaneous tissue may also be sutured.
Close the skin incision with non-absorbable suture material.	Skin may be closed with a stainless steel skin staple device or non-absorbable monofilament skin suture such as polypropylene or nylon suture material.
Processing of sample.	Samples should be submitted by expedited shipping according to laboratory specifications.

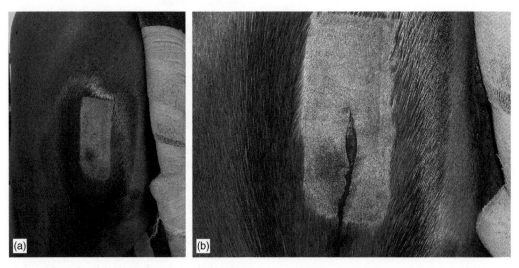

Figure 31.5 Collection of incisional muscle biopsy. (a) Local anesthetic injected in the form of an inverted L in the center of the area that was previously clipped and scrubbed. (b) Skin incised after local anesthesia.

31.6 Procedure: Needle Muscle Biopsy

Technical action	Rationale
Locate the appropriate site (Table 31.1).	Knowledge of the anatomy is important.
Clip the hair in the area of the biopsy.	Removal of hair is necessary for appropriate aseptic technique.
Aseptically prepare the site.	A detailed description of aseptic technique is given in Chapter 10.
Anesthetize the area by injecting a bleb of 2% lidocaine or other local anesthetic agent subcutaneously at the site of the stab incision.	Avoid injecting anesthetic agent directly into the muscle tissue to be sampled in order to avoid distortion of the tissue.
Perform a stab incision (approximately 1–1.5 cm) into the skin and muscle fascia for the insertion of the biopsy needle.	The small stab incision must be sufficiently long to insert the biopsy needle.
Insert the biopsy needle through the stab incision, 6–8 cm into the muscle (Figure 31.6). After inserting the needle, partially withdraw the internal cutting cylinder and expose the window in the needle. Press the biopsy needle firmly against the muscle to trap a piece of muscle within the window, then depress the cylinder to excise a piece of the muscle that moved into the hollow cylinder. Repeat it several times.	The chopping motion is repeated several times before withdrawing the needle.
Withdraw the needle containing the sample. Remove the sample from the biopsy needle carefully.	Avoid crushing muscle tissue with instruments during manipulation to prevent morphological artifacts. Use a small hypodermic needle to remove the samples from the needle.
Wrap the core of tissue in slightly damp (with saline) gauze and refrigerate it (do not freeze).	Biochemical tests are performed on fresh muscle sample. Special processing is required before freezing.
Closure of muscle incision is not necessary.	
Close the skin incision with non-absorbable suture material.	Skin may be closed with a stainless steel skin staple device and/or non-absorbable monofilament skin suture such as polypropylene or nylon suture material.
Processing of sample.	Samples should be submitted by expedited shipping according to laboratory specifications.

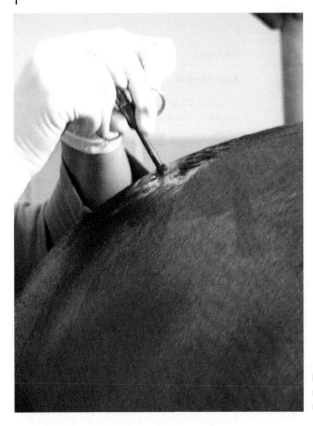

Figure 31.6 Insertion of the Bergström needle through the stab incision and into the muscle for collection of the muscle sample.

Further Reading and Bibliography

Aleman, M. UCD Neuromuscular Disease Laboratory. http://www.vetmed.ucdavis.edu/vsr/neurology/Downloads/Equine Muscle Biopsy.pdf

Bergstorm, J. (1962) Muscle electrolytes in man: Determined by neutron activation analysis on needle biopsy specimens: a study in normal subjects, kidney patients, and patients with chronic diarrhea. *Scandinavian Journal of Clinical Laboratory Investigations*, **14** (68), 1–100.

Divers, T.J., De Lahunta, A., Hintz, H.F., Riis, R.C., Jackson, C.A., and Mohammed, H.O. (2001) Equine motor neuron disease. *Equine Veterinary Education*, **3**, 89–93.

Horse Report (2005); "Neuromuscular diseases in horses". Center for Equine Health, 23 (2) 1-7; www.vetmed.ucdavis.edu/ceh/local_resources/pdfs/pubs-HR23-2-bkm-sec.pdf

Ledwith, A. and McGowan, C.M. (2004) "Muscle biopsy: a routine doagnostic procedure". *Equine Veterinary Education* 6 (2) pp. 84-93.

Schumacher, J. and Moll, H.D. (2006) Muscle biopsy, in *Manual of Equine Diagnostic Procedures*, Teton NewMedia, Jackson, WY, pp. 140–145.

Snow, D.H. and Guy, P.S. (1980) Muscle fiber type composition of number of limb muscles in different type of horse. *Research in Veterinary Science*, **28**, 137–144.

Valberg, S.J. (2012) Muscling in on the cause of tying-up. Frank J. Milne State-of-the art Lecture, *Proceedings of the Annual Convention of the American Association of Equine Practitioners*, **58**, 85–123.

Valberg, S.J. (2014) Obtaining and Submitting Muscle Sample for Biopsy. https://cvm.msu.edu/research/faculty-research/valberg-laboratory/for-veterinarians. Equine Neuromuscular Diagnostic Laboratory.

Valentine, B.A., Credille, K.M., Lavoie, J.-P., Fatone, S., Guard, C., Cummings, J.F., and Cooper, B.J. (1997) Severe polysaccharide storage myopathy in Belgian and Percheron draught horses. *Equine Veterinary Journal*, **29**, 220–225.

Valette, J.P., Barrey, E., Jouglin, M., Courouce, A., Aurinet, B., and Flaux, B. (1999) Standardization of muscle biopsy of gluteus medius in French trotters. *Equine Veterinary Journal*, Supplement, **30**, 342–344.

32

Examination of Foot Conformation and Balance

Colin Mitchell

32.1 Purpose

- To evaluate the hoof and identify any structural or hoof balance abnormalities that can potentially cause lameness or foot pain. Table 32.1 lists pertinent terminology of the equine foot and descriptions of common foot abnormalities.

32.2 Complications

None

32.3 Equipment Required

Equipment required for examination of the equine foot are depicted in Figure 32.1.

- Hoof pick
- Hoof brush
- Hook knives
- Rasp
- Hoof testers

32.4 Restraint and Positioning

- The horse should preferably be standing on a firm, flat surface to allow visualization of the hoof from all angles.

Table 32.1 Terminology of the equine foot and description of common foot abnormalities

	Description
Hoof–pastern axis	Viewed from the side and front by drawing an imaginary line passing through the center of the pastern and the center of the foot (Figure 32.5)
Ideal hoof angulation	When the hoof–pastern axis, the phalangeal alignment, and the heel angle are parallel (Figures 32.5 and 32.6)
Functional foot	Term used to indicate the features of a sound equine foot: parallel hoof–pastern axis, thick hoof wall, adequate depth of the sole (>15 mm), adequate heel base conformation, and growth rings of equal size
Breakover	The phase of the stride between the time the horse's heel lifts off the ground and the time the toe lifts off the ground
Weak or underrun heels	Hoof distortion where the hoof angle measure at the heel is greater than 5° lower than the hoof angle measured at the toe
Broken-back hoof–pastern axis	When the line in the center of the pastern is not parallel with the line in the center of the hoof (Figure 32.10)
Broken forward hoof–pastern axis	When the line in the center of the pastern is not parallel with the line in the center of the hoof (Figure 32.9)
Sheared heels	Hoof capsule distortion where one heel bulb is displaced proximally relative to the adjacent heel bulb (Figure 32.13b)

Manual of Clinical Procedures in the Horse, First Edition. Edited by Lais R.R. Costa and Mary Rose Paradis.
© 2018 John Wiley & Sons, Inc. Published 2018 by John Wiley & Sons, Inc.

- This can be performed in a stall without shavings or bedding (as bedding can hamper evaluation), or another area where there is enough clearance around the horse to evaluate the limbs from the front, side, and rear.

- The horse should be held, no other chemical or physical restraint is usually necessary. Keeping the horse standing square and comfortably is all that is required.

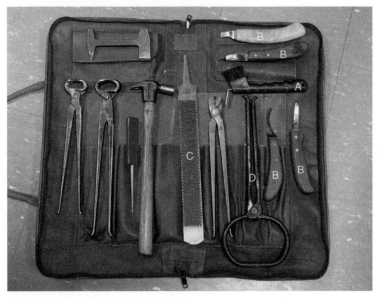

Figure 32.1 Equipment required for examination of the equine foot: (A) hoof pick and brush, (B) hoof knives, (C) rasp, and (D) hoof testers.

32.5 Procedure: Foot Examination

Technical action	Rationale
Obtain a brief but complete health history, making sure to include details on foot care, type of work, type of ground where the horse is exercised, amount of exercise, diet and supplements.	Foot abnormalities are not always associated with overt lameness. Lameness examination is discussed in Chapter 27. Nutrition and exercise are important in the health of the foot. And a number of medical conditions affect the health of the foot (e.g. pituitary pars intermedia dysfunction and equine metabolic syndrome).
Perform a brief, but thorough physical examination, paying particular attention to the horse's body condition and conformation.	The foot conformation generally reflects the conformation of the limbs.
The horse should be observed from outside the stall without a handler, as it moves around and stands still.	This allows a brief evaluation of the conformation of the horse's limbs. In cases of severe foot abnormalities, this will help identify the limb that is causing or contributing to the lameness.
Inspect all four feet while weight-bearing, paying special attention to the size and shape of each foot (Figure 32.2).	Any gross discrepancies between size of feet or hoof shape (Figure 32.3) can often be identified initially and investigated more closely as the examination continues. If present, prominent rings in the hoof wall should be noted.
The horse should be taken to an area where the feet can be examined. A clean, hard, and dry surface with no bedding is ideal. Picking out the horse's feet prior to moving them is helpful to minimize contamination of the examination area.	Examining the feet can be difficult if the horse is standing in shavings, on soft ground or on other surfaces that either yield to or mask the hoof capsule.

Technical action	Rationale
The front feet should be examined with the horse standing as square as possible. Getting down on the ground allows evaluation of the size of the foot, the mediolateral balance (by examining the coronary band, which should be parallel to the ground; Figure 32.4a), as well as closer evaluation to identify any hoof cracks or defects. Rotational abnormalities can be related to conformation or to mediolateral imbalance (Figure 32.4b).	Mismatched feet indicate a chronic lack of use (usually secondary to some lameness) and any mediolateral balance issues are present if the coronary band is higher medially or laterally compared to the contralateral side. Hoof symmetry and how centered the hoof is on the limb can also be evaluated. Horses with any of these issues often have some degree of foot pain due to the foot being unevenly loaded.
The front feet should be viewed from the lateral side. This allows evaluation of the hoof–pastern axis (Figure 32.5), hoof angulation, the phalangeal alignment, and the heel angle (Figure 32.6). Comparing the angle of the dorsal hoof wall and the palmar wall (i.e., heel angle) will allow identification of abnormalities: weak or underrun heels, flexural deformities of the distal interphalangeal joint (Figure 32.7), excessive toe length (Figure 32.8), and abnormal hoof–pastern axis (Figures 32.9 and 32.10, Table 32.1). Shoe placement can also be evaluated, with regard to breakover and heel support (Figure 32.11).	Abnormalities in the angle of either the dorsal or palmar hoof wall can result in increased stress over the heel region, resulting in heel pain and, potentially, chronic lameness. If the horse is shod, the shoe should extend far enough caudally to support the heel.
The foot should be picked up so that it can be examined from the caudal aspect. The limb is held on the dorsum of the cannon bone, maintaining the cannon bone parallel to the ground and allowing the distal limb to relax. The heel region can then be examined by viewing it from above without getting underneath the horse into a potentially dangerous position.	Abnormalities of the heel region can be observed and evaluated. Mediolateral balance can be assessed by evaluating if the ground-bearing surface of the foot is flat and perpendicular to the long axis of the cannon bone (Figure 32.12). Sheared heels are a significant cause of lameness and are easy to diagnose from this angle (Figure 32.13).
The leg should now be supported between the examiner's legs (see Chapter 1) by gripping the pastern region with the knees to allow the solar surface to be evaluated. The solar surface or sole callus may need to be cleaned with a hoof brush or pick, or sparingly trimmed with a hoof knife.	Supporting the limb with your legs frees up both hands to manipulate instruments or to examine the sole (Figure 32.14).
The bottom of each foot should be carefully inspected (Figure 32.15a). Cleaning the foot is necessary to allow the frog, central, and collateral sulci to be clearly visualized and examined. The front feet tend to have a rounder shape, whereas the rear feet are more oval shaped (Figure 32.15b) when viewed from the solar aspect.	Removal of debris or sole callus should be performed as this may make identification of problems or sensitivity to hoof tester application more apparent.
Hoof testers should be methodically applied to the solar surface and hoof capsule. An eight-point pressure technique is applied around the hoof wall to determine if there is response to pressure applied to the hoof (Figure 32.16 and Figure 27.11 on page 269). Start with minimal force and increase pressure gradually. After the whole foot has been assessed, return to the sensitive places to determine if the sensitivity is repeatable.	To properly apply the hoof testers, the examiner needs both hands free and the horse's leg supported by the examiner's leg (Figure 32.14) make sure hoof testers are not applied to the coronary band, only hoof.
While inspecting the solar surface of the foot, if the foot is shoed the fit of the shoe can be evaluated (Figure 32.17).	

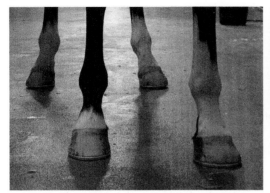

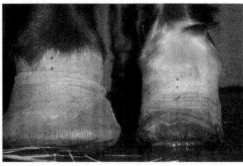

Figure 32.2 The horse is standing on a firm surface, with no bedding. All four feet can be clearly seen and the observer has space to move around the horse safely.

Figure 32.3 Inspection of the foot from the front. This horse is chronically laminitic and the left fore (on the right of the image) has been the most severely affected. This has affected growth and decreased weight bearing, resulting in the foot being smaller than the contralateral hoof. In addition, prominent rings in the hoof wall can be noted.

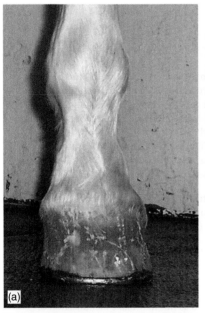

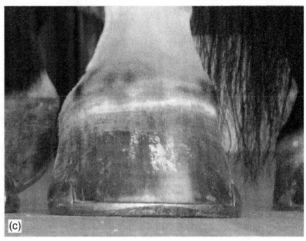

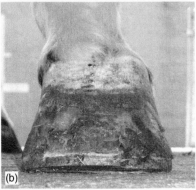

Figure 32.4 The hoof is observed from the front. (a) The coronary band appears parallel to the ground and the mediolateral balance of this foot is good. (b) The coronary band appears parallel to the ground, indicating that the mediolateral balance of this foot is good, but the horse is toe-in due to a rotational deformity proximal in the limb. (c) The coronary band is not parallel to the ground, indicating the mediolateral imbalance.

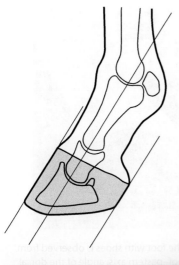

Figure 32.5 The hoof–pastern axis is observed from the side. Assessment of the hoof–pastern axis by drawing an imaginary line passing through the center of the pastern and the center of foot. O'Grady and Poupard (2003). Reproduced with permission of Elsevier.

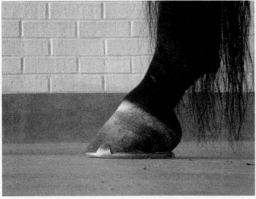

Figure 32.6 Ideal hoof angulation of a rear foot. When the hoof–pastern axis, the phalangeal alignment, and the heel angle are parallel.

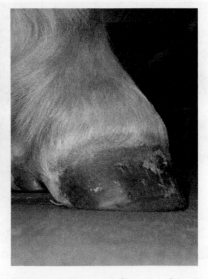

Figure 32.7 Flexural deformities of the distal interphalangeal joint.

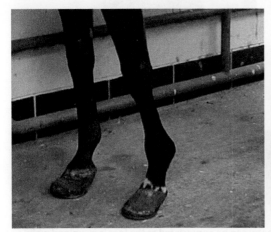

Figure 32.8 Excessive toe length. Courtesy of Dr. Lais R.R. Costa.

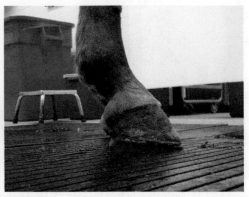

Figure 32.9 Abnormal hoof–pastern axis: broken forward hoof–pastern axis.

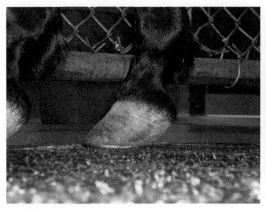

Figure 32.10 Abnormal hoof–pastern axis: broken back hoof–pastern axis.

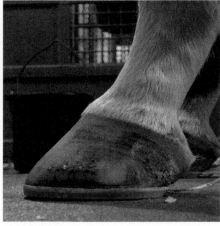

Figure 32.11 The foot with shoes is observed from the side. The hoof–pastern axis, angle of the dorsal hoof wall, and heel region can be evaluated. Ideally the shoe extends slightly behind the heel to provide appropriate support to the region.

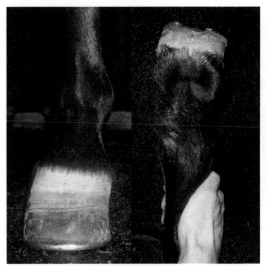

Figure 32.12 Evaluation of foot balance: (a) front view of the right fore foot and (b) palmar view of the right fore foot. From the front view, the lateral (left side of image) coronary band appears higher than the medial side. This is confirmed when the hoof is viewed from the palmar aspect, as the lateral hoof wall appears longer, which is contributing to this horse's toed in conformation. Ideally on this view, the weight-bearing surface of the foot should be perpendicular to the long axis of the cannon bone and phalanges.

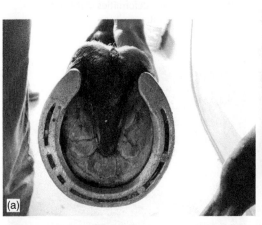

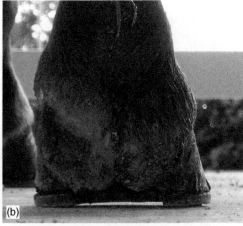

Figure 32.13 Evaluation of foot balance. (A) Heel symmetry can be appreciated as the foot is examined while holding it up by the cannon bone. (b) This right rear foot has a sheared heel on the medial side (left of image). Sheared heel frequently results in lameness or decreased performance.

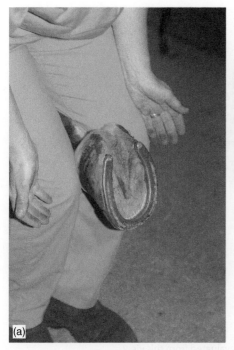

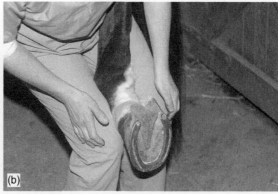

Figure 32.14 Support the limb with your legs to free up both hands and allow manipulation of instruments or to examine the sole of the foot. (a) Front limbs are placed between the knees. (b) When examining the rear foot, instead of holding the limb between your legs (as when applying hoof testers to a fore foot), the dorsum of the horse's rear fetlock is rested on the examiner's knee, leaving both hands free to examine the foot.

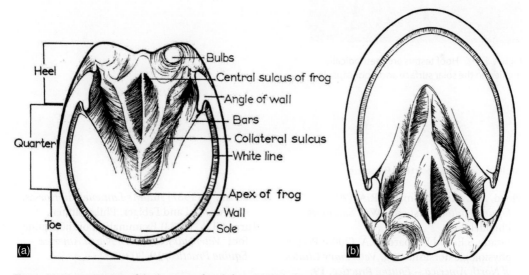

Figure 32.15 Inspection of the bottom of each foot. (a) With the structures appropriately labeled, the solar aspect of the front feet tends to have a rounder shape. (b) The solar aspect of the rear feet is more oval shaped. Stashak (1987). Reproduced with permission of Lea and Febiger.

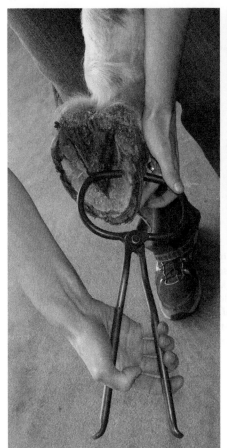

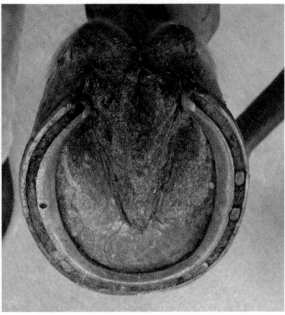

Figure 32.17 The solar surface of the foot and the fit of the shoe can be evaluated from this view.

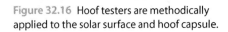

Figure 32.16 Hoof testers are methodically applied to the solar surface and hoof capsule.

Bibliography and Further Reading

Floyd, A.E. and Mansmann, R.A. (2007) *Equine Podiatry*, 1st edn, W.B. Saunders, Philadelphia.

O'Grady, S.E. and Poupard, D.A. (2003) Proper physiologic horseshoeing. *Veterinary Clinics of North America – Equine Practice*, **19**, 333–351.

Stashak, T. (1987) *Adam's Lameness in Horses*, 4th edn, Lea and Febiger: Philadelphia.

Turner, T.A. (2003) Examination of the equine foot. *Veterinary Clinics of North America – Equine Practice*, **19**, 309–332.

33

Limb Bandages and Splints

Daniel J. Burba

33.1 Purposes

- To cover and protect wounds of the limbs.
- To reduce swelling associated with soft tissue injury and trauma of the limbs.
- To reduce swelling of tendonitis.
- To reduce weight-bearing injuries to the limbs.
- To support soft tissue structures, especially tendons, during excessive weight bearing on a limb due to severe lameness of the contralateral limb.
- To protect limbs from potential external trauma (e.g., during transportation and certain competitions).

33.2 Complications

- Tissue edema and skin necrosis may occur when bandages are applied too tightly or unevenly. Bandages should be monitored closely, at least twice daily, and changed as needed.

33.3 Equipment Required

- There are various materials for use as bandages. Commonly used materials are (Figure 33.1):
- non-adherent wound dressing
- conforming rolled gauze (kling)
- elastic adhesive tape (Elastikon®, Johnson & Johnson, New Brunswick, NJ)
- elastic self-retaining wrap (e.g., Vetrap®, 3M, St. Paul, MN)
- elastic reusable bandage (e.g., ACE™,3M, St. Paul, MN)
- cotton combine
- white tape
- brown reinforcing gauze
- polo wrap
- rolled cotton
- military field bandage
- sheet cotton
- quilted cotton wrap

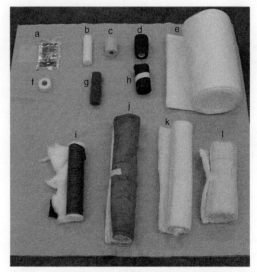

Figure 33.1 Various bandage materials: (a) non-adhering wound dressing, (b) kling rolled gauze, (c) adhesive elastic bandage (Elasticon®), (d) self-klinging wrap (Vetrap®), (e) combined cotton roll, (f) white tape, (g) brown gauze, (h) polo wrap, (i) rolled cotton, (j) military field bandage, (k) sheet cotton layers rolled together, and (l) quilted wrap.

Manual of Clinical Procedures in the Horse, First Edition. Edited by Lais R.R. Costa and Mary Rose Paradis.
© 2018 John Wiley & Sons, Inc. Published 2018 by John Wiley & Sons, Inc.

33.4 Restraint and Positioning

- Minimal restraint is usually needed to apply bandages to the front limbs of a horse.
- Usually one person is needed to hold the horse on a lead shank while another applies the bandage.

- Some horses object to having their hock wrapped by kicking out so it is important to use caution when applying a bandage to the hock.
- An assistant may need to apply a lip twitch, hold up a front limb or give sedation if the horse strongly objects a hind limb bandage.

33.5 Procedures

33.5.1 *Lower Limb Wound Bandage*

To cover a wound on a limb distal to the carpus or tarsus, primarily the metacarpus or metatarsus, or provide the lower limb with a support bandage.

Technical action	Rationale
After cleaning and drying the wound, apply topical antimicrobial ointment.	Topical antimicrobials such as neomycin-containing ointment will reduce bacterial growth in the wound.
Place a non-adherent dressing directly over the wound (Figure 33.2).	This prevents the bandage from adhering to the underlying wound, which may cause bleeding and disrupt healing.
Secure the wound dressing to the limb with rolled conforming gauze (kling) (Figure 33.3). The gauze should be wrapped proximal and distal to the wound edges approximately 2–4 cm using light pressure, overlapping the edges with no wrinkles. When applying any rolled bandage material onto the horse's limb, it should be wrapped from cranial to caudal on the limb when viewing the limb from the lateral side.	Tightly wrapped gauze can become even tighter if swelling occurs at the wound site. This could result in the formation of pressure lines and necrosis. By applying the rolled bandage material from cranial to caudal, tension is not applied to the flexure tendons, thus preventing bandage-induced tendonitis.
Apply a padded layer. Wrap the padded layer around the limb (Figure 33.4). It should cover from just below the carpus/tarsus to the coronary band. Apply with as few wrinkles as possible.	The padded layer can be composed of cotton sheets cut from a roll, layered cotton sheets, quilted leg wraps, a military field bandage or a combination of the above.
Secure the padded layer to the limb with another roll of gauze, preferably brown gauze (Figure 33.5).	Brown gauze works best for this as it molds well to the limb when applied tightly, thus avoiding wrinkles.
Apply the outer shell using elastic self-retaining wrap (Vetrap®), elastic adhesive tape (Elastikon®), a re-usable elastic bandage (ACE™) or a track bandage (Figure 33.6).	If an ACE™ bandage or track wrap is used, it is secured with white tape cut into strips or placed around the bandage in a "barber pole" fashion (Figure 33.7).
Place elastic adhesive tape (Elastikon®) around the top and bottom of the bandage, with half of the tape sticking to the wrap and half to the skin (Figure 33.7).	This prevents slippage and keeps debris (e.g., bedding) from getting inside the bandage.

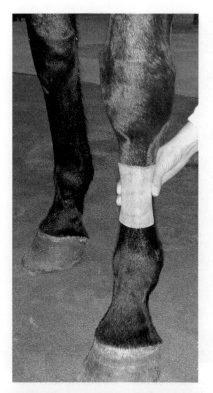

Figure 33.2 Application of a non-adhering wound dressing over a metacarpal wound.

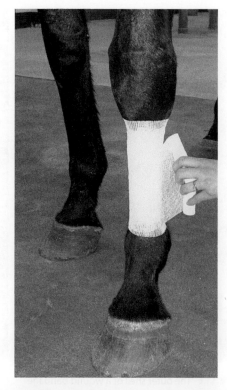

Figure 33.3 Application of kling rolled gauze to secure a wound dressing to a limb.

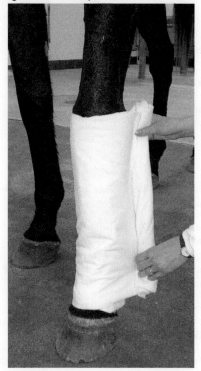

Figure 33.4 Application of the padded layer of a wound bandage.

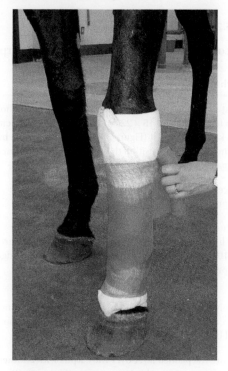

Figure 33.5 Application of brown gauze to secure the cotton padded layer of a wound bandage.

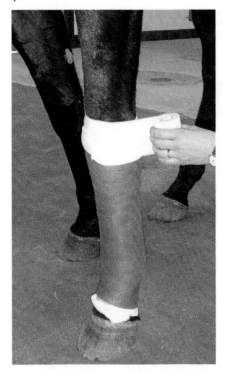

Figure 33.6 The outer shell of a wound bandage and application of elastic adhering tape to the top and bottom of a wound dressing.

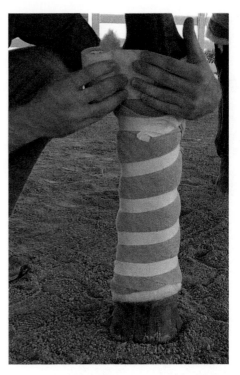

Figure 33.7 Use of an ACE™ wrap as the outer shell of a wound bandage. Notice it is secured with white tape applied in a barber pole fashion.

33.5.2 Carpal Bandage

To cover a wound over the dorsum of the carpus or post-arthroscopic surgery.

Technical action	Rationale
First make a "doughnut" pad by cutting a fusiform hole in a folded sheet of 15 × 22 cm combine or ½″ (1.5 cm) thick orthopedic felt (Figure 33.8). Place it over the back of the carpus and position the hole over the accessory carpal bone (Figure 33.9).	This reduces the chances of pressure necrosis over the accessory carpal bone.
Place non-adherent dressing over the wound of the carpus.	This prevents the bandage from adhering to the wound.
Secure the wound dressing and doughnut pad over the limb with rolled conforming gauze (kling) (Figure 33.10). Wrap it proximal and distal to the wound edges (approximately 4 cm).	The kling can be wrapped in a figure-of-eight configuration above and below the accessory carpal bone (Figure 33.11). This allows the bandage to move better with the flexion of the joint.
Apply the padded layer. Wrap the padded layer around the carpus. It should cover approximately 10 cm above and below the carpus.	Combine cotton sheets cut from a roll, rolled cotton, or layered cotton sheets can be used but bulky material should be avoided.
Secure the padded layer over the carpus with another roll of gauze, preferably brown gauze (Figure 33.12).	Refer to section 33.5.1 on lower wound bandages.

Technical action	Rationale
Apply the outer shell using elastic self-retaining wrap (Vetrap®) or elastic adhesive tape (Elastikon®).	Refer to section 33.5.1 on lower wound bandages.
Place elastic adhesive tape (Elastikon®) around the top and bottom of the bandage, with half of the tape sticking to the wrap and half to the skin, to prevent slippage.	Refer to section 33.5.1 on lower wound bandages.
A support bandage (see section 33.5.1 and Figures 33.4 to 33.7) can be placed below the carpal bandage.	This is an additional measure to prevent slippage of the carpal bandage.

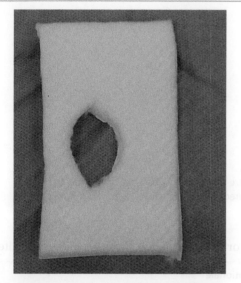

Figure 33.8 Construction of a "doughnut" pad from orthopedic felt.

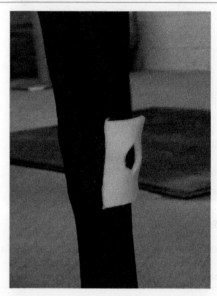

Figure 33.9 Placement of a "doughnut" pad over the accessory carpal bone.

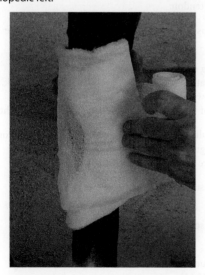

Figure 33.10 Application of a wound dressing on the dorsum of the carpus. Kling rolled gauze used to secure the wound dressing. This is the view from the back of the limb, showing the "doughnut" pad on the back of the carpus.

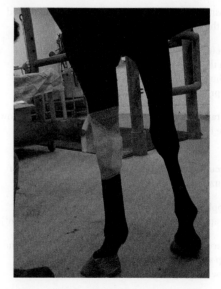

Figure 33.11 Kling rolled gauze placed over the carpus in a figure-of-eight pattern to allow more flexibility of the dressing during flexion of the joint.

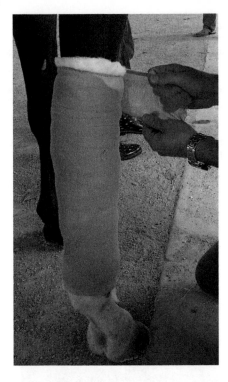

Figure 33.12 The padded layer of a carpal bandage secured with brown gauze.

33.5.3 Hock Bandage

To cover a wound over the dorsum of the tarsus or to protect a post-arthroscopic surgery site.

Technical action	Rationale
Place a strip of padding over the tendons leading to the point of the hock (Figure 33.13).	This reduces the chances of pressure sores over the Achilles tendon.
Position a non-adherent dressing over the wound of the tarsocrural joint.	This helps to prevent adhesion of the bandage to the wound.
Secure the wound dressing and tendon padding on the limb with rolled conforming gauze (kling) (Figure 33.13). Wrap it distal to the joint approximately 2–4 cm.	The kling can be wrapped in a figure-of-eight configuration above and below the point of the hock. This allows the bandage to move better with the flexion of the joint. Be careful not to get this too tight.
Wrap the padded layer approximately 10 cm below the tarsus (Figure 33.14).	Avoid bulky material. Typically, cotton sheets cut from a roll (Figure 33.1a) or layered cotton sheets (Figure 33.1k) are recommended.
Secure the padded layer to the limb with a roll of gauze, preferably brown gauze (Figure 33.14).	Refer to section 33.5.1 on lower wound bandages.
Apply the outer shell using elastic self-retaining wrap (Vetrap®) or elastic adhesive tape (Elastikon®).	Refer to section 33.5.1 on lower wound bandages.
Place elastic adhesive tape (Elastikon®) around the top and bottom of the bandage, with half of the tape sticking to the wrap and half to the skin.	This reduces the chances of slippage of the bandage (Figure 33.15).
A support bandage (see section 33.5.1 and Figures 33.4 to 33.7) can be placed below the hock bandage.	This is an additional measure to prevent slippage of the hock bandage.

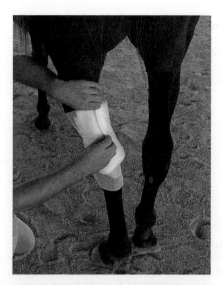

Figure 33.13 Hock bandage: application of cotton padding over the tendons leading the hock.

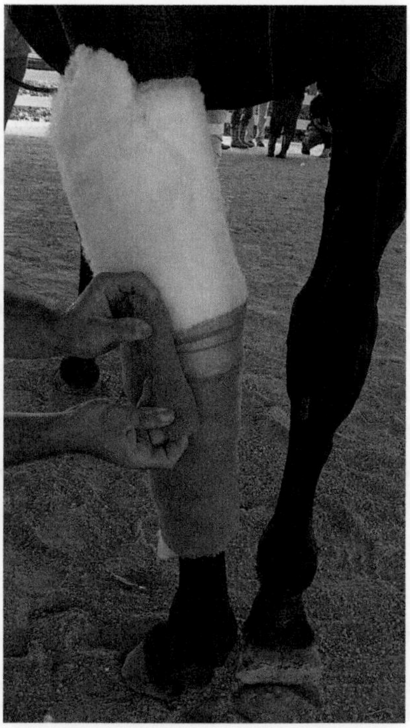

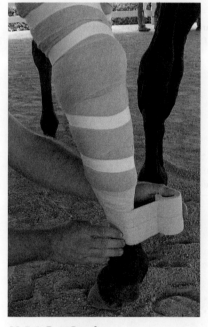

Figure 33.14 Application of the padded layer of a hock bandage with brown gauze.

Figure 33.15 A reusable elastic (ACE™) bandage used as the outer shell of a hock bandage. Notice it is secured with white tape applied in a barber pole fashion. Elastic adhering tape is used to seal the top and bottom of the bandage.

33.5.4 Foot Bandage

To cover an open (puncture) wound to the sole of the foot or to cover an opened subsolar abscess.

Technical action	Rationale
Make a 30 × 30 cm square shell by cross-lapping strips of duct tape (Figure 33.16).	This is constructed before being applied to the hoof.
The wound or opened abscess is cleaned and the hoof is dried.	Refer to another source regarding treatment of subsolar or solar wounds.

(continued)

Technical action	Rationale
Pick up the foot.	See Chapter 2 for detailed instructions on picking up the front feet (Figure 2.20) and hind feet (Figure 2.21).
Front foot: Place a hand on the horse's shoulder, facing the horse's rump. Bend forward, pushing your shoulder against the horse's shoulder/forearm. Slide one hand distally down the leg, gently squeeze the flexor tendons or the chestnut, and pick the leg up, holding on by the cannon bone.	
Hind foot: Stand by the horse's torso, facing the rear of the horse and touching the horse's rump. Bend gradually and slide one hand distally down the leg, picking the hind limb up when the horse lifts it off the ground. Hold the dorsal aspect of the pastern.	
Place a clean diaper with medication over the sole of the foot (Figure 33.17).	A diaper works well as a sole bandage to hold medication on the sole. Alternatively a square piece of rolled cotton is applied to the bottom of the foot, followed by wrapping the foot with brown gauze. This can be utilized instead of the diaper.
Center the duct tape shell over the bottom of the foot.	
Set the foot on the ground and make four relief cuts in the duct tape around the foot (Figure 33.18). The relief cuts are made at the corners of the shell and directed toward the center.	The relief cuts allow the shell to conform better to the shape of the foot.
Pull the edges of the duct tape up and around the hoof (Figure 33.19).	
Trim the corners of the duct tape.	
Place a strip of elastic adhesive tape (Elastikon®) around the bandage (Figure 33.20).	Be sure the tape sticks to the skin to seal the top of the bandage. This will prevent debris from getting down inside the bandage.

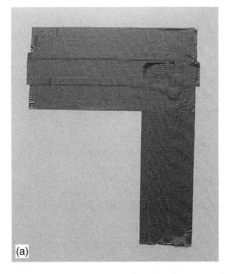
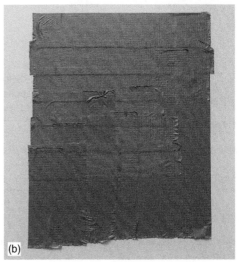

(a)   (b)

Figure 33.16 Construction of a foot bandage out of duct tape. The tape is cross-hatched to form a square.

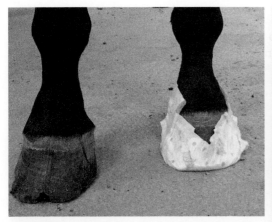

Figure 33.17 Application of a diaper containing foot medication to the sole.

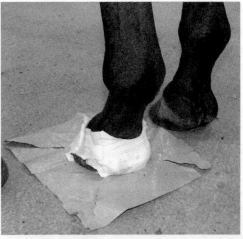

Figure 33.18 Placement of the foot over a cross-hatched duct tape bandage. Notice the splits cut at each corner.

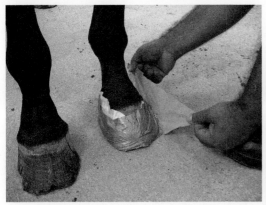

Figure 33.19 Application of a foot bandage. The flaps are brought up and stuck to the hoof wall.

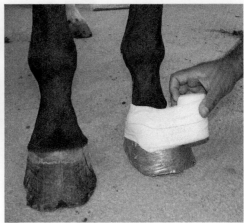

Figure 33.20 The top of the foot bandage is sealed with elastic adhesive tape.

33.5.5 *Distal Limb Support Bandage*

This bandage is applied in the same manner and with same materials as a distal limb wound bandage except that the wound dressing layer is not used (see section 33.5.1 and Figures 33.4 to 33.7). Its purpose is to support of soft tissue structures (i.e., flexor tendons and ligaments) of the distal limb.

33.5.6 *Forelimb Stack Bandage*

This bandage is used to support an upper limb fracture or luxation in conjunction with a rigid external coaptation (splint) or to provide coverage of a large upper limb wound.

Technical action	Rationale
Place a "doughnut" pad over the back of the carpus and secure it over the limb with rolled conforming gauze.	Refer to section 33.5.2 on carpal bandages.
Place a support bandage on the bottom half and then the top half of the limb (Figure 33.21).	Multiple layers can be added as needed for support (Robert–Jones bandage).

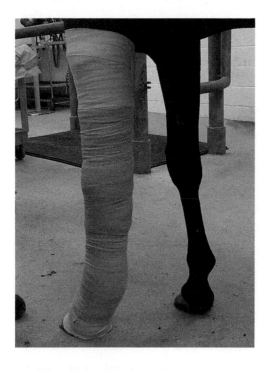

Figure 33.21 Full-limb stack bandage applied to the right front limb.

33.5.7 *Half-limb Splint*

A splint provides rigid support of the distal limb in the case of a P1 or P2 fracture, flexor tendon laceration or luxation/subluxation of the metacarpophalangeal or interphalangeal joints.

Technical action	Rationale
Apply a Robert–Jones bandage to the distal limb.	A Robert–Jones bandage is a multiple-layered distal limb support bandage.
Place rigid splint material (e.g., split PVC pipe) on the flexor surface of the limb, from just below the carpus/tarsus to the ground (Figure 33.22).	Be sure ends of the rigid splint material are padded and that the Robert–Jones bandage goes farther proximal on the limb than the splint material.
	This reduces the chance of pressure sores developing under the ends of the splint.
Secure the splint to the bandage by firmly wrapping with non-elastic tape (duct tape) (Figure 33.22).	

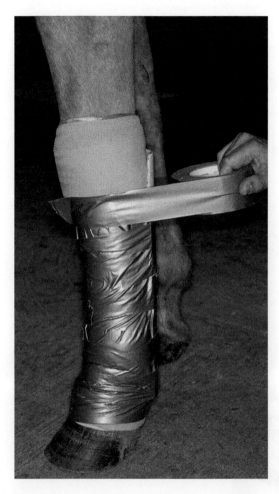

Figure 33.22 Application of a linear portion of heavy duty PCV pipe used as a half-limb splint along the flexor surface of the front limb.

33.5.8 Full-limb Splint

This bandage provides support of an upper limb in cases of fracture or luxation of the carpal or tarsal joints in conjunction with a rigid external coaptation (splint).

Technical action	Rationale
Apply a stack Robert–Jones bandage to the entire limb.	A Robert–Jones bandage is a multiple layered full-limb splint.
Front limb: Secure splint material to the flexor surface of the limb, from just below the olecranon to the ground (Figure 33.23a) with non-elastic tape (duct tape) (Figure 33.23b).	
Hind limb: Secure the splint on the lateral and medial aspects of the limb with non-elastic tape (Figure 33.24).	It is very difficult to splint the entire limb.

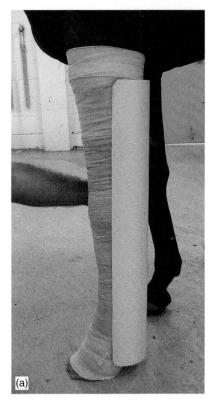
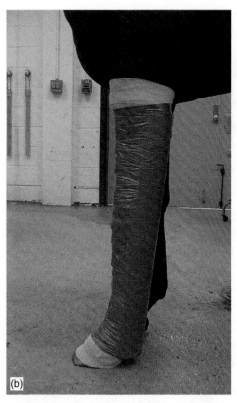

Figure 33.23 Application of a long linear piece of heavy duty PCV pipe used as a full-limb splint over the top of a full-limb stack bandage. (a) Notice that the splint is placed along the flexor surface of the front limb. (b) The splint is secured to the limb with duct tape.

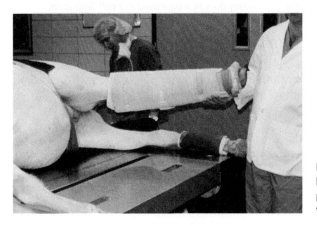

Figure 33.24 Splint being removed from a hind limb. Notice that the rigid material was placed medial and lateral. The horse had a tarsal luxation.

Bibliography and Further Reading

Hosgood, G. and Burba, D.J. (2010) Wound healing, wound management, and bandaging, in *McCurnin's Clinical Textbook for Veterinary Technicians*, 7th edn (eds J.M. Bassert and D.M. McCurnin), Saunders Elsevier, St Louis.

Southwood, L.L. (2008) Bandaging of the limb, in *The Equine Hospital Manual*

(eds K. Corley and J. Stephen), Blackwell, Oxford, pp. 100–106.

Stephen, J.O. (2008) Application of spints, in *The Equine Hospital Manual* (eds K. Corley and J. Stephen), Blackwell, Oxford, pp. 106–108.

34

Cast Application

Daniel J. Burba

34.1 Purpose

- To provide immobilization and external coaptation for fractures of the distal limb, from the hoof to the proximal metacarpus or metatarsus.

34.2 Complications

- Pressure sores resulting from casts that are placed without correct padding or that are placed too loosely.

34.3 Equipment Required

Supplies needed for cast application (Figure 34.1):

- broom handle
- heavy duty wire (approximately 30 cm)
- drill with 1/8″ bit and drill
- hoof rasp
- shoe pullers
- hoof knife and pick
- wooden heel block
- wire cutters
- fiberglass cast tape
- foam orthopedic padding
- orthopedic felt
- orthopedic stockinette (3″)
- orthopedic padding
- white medial tape (1″ or 2″)
- towel clamps
- bandage scissors
- examination gloves
- polymethylmethacrylate
- bucket of water.
- elastic adhesive tape (Elasticon®, Johnson & Johnson, New Brunswick, NJ)
- optional materials (in case of wound present):
  - non-adherent dressing
  - conforming gauze (i.e., kling)
  - elastic self-retaining wrap (e.g., Vetrap®, 3M, St. Paul, MN)

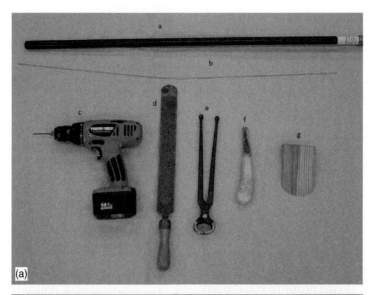

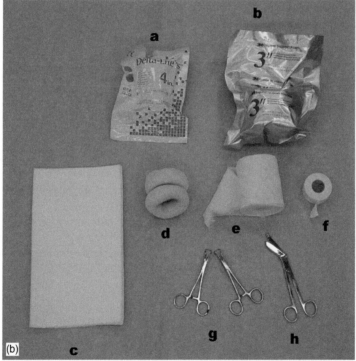

Figure 34.1 Supplies necessary for cast application. (A) Equipment: (a) broom handle, (b) wire, (c) drill and 1/8″ bit, (d) hoof rasp, (e) shoe pullers, (f) hoof knife, (g) wooden heel wedge. (B) Casting materials: (a) fiberglass casting tape, (b) foam cast padding, (c) orthopedic felt, (d) orthopedic stockinette, (e) cast padding, (f) white tape, (g) towel clamps, (h) bandage scissors.

34.4 Restraint and Positioning

- For proper application of a lower limb cast that includes the hoof, general anesthesia is optimal (see Chapter 76).

34.5 Procedure

Technical action	Rationale
Place the horse in lateral recumbency with the affected limb up (Figure 34.2).	This allows easier application of the cast.
Remove splint if there is one on the affected limb.	Splints are used on horses for transportation and movement of the horse until a cast is applied.
Clean debris from the sole and trim the hoof if the hoof wall and toe are excessively long (Figure 34.3).	
Thoroughly scrub and disinfect the sole of the foot.	This will reduce the amount of bacterial contamination and reduce the bacterial growth under the cast.
Place the affected limb in the extended position, perpendicular to the body.	This reduces angulation to the cast as it is being applied.
Drill two holes in the hoof wall, 5 cm apart, on either side of the toe (Figure 34.4).	Drill in the same direction as driving a horseshoe nail so that you do not quick the horse.
Place the ends of a wire through the holes (Figure 34.5) and twist the ends together to form a large loop.	This will be used to apply traction while applying the initial layers of the casting material.
Pack the frog with povidone-iodine impregnated gauze sponges.	This will reduce the amount of bacterial contamination and bacterial growth under the cast.
If a wound is present, apply a wound bandage consisting of a non-adherent dressing, conforming gauze (i.e., kling), and elastic self-retaining wrap.	See Chapter 33, Figures 33.2 and 33.3.
Measure out a length of 3″ orthopedic stockinette by taking the distance from the carpus/tarsus to the toe, double this length, and add approximately 40 cm.	This will provide you with enough stockinette to apply a double layer on the leg and an excess at the proximal end of the cast.
Fold the stockinette in half and mark the middle. Roll one end outward and the other end inward until they meet at the midpoint (Figure 34.6).	This will give two equal lengths of stockinette such that when the outward and inward stockinette is unrolled there will be two equal lengths of stockinette left at the proximal aspect of the cast.
Pull the stockinette over the wire and put the leg in traction by placing a broom handle through the wire loop (Figure 34.7). Starting at the toe, unroll the outward stockinette, rolling it up the leg.	Orthopedic stockinette is used to keep the cast material from adhering to the limb.
Place a twist in the stockinette just beneath the toe (Figure 34.8) and unroll the inward roll.	
Pull the stockinette tight over the limb and secure both layers to the limb above the carpus/tarsus with a towel clamp placed laterally and medially (Figure 34.9).	Be careful not to penetrate a tendon sheath or vessel with the towel clamp. Smooth any wrinkles out of the stockinette.
Cut a 7 cm wide strip of orthopedic felt, enough to provide coverage of the circumference of the limb just below the carpus/tarsus. Secure the ends of the strip of orthopedic felt with 1″ white tape (Figure 34.10).	The felt will aid in the prevention of pressure sores at the top of the cast.

(continued)

Technical action	Rationale
Place a couple layers of 4″ wide orthopedic padding around the fetlock and coronary band (Figure 34.11).	These areas are most vulnerable to cast sores.
Put on examination gloves. Submerge a 3″ roll of fiberglass casting tape until most of the air bubbles dissipate from the roll (Figure 34.12).	Use water at room temperature. Warm water will cause the resin in the cast tape to cure too fast.
Start at the level of the fetlock and carefully apply the casting tape by working distally and then proximally (Figure 34.13).	Be very careful not to allow wrinkles to develop in the casting tape as it is being applied.
Overlap the cast material by 1/3 to ½ (1–1.5 cm). Leave half the width of the orthopedic felt at the top of the cast exposed (Figure 34.14).	Leaving half of the felt exposed will reduce the chances of a cast sore developing.
Cut the traction wires once you have incorporated the foot in the initial layers of the cast.	Once the wires are cut, an assistant will need to continue holding the limb by grasping the foot (Figure 34.15).
Continue adding layers of casting tape. Add the 3″ casting tape first (approximately four rolls).	In total approximately four rolls of 3″ casting tape and four to six rolls of 4″ casting tape are required.
Before applying the 4″ rolls of casting tape, place a roll of 4″ casting tape (Figure 34.16a) or wooden wedge block (Figure 34.16b) under the heels and incorporate it in the cast with the remaining rolls of 4″ casting tape.	A heel wedge incorporated in the cast allows the horse to walk more easily while wearing a cast by decreasing the breakover force, reducing pressure on the dorsal proximal limits of the cast on the metacarpus or metatarsus, and allowing more even axial weight bearing down through the cast.
Before the last couple of rolls are added, the top of the stockinette is turned down over the cast and incorporated into it.	This flares the orthopedic felt over the top of the cast to reduce cast sore formation.
Cap the bottom of the cast with polymethylmethacrylate (PMMA) (Figure 34.17). This is accomplished by mixing PMMA ingredients in a disposable bowel and applying the mixture with a wooden tongue depressor like cake icing.	PMMA adds strength to the bottom of the cast and helps to prevent wearing of the cast material as the horse walks on it.
Seal the top of the cast by applying elastic adhesive tape Elasticon®) to it and the skin (Figure 34.18).	This will prevent debris from getting down inside the bandage.

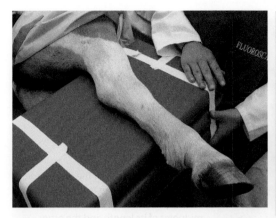

Figure 34.2 Horse positioned in lateral recumbency with the affected limb uppermost for application of a cast.

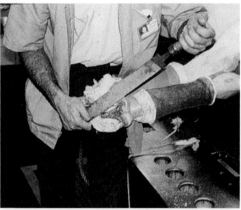

Figure 34.3 Prior to application of a cast the hoof should be trimmed and thoroughly cleaned with a disinfectant.

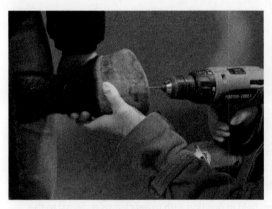

Figure 34.4 Two holes are drilled in the toe of the hoof just outside the white line for insertion of a traction wire for cast application.

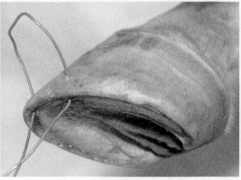

Figure 34.5 Insertion of a traction wire through the two holes drilled in the toe of the hoof.

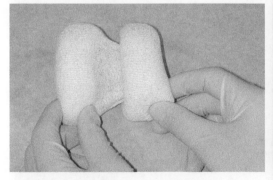

Figure 34.6 Orthopedic stockinette used under a limb cast. In preparation for placement, half of the stockinette is rolled to the outside and half is rolled to the inside until they meet at the midpoint of the length of stockinette.

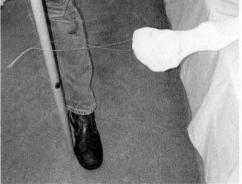

Figure 34.7 Once the orthopedic stockinette in placed on the limb, a loop is made in the traction wire placed through the broom handle in preparation for a cast application.

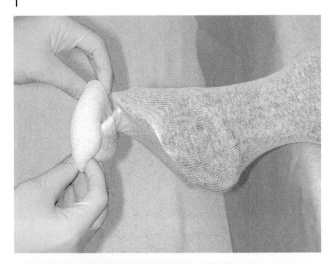

Figure 34.8 One end of the orthopedic stockinette is rolled up the limb. A twist is placed in the stockinette at the midpoint of its length and the other end is rolled up the limb prior to cast application.

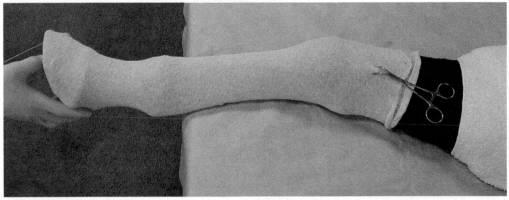

Figure 34.9 The orthopedic stockinette is stretched and held in position with towel clamps proximal to the area to be casted.

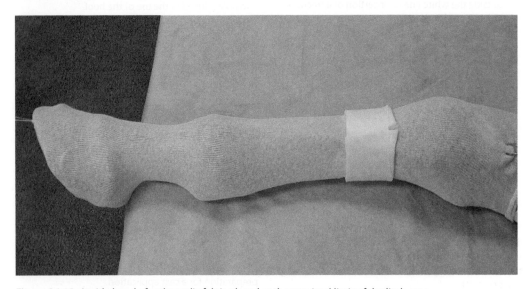

Figure 34.10 A wide band of orthopedic felt is placed at the proximal limit of the limb cast.

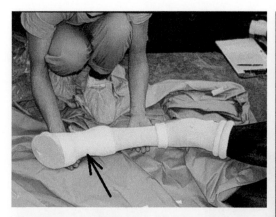

Figure 34.11 Cast padding is applied around the fetlock and coronary band.

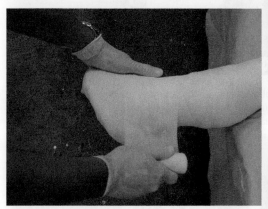

Figure 34.13 Application of the fiberglass casting tape to a limb of a horse, starting at the level of the fetlock and working distally and then proximally. Care is taken to ensure a smooth application.

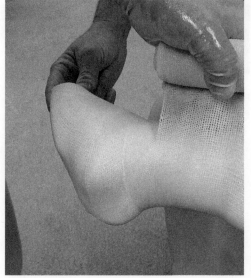

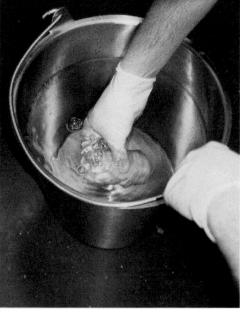

Figure 34.12 The roll of fiberglass casting tape must be wetted prior to application.

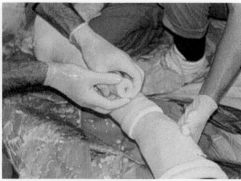

Figure 34.14 A portion of the orthopedic felt placed at the proximal limit of the cast is left exposed to provide padding at the top of a limb cast.

Figure 34.15 Once the traction wires have been cut, the toe is held by an assistant while the remaining layers of cast material are applied.

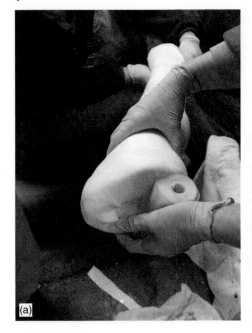

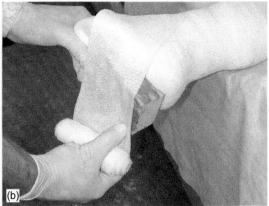

Figure 34.16 Incorporate a heel wedge in the cast to allow the horse to walk more easily while wearing the cast by decreasing the breakover force, reducing pressure on the dorsal proximal limits of the cast on the metacarpus or metatarsus, and allowing more even axial weight bearing down through the cast. (a) Use of a roll of fiberglass casting tape as a heel wedge during application of a cast. (b) Alternatively, a wooded heel wedge is incorporated into a limb cast on a horse.

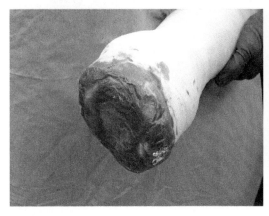

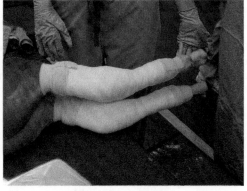

Figure 34.17 The bottom of a completed limb casted is capped with acrylic.

Figure 34.18 The top of a limb cast is sealed with elastic adhesive tape (Elasticon®).

Bibliography and Further Reading

Hosgood, G. and Burba, D.J. (2010) Wound healing, wound management, and bandaging, in *McCurnin's Clinical Textbook for Veterinary Technicians*, 7th edn (eds J.M. Bassert and D.M. McCurnin), Saunders Elsevier, St Louis.

Part V

Clinical Procedures by Body Systems: Reproductive System

35

Reproductive Evaluation of the Stallion

Carlos R. F. Pinto

35.1 Purpose

- Reproductive evaluation of stallions constitutes a routine pre-breeding examination to be performed prior to the beginning of the breeding season. It is also part of a pre-purchase examination of a stallion, especially if the stallion is being purchased as breeding stock.
- Reproductive evaluation is indicated for the investigation of the cause of reproductive failure of a stallion.
- The reproductive examination of the stallion includes:
  - examination of the integrity of the external genitalia, evaluating the testes within the scrotum, the penis, and the prepuce
  - measurement of testes, testicular examination by manual palpation, and ultrasonography
  - obtaining a semen sample for complete analysis and estimation of breeding capacity and fertility potential
  - obtaining swab samples from the penis, glans penis, and urethra (before and after ejaculation) for microbiology analysis (culture and sensitivity).

35.2 Complications

- Trauma to the penis, prepuce or scrotum/testes during semen collection using an artificial vagina or inflicted by kicks if using a teaser mare.

- Generalized body injuries following a fall from the breeding phantom.
- Iatrogenic rectal tears following examination of the internal genitalia by palpation per rectum.

Note: Examination of the stallion's internal genitalia using palpation per rectum is not routinely performed in every breeding soundness evaluation owing to the perception that stallions may resent the examination per rectum more than mares, thus subjecting them to increased risk for rectal tears. Because palpation per rectum and ultrasonography of the stallion's accessory sex glands (bulbourethral, prostate, vesicular glands, and ampullae) may provide valuable information, equine practitioners should use this potential diagnostic approach if a thorough reproduction evaluation is warranted.

35.3 Equipment Required

- Non-sterile shoulder-length obstetrical sleeve for palpation per rectum.
- Non-sterile and sterile non-spermicidal isosmotic lubricants for rectal palpations and artificial vagina, respectively.
- Roll cotton for cleaning the penis.
- Bucket with disposable liner to hold water for washing the penis (Figure 35.1).
- Calipers for measuring total scrotal width or individual testis.
- Culture swabs and transport media.

Manual of Clinical Procedures in the Horse, First Edition. Edited by Lais R.R. Costa and Mary Rose Paradis.
© 2018 John Wiley & Sons, Inc. Published 2018 by John Wiley & Sons, Inc.

- Portable ultrasound unit equipped with a 5 or 7.5 MHz linear transducer
- Artificial vagina (AV) and related supplies (Figure 35.2a):
  - liners (disposable or latex)
  - semen collection bottles and filters
  - thermometer (Figure 35.2b).
- Breeding phantom (optional) plus plastic cling film wrap for breeding phantom (Figure 35.2c)
- Teaser mare
- Helmets for protection of personel
- Cotton lead rope with chain for proper handling and restraint of the stallion.
- Hobbles for the mare, if using the teaser mare as a "jump mare".

Semen analysis equipment and supplies

- Automated semen densimeter (Figure 35.3) or hemocytometer (Neubauer chamber) for sperm count.
- Phase-contrast microscope
- Glass slide warmer stage
- Glass slides and coverslips
- Water bath

- Warming incubator
- Semen extenders
- Pipettors, pipette tips, etc.

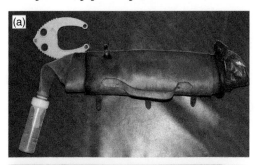

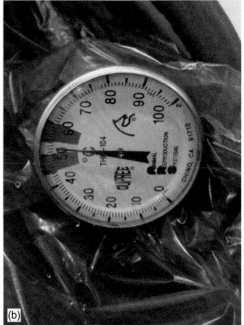

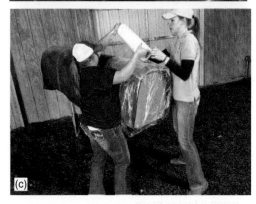

Figure 35.2 Equipment and resources include (a) artificial vagina with liner and semen collection bottles with filter, (b) thermometer, and (c) breeding phantom covered with plastic cling film wrap.

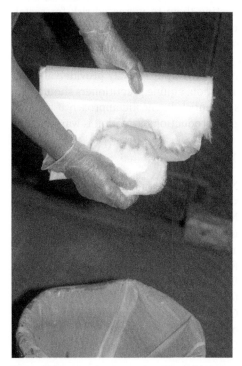

Figure 35.1 Use a bucket with a disposable liner to hold warm water and pledgets of rolled cotton for washing the stallion's penis.

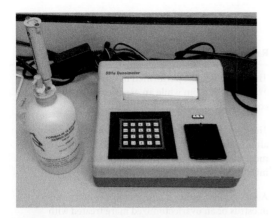

Figure 35.3 The use of an automated semen densimeter is highly recommended.

Note: Specialized equipment designed for stallion semen analyses is available and indicated if the veterinary practice often performs stallion reproductive examinations. Examples of these types of equipment are:

- computerized automated semen analyzers (CASA) to perform sperm count and motility analyses.
- nuclecounters (Figure 35.4) utilizing molecular probes to perform a sperm count and determination of viable sperm (membrane integrity).

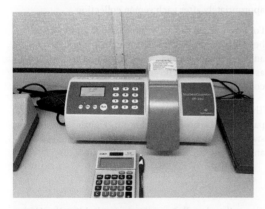

Figure 35.4 The use of nuclecounters is recommended. The nucleocounter utilizes molecular probes to perform sperm count and determination of viable sperm by detecting membrane integrity.

35.4 Restraint and Positioning

- For many parts of the reproductive evaluation of a stallion it is important to have a handler accustomed to handling stallions. A lip chain (with a cotton lead rope) must be applied and used as necessary (see Chapter 2).
- The initial physical examination is preferably performed in the stall or in an examination room. Once a thorough physical examination has been performed, it is best to proceed with the preparation for semen collection.
- The semen collection is performed at a breeding shed and requires a handler to lead the stallion, a handler to lead the teaser mare, the examiner, and an assistant to help with washing the penis once in full erection. During the washing of the penis, the examiner can evaluate the penis.
- For semen collection it is highly recommended that the person handling the artificial vagina and the assistant wear helmets.
- If a teaser mare is used as the "jump mare" rather than using a phantom, the mare should be hobbled to prevent her from kicking the stallion or a person.
- After ejaculation, the handler leads the stallion to restraint stocks for testicular measurement and completion of the reproductive examination.
- If a complete evaluation is warranted, palpation per rectum and ultrasonography is required for evaluation of the internal genitalia. Because stallions are not commonly subjected to this modality of reproductive examination, in contrast with brood mares, it is prudent to provide appropriate physical restraint (e.g., placing the stallion in stocks) and chemical restraint (sedation with an alpha-2 agonists is highly recommended, see Chapter 9).

35.5 Procedure: Reproductive Evaluation

Technical action	Rationale
Perform a general physical examination to ensure that the stallion is well enough to perform the breeding.	This might be best performed in the stall or an examination room while an experienced handler controls the stallion.
Once the physical examination has been performed, proceed with the preparation for semen collection.	The evaluation of the external genitalia is performed after semen collection because the stallion will be more cooperative then. If indicated, the evaluation of internal genitalia is performed last.
Expose the stallion to the teaser mare to sexually stimulate it (Figure 35.5).	A teaser mare, either a reproductively intact mare in estrus or an ovariectomized mare treated with injectable estrogens, is typically needed to sexually stimulate the stallion. The mare's tail should be wrapped to avoid tail hairs from traumatizing the penis.
Once the stallion achieves full erection, begin to wash the penis using large pieces of roll cotton and clean warm (around 42°c) water (Figure 35.6). Do not use disinfectants. Special attention should be given to the cleansing of the fossa glandis (removal of the "bean" = dried smegma). The penis should be carefully dried with clean paper towels.	Use a disposable plastic liner for the water bucket to avoid potential contamination between stallions. Use of disinfectants may disrupt the normal flora and therefore their use should be avoided. It is prudent to have an assistant hold the bucket with water to assist the person washing the stallion's penis.
While performing the washing of the penis, the reproductive examination begins with inspection and palpation of the penis.	Stallions generally do not resent this examination at this time.
Meanwhile, prepare the artificial vagina (AV) for collection of the semen. Attention should be paid to the temperature and pressure within the AV: the internal temperature should be 45°- 48°C (in some cases, the temperature might be set to 50°C). While wearing a sterile plastic sleeve, apply warm, sterile, water-soluble, non-spermicidal lubricant to the upper two-thirds of the AV; remove the hand, leaving the sleeve in place to prevent the lubricant from drying out.	The AV should be equipped with a disposable liner. If a latex/rubber liner is used instead of a disposable liner, the liner must be cleaned and maintained appropriately after each semen collection. For appropriate care, the latex/rubber liners should be completely washed with abundant running water and an appropriate detergent or disinfectant, such as chlorhexidine or Tergazyme™, after the semen collection is completed.
Once the penis is fully erect, the stallion is led to mount either the teaser mare or a breeding phantom so that semen collection can be performed using an AV. Depending on the level of stallion training to jump a breeding phantom, the teaser mare may or not be placed near the phantom.	The teaser mare is typically placed on the right side, parallel to the breeding phantom (Figure 35.7). The stallion is led to approach the phantom at a 20–30° angle on the left side of the breeding phantom.
Once the stallion jumps the breeding phantom, the loose plastic sleeve placed with the lubricant is removed from the artificial vagiva, and penis is quickly guided to engage into the AV (Figure 35.8).	The stallion handler and the person holding the AV must stay on the left side of the stallion and phantom.
Ejaculation is confirmed by: • observing the semen going into the collection bottle • observing the stallion flagging its tail • palpating the rhythmic urethral ejaculatory pulses when placing one hand in the ventral shaft of the penis.	If the stallion successfully ejaculates, the semen secretion at the tip of the urethral opening in the glans penis will appear frothy (Figure 35.9).

Technical action	Rationale
The semen sample is then taken immediately to the laboratory for semen evaluation and processing if needed.	Protect the semen from cold shock, water, and sunlight.
The filter previously fitted into the semen collection bottle must be quickly discarded immediately after the stallion completes the ejaculation process.	The filter with gel should be immediately discarded. Semen analysis and artificial insemination are best performed with gel-free semen samples.

Evaluation and processing of the semen:
• Record the **volume of semen**.
• Obtain an aliquot of the semen for evaluation.
  – Immediately determine the **sperm motility**.
  – Determine the **sperm concentration**.
  – Analyze **sperm morphology**.
• The remaining semen can be mixed with a Kenney's type semen extender for:
  – longevity analysis
  – further processing for artificial insemination.
	The semen sample to be analyzed can be left at room temperature.
	
	The goal of the semen evaluation is to calculate the total number of motile and morphologically normal sperm (Figure 35.10).

Determine the **sperm motility** as soon as possible. Prepare a wet mount of the semen sample (a small droplet with 5 or 10 µl of semen) and observe it using phase contrast microscopy at 200× or 400× magnification.	Alternatively, computer-automated sperm analyzers are available for determining the motility and concentration of stallion sperm.
Determine the **sperm concentration** (number of sperm per milliliter) using a hemocytometer or a commercial densimeter for stallion semen analysis. If using a hemocytometer, dilute the semen 1:100 (10 µl of semen to 990 µl of formol-saline), fill the hemocytometer chamber and wait a few minutes, so the sperm can settle to the bottom of the chamber. Count the sperm heads in the 5 x 5 squares (large central squares surrounded by triple line). Sperm heads that are on the edge of the squares should only be counted if on top and left sides (not bottom and right sides). The number obtained is multiplied by 106 to give the number of sperm per milliliter.	Typically, the total sperm number of an ejaculate averages 8.0 x 109, but seasonal variation occurs. For samples with very low concentration, the sample is diluted 1:10 rather than 1:100 and the count obtained is multiplied by 105 to give the number of sperm per milliliter. Alternatively, computerized automated semen analyzers or nucleocounters might be used. There are several models available commercially.
Lastly, analyze the **sperm morphology**: • Prepare a dry mount by making a semen smear mixed with a eosin-nigrosin stain (Hancock's stain). • Evaluate microscopically (bright field) at 1000× magnification under immersion oil. • Alternatively, dilute the semen 1:10 and examine an aliquot under phase contrast microscopy at 1000× magnification under immersion oil. The percentage of sperm membrane integrity can be determined by using the hypo-osmotic sperm swelling test (HOST). Add 10 µl of semen to 90 µl of a 100 mmol hypoosmotic sucrose solution and prepare a wet mount to be evaluated microscopically with phase contrast at 400× magnification.	The smear is used to count and document the sperm morphological characteristics. Typically 200 sperm (at least a minimum of 100 sperm) should be counted. The eosin-nigrosin smear can also be utilized to determine the percentage of live-dead sperm (dead sperm will take up the eosin stain and appear lightly red or pinkish). A nucleocounter employing the molecular probe propidium iodide is available commercially to determine the sperm concentration of total and viable (intact membrane) sperm.
Calculate the **total number of motile and morphologically normal sperm**: volume × sperm concentration × % of progressively motile sperm × % of morphologically normal sperm	For the calculation use: • the total volume of gel-free semen collected • the sperm concentration (millions of sperm per ml) • the % progressively motile sperm (from the wet mount) • % of morphologically normal sperm (from the dry mount).

(continued)

Technical action	Rationale
A complete breeding soundness evaluation should include the determination of daily sperm output (DSO).	The fertility potential and serving capacity of the stallion can be predicted based on the estimation of the DSO.
An accurate determination of the DSO requires that the extragonadal reserves be stabilized by daily collections over a period of 5–7 days. This is rarely feasible.	The DSO is determined accurately by averaging the total sperm count from ejaculates obtained on a further three consecutive days. This approach is time consuming.
DSO can also be estimated by collecting the semen from the stallion on two occasions 1 hour apart.	The total sperm count obtained in the second collection is representative of the stallion daily sperm output.
The DSO can also be estimated from the testicular measurements obtained with the use of calipers or ultrasonography.	The total sperm count in the second collection is typically half of that obtained in the first collection and should be at least 1 billion.
These measurements are then used to calculate the testicular volume.	Formulas for calculation of DSO based on testicular measurements:
Testicular volume is subsequently used to estimate the DSO.	testicular volume = 0.5233 × height × length × width (cm)
	predicted DSO = [0.024 × (volume left testis + volume right testis)] − 0.76

After semen collection, the stallion is led to restraint stocks for completion of the physical reproductive examination of the external genitalia:
 	
• measurement of the testes
• examine the testes by:
  – manual palpation
  – ultrasonography (Figure 35.11)
	Most stallions do not resent the examination of penis and scrotum/testes if this is conducted immediately after they have ejaculated.

Examination of the internal genitalia via palpation per rectum might be performed. This is an optional procedure, not always performed because of the risk of rectal tear.	Rectal palpation of the stallion generally requires sedation with an alpha-2 agonist (see Chapter 9).

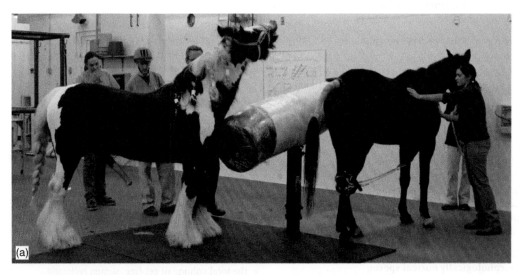

Figure 35.5 Sexually stimulate the stallion by exposing him to the teaser mare. A teaser mare can be (a) a reproductively intact mare in estrus or (b) an ovariectomized mare treated with injectable estrogens. In either case it is best to keep the phantom between the stallion and the teaser mare.

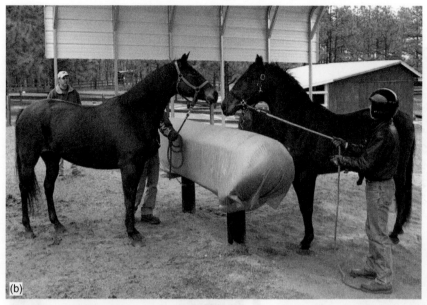

Figure 35.5 *Continued*

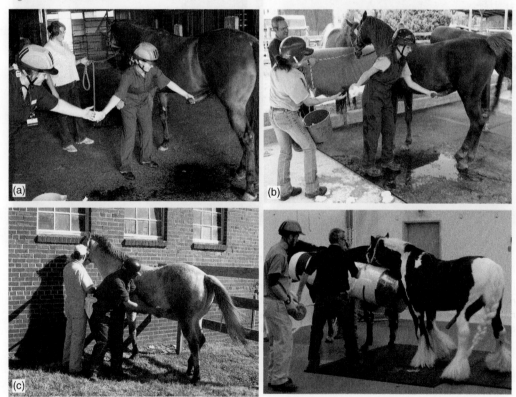

Figure 35.6 Once fully erect, the penis is washed using large pieces of roll cotton and clean water. Do not use disinfectants. Examination of the penis is performed at this time. Note these three different scenarios showing how the stallion might be restrained for this step of the procedure.

Figure 35.7 The teaser mare is typically placed on the right side and parallel to the breeding phantom, while the stallion is led to approach the phantom at a 20–30 degree angle on the left side of the breeding phantom.

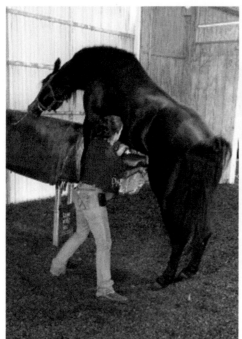

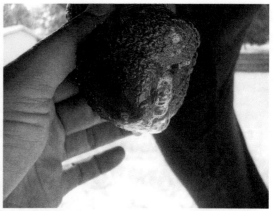

Figure 35.9 Examination of the tip of the urethral opening in the glans penis, after a successfully ejaculation by the stallion, should reveal semen secretion with frothy appearance.

Figure 35.8 Once the stallion jumps on the phantom, the penis is quickly guided to engage in the artificial vagina.

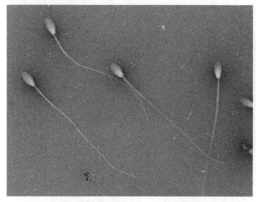

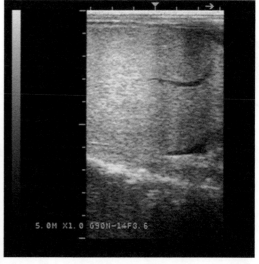

Figure 35.10 Microscopic picture of morphologically normal sperm. Calculation of the total number of motile and morphologically normal sperm is the goal of the semen evaluation.

Figure 35.11 Ultrasonographic evaluation of a normal testicle, showing the central vein. This is performed after collection of the semen because the stalion will be much more cooperative at this time. The stallion is led to restraint stocks and the external genitalia is carefully examined. The examination includes performing manual palpation and ultrasonography of the testicles.

Bibliography and Further Reading

Brinsko, S.P. Blanchard, T.L., Varner, D.D., Schumacher, J., Love, C.C., Hinrichs, K., and Hartman, D.L. (2011) *Manual of Equine Reproduction*, 3rd edn, Mosby Elsevier, Maryland Heights, MO.

Pinto, C. (2010) Genital diseases, fertility and pregnancy, in *Diagnostic Techniques in Equine Medicine*, 2nd edn, W.B. Saunders, Philadelphia, pp. 117–143.

Samper, J. (2009) Equine Breeding Management and Artificial Insemination, 2nd edn (eds F.G.R. Taylor, T.J. Brazil, and M.H. Hillyer), Saunders Elsevier, St. Louis.

36

Reproductive Evaluation of the Mare

Carlos R. F. Pinto

36.1 Purpose

- To evaluate the mare for breeding soundness.
- Examination includes inspection of the perineal conformation and caudal reproductive tract, palpation per rectum and transrectal ultrasonography to examine the uterus and ovarian structures, and collection of samples for endometrial culture, cytology, and biopsy to determine the status of uterine health and formulate a prognosis for the potential for fertility.
- Reproductive examination of the mare is important for pre-breeding assessment, for pre-purchase examination if the mare is expected to be a broodmare, for investigation of causes for reproductive failure, and for identification of reasons for changes in behavior.
- To record the reproductive history and examination findings following a systematic approach (Figure 36.1, Table 36.1 and 36.2).

36.2 Complications

- Iatrogenic rectal tears (see Table 16.1, page 182).

36.3 Equipment Required

- Non-sterile and sterile shoulder-length obstetrical sleeve for palpation per rectum and per vaginal, respectively.
- Non-sterile and sterile lubricants
- Roll cotton for perineal asepsis
- Betadine scrub
- Bucket with disposable liner to hold water for perineal asepsis.

- Disposable vaginal speculum
- Pen light or any other light source suitable for illuminating the vaginal speculum
- Uterine culture swabs, double guarded
- Uterine cytology brushes
- Glass slides
- Portable ultrasound unit equipped with a 5 or 7.5 MHz linear transducer
- Large alligator-jaw forceps for endometrial biopsy
- Bouin's fixative solution or 10% phosphate-buffered formalin to preserve the biopsy specimen.

36.4 Restraint and Positioning

- The reproductive examination should preferably be conducted with the mare restrained in stocks.
- The degree of restraint will depend on the disposition of the mare and whether the mare has been previously subjected to serial examinations per rectum.
- Application of a nose twitch might be indicated if the mare appears to resent the examination.
- Administration of alpha-2 agonists (xylazine, detomidine, etc.) or acepromazine are good options for sedating mares that are nervous or unfamiliar with the examination (see Chapter 9).
- For mares that strain excessively, the administration of an anti-spasmodic drug (Buscopan™, N-butylscopolammonium bromide at the label dose of 0.3 mg/kg body weight, slowly IV) may prove of benefit.

Manual of Clinical Procedures in the Horse, First Edition. Edited by Lais R.R. Costa and Mary Rose Paradis.
© 2018 John Wiley & Sons, Inc. Published 2018 by John Wiley & Sons, Inc.

Equine Individual Reproductive Record -   **Year:** _____

Month	Day 01	02	03	04	05	06	07	08	09	10	11	12	13	14	15	16	17	18	19	20	21	22	23	24	25	26	27	28	29	30	31
Jan																															
Feb																															
Mar																															
Apr																															
May																															
Jun																															
Jul																															
Aug																															
Sep																															
Oct																															
Nov																															
Dec																															

■	•	O	✓	E	CH	CL	◪	◹
Foaled	Pregnant	Open	Check	Estrus	<72 h	C luteum	Mated	A.I.

_____   _____

Stallion name   Stud farm

_____   _____   _____

Contact information   Collection schedule   Mare name

(a)

DATE	EXAMINATION	DATE	EXAMINATION

LO, left ovary; RO, right ovary; C, cervix; U, uterus; E, edema.
Grading system: 1, 2, 3, 4 (for cervix and follicle, 1 = firm and 4 = very
soft; for edema, 1 = ± edema and 4 = very strong).

(b)

Figure 36.1 Example of a two-page form for recording findings during reproductive evaluation of a mare: (a) front page and (b) back page.

Table 36.1 Relevant history information prior to breeding soundness examination in the mare

General	Reproductive specific
Age	Duration of estrus
When and why termination of performance career	History of vulvar discharge
Medications received during performance career	History of behavior during anestrus
History of abdominal surgery	History of behavior during breeding season
History of hindlimb lameness	Method of breeding: natural cover, artificial insemination with fresh, cooled or frozen semen
History of trauma	Number of pregnancies
Vaccination history	Number of foals delivered
Diet	Number of abortions
Medical problems in general	Number of early embryonic death
	Number of stillbirths
	Number of twin pregnancies
	Number of neonatal deaths
	History of dystocia

Table 36.2 Systematic approach to a complete breeding soundness examination in the mare

Steps	Purpose
Examination of the vulva and perineal region	Evaluation of anatomical relationships provides information concerning the risk of reproductive problems (see Table 36.3)
Clitorial swabbing	Required by regulatory bodies for screening for contagious equine metritis (CEM)
Manual examination of the internal genital tract per rectum	Rectal palpation of the ovaries and uterus provides important information concerning the mare's reproductive status
	Most importantly is the determination of whether or not the mare is pregnant
Transrectal ultrasonography	Ultrasonographic examination of the ovaries and uterus provides further refinement of the information obtained by rectal palpation
	Ultrasonographic confirmation that the mare is not pregnant prior to any vaginal, cervical or intrauterine procedures is critical
Vaginal examination	Useful in identifying the stage of the cycle of the mare, as well as the presence of anatomical, and possibly pathological, abnormalities.
Digital examination of the vagina and cervix	Allows detection of lesions in the vagina or cervix, including tears and adhesions
Endometrial culture swabbing	Obtain a sample for microbial culture and sensitivity
	Endometrial cytology should be performed concurrently to aid the interpretation of the culture results
Endometrial cytology	Detection and evaluation of uterine inflammation
Endometrial biopsy	Prognosticate the mare's reproductive potential

36.5 Procedure: Breeding Soundness Examination of the Mare

Technical action	Rationale
Obtain a brief, but complete, history of the mare's general health and reproductive career. Make sure to include all relevant details.	Important historical information is outlined in Table 36.1 and in the reproductive examination form in Figure 36.1. Proper identification of the mare is critical in cases of sale/purchase.
Perform a brief physical examination, paying particular attention to the mare's general health appearance and body condition score.	Note any signs that might be indicative of overt medical abnormalities. Note any ambulatory/locomotor problems that might impact the ability of the mare to sustain a pregnancy.
Perform a systematic breeding soundness examination following the sequential steps described in Table 36.2.	A systematic approach is important to avoid compromising the interpretation of a procedure because of interference from an earlier one. Considerations concerning reproductive procedures in the mare are listed in Table 36.3.
Perform an examination of the vulva and perineal region prior to administration of any sedative or spasmolytic drugs to the mare.	Sedation can lead to relaxation of the perineal area and interference with the functions of the vulvar lips and vaginovestibular fold.
Examine the vulva and perineal region to determine the mare's conformation. 1. Assess the integrity and seal of the vulvar lips (or labia) (Figure 36.2). 2. Evaluate the vulvar vertical inclination (Figure 36.3). 3. Evaluate the anatomical relation between vulva and pelvic brim (Figure 36.4). 4. Evaluate the vestibule and the vaginovestibular fold function (Figure 36.5). 5. Perform the "windsucker" test by parting the vulvar lips (labia) and listening for a sound of inrush of air. 6. Evaluate the floor of the vagina for the presence and appearance of fluid.	See Table 36.4 for details on examination of the vulva and perineal region. 1. The vulvar lips should be closely apposed to each other to minimize contamination of the vestibule and possibly the vagina and uterus. 2. The vulva should be vertically straight and have a cranial to caudal slope of no more than 10°. 3. At least two-thirds of the vulva should lie below the floor of the pelvis. 4. The vaginovestibular fold functions as a sphincter (and is often referred as the "vaginal vestibular sphincter"). 5. The "windsucker" test evaluates the integrity of the vaginal vestibular sphincter. 6. Accumulation of frothy fluid in the cranial vagina is indicative of pneumovagina. Older mares that are thin often have atrophy of vulvar lips and flat croup, making them more prone to pneumovagina.
Before examining the mare per rectum, the tail should be bandaged or wrapped and tied around the mare's neck (Figure 36.6).	The mare's tail hairs can irritate the rectum mucosa if inadvertently introduced into the anus during palpation. Never tie the tail to an object (e.g., the poll of the restraint stocks).

Technical action	Rationale
If the mare is uncooperative and unfamiliar with reproductive examination, or if the mare is straining excessively, administration of sedative or spasmolytic drug is indicated.	Routinely, mares do not need to be given any drugs for breeding soundness examination. Exercise caution when working with maiden mares.
If indicated, a clitoral swab should be collected at this time.	The vulva should not be washed or scrubbed prior to collection of a clitoral swab.
1. Any gross contamination of the vulva must be wiped with a dry paper towel prior to clitoral swab.	Clitoral swabs are collected for the sole purpose of testing for *Taylorella equigenitalis* (causative agent of contagious equine metritis, CEM).
2. With a gloved hand, expose the clitoral area, parting the vulvar lips.	After collection of the clitoral swabs and placement into the transport medium, they should be kept at 4 °C.
3. Evert the clitoral area by placing the index finger below the vulvar lips (Figure 36.7).	The swab in transport medium should be submitted to an approved laboratory as soon as possible to ensure that it arrives within 48 hours from the time of collection.
4. Use a narrow-tipped swab to sample the central and, if present, the lateral sinuses.	
5. Use a standard-type swab to sample all other areas of the clitoral fossa.	
6. Place both swabs in Amies charcoal-based transport medium.	

Table 36.3 Considerations concerning manipulations involving entry into the uterus

Consideration	Explanation
Perform thorough rectal palpation and ultrasonography of the uterus and ovaries prior to any procedure involving entry into the genital tract	Withhold any vaginal, cervical or intrauterine examination until it has been confirmed that the mare is not pregnant
Manipulations involving entry into the uterus are best performed during estrus	It is inevitable that resident populations of microorganisms from the vestibule and vagina will gain entry to the uterus
	Mares can best eliminate this contamination during estrus
	If a procedure involving entry into the uterus is performed during diestrus, the mare should be treated with a luteolytic dose of prostaglandin F2-alpha to minimize the chances of endometritis
Digital examination of the cervix during diestrus is only indicated if there is concern about cervical integrity	During diestrus the cervix should be tightly closed
	If it is not, then the cervical integrity is most likely compromised
If a procedure involving entry into the uterus is performed during diestrus, the mare should be treated	The mare should be given a luteolytic dose of prostaglandin F2-alpha
	This will bring the mare into estrus, which will help to eliminate any contamination

(continued)

Consideration	Explanation
Do not collect an endometrial culture swab from mares without clinical signs of endometritis	The risk of a false positive culture is high
	Only after evidence of endometritis has been established by ultrasonography should an endometrial swab be collected because of the risk of contamination of the uterus during the collection of the endometrial culture swab.

Table 36.4 Examination of the vulva and perineal region, and anatomical relationships

Anatomical relationships	Guidelines
Seal of the vulvar lips	Integrity of the vulvar lips and the proper anatomical relationship with the anus are essential because they provide the first barrier for contamination of external organisms to the uterus
Vulvar vertical inclination	The vulva should be vertical and the cranial to caudal slope should be no more than 10°
	Conformation that deviates from that is considered undesirable because it will predispose the mare to development of endometritis
Anatomical relation between vulva and pelvic brim	At least two-thirds of the vulva should lie below the pelvic brim (i.e., the floor of the pelvis)
	If not, the mare will be predisposed to contamination of the vagina with feces
Evaluate the vestibule (the area that separates the vulva and clitoris from the vagina proper)	At the cranial border of the vestibule is a folded muscular membrane, the vaginovestibular fold
	The vaginovestibular fold functions as a sphincter, acting as a second physical barrier between the uterus and the external environment
	A poor vaginovestibular seal will predispose the mare to development of endometritis
"Windsucker" test	To test the adequacy of the vaginovestibular fold as a physical barrier to external contaminants
Evaluate the vagina for the presence and appearance of fluid	Accumulation of frothy fluid in the cranial vagina is indicative of pneumovagina
Determine the presence of pneumovagina, which is a consequence of improper functioning of the first (vulva) and second (vaginovestibular fold) barriers	Constant or frequent entry of air into the vagina facilitates the entry of debris and contaminants into the caudal reproductive tract, leading to decreased fertility
	The presence of pneumovagina prompts the clinician to further evaluate the uterus to determine the presence of pneumouterus

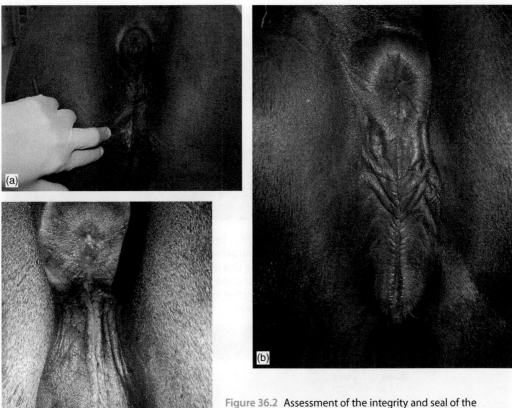

Figure 36.2 Assessment of the integrity and seal of the vulvar lips. (a) Good seal of the vulvar lips is noted when pulling one of the sides away. (b) An example of good perineal conformation showing the vulvar lips closely apposed to each other. (c) Poor vulvar lip integrity noted by the presence of visible mucosa (pink), indicating poor vulvar lip seal.

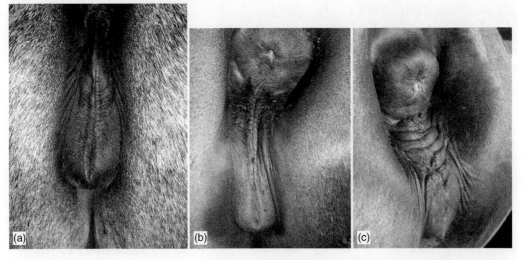

Figure 36.3 Evaluation of vulvar vertical inclination. (a) An example of good conformation showing that the vulva is vertically straight and has a cranial to caudal slope of no more than 10°. (b) An example of poor vulvar inclination showing a curved/crooked vulva. (c) Another example of poor vulvar inclination showing cranial to caudal slope greater than 10°.

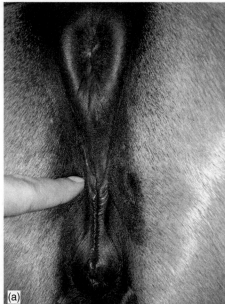

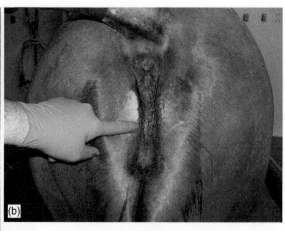

Figure 36.4 Evaluation of the anatomical relation between vulva and pelvic brim. (a) An example of good conformation showing that more than two-thirds of the vulva lies below the floor of the pelvis. (b) An example of poor conformation showing that more than one-third of the vulva lies above the pelvic brim.

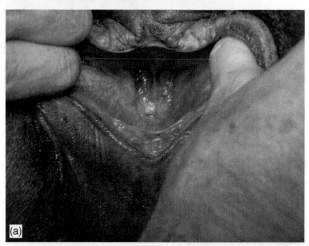

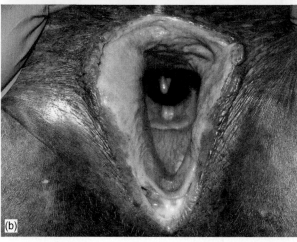

Figure 36.5 Evaluation of the vestibule and the vaginovestibular fold seal: (a) a normal vaginovestibular fold seal and (b) an inadequate vaginovestibular fold seal.

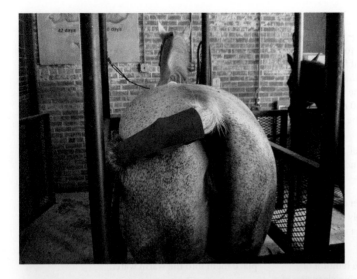

Figure 36.6 Wrap the tail with neoprene tail wrap (or brown gauze) and tie it around the mare's neck before proceeding with rectal examination of the mare.

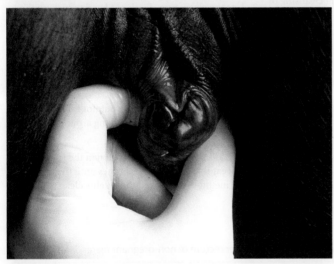

Figure 36.7 Evert the clitoral area to perform the clitoral swabbing. The clitoreal area is exposed by parting the vulvar lips and placing the index finger below them, as shown. This procedure requires sterile gloves to be worn.

Technical action	Rationale
The rectal examination should be done before proceeding with aseptic procedures. Aseptic procedures include vaginal examination and intra-uterine collection of endometrial samples.	Pregnancy should always be ruled out before performing procedures that will invade the cervix and uterus.
Wearing a non-sterile sleeve, adequately lubricated, the arm is introduced into the rectum and any fecal material within arm's reach should be removed prior to attempting to palpate the uterus and ovaries.	The presence of fecal balls can make palpation of reproductive structures difficult while also increasing intra-rectal pressure.

(continued)

Technical action	Rationale
The cervix should be palpated for its tone and length. The uterus should be palpated for tone, symmetry, and presence of intraluminal fluid The ovaries should be palpated for the presence of preovulatory follicles (typically <30 mm in diameter). The ovarian fossa should be identified.	A careful examination of the internal reproductive tract is very important and it prepares the way for conducting an objective examination using transrectal ultrasonography. See Table 36.5 for details on manual examination of the internal genital tract of a non-pregnant mare.
Proceed to performing the transrectal ultrasonography. The whole uterus and ovaries should be carefully scanned.	Documentation using video recording or still pictures is instrumental in recording the reproductive findings (Figure 36.8).
Once the rectal examination has been completed, scrub the mare's perineum thoroughly (Figure 36.9) using cotton, clean warm water, and a non-residual soap or povidone-iodine. Use one hand ("clean") to transfer the handful of cotton to the other hand ("dirty") during cleansing of the perineum. Scrub several times, at least three times, or until no visible debris is obtained in the cotton.	1. Place the warm water in a bucket with a disposable plastic liner to avoid contamination among horses through fomites. 2. Rip tufts of cotton from a clean rolled cotton and place them into the warm water. 3. Use the clean, non-dominant hand to pick up the cotton from the warm water bucket, squeeze out the excess water, and transfer the cotton to the dominant hand. 4. Have an assistant pour about a tablespoon of betadine scrub onto the center of the cotton. 5. Scrub the perineum firmly (but not forcefully), starting at the vulva and working around in a circle towards the periphery.
After the perineum is visibly clean, rinse it thoroughly with warm, clean water and dry the area with clean paper towels.	6. Discard the used piece of cotton in the garbage. Repeat these steps several times until the perineum is visibly and thoroughly clean.

Table 36.5 Manual examination of the internal genital tract per rectum of non-pregnant mares

Stage of the estrus cycle	Anatomical structure (on rectal palpation)		
	Cervix	Uterus	Ovaries
Estrus	Edematous and relaxed	Edematous and flaccid	Presence of follicle >25 mm
Diestrus	Firm and narrow	Increased tone tubular	Multiple small follicles or a follicle <25 mm
Anestrus	Moderately firm or thin and open	Flaccid	No palpable structures
Transitional	Not tightly closed until first ovulation	Flaccid	Multiple follicles, some can be >30 mm

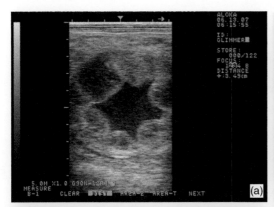

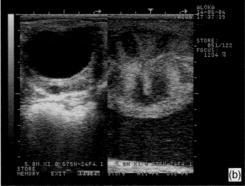

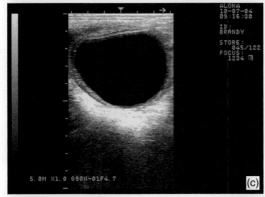

Figure 36.8 Transrectal ultrasonography is an important part of the reproductive examination of the mare. While wearing a non-sterile sleeve, adequately lubricated, introduce the arm with the rectal probe into the rectum after the rectum has been emptied of feces. The reproductive organs (uterus and ovaries) are scanned. (a) Ultrasonographic image of the uterus showing persistent post mating accumulation of fluid in a case of endometritis. (b) Ultrasonographic image during estrus showing the ovary with mature preovulatory follicle (left) and the uterus with normal edematous walls (right). (c) Ultrasonographic image of the ovary during estrus (note the mature preovulatory follicle measuring more than 25 mm in diameter).

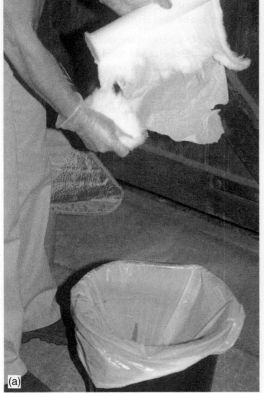

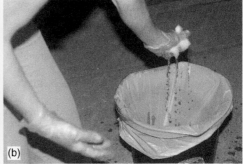

Figure 36.9 The sequence of steps for cleaning the mare's perineum thoroughly. (a) Place warm water into a bucket with a disposable plastic liner. Rip large tufts of cotton from the rolled cotton and place them in the warm water. (b) Use the clean, non-dominant hand to pick up the cotton from the warm water bucket and squeeze out the excess water. (c) Transfer the wet cotton tufts to the dominant hand. (d) Have an assistant pour about a tablespoon of betadine scrub onto the center of the cotton. (e) Scrub the perineum firmly (but not forcefully), starting at the vulva and working around in a circle towards the periphery. Discard the used piece of cotton in the garbage. Repeat these steps several times until the perineum is visibly and thoroughly clean. Courtesy of Dr. Lais R.R. Costa.

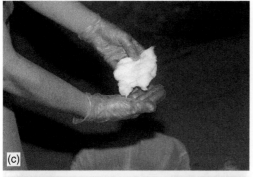

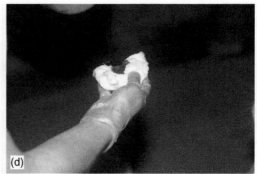

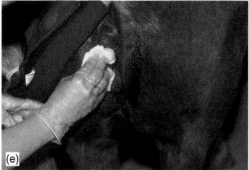

Figure 36.9 (*continued*)

Technical action	Rationale
Perform a vaginal examination. • Apply sterile lubricant onto the disposable vaginal speculum (Figure 36.10a) • Part the labia and introduce the speculum initially at a 30° angle (Figure 36.10b). • Once passed the vestibular area, advance the speculum horizontally (Figure 36.10c). • Use the light source to inspect the vaginal mucosa and floor, and the cervix. • Observe the appearance of the cervix (and interpret your findings considering the normal cyclical changes), gathering information concerning the mare's current reproductive status.	Alternatively a sterile, reusable autoclavable speculum can be used (Figure 36.11). A resistance to advancing the speculum at the level of the vaginovestibular fold should be felt. This is normal as the fold works as a second physical anatomical barrier to protect the uterus from contaminants. The cervix position in relation to the vaginal floor changes significantly according to the stage of the estrous cycle. See Table 36.6 for cyclical changes in the cervix observed during speculum or digital examination.
Perform a digital examination of the vagina and cervix using a sterile shoulder length glove and water-soluble sterile lubricant.. Palpate all around the vagina and cervix, feeling for the presence of lesions such as tears and adhesions. If endometrial culture and endometrial cytology samples are to be collected, they should be collected sequentially right after vaginal examination.	See Table 36.3 for important considerations concerning manipulations involving entry into the uterus.
For endometrial culture collection, wear a sterile shoulder-length sleeve lubricated with sterile lubricant gel and introduce the arm into the mare's vagina holding the endometrial double-guarded culture swab (Figure 36.12). With the index finger,	The double-guarded swab minimizes the risk of contamination with flora from the caudal reproductive tract. The sample may be taken from the uterine body or from the base of one of the uterine horns.

Technical action	Rationale
locate the caudal cervical os and introduce the double-guarded uterine culture swab into the uterus. Once inside the uterus, the inner protective casing is pushed through the outer casing, then the cotton swab is pushed into the uterus. Expose the swab for at least 30 seconds to allow contact with the endometrium. Once uterine sampling has been performed, the cotton swab is retracted into the inner casing, and the inner casing is retracted into the outer casing. Then, the double-guarded swab is withdrawn through the vagina. Once out of the mare, carefully expose the cotton tip swab without contaminating it, and place it in a tube with transport media. Break off the hand-contaminated end of the swab rod and discard it.	There are many options of transport media for endometrial culture swabs, BBL™ Port-A-Cul™ tubes work very well in preserving the samples up to 72 hours at room temperature.
For collection of an endometrial cytology sample use a cytology brush guided through the double-guarded endometrial swab (Figure 36.13). Place a double-guarded culture swab into the uterus as described above. Remove the cotton swab itself, leaving the outer guard of the culture swab in the mare's uterus. Carefully introduce the cytologic brush into the guard until it reaches the uterus. Rotate the shaft of the cytology brush a couple of times to ensure the brush bristles harvest endometrial epithelial cells. Prepare a smear using the sample collected from the cytology brush. Air dry and heat fix the smear, then stain with Romanowski, Giemsa or Diff-Quik (Baxter Healthcare Ltd, Thetford, UK) staining techniques.	The cytology brush is a very effective method for collecting sufficient epithelia cells for endometrial cytology. Care should be taken to not vigorously rotate the brush inside the mare's uterus as the 10 cm long cytobrush that is glued to an 18″ long plastic shaft may break off within the mare's uterus.

Alternatively, the endometrial cytology sample may be collected using a standard single or double-guarded endometrial swab. There are some instruments available for collection of both culture swab and cytology all in one.

Endometrial cytology should be collected during early and mid-estrus. The presence of neutrophils during the postpartum period is considered normal. |
| Evaluate the endometrial cytology under a light microscope. | Figure 36.14 depicts examples of endometrial cytologic findings. |
| Finally, if obtaining an endometrial biopsy is indicated, this procedure would be performed last. | See Table 36.3 for important considerations concerning endometrial biopsy. |
| An endometrial biopsy can be obtained using a long large alligator-jaw biopsy forceps (Figure 36.15).

The collection procedure is illustrated in Figure 36.16.

Introduce the arm wearing a lubricated sterile shoulder-length sleeve into the mare's uterus while holding the biopsy forceps, making sure to protect the forceps within the palm of your hand. Once in the vagina the forceps are guided through the cervix by the index finger and advanced until they reach the body of the uterus. The hand is then withdrawn and inserted into the rectum. The jaws of the forceps are kept closed until they are located in the uterus by the hand in the rectum. The jaws should be positioned sideways (horizontally) and then opened. The uterine endometrium is pushed down into the jaws, which are then closed. Withdraw the forceps and place the specimen into a tube or jar with a fixative solution at a ratio of at least 1:10 (specimen:fixative solution). | The specimen should be carefully removed from the forceps jaws with a fine needle (25-gauge) to avoid tissue damage and potential artifacts. Check in advance with the pathology laboratory you are using to find out what fixative solution they prefer or recommend. Tissue in Bouin's should be processed within 24 hours of collection. If the biopsy is not likely to reach the laboratory within 24 hours, it should be transferred to 70% alcohol on the day after collection. Alternatively, the specimen may be placed in 10% phosphate-buffered formalin, which is the preferred fixative of several histopathology laboratories. |

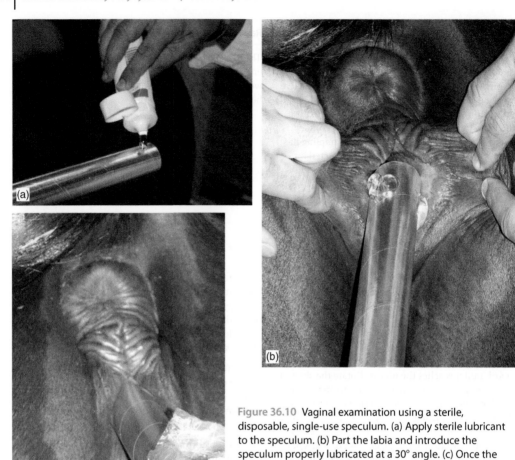

Figure 36.10 Vaginal examination using a sterile, disposable, single-use speculum. (a) Apply sterile lubricant to the speculum. (b) Part the labia and introduce the speculum properly lubricated at a 30° angle. (c) Once the vestibular area has been passed, the speculum is advanced in a horizontal position.

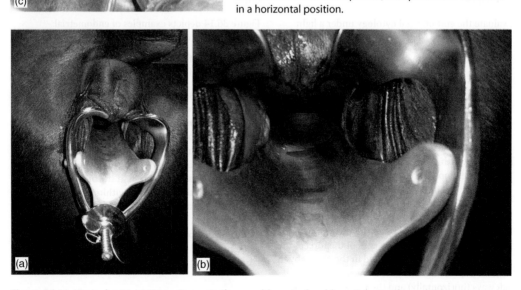

Figure 36.11 Vaginal examination using a sterile, reusable, autoclavable metal speculum, also known as Caskick's speculum or Polanki's speculum. This speculum is especially useful during post-foaling evaluations of vagina and cervix for detection of lacerations or tears that may have occurred during foaling. (a) Apply the speculum in the retracted position separating the labia. (b) Crank the knob to widen the speculum and expand the opening to allow examination of the vaginal mucosa and floor, and the cervix.

Table 36.6 Cyclical changes in the cervix visualized during speculum or digital examination

	Estrus	Diestrus	Anestrus	Pregnancy
Diameter of the cervix (number of fingers)	≥3	1	1–3	1
Color of the cervical mucosa	Red	Pale grey or yellow	Pale white	White
Overall appearance of the cervical os	Glistening, edematous, slit-like	Dry, closed	Dry, atonic, possibly open	Dry, closed
Position of the cervix	On the floor of the vagina	Midway in rostral wall of vagina	Midway in rostral wall of vagina	Midway in rostral wall of vagina

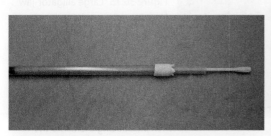

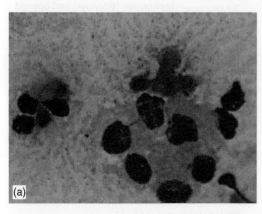

Figure 36.12 Instrument for the collection of endometrial swabs. Close-up of the tip of the double-guarded uterine culture swab showing the outer and inner protective layers and the cotton tip exposed.

Figure 36.13 Instrument for the collection of the endometrial cytologic sample. The endometrial cytology brush is inserted through the outer guard of the culture swab.

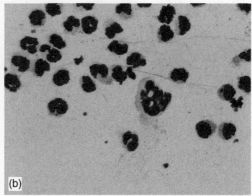

Figure 36.14 Example of endometrial cytology findings: (a) endometrial cells and (b) numerous degenerative polymorph nuclear cells/neutrophils in endometritis.

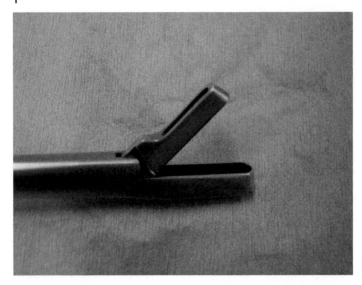

Figure 36.15 Large alligator-jaw forceps.

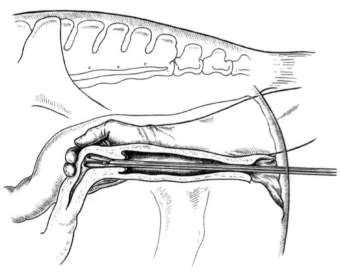

Figure 36.16 Schematic drawing demonstrating how the endometrial biopsy is collected. Wearing a lubricated sterile shoulder-length sleeve, protect the biopsy forceps when introducing them into the mare's uterus. Once the biopsy forceps is in the uterus, the hand is then inserted into the rectum. The alligator-jaw forceps is kept closed until it is located by the hand in the rectum. The jaws are positioned horizontally (sideways), and opened while the hand in the rectum applies gentle pressure on the uterine wall, pushing the endometrium tissue to be biopsied. The endometrial biopsy is obtained as shown. LeBlanc *et al.* (2000). Reproduced with permission of Elsevier.

Bibliography and Further Reading

LeBlanc, M.M., Rose, R.J., and Hodgson, D.R. (2000) Reproduction, in *Manual of Equine Practice*, 2nd edn (eds R.J. Rose and D.R. Hodgson), W.B. Saunders, Philadelphia, pp. 341–379.

Pinto, C. (2010) Genital disease, fertility and pregnancy, in *Diagnostic Techniques in Equine Medicine*, 2nd edn, W.B. Saunders, Philadelphia, pp. 117–143.

37

Artificial Insemination

Carlos R. F. Pinto

37.1 Purpose

- To place an adequate dose of semen, appropriately processed, into the uterus of a mare using non-surgical transvaginal catheterization of the cervix for delivery of the semen.

  Note: Artificial insemination must be done in conjunction with proper breeding management to ensure optimal chances for fertility.

- To inseminate mares with fresh semen when several mares are to be bred to the same stallion on a given day.
- To inseminate mares with shipped cooled semen when stallions and mares are in different geographical locations.
- To inseminate mares with frozen–thawed semen when the stallion is deceased, or not available for mating, or when semen sample can't be delivered by overnight transport.

37.2 Complications

- Iatrogenic cervical or uterine injury at the time of insemination
- Inadvertent catheterization of the bladder (rare).
- Unsuccessful conception

37.3 Equipment Required

- Non-sterile shoulder-length obstetrical sleeve for palpation per rectum.
- Non-sterile lubricants for rectal palpation

- Sterile shoulder-length obstetrical sleeve for the insemination.
- Sterile lubricants for the insemination
- Roll cotton for perineal asepsis
- Povidone-iodine scrub
- Bucket with disposable liner to hold water for perineal asepsis.
- Disposable artificial insemination rods (pipettes), 21–25″ in length
- Disposable plastic syringes, preferably all plastic, latex-free syringes (e.g., Norm-Ject®).
- Portable ultrasound unit equipped with a 5 or 7.5 MHz linear transducer for reproductive examination prior to performing the artificial insemination (ultrasonography is important to document follicle diameter, presence of uterine edema, etc.).
- Semen of choice (fresh, cooled or frozen–thawed semen)

37.4 Restraint and Positioning

- The artificial insemination procedure should preferably be conducted with the mare restrained in stocks.
- The degree of restraint will depend on the disposition of the mare and whether the mare has been previously subjected to reproductive procedures.
- Administration of alpha-2 agonists (xylazine, detomidine, etc.) or acepromazine are good options for sedating or tranquilizing mares, especially if working with maiden mares (see Chapter 9).
- Application of a nose twitch might be indicated.

Manual of Clinical Procedures in the Horse, First Edition. Edited by Lais R.R. Costa and Mary Rose Paradis.
© 2018 John Wiley & Sons, Inc. Published 2018 by John Wiley & Sons, Inc.

37.5 Procedure: Artificial Insemination

Technical action	Rationale
Place the mare in the stocks.	This will provide ideal restraint.
Apply a bandage (Figure 37.1a) or wrap (Figure 37.1b) to the tail. Tie a rope or brown gauze to the tail and bring it toward the mare's neck (Figure 37.2a) so the tail is pulled to the side and not over the perineal area (Figure 37.2b,c). Never tie the tail to an object.	The mare's tail hairs can irritate the rectum mucosa if inadvertently introduced into the anus during palpation. Tying back the tail also keeps the tail hairs away from the perineal area and vulva during aseptic preparation for the insemination procedure.
If necessary, administer sedation or tranquilization: • alpha-2 agonists (xylazine, detomidine, etc.) or • acepromazine	This will reduce the mare's reaction to the procedure.
Empty the rectum. Introduce the arm protected by a non-sterile shoulder-length sleeve, adequately lubricated, into the rectum (Figure 37.3a). Remove any fecal ball within arm's reach (Figure 37.3b).	This will avoid defecation during the insemination procedure.
It is very important to ensure mares are inseminated only when in estrus. If teasing the mare to a stallion is not available, the use of sequential reproductive ultrasonography may prove useful.	Remember that the sole presence of a follicle of preovulatory size does not guarantee the mare is in estrus. Other signs or evidence of estrus must be present.
Once the rectal examination has been completed, the time is deemed appropriate for insemination. Proceed to scrubbing the mare's perineum.	Antiseptics such as povidone-iodine can be as safe as the so-called mild soaps to cleanse the perineal area and vulvar lips. Regardless of the cleansing agent, it is important to rinse the perineal area very well and blot it dry to avoid inadvertent contamination of the insemination pipette and semen with chemicals.
Scrub the mare's perineum thoroughly, using cotton, water, and a non-residual soap or povidone-iodine. Use one hand (the "clean" hand) to transfer the handful of cotton to the other hand (the "dirty" hand) during cleansing of the perineum. Scrub several times, at least three times, or until no visible debris is obtained in the cotton. Once the perineum is visibly clean, rinse it thoroughly with warm, clean water and dry the area with clean paper towels.	Place the warm water in a bucket with a disposable plastic liner to avoid contamination among horses through fomites. Place tufts of cotton in the warm water. (Figure 37.4a). Use the clean, non-dominant hand to pick up the cotton for the warm water bucket, squeeze out the excess water, and transfer the cotton to the dominant hand (Figure 37.4b). Have an assistant pour about a tablespoon of betadine scrub onto the center of the cotton (Figure 37.4c). Scrub the perineum firmly (but not forcefully), starting at the vulva and working around in a circle towards the periphery (Figure 37.4d). Discard the used piece of cotton in the garbage. Repeat these steps several times until the perineum is visibly and thoroughly clean. Rinsing thoroughly with warm is very important. Dry well.

Technical action	Rationale
Proceed to the insemination. • Wear the sterile sleeve and adequately lubricate it with a sterile, non-spermicidal lubricant. • Introduce the arm holding the insemination pipette into the vagina. • Identify the caudal cervical os. • Introduce the insemination pipette carefully into the cervix just along and beneath the index finger. • Keep the index finger inside the cervix to guide the path of the pipette through the cervical lumen until it reaches the uterine body. • Deliver the semen by pressing the syringe plunger carefully.	Although the introduction of the insemination pipette into the uterus is straightforward, occasionally it may be difficult to ensure the pipette is correctly introduced in the uterine body. In these instances, one alternative is to withdraw the inseminating arm from the vagina and introduce the arm into the rectum to aid in the correct positioning of the pipette within the uterus. This approach is particularly helpful when deep (horn) intrauterine insemination is being performed to deposit relatively low insemination doses.
Treat the mare with an ovulation-inducing agent, such as human chorionic gonadotropin or an appropriate gonadotropin releasing hormone (GnRH) analogue (deslorelin or histrelin).	Treatment with an ovulation-inducing agent is recommended to minimize the number of insemination procedures performed in a given cycle. Most mares ovulate within 48 hours from the induction of ovulation.
Monitor the mare regularly to document the time of ovulation and the number of ovulating follicles.	Monitoring the number of ovulating follicles is important to identify the greater risk of twin pregnancy.
Check the mare 12 days after ovulation. Perform rectal palpation and transrectal ultrasonography to check if the mare has become pregnant, and to rule out twin pregnancy.	This is especially important if there was more than one ovulating follicle as the chance of twin pregnancy is greater. Twin pregnancy should be always ruled out even if only one ovulation is detected (as monozygotic twinning in horses has been reported).
If twin pregnancy is diagnosed (Figure 37.5) manual crush of one vesicle can be done at that time.	Twin pregnancy is best managed between days 12 and 15, before implantation takes place around day 16 or 17.

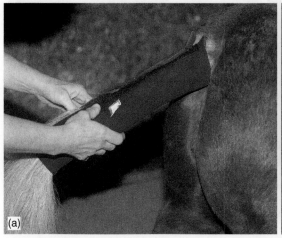
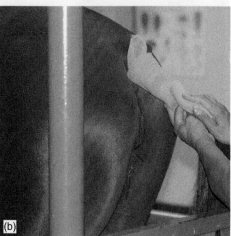

Figure 37.1 Apply a bandage or wrap to the tail: (a) brown gauze wrap around the base of the tail and (b) neoprene tail. Courtesy of Dr. Lais R.R. Costa.

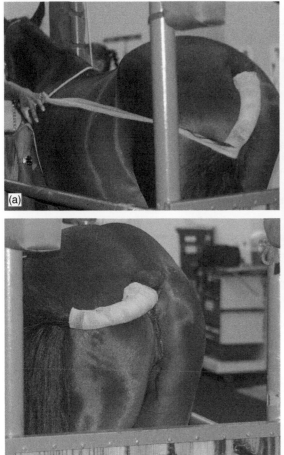

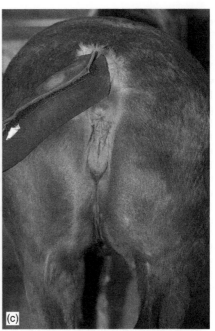

Figure 37.2 Tie a rope or brown gauze to the end of the tail and bring it towards the mare's neck, so the tail is pulled to the side and not over the perineal area. (a) After the base of the tail has been wrapped with brown gauze, the brown gauze is tied around the mare's neck. (b) The base of the tail wrapped with brown gauze is pulled to the side to free the perineal area. (c) The base of the tail, wrapped with neoprene, is pulled to the side to free the perineal area. Courtesy of Dr. Lais R.R. Costa.

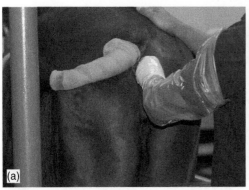

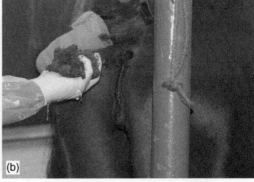

Figure 37.3 Empty the rectum to avoid defecation during the sterile insemination procedure. (a) Introduce the arm protected by a non-sterile shoulder-length sleeve, adequately lubricated, into the rectum. (b) Remove any fecal ball within arm's reach. Courtesy of Dr. Lais R.R. Costa.

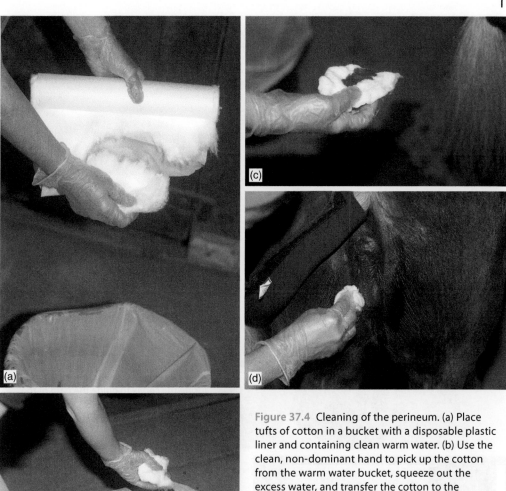

Figure 37.4 Cleaning of the perineum. (a) Place tufts of cotton in a bucket with a disposable plastic liner and containing clean warm water. (b) Use the clean, non-dominant hand to pick up the cotton from the warm water bucket, squeeze out the excess water, and transfer the cotton to the dominant hand. (c) Have an assistant pour about a tablespoon of betadine scrub onto the center of the cotton. (d) Scrub the perineum firmly (but not forcefully), starting at the vulva and working around in a circle towards the periphery. Discard the used piece of cotton in the garbage. Courtesy of Dr. Lais R.R. Costa.

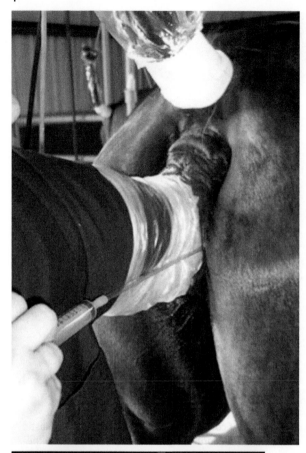

Figure 37.5 Insemination procedure: wearing sterile sleeve adequately lubricated with a sterile, non-spermicidal lubricant, introduce the arm holding the insemination pipette into the vagina, introduce the insemination pipette carefully into the caudal cervical os just along and beneath the index finger keeping the index finger inside the cervix to guide the path of the pipette through the cervical lumen until it reaches the uterine body, and deliver the semen by pressing the syringe plunger carefully (Courtesy of Dr. G. A. Dujovne).

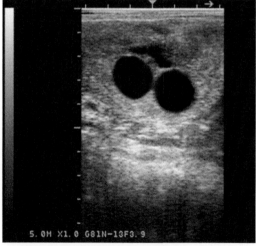

Figure 37.6 Twin pregnancy diagnosed by ultrasonography. Management of twin pregnancy is best performed between days 12 to 15, before implantation takes place, by manually crushing one vesicle.

Bibliography and Further Reading

LeBlanc, M.M., Rose, R.J., and Hodgson, D.R. (2000) Reproduction, in *Manual of Equine Practice*, 2nd edn (eds R.J.Rose and D.R. Hodgson), W.B. Saunders, Philadelphia, pp. 341–379.

Pinto, C. (2010) Genital disease, fertility and pregnancy, in *Diagnostic Techniques in Equine Medicine*, 2nd edn, W.B. Saunders, Philadelphia, pp. 117–143.

38

Placement of Caslick's Suture

Catherine Renaudin and Carlos R. F. Pinto

38.1 Purpose

- For the treatment of pneumovagina and infertility of the mare due to ascending infection of the genital tract.
- Correction of pneumovagina leads to reestablishment of normal defense mechanisms of the mare's genital tract, ultimately resulting in resolution of endometritis.
- To prevent infertility secondary to pneumovagina in mares who present with poor perineal conformation, specifically with the dorsal vulvar commissure located more than 4 cm dorsal to the pelvic floor.

38.2 Complications

- Fistula (gaps) at the surgical site may be managed at suture removal.
- Local infection (which can be prevented by topical application of antibiotic spray at the end of the procedure and for several days thereafter).
- Urovagina may occur with excessive closure of the vulvar cleft.

38.3 Equipment Required

- Brown gauze to wrap the tail or a clean neoprene tail wrap
- A rectal sleeve and lubricant
- A bucket with a clean plastic bag, cotton, non-residual soap or povidone-iodine.

- A clean towel
- A pair of surgical gloves
- A pair of sharp scissors or a scalpel blade.
- A needle holder
- Tissue forceps
- Non-absorbable monofilament sutures such as nylon or polypropylene or absorbable 0 catgut
- Local anesthetic:
  - 2% lidocaine or mepivacaine
  - 22-gauge or smaller needles and 20 ml syringe
- Sedation (optional): detomidine, xylazine or acepromazine
- A twitch

38.4 Restraint and Positioning

- The placement of Caslick sutures should be conducted with the mare restrained in stocks.
- Additional restraint will depend on the disposition of the mare.
- Administration of sedative such as alpha-2 agonists (xylazine, detomidine, etc.) is indicated. Alternatively, acepromazine is a good option for tranquilization (see Chapter 9).
- Application of a nose twitch might be indicated.

Manual of Clinical Procedures in the Horse, First Edition. Edited by Lais R.R. Costa and Mary Rose Paradis.
© 2018 John Wiley & Sons, Inc. Published 2018 by John Wiley & Sons, Inc.

38.5 Procedure

Technical action	Rationale
Place the mare in the stocks.	This will provide ideal restraint.
Apply a bandage using brown gauze (Figure 38.1) or apply a wrap to the base of the tail (Figure 38.2). Pull the tail to one side (Figure 38.3). Tie the rope or brown gauze around the mare's neck.	This will stop hair from entering the surgical field. Never tie the tail to an object or the stocks.
Empty the rectum. • Introduce the arm protected by a non-sterile shoulder length sleeve and, adequately lubricated, into the rectum. • Remove any fecal ball within arm's reach.	This will avoid defecation during the surgical procedure.
Administer sedation or tranquilization using: • alpha-2 agonists (xylazine, detomidine, etc.) or • acepromazine. Alternatively apply a twitch to the upper lip.	This will reduce the mare's reactions during tissue resection and suturing, ensuring a better apposition of the edges.
Scrub the mare's perineum thoroughly, using cotton, water and a non-residual soap or povidone-iodine. • Use the non-dominant hand as the "clean" hand to pick up the cotton from the warm water bucket and squeeze out the excess water (Figure 38.4a). Transfer the handful of cotton to the other hand (the "dirty" hand) (Figure 38.4b). Clean the perineum with the cotton in the "dirty" hand. • Have an assistant pour about a tablespoon of betadine scrub onto the center of the cotton (Figure 38.4c). • Scrub the perineum firmly (but not forcefully) starting at the vulva and working around in a circle towards the periphery. Discard the used piece of cotton in the garbage. • Repeat these steps several times until the perineum is visibly and thoroughly clean. • After the perineum is visibly clean, rinse it thoroughly with warm, clean water and dry the area with clean paper towels. • Place a clean towel over the top of the stock door.	• Place the warm water in a bucket with a disposable plastic liner to avoid contamination among horses through fomites. • Maintaining the use of the clean, non-dominant hand to pick up the clean cotton from the bucket, squeeze out the excess water, and transfer the cotton to the dominant hand will prevent contamination of the water and cotton during the cleaning procedure. • Having an assistant pour the betadine scrub will avoid contaminating from the hand while picking up the bottle of antiseptic soap. • Scrub several times, at least three times, or until no visible debris is obtained in the cotton. • Once the mare's perineum has been scrubbed, placing a clean towel on the door will prevent contamination of the suture and the surgical site if the mare sits on the door of the stocks.
Infiltrate the labial margins with about 10-20 ml of local anesthetic (2% lidocaine or mepivacaine) using a 22-gauge or smaller gauge needle (Figure 38.5a).	The infiltration of local anesthetic should cause sufficient distension of the tissues to stretch the skin along the labial margins (Figure 38.5b).
Create a raw margin for union of the two sides of the vulva, making sure an uninterrupted raw surface is obtained. Using a pair of scissors, remove an 8-mm strip of mucosa and skin along the mucocutaneous junction, starting at about 1 cm ventral to the pelvic floor, dorsally, including the dorsal commissure.	Considering the procedure will have to be repeated throughout the mare's reproductive life, it is important to remove the minimal amount of tissue (no more than an 8- to 10-mm strip of mucosa and skin) from the stretched labial margin during the initial procedure or just incise both vulvar lips 1 cm deep at the muco-cutaneous junction. Otherwise,

Technical action	Rationale
Alternatively, using a scalpel blade, make a deep incision (1 cm) along the muco-cutaneous junction, starting at the dorsal commissure and finishing about 1 cm ventral to the pelvic floor.	with repetitive placement of the Caslick suture there will be excessive scarring and loss of plasticity of the perineal tissues. Removal of a strip narrower than 8 mm may lead to gaps.
Place a suture along the raw edges of the right and left labia, bringing them together. Start at the dorsal vulvar commissure and move downwards.	Various suture patterns are possible, including simple-continuous, interrupted, and vertical mattress.
When finished insert a finger in the vulva under the suture.	Alternatively, staples may be placed instead of sutures (Figure 38.6). Make sure there are no gaps and no additional suture is needed.
It is very important to remove the sutures and reopen the vulvar cleft at the time of foaling to prevent laceration of the vulva.	Removal of the suture and reopening of the vulvar cleft might also be indicated at the time of breeding.

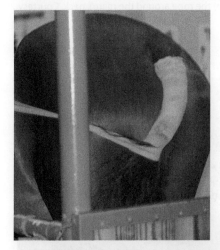

Figure 38.1 Apply a bandage using brown gauze to the base of the tail. Courtesy of Dr. Lais R.R. Costa.

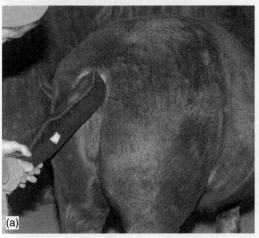

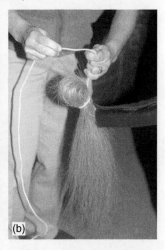

Figure 38.2 To tie the tail around the neck (a) apply a neoprene wrap to the base of the tail and (b) tie a rope at the end of the tail. Courtesy of Dr. Lais R.R. Costa.

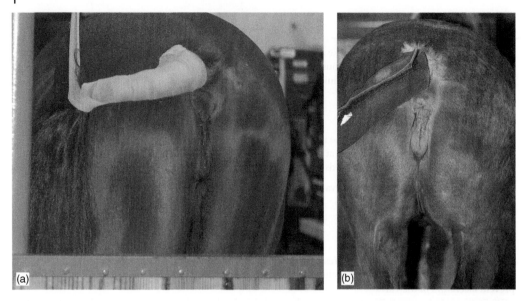

Figure 38.3 Pull the tail to one side to tie (a) the brown gauze or (b) the rope around the mare's neck. Courtesy of Dr. Lais R.R. Costa.

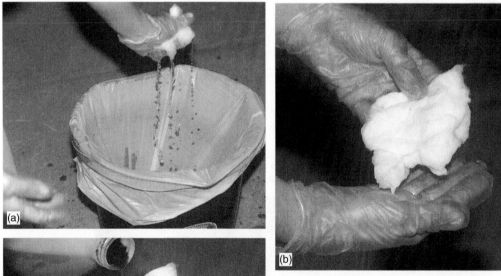

Figure 38.4 To scrub the mare's perineum thoroughly, use the clean hand/dirty hand technique. (a) Use the non-dominant hand as the "clean" hand to pick up the cotton from the warm water bucket and squeeze out the excess water. (b) Transfer the handful of cotton to the other hand (the "dirty" hand). (c) Have an assistant pour about a tablespoon of betadine scrub onto the center of the cotton, and use it to clean the perineal area in circular motions starting at the center and moving to the periphery. Courtesy of Dr. Lais R.R. Costa.

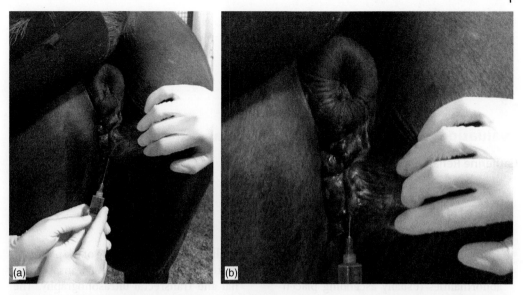

Figure 38.5 Infiltration of the vulvar labial margins with about 20 ml of local anesthetic, either 2% lidocaine or mepivacaine. (a) Inject subcutaneously using a 22-gauge needle. (b) Note the slight bulging of the subcutaneous tissue.

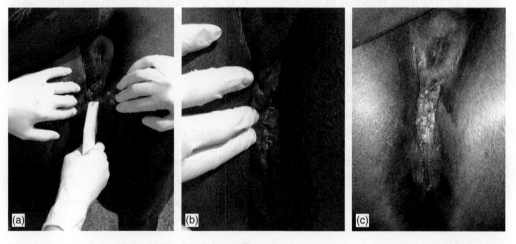

Figure 38.6 Placement of the staples. (a) Bring together the raw edges of the right and left labia using a staple gun. (b) When finished evaluate the apposition of the margins. (c) After healing, the staples are removed.

Bibliography and Further Reading

Bradecamp, E.A. (2011) Pneumovagina, in *Equine Reproduction*, 2nd edn, Wiley Blackwell, Chicester, pp. 2537–2544.

Trotter, G.W. (1993) Surgery of the perineum in the mare, in *Equine Reproduction*, Lea and Febiger, Philadelphia, pp. 417–427.

39

Evaluation and Monitoring of the Pregnant Mare

Catherine Renaudin

39.1 Purpose

- To evaluate fetal well-being and growth.
- To document and monitor placental abnormalities (usually ascending placentitis).
- Once abnormalities are identified, mares can be placed on appropriate therapy as soon as possible (Leblanc 2010) and monitored for treatment response in the hope of maintaining the pregnancy.
- Monitoring of pregnancy by ultrasonography, using the transrectal and transabdominal approaches, once a month starting at 7 months of gestation increases fetal and neonatal survival in both normal and high-risk mares (Carrick *et al.* 2010).
- To monitor mares at risk of abortion, those include mares with:
  - poor perineal conformation (risk of ascending infection, especially if not "Caslicked" (see Chapter 38)
  - vaginal discharge
  - premature lactation/mammary development
  - systemic disease
  - recent anesthesia/surgery
  - concern for twins
  - enlarged abdomen for stage of gestation (concern for twins or hydrops)
  - prolonged gestation
  - history of previous abortion.
- To know or confirm the sex of the fetus (not described here).

39.2 Complications

- Evaluation and monitoring of the pregnant mare is mainly done using transabdominal and transrectal ultrasonography. The ultrasonographic examination by itself is very safe for the fetus and the mare. The transrectal approach has the same risk of rectal tear as for a non-pregnant mare.
- If a speculum examination is indicated, in cases of bloody or mucopurulent vaginal discharge, care should be taken not to touch the cervix as it could induce abortion.

39.3 Equipment Required

Document all your findings (Figure 39.1)

Rectal examination

- Sleeve and lubricant
- Portable, good-quality ultrasound machine equipped with a 5–7 MHz linear transducer.

Transabdominal examination

- Same ultrasound machine also equipped with a 3.5 MHz curved linear transducer.
- Ultrasonic coupling gel: 1 gallon
- Clippers with #40 blade
- Alcohol spray or pressurized garden sprayer
- Chair

Manual of Clinical Procedures in the Horse, First Edition. Edited by Lais R.R. Costa and Mary Rose Paradis.
© 2018 John Wiley & Sons, Inc. Published 2018 by John Wiley & Sons, Inc.

Speculum examination

- Brown gauze to wrap the tail or a clean neoprene tail wrap
- Bucket with a clean plastic bag, cotton, non-residual soap or povidone-iodine
- Clean towel
- Speculum
- Sterile lubricant
- Flashlight

Culture

- Long guarded swab, culturette

39.4 Restraint and Positioning

- The evaluation should be conducted with the mare restrained in stocks.
- To keep the mare busy, it is best to provide hay in a hay net in front of the mare.
- Additional restraint will depend on the disposition of the mare, but sedation should be avoided because it will affect the parameters of the biophysical profile (decrease fetal activity and fetal heart rate).

FETAL - PLACENTAL EVALUATION

MARE:
Gestation length: Date of examination:
History:

RECTAL PALPATION: Cervix: Tight ☐   Relaxed ☐
                     Fetal Activity: 0 1   2   3

TRANRECTAL US: Fetal Activity: 0 1   2   3
                     CTUP =
                     Placental Contact:
                     Echogenicity: Amniotic Fluid Grade 1 2 3 4   Allantoic Fluid Grade 1 2 3 4
                     BPD =
                     eyeL =   eyeD =   eyeV =
                     Fetal Presentation: Anterior ☐   Posterior ☐   Transverse ☐

TRANSABDOMINAL US: Fetal Activity: 0   1   2   3
                     CTUP =
                     Placental Contact:
                     HRR =   HRM =
                     AllMD =   AmnMD =
                     Fetal Presentation: Anterior ☐   Posterior ☐   Transverse ☐
                     Biometry: BPD =
                                  AortD =
                                  eyeL =   eyeD=   eyeV=
                                  FemurL =
                     Sex: M   F

        Fetal Activity: 0 (immobile); 1 (<33% exam); 2 (33-66% exam); 3 (> 66% exam)
               Normal: from 100 to 250 d = 2 to 3
                             from 250 to 320 d = 1 to 3
                             from > 320 d = 1 to 2

        Fetal Heart Rate: HR @ rest (HRR) and HR after movement (HRM)
               HRR: from 100 to 250 d : > 100 bpm (145 to 100 bpm)
                      from 250 to 300 d : > 80 bpm
                      from > 300 d: 60 bpm
               HRM: > 15 - 20 bpm above HRR

Figure 39.1 Fetoplacental form (C.D. Renaudin, unpublished data). The abbreviations are as follows: CTUP (Combined Thickness of the Uterus and Placenta); BPD (Biparietal Diameter, i.e. cranium diameter); eyeL (eye Length); eyeD (eye Depth); eyeV (eye Volume) which is calculated with the formula eyeV = eyeL × eyeL × eyeD; AortD (Aorta Diameter); FemurL (Femur Length); AllMD (Allantoic fluid Maximal Depth); AmnMD (Amniotic fluid Maximal Depth); HRR (Heart Rate at Rest), HRM (Heart Rate after Fetal Movement); bpm (beats per minute); M (Male); F (Female); d (days).

Procedure: Transrectal Evaluation

Technical action	Rationale
The mare should be evaluated by means of a thorough physical examination.	See Chapter 3. Document all physical exam findings.
Enter the initial information in the Fetoplacental form.	Document all your findings, preferably using a form, so no information is forgotten (Figure 39.1).
Place the mare in the stocks.	This will provide ideal restraint (see Chapter 2).
Empty the rectum (see Chapter 38).	Take this opportunity to examine the perineal area.
Perform transrectal palpation, taking time to evaluate the following: • The fetus and the uterus: The fetus can usually be felt by its bony structures. It should be moving if it is alive but may be sleepy for as long as 60 minutes in late pregnancy. • Broad ligaments are located on either side of the uterine body and horns. • Cervix: Gently palpate the cervix through the rectal wall. During pregnancy the cervix should feel tight like a pencil and long (the length of your index finger).	If the foal cannot be felt, it may be located too deep in the mare's abdomen (which is normal) or may be surrounded by an increase amount of fetal fluids in case of hydrops (which is abnormal). Ensure there is no uterine torsion. If there is uterine torsion, which usually occurs in the last third of gestation, the mare would be colicky. An open relaxed cervix is abnormal during pregnancy except close to parturition.

Perform a transrectal scan of the placenta.
 	
• Locate the placento-cervical junction where there is absence of fetal contact with the placenta (Figure 39.2).
• Measure the combined thickness of the uterus and placenta (CTUP) in three different areas:
  – calculate the mean
  – compare to normal ranges according to gestational age (see Table 39.1).
• Assess the placental contact.
	Fetal contact with the placenta puts pressure on it and minimizes its thickness.
	
	Transrectally measured CTUP plateaus from 4 to 9 months of gestation and progressively increases afterwards
	
	The placenta and uterus should be in contact (Figure 39.2). The placenta and uterus are always indistinguishable except after 300 days of gestation (Figure 39.3).

• Interpret the findings.	An increase in the CTUP (see Table 39.1) and/or a placental detachment are considered abnormal and consistent with ascending placentitis and placental separation, respectively (Figures 39.4 and 39.5).
• Assess the echogenicity of fetal fluids (Figure 39.6). The allantoic fluid should look less echogenic with less free floating particles (Grade III) than the amniotic fluid (Grade II–III) (Table 39.2).	Appropriate treatment must be initiated promptly. Close monitoring by serial ultrasonography is necessary to assess response to treatment and maintenance of pregnancy. Table 39.2 depicts the grading of fluid echogenicity and normal findings according to gestational age. Increased echogenicity (Grade I) is abnormal and may be associated with the passage of meconium in utero, hemorrhage or inflammatory debris, which may reflect fetal hypoxia, placental detachment or placental infection, respectively.

Technical action	Rationale

Perform a transrectal scan of the fetus.

If the fetus is in an anterior presentation, the fetal head and eye will be readily seen, thus measurements can be obtained as listed below.

1. Measure the biparietal diameter (BPD) = cranium diameter (Figure 39.7). The cranium is imaged in cross-section (oval shape) and the maximal diameter is measured using caliper cursors positioned from the outer margin of the skull nearest to the transducer to the inner margin of the skull furthest away from the transducer.

1. The BPD has a linear relationship with days of gestation: $y = 1.26 + 0.29x$, where x = days of gestation and y = BPD in mm. Measurement is compared with the BPD calculated with the equation or Table 39.3. Measurements corresponding to a month smaller than established suggest intrauterine growth retardation (IUGR) or small-size fetus for gestational age.

2. Measure eye length and eye depth (also referred to as eye width). The eye is imaged in cross-section, visualizing the anterior and posterior portions of the capsule of the lens (Figure 39.8). The image is frozen when the maximal cross-sectional diameter of the vitreous body is obtained. Eye length (eyeL) is the maximum length of the inner margins of the vitreous body and eye depth (eyeD) is measured from the margin of the anterior portion of the capsule of the lens to the inner portion of the optic disc. EyeL and eyeD are measured and the approximate eye volume (eyeV) is calculated: eyeV = eyeL × eyeL × eyeD.

2. The eyeV has a linear relationship with days of gestation: $y = -8175.59 + 91.73x$, where x = days of gestation and y = eyeV in mm^3.

Compare the calculated eyeV using the equation and the numbers in Table 39.3.

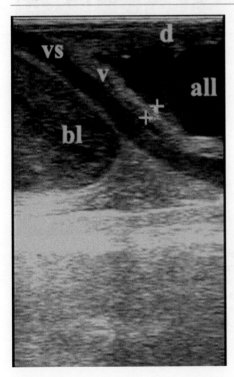

Figure 39.2 Normal echographic appearance of the placenta at the placenta–cervical junction of a mare at 232 days of gestation (5 MHz linear transducer). The combined thickness of the uterus and placenta (CTUP) (+) is 4 mm recorded from the ventral aspect of the uterine body, close to the cervix. The borders of the uterus, placenta and vascular space are visualized. The chorioallantois and uterus are indistinguishable. d = dorsal aspect of the uterine body, v = ventral aspect of the uterine body, all = allantoic fluid, vs = vascular space, bl = bladder.

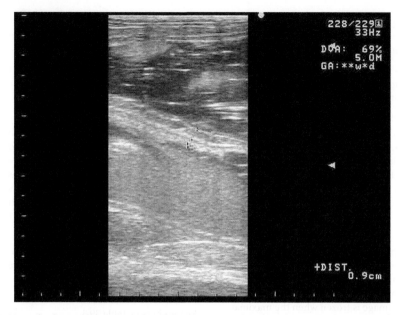

Figure 39.3 Normal echographic appearance of the placenta at the placenta–cervical junction of a mare at 319 days of gestation (5 MHz linear transducer). The uterus and placenta are in contact but are distinguishable after 300 days of gestation.

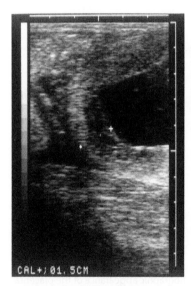

Figure 39.4 Abnormal echographic appearance of the placenta at the placenta–cervical junction in a mare at 319 days of gestation (5 MHz linear transducer). Note CTUP is increased (15 mm). The placenta and uterus are in contact. Renaudin *et al.* (1999). Reproduced with permission of John Wiley & Sons, Inc.

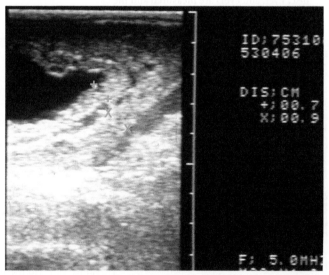

Figure 39.5 Abnormal echographic appearance of the placenta at the placenta–cervical junction in a mare with placentitis (5 MHz linear transducer). Note CTUP is increased (16 mm), chorioallantois is 7 mm (+) and uterus is 9 mm (x). Hyperechoic fluid is present in the space where the chorioallantois detached from the uterus. Renaudin *et al.* (1999). Reproduced with permission of John Wiley & Sons, Inc.

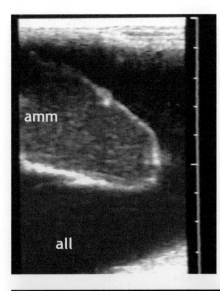

Figure 39.6 Transrectal imaging of amniotic (amn) and allantoic (all) fluid at 6 months of gestation. The allantoic fluid is anechoic with few free-floating particles (Grade III = dark grey) and the amniotic fluid is semi-echoic but not totally hyperechoic (Grade II = light grey) containing more free-floating particles than the allantoic fluid. Adapted from Renaudin *et al.* (1997).

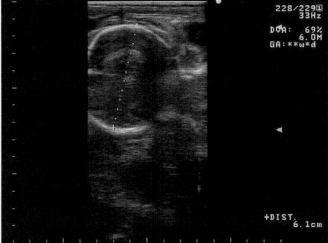

Figure 39.7 Cross-sectional view of a fetal cranium (195 days of gestation) by transrectal ultrasonography using a 5 MHz linear transducer. The biparietal diameter (BPD) is measured using caliper cursors positioned from the outer margin of the skull nearest to the transducer to the inner margin of the skull furthest away from the transducer (distance between the two + = 61 mm). The falx cerebri separates the two hemispheres symmetrically.

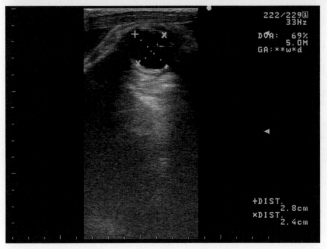

Figure 39.8 Cross-section of a fetal eye (266 days of gestation) by transrectal ultrasonography (5 MHz linear transducer). The anterior and posterior portions of the capsule of the lens are visualized. The image is frozen when the maximal cross-sectional diameter of the vitreous body is obtained. Eye length (eyeL) (maximum length of the inner margins of the vitreous body between the two +) and eye depth (eyeD) (margin of the anterior portion of the capsule of the lens to the inner portion of the optic disc between the two ×) are measured. Eye volume (eyeV) is calculated: eyeL (28 mm) × eyeL (28 mm) × eyeD (24 mm) = 18,816 mm^3, corresponding in Table 39.3 to about 250 days of gestation.

Table 39.1 Normal and suggested abnormal values of the combined thickness of the uterus and placenta (CTUP) from 4 months of gestation to term using the transrectal ultrasound approach in quarter-horse-type horses.

Month of gestation (days)	Mean CTUP (mm)	95% CI (mm)		Abnormal CTUP (mm)
		Lower limit	Upper limit	
4 (91–120)	3.98	3.81	4.47	>7
5 (121–150)	3.58	3.50	3.81	>7
6 (151–180)	3.84	3.78	4.04	>7
7 (181–210)	3.91	3.86	4.07	>7
8 (211–240)	4.33	4.21	4.69	>7
9 (241–270)	4.38	4.28	4.66	>7
10 (271–300)	5.84	5.53	6.77	>8
11 (301–330)	7.35	6.93	8.54	>10
12 (331–360)	9.52	8.51	11.77	>13

CI, confidence interval.
Adapted from Renaudin *et al.* (1997).

Table 39.2 Grade of normal allantoic and amniotic fluid echogenicities from 4 months of pregnancy to term

Month of gestation (days)	Allantoic fluid echogenicity	Amniotic fluid echogenicity
4 (91–120)	III	II or III
5 (121–150)	III	II or III
6 (151–180)	III	II or III
7 (181–210)	III	II or III
8 (211–240)	III	II or III
9 (241–270)	III	II or III
10 (271–300)	III	II or III
11 (301–330)	III	II
12 (331–360)	III	II

Grade I, white (strongly echogenic or hyperechoic medium); Grade II, light grey (semi-echogenic or hyperechoic medium); Grade III, dark grey (hypoechoic – few hyperechoic foci suspended in anechoic medium); Grade IV, black (anechoic medium).

Table 39.3 Predicted equine fetal measurements at specific gestation days in quarter-horse-type horses

Days	AortD (mm)	EyeV (mm³)	BPD (mm)	FemurL (mm)
110	3.98	2668.67	30.78	20.07
120	4.95	3814.75	34.65	25.84
130	5.92	4960.82	38.4	31.61
140	6.9	6106.9	42.04	37.39
150	7.89	7252.98	45.57	43.16
160	8.85	8399.05	48.99	48.93
170	9.82	9545.13	52.29	54.7
180	10.79	10691.2	55.48	60.48
190	11.77	11837.28	58.57	66.25
200	12.74	12983.36	61.54	72.02
210	13.72	14129.43	64.39	77.8
220	14.69	15275.51	67.14	83.57
230	15.67	16421.58	69.78	89.34
240	16.64	17567.66	72.3	95.11
250	17.61	18713.73	74.71	100.89
260	18.59	19859.81	77.01	106.66
270	19.56	21005.89	79.2	112.43
280	20.54	22151.96	81.27	
290	21.51	23298.04	83.24	
300	22.49	24444.11	85.09	
310	23.46	25590.19	86.83	
320	24.43	26736.27	88.46	
330	25.41	27882.34		
340	26.38	29028.42		
350	27.36	30174.49		

C.D. Renaudin, unpublished data.

39.5 Procedure: Transabdominal Evaluation

Technical action	Rationale
Prepare the mare.	
• Clip (#40 blade) the ventral abdomen from the mammary glands to the xyphoid and laterally up to the level of the stifle (Figure 39.9). • Alcohol may be sprayed, preferably with a pressurized garden sprayer, for maximal ventral saturation. • After cleaning the ventral abdomen with water and drying it with a towel, apply ultrasound coupling gel to the abdomen.	Ultrasound does not go through air located between the skin and hairs. Clipping the hair of the ventral abdomen increases image quality tremendously. If clipping is not appropriate because of a coming sale, alcohol saturation of the hair coat on the ventral abdomen is helpful but less optimal.
• Sit on a chair on the side of the mare, facing the mare's head with the ultrasound placed at eye level (Figure 39.10).	It is best to sit on a chair on same side of mare as the fetus to prevent shoulder fatigue.
Locate the fetus.	The resting fetus is in the dorso-pubic position but commonly lies in left or right lateral recumbency.
• Place the transducer (5 or 3.5 MHz) at midline on the ventral abdomen cranial to the mammary glands in a longitudinal plane and go down the abdomen until fetal parts are identified (ribs, heart, scapula). • Look for twins by screening the entire ventral abdomen (head, neck, thorax, abdomen should be connected).	The transabdominal ultrasound approach is the best way to diagnose twins after 100 days of gestation.
Identify fetal presentation. Know the direction of the image (e.g., the right side of the image is toward the mare's head). The fetus should be in anterior presentation after 220–240 days of gestation (C.D. Renaudin, unpublished data; Bucca 2005).	Before 220–240 days, a fetus may be in anterior, transverse or posterior presentation. After 240 days, all fetuses should be in anterior presentation. There is no room for the fetus to rotate about its short axis anymore after 240 days of gestation. Mares with a fetus in abnormal presentation after 240 days of gestation are prone to dystocia and should foal at a veterinary hospital.
Evaluate the CTUP and placental contact. This is preferably done using a 5 MHz probe; in many areas without fetal contact (Figure 39.11).	The feto-placental unit is best evaluated with a high frequency probe because the placenta is located near the ventral abdomen.
	It is recommended that measurements are obtained from six quadrants of the uterus (left cranial, mid, caudal and right cranial, mid and caudal). These measurements should be similar or thinner than the one obtained at the placenta–cervical junction.
	Increased CTUP or placental separation are abnormal and suggest the presence of placentitis (hematogenous or nocardioform in origin).
Evaluate fetal activity during a minimum examination time of 30 minutes. Fetal activity includes any fetal movements (extension and flexion of limbs, whole-body rotations around the fetal long axis, spinning and translation). Fetal activity is graded on a scale from 0 to 3 (as listed in Figure 39.1).	Fetal activity declines as gestation advances. Normal values are (Figure 39.1): 100–250 days: 2–3 250–320 days: 1–3 >320 days: 1–2 (rarely 3). Resting periods of 10–60 minutes are common. Re-evaluate later.

Technical action	Rationale
0: No movement detected during the examination period. 1: Small amount of movement detected during the examination period (<33% of the examination time). 2: Fetus fairly active (>33–<66% of the examination time). 3: Fetus very active, few or no quiet periods detected (>66% of the examination time).	Fetal activity reflects central nervous system (CNS) function and development; such that a depressed CNS function results in decrease activity. Abnormal fetal activity is suggestive of poor fetal outcome and includes prolonged hyperactivity or inactivity. In that case evaluate fetal heart rate to ensure the fetus is alive.
Evaluate the fetal heart rate at rest and after fetal movement. It can be obtained either by using a stopwatch (B-mode ultrasonography) or utilizing M-mode (Figure 39.12). The M-mode cursor is moved so that it intersects the heart (in B-mode). The M-mode image is activated and shows movement of the heart over time. Measure the distance between heartbeats to calculate the fetal heart rate with ultrasound machine software. The heart rate should be regular. • Heart rate at rest (HRR): decreases as gestational age progresses (Figure 39.1) and accelerations generally occur in response to activity. • Heart rate after movement (HRM): obtained immediately after the fetus has moved. HRM is generally 15–20 beats/minute higher than HRR and last 20–40 seconds.	M-mode analysis is more accurate in assessing fetal heart rate than the stopwatch method. Abnormal heart rate includes persistent fetal bradycardia, tachycardia, and cardiac arrhythmias. Fetal tachycardia has been observed preceding abortion and stillbirth. Transient fetal heart rate elevation above normal for gestational age is not threatening unless it fails to return to baseline. Maternal anxiety or pain may sometimes be the underlying cause. Fetal bradychardia is the most reliable indicator of impending fetal demise. Fetal asystole ultimately identifies fetal demise.
Evaluate fetal growth. Different biometric measurements may be obtained. • BPD and eyeV: The BPD and eye length and depth may be measured as described with the transrectal approach (see above).	When fetuses are located low in the abdomen or in a posterior presentation, the transabdominal approach is the best way to measure the BPD or the eye length and eye depth.
• Fetal aortic diameter (aortD): The fetal aorta is observed in longitudinal section. The image is frozen when the most anterior portion of the aorta (as it emerges from the heart) is seen in systole (maximum dilation of the diameter of the aorta). The diameter of the aorta is measured by placing two caliper cursors on the vessel margins (Figure 39.13).	The aortD has a linear relationship with days of gestation: $y = -6.74 + 0.09x$, where x = days of gestation and y = aortD in mm. Measurement is compared with the aortD calculated with the equation or to Table 39.3. The aortD is the measurement most closely associated with birth weight. Lower than expected aortD has been correlated with low birth weight. Generally, if aortD is less than 18.5 mm (after 300 days of gestation, in a regular size horse), IUGR is very likely to be present. AortD and eye measurements are the only biometric parameters consistently measurable from 100 days of gestation to term.

(continued)

Technical action	Rationale
• Femur length (femurL): The longest view of the ossified portion of the femur must be obtained. Femur length is then measured (Figure 39.14). Femur length can be measured up to 270 days of gestation.	The femurL has a linear relationship with days of gestation: $y = -43.43 + 0.58x$, where x = days of gestation and y = femurL in mm). Measurement is compared with the femurL calculated with the equation or to Table 39.3. Femur length becomes impossible to measure after 270 days of gestation due to the increased size of the femur.
Evaluate the maximum fluids depth Generally the largest fluid depths are located around the fetal thorax in the region of the elbow.	Hydrallantois and hydramnios are rare conditions that occur in the last third of pregnancy.
• Allantoic maximum depth (AllMD) is measured by placing one cursor on the edge of the placenta in contact with the allantoic fluid and the other cursor on the amniotic membrane so that the connecting line is perpendicular to the placental surface (Figure 39.15). As the amniotic membrane floats, the image should be frozen once the amniotic membrane gets to its lowest point.	Normal reported AllMD is between 47 and 221 mm in term mares. Hydrallantois is more common than hydramnios and is often associated with growth-retarded fetuses. Reduced amounts of allantoic fluid are associated with poor fetal outcome.
• Amniotic maximum depth (AmnMD) is measured by placing one cursor on the amniotic membrane (at its highest point) and the other cursor on the fetal skin with the connecting line perpendicular to the placental surface.	Normal reported AmnMD is between 8 and 149 mm in term mares. Hydramnios is usually associated with a congenitally abnormal fetus. Markedly reduced amounts of amniotic fluid have been observed in mares with severe systemic illness.
Evaluation of fetal fluid echogenicity should only be performed with the transrectal approach.	Fetal fluids are best viewed transrectally because of the excellent image quality and their vicinity to the probe.

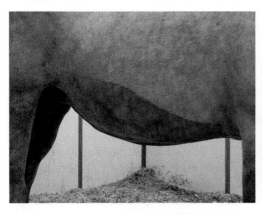

Figure 39.9 Clipping (#40 blade) of the ventral abdomen from the mammary glands to the xyphoid and laterally up to the level of the stifle is best to obtain maximum image quality.

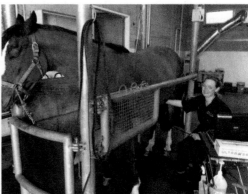

Figure 39.10 The ultrasonographer should sit on a chair at the side of the mare, facing the mare's head to be comfortable scanning via the transabdominal approach. The mare is restrained in the stocks.

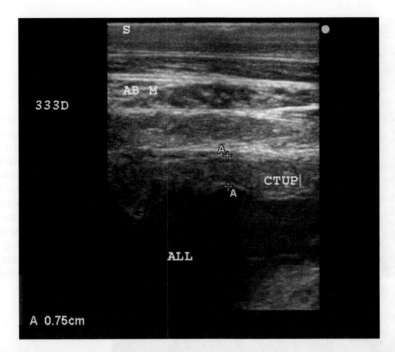

Figure 39.11 Normal echographic appearance of the placenta and uterus seen via the transabdominal approach in a mare at 333 days of gestation. The CTUP is measured between the two A+ and measures 7.5 mm. The skin of the ventral abdomen of the mare is at the top of the image (S). AB M, abdominal muscle; ALL, allantoic fluid.

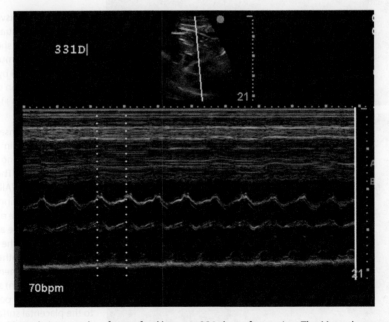

Figure 39.12 M-mode image taken from a fetal heart at 331 days of gestation. The M-mode cursor intersects the heart (in B-mode) at the top of the image. The M-mode image shows movement of the heart over time. The distance between heartbeats (vertical dotted cursors) is measured and the fetal heart rate is calculated here as 70 beats per minute (bpm) with the ultrasound machine software.

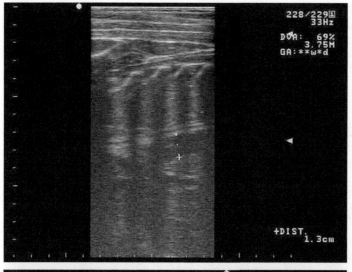

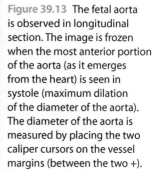

Figure 39.13 The fetal aorta is observed in longitudinal section. The image is frozen when the most anterior portion of the aorta (as it emerges from the heart) is seen in systole (maximum dilation of the diameter of the aorta). The diameter of the aorta is measured by placing the two caliper cursors on the vessel margins (between the two +).

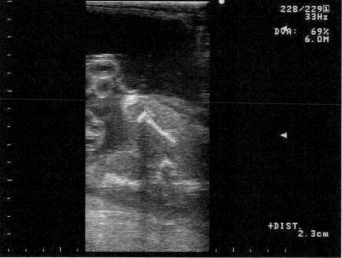

Figure 39.14 Transverse view of the hind quarter of a 114-day-old fetus showing the two thighs and femurs. Femur length is obtained by measuring the ossified portion of the femur (between the two +).

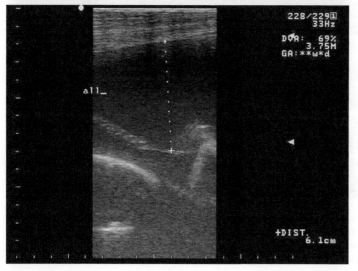

Figure 39.15 Transabdominal ultrasonographic image of the fetal fluids using a 5 MHz linear transducer. The allantoic maximum depth (AllMD) is measured by placing one cursor on the edge of the placenta in contact with the allantoic fluid (+ cursor at the top of the picture) and the other cursor on the amniotic membrane (+ cursor lower down) so that the connecting line is perpendicular to the placental surface. As the amniotic membrane floats, the image should be frozen once the amniotic membrane gets to its lowest point.

39.6 Procedure: Vaginal Evaluation

Technical action	Rationale/amplification
Speculum examination is performed in cases of suspicious vaginal discharge.	It will help identify the source of the discharge.
Prepare for vaginal evaluation. • Wrap and tie the tail. • Scrub the mare's perineum.	See description in Chapter 38.
Lubricate the vaginal speculum (metal or cardboard) with sterile lubricant.	Lubricant facilitates the introduction of the speculum.
Introduce the speculum in the vagina initially directed slightly upward to avoid the opening of the urethra and then straight. Do not touch the cervix.	Try not to disturb the cervix as this may induce abortion.
Locate the external os of the cervix and explore the entire vagina. The cervix should be tight and above the floor of the vagina. No secretion should be observed.	An open cervix and/or purulent or bloody secretions coming from the external os of the cervix are abnormal during gestation. Close to parturition, it is normal to find a relaxed cervix.
Collect samples for culture and cytology when a suspicious discharge is identified via speculum examination: Collect two samples using long guarded cotton swabs introduced through the speculum and guided into the exudate. The first swab should be submitted for bacterial/fungal culture. A second swab is used to collect a sample for cytologic examination.	A positive culture allows an antibiogram to guide the appropriate antimicrobial treatment. Cytology showing large number of neutrophils or lymphocytes are indicative of inflammatory response. Lymphocytes are seen in chronic inflammation. Presence of bacteria (rods and/ or cocci) or hyphae (fungal elements) are suggestive of infectious process.

Bibliography and Further Reading

Bucca, S. (2011) Ultrasonographic monitoring of the fetus, in *Equine Reproduction*, 2nd edn, pp. 39–54.

Carrick, J.B., Begg, A.P., Perkins, N., and O'Meara, D. (2010) Ultrasonographic monitoring and treatment of pregnant mares at risk for placentitis. *Animal Reproduction Science*, **121S**, S331–S333.

Leblanc, M.M. (2010) Ascending placentitis in the mare: an update. *Reproduction in Domestic Animals*, **45** (suppl. 2), 28–34.

Renaudin, C.D., Troedsson, M.H.T., Gillis, C.L., King, V.L., and Bodena, A. (1997) Ultrasonographic evaluation of the equine placenta by transrectal and transabdominal approach in the normal pregnant mare. *Theriogenology*, **47**, 559–5573.

Renaudin, C.D., Liu, I.K.M., Troedsson, M.H.T., and Schrenzel, M.D. (1999) Transrectal ultrasonographic diagnosis of ascending placentitis in the mare: a report of 2 cases. *Equine Veterinary Education*, **11**, 69–74.

Renaudin, C.D., Gillis, C.L., Tarantal, A.F., and Coleman, D.A. (2000) Evaluation of equine fetal growth from day 100 of gestation to parturition by ultrasonography. *Journal of Reproduction and Fertility Supplement*, **56**, 651–660.

40

Impending Parturition and Delivery

Catherine Renaudin

40.1 Purpose

- To describe signs of impending parturition so that foaling can be most likely observed. Gestational length is highly variable in the mare, ranging from 330 to 360 days (315–350 in pony breeds).
- To describe the three stages of foaling in order to recognize abnormalities and intervene early if a problem arises.
- To describe the many kinds of dystocia that can be corrected at the farm and those that should be referred at once to an equipped facility to increase the chance of delivering a live foal.

40.2 Complications

- It is important to observe each foaling. Even though dystocia is not a common occurrence in the mare, when it does occur it can be life threatening for the foal as well as the mare.

40.3 Equipment Required

- Brown gauze to wrap the tail or a clean neoprene tail wrap
- Sterile rectal sleeves (optional)
- Bucket with a clean plastic bag, cotton, non-residual soap or povidone-iodine
- Lubricant:
  - sterile obstetrical lubricant for vaginal examination
  - volume-expanding lubricant for manipulation and traction (e.g., carboxymethylcellulose)
- Nasogastric tube and pump
- Obstetrical chains or nylon ropes and handles
- Obstetrical snare

40.4 Restraint and Positioning

- For monitoring impending signs of delivery, the mare is handled and observed in her stall.
- To apply the tail wrap, clean the perineum and remove the Caslick suture, the mare should be placed in the stocks. Application of a nose twitch or flexion of a forelimb might be indicated.
- For delivery, the mare should be in a clean, large, well bedded stall or a small grassy paddock to ensure safety for all personel involved.
- In case of dystocia, chemical restraint with a xylazine-butorphanol combination may be considered. Moreover, injectable tocolytic agents (Table 40.1) may be indicated to induce uterine relaxation and permit repulsion and mutation of the fetus. Epidural is often not recommended because the time involved in administering effective epidural anesthesia is too long for the delivery of a live foal.

Manual of Clinical Procedures in the Horse, First Edition. Edited by Lais R.R. Costa and Mary Rose Paradis.
© 2018 John Wiley & Sons, Inc. Published 2018 by John Wiley & Sons, Inc.

Table 40.1 Injectable tocolytic agents

Active ingredients	Trademark	Dose	Route
Clenbuterol hydrochloride	Planipart (not USA)	2 ml/100 kg	IV slowly
	Ventipulmin solution (not in USA)	0.17–0.35 mg/454 kg	
N-butylscopolammonium bromide	Buscopan	0.3 mg/kg or 0.14 mg/lb = 1.5 ml/100 kg or 1.5 ml/220 lb	IV slowly
Isoxuprine	Duphaspasmin (not USA)	178 mg/animal or 20 ml/animal	IM or IV (slowly after dilution)

40.5 Procedure: Monitoring and Preparing the Mare for Parturition

Technical Action	Rationale
Move the mare 4–6 weeks prior to her due date to a large and clean (disinfected), well-bedded and well-ventilated stall. The mare can be turned out during the day.	The mare will have time to develop antibodies to organisms present in the foaling area and will then transfer them to the foal through the colostrum.
Vaccinate and deworm.	
• Vaccination against tetanus, Eastern/Western equine encephalomyelitis (EEE/WEE), West Nile virus (WNV), influenza, equine herpes virus and rabies 4–6 weeks pre-partum. Based on risk factors (endemic areas), mares may be vaccinated against rotavirus, strangles, potomac horse fever and botulism. Inactivated vaccines are the safest. Parenteral vaccines are more effective than intranasal ones for stimulating high levels of IgG.	Vaccination will protect the dam, fetus, and newborn foal. A booster 1 month prior to foaling will increase the antibody level in the mares colostrum. Use killed vaccines and avoid modified live vaccines. Use multivalent vaccines to avoid multiple vaccines.
• Deworming 2 weeks prior to the due date with approved safe dewormers for use during pregnancy: ivermectin, pyrantel pamoate and tartrate, thiabendazole, fenbedazole, or piperazine.	The mare will be the primary source for infecting her foal with parasites.
Open the Caslick suture.	Prevent laceration of the vulva at foaling.
• Place the mare in the stocks if possible. Otherwise, have a handler properly restrain the mare.	With mares prone to ascending placentitis, the vulva should be reopened close to parturition.
• Clean the perineal area as described in Chapter 39.	
• Block the vulva with lidocaine from the dorsal opening to the normal upper commissure of the vulva.	
• Place two fingers in the vagina and put tension in the area to be opened.	
• Open with scissors or a scalpel blade from bottom to top.	
Monitor physical changes associated with impending parturition.	During the last month before foaling the mare should be examined frequently for physical changes.
• Filling of the udder: 2–4 weeks pre-foaling.	Maiden mares often do not show any of the physical changes described.
• Distension of the teats: 4–6 days pre-foaling (Figure 40.1a).	

(continued)

Technical Action	Rationale
• Waxing of the teats: 1–4 days pre-foaling (Figure 40.1b) • Dripping of milk	Mares eating endophyte-contaminated fescue often develop agalactia and do not show the normal development of the udder (Figure 40.1c).
• Ventral edema 2–4″ thick may develop due to the weight of the gravid uterus impairing lymphatic and venous drainage (Figure 40.2).	Ventral edema should be differentiated from ventral body wall rupture (pre-pubic tendon rupture, ventral hernia) (Figure 40.3). Ultrasonography will show tearing and edema within the musculature. Mammary secretion will often contain blood.
Observe for more subtle changes: • Softening of the sacrosciatic ligaments • Relaxation and lengthening of the vulva	These subtle changes may not be detected until foaling is imminent.
Monitor mammary secretions for changes associated with impending parturition: Monitoring should be done once a day, preferably in the evening.	A rise in calcium concentration will provide an accurate estimation of impending parturition. Calcium rises late in the day.

• Clean the udder: wipe the udder with a clean dry soft paper towel.
• Collect a 2–5 ml sample of mammary secretion by gently stripping a small amount from each teat.
• Measure the electrolytes level:
  – Using a laboratory chemistry analyzer or spectrophotometry gives a precise measure. Close to parturition Ca^{++} and K^+ increase, and Na^+ decreases. When:
    $Ca^{++} > 40$ mg/dl
    $K^+ > 35$ mEq/l and
    $Na+ < 30$ mEq/l
    (time of inversion Na^+/K^+) mares tend to foal 24–36 hours later.
  – Stall-side tests to measure:
    Ca^{++} content in ppm:, Predict-A-Foal test (www.ahcpi.com/products/ predict-a-foal), Mare Foaling Predictor Kit (datasheets.scbt .com/sc-359871_mfr.pdf);
    Ca^{++} carbonate: Foal Watch test kit (www.foalwatch.eu/).
	This will reduce sample contamination and mastitis. When using water hardness tests, it is important not to use water but a dry towel.
	
	These electrolyte changes are used to predict readiness for birth. They are not a reliable indicator of fetal maturity if placental abnormality is present (e.g., placentitis, twin).
	
	Multiparous mares show more consistent changes in electrolytes prior to foaling than maiden mares.
	
	If induction of parturition is performed, the Na^+/K^+ inversion is one of the main criteria to consider.
	
	Stall-side tests are helpful in determining on which day the mare will *not* foal and in reducing the number of sleepless nights.
	
	With the Foal Watch test kit most mares (98%) with $Ca^{+++} < 200$ ppm will not foal within 24 hours of the test while 99% of mares with $Ca^{++} > 200$ ppm will foal within 72 hours.

Use a birth alarm system that is connected to a receiver that sounds the alarm and/or dials a phone.	
Some alarms are attached to the mares halter and are activated when a mare is in lateral recumbency for at least 15 seconds (e.g., Breeder Alert (https:// www.breederalert.com/), EquiFone system (www .foalingalarm.com/equifone.htm)).	During the first stage of labor, the mare gets up and lies down for a longer time than usual. There is a risk of false alarm with late pregnant mare lying down when they are sleeping or resting but not in labor.
Some alarms are composed of a surcingle and breastplate that detect sweat (e.g., Wyke Foaling Alarm system (www.wyke-equine.co.uk/foaling-alarm/Foal Alert system. foalert.com/)).	During the first stage of labor the mare sweats profusely. Environmental heat and some conditions like colics will activate the receiver and induce a false alarm.
Some alarms detect when the foals feet emerge through the vulva (e.g., Foal Alert system; Figure 40.4). The magnet and transmitter are both sutured into the vulvar lips and the magnet is inserted into the transmitter.	Once the feet emerge from the birth canal, they pull the magnet out of the transmitter, which sends a signal to the receiver. There is very little chance of a false alarm unless there is a dystocia, with the front feet not emerging from the birth canal.

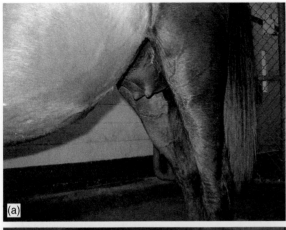

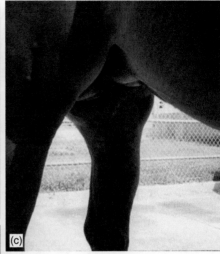

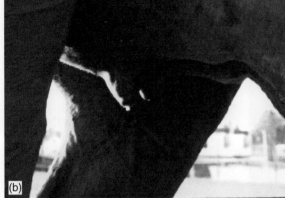

Figure 40.1 Signs of impending parturition.
(a) Enlargement of the udder and teats.
(b) Waxing of the teat end usually occurs
1–4 days before foaling, and sometimes as
early as 2 weeks prior to parturition. (c) Lack
of mammary gland development near foaling
date in a mare fed endophyte-contaminated
fescue. Courtesy of
Dr. Lais R.R. Costa.

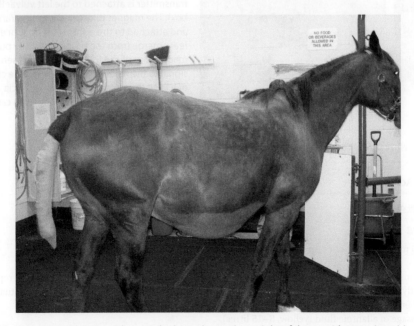

Figure 40.2 Late pregnant mare with ventral edema due to the weight of the gravid uterus impairing
lymphatic and venous drainage. Courtesy of Dr. Lais R.R. Costa.

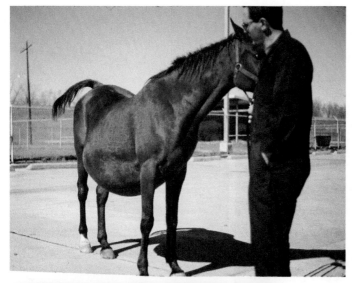

Figure 40.3 Pre-pubic tendon rupture in a late pregnant mare due to the increased weight of the uterus. It is a critical condition as opposed to ventral edema. Courtesy of Dr. Lais R.R. Costa.

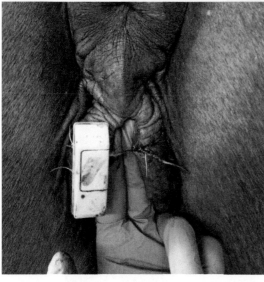

Figure 40.4 Foal Alert system in place. The transmitter is attached to the left vulvar lip (blue box). The magnet is inserted into the transmitter and attached to the right vulvar lip. Once the feet emerge from the birth canal, they pull the magnet out of the transmitter, which sends a signal to the receiver. There is very little chance of a false alarm unless there is a dystocia with the front feet not emerging from the birth canal.

40.6 Procedure: Foaling

Technical Action	Rationale
First Stage of Labor.	
Description	
• Lasts 30 minutes to 4 hours (in rare instances a few days).	
• Colic signs (restless, lying down and getting up frequently, rolling, sweating, pollakiuria).	Rolling and uterine contractions help reposition the foal from the dorso-pubic to eventually the
• Ends when the choriallantois ruptures ("water breaks"), with passage of allantoic fluid (yellow, 8–15 litres).	dorsosacral position.

Technical Action	Rationale

Mare preparation

- Once the mare is in first stage of labor, the tail is wrapped, the perineal area is scrubbed and dried, and the mammary glands are cleaned.
- Do not intervene unless a velvety "red bag" (non-ruptured choriallantois) appears at the vulvar lips (Figure 40.5a). The velvety "red bag" or choriallantois should be ruptured with scissors at once. Gentle traction in unison with the mares abdominal contractions will help deliver the neonate as quickly as possible.

A "red bag" is an emergency. The mares owner should rupture it because the choriallantois is separated from the endometrium, impairing fetal oxygenation.

Asynchronous forceful traction may create laceration or rib fracture in an incompletely dilated cervix.

Second Stage of Labor (Delivery of the Fetus).

Description

- Lasts 20–30 minutes.
- Mare in lateral recumbency with strong abdominal contractions, and within 5 minutes the amnion protrudes at the vulva (Figure 40.5b).
- One front foot followed by the second one visible at the vulva with the sole of the hooves directed downward.
- Nose follows with the head resting on top of the canon bones.
- Amnion breaks at the passage of the shoulder and the neonate starts breathing air.
- Hips pass through the maternal pelvic canal (Figure 40.5c).
- Mare rests for 15–20 minutes.
- The umbilical cord ruptures once the foal or mare stands (Figure 40.5d).

This ensures that one shoulder is advanced in front of the other and that both limbs are extended. If the hooves are directed upward suspect posterior presentation (hindlimbs) or anterior presentation with dorsopubic position.

Avoid cutting the umbilical cord, thus allowing natural rupture of the umbilical cord.

Decision for intervention during second stage.

If there is absence of strong contractions or no progress within 10 minutes of chorioallantois rupture, vaginal examination is warranted. The mare's tail is wrapped and the perineal area scrubbed and dried, if this was not done earlier. The arms and hands of the person performing the intervention should be scrubbed too. Sterile sleeves are optional.

Contamination of the genital tract should be avoided to prevent post-parturient metritis.

Vaginal examination allows determination of abnormal presentation or posture or malposition.

Use of copious amounts of sterile lubricant is essential.

Vaginal examination and palpation helps determine:

- the presence of lacerations, lesions, and contusions of the genital tract
- the presence of pelvic abnormalities or feto-pelvic disproportion
- the degree of cervical relaxation
- fetal viability by pinching the coronary band or nose or anus or using transabdominal ultrasound to check the heart beat

Abundant lubrication is important because the cervix and vagina are easily traumatized. Adhesions and fibrosis may develop and jeopardize the mares future fertility.

Pelvic abnormalities may impede passage of the fetus.

Traction should not be attempted if the cervix is not fully relaxed.

If the fetus is alive, the decision needs to be made quickly whether to correct the dystocia with brief manipulation at the farm or refer it to a well-equipped facility.

(continued)

Technical Action	Rationale
• fetal presentation, position, and posture: forelimb (fetlock and carpus flex in the same direction) should be differentiated from hindlimb (fetlock and hock flexed in the opposite direction).	Some dystocias are known to be relatively easily corrected; others should be referred at once for general anesthesia and controlled vaginal delivery with hoisted hindlimb or C-section.

Intervention.

Pump 1–2 gallons of warm obstetrical lubricant into the uterus and around the fetus before attempting mutations if the uterus is intact.

If the foal is in a normal presentation, position, and posture, place chains or ropes around the fetlock (Figure 40.6) and pull the foal while the mare pushes.

Some manipulations may be attempted at the farm. Have a person keep track of time while manipulations are attempted. If attempts are unsuccessful for 10 minutes, refer the case right away.

Abundant lubrication helps prevent vaginal and cervical lacerations, and facilitates manipulations. In case of uterine rupture (uterine body or tip of the horn) pumping lubricant increases the risk of peritonitis.

1. Two forelimbs and nose at the vulva but upward hooves (dorsopubic or dorsoilial position): rotate the foal by applying lateral pressure over the shoulder then pull the foal.

1. Lack or insufficient repositioning of the foal during stage 1 of labor (due to uterine inertia, or a sick or dead foal).

2. Two forelimbs and nose appearing at the same time and at same level (bilateral elbow lock/shoulder lock): repel the fetus, extend the elbows/shoulders, and pull the fetus with one shoulder in front of the other.

2. In horses, the widest part of the fetus is the shoulder. Both elbows and shoulders should be extended with one shoulder advanced in front of the other to pass through the pelvic canal.

3. Incomplete extension of a forelimb with the nose at the fetlock (unilateral elbow/shoulder lock; Figure 40.7): repel the fetus, extend the elbow/shoulder, and pull the fetus with one shoulder in front of the other.

4. One or both forelimbs over the head (foot–nape posture; Figure 40.8): repel the fetus, lift the limb off the neck, and pull the fetus.

4. The limb over the head increases the diameter across the fetal chest, impairing fetal delivery. There is a high risk of rectovaginal fistula or third-degree perineal laceration if the limb is not repositioned immediately. This is more likely in maiden mares due to insufficient laxity of vaginal and vestibular tissues.

It is important to cup the fetal hooves while rotating the limb to protect the reproductive tract from injury.

5. Nose with only one or no forelimbs visible at the vulva (unilateral or bilateral carpal flexion): repel the fetus, rotate the carpus dorsolaterally with one hand, while with the other hand cupped over the fetal hoof rotate the fetlock medially and caudally into the birth canal, extend the limb, and pull the fetus.

5. Most carpal flexions are relatively easy to correct. If not, suspect contracted tendons/ limb deformities.
If mutations is impossible within 10 minutes, refer the case.
If the fetus is dead, one-cut fetotomy (at the level of the distal row of the carpal bones) permits atraumatic extraction within minutes.

Technical Action	Rationale
6. Two forelimbs without nose at the vulva but ventral deviation of the head (vertex or poll posture; Figure 40.9): rotate the head laterally then move the muzzle up over the pelvic brim.	6. Vertex or poll posture is relatively easy to correct. If the neck is tucked down between the forelimbs (nape posture), mutation is more difficult and may be referred quickly.
7. Two hindlimbs at the vulva with upward hooves (posterior presentation with both extended hindlimbs; Figure 40.10): gently put traction on the hindlimbs in conjunction with mares uterine/abdominal contractions.	7. Due to compression of the umbilical cord and the increased risk of fetal hypoxia, the fetus should be extracted quickly. Fetal death may occur after premature rupture of the umbilical cord.

Dystocia that should be referred.

1. Dystocia not corrected within 10–15 minutes with the mare standing.	1. The survival rate of a foal decreases rapidly if the foal is delivered 45-60 minutes post chorioallantois rupture.
2. Two forelimbs and nose protruding at the vulva with bilateral hip flexion, also referred to as "dog-sitting posture" (Figure 40.11) or unilateral hip flexion ("hurdling posture").	2. Manipulations are difficult as the hindlimbs are often out of reach. Because of the high risk of laceration or perforation of the uterus, C-section is the best form of delivery.
3. Two forelimbs, no nose at the vulva, with lateral deviation of the neck and head (Figure 40.12).	3. Due to the long neck, the head is hard to reach. Possibility of wry neck.
4. One or no forelimb and nose at the vulva with shoulder flexed (Figure 40.13).	4. Correction difficult due to long extremities and access to the retained limb.
5. Nothing protruding at the vulva with the tail in the birth canal and hock flexed or hips flexed (breech) (Figure 40.14).	5. Very difficult to correct and high risk of laceration or rupture of the uterus. C-section is best.
6. Nothing protruding at the vulva with the spinal column in the birth canal: dorso-transverse (rare occurrence = 1 in 1,000).	6. Impossible to correct. C-section is required.
7. Four feet at the vulva: ventro-transverse presentation (rare) or twins (Figure 40.15).	7. Very difficult to correct. High incidence of large foal and fetal malformation. Cesarean section is best.
8. Fetal oversize (rare): gentle traction with copious lubrication may not progress.	8. Occurs more often in maiden mares. May be complicated by a tight vaginovestibular sphincter. Cesarean section is best.

Third Stage Labor **(Expulsion of the Fetal Membranes).**

Duration: the placenta is typically expelled within 30 minutes to 3 hours.

Intervention.

Once the mare rises, the placenta can be tied to itself to avoid being stepped on. It also adds some weight, facilitating fetal membrane expulsion.	
3 hours post partum, if the fetal membranes are not passed they are considered retained.	Retained fetal membranes in mares is considered an emergency. Treatment for retained fetal membranes should be initiated as soon as possible in order to prevent severe complications such as metritis, laminitis and septicemia (see Chapter 41).

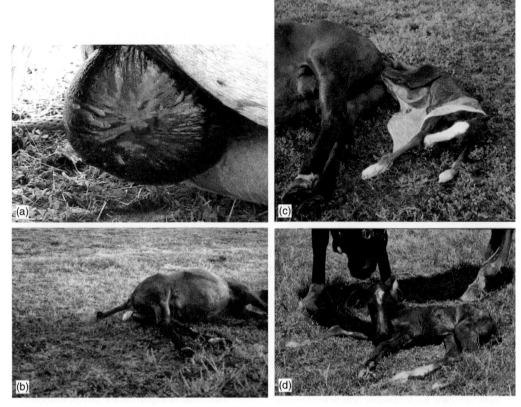

Figure 40.5 Normal and abnormal second stage of delivery. (a) Velvety "red bag" protruding at the vulvar lips corresponding to a non-ruptured chorioallantois with an intact cervical star (courtesy of Dr. Dale Paccamonti). In an emergency it may be ruptured with scissors. The chorioallantois separated from the endometrium impairs fetal oxygenation. (b) During normal delivery, the amnion protrudes at the vulva (courtesy of Dr. Lais R.R. Costa). (c) During normal delivery, the hips pass through the maternal pelvic canal and the hindlimbs remain within the vaginal canal (courtesy of Dr. Lais R.R. Costa). (d) During normal delivery, the umbilical cord ruptures once the mare stands (courtesy of Dr. Lais R.R. Costa).

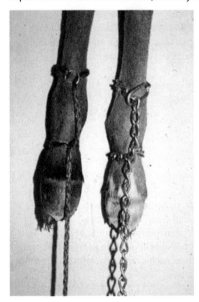

Figure 40.6 Obstetric strap and chain placed on the dorsal part of the distal front limbs (*not* on the plantar surface to avoid injury to the digital tendons) with the first loop encircling the distal canon bone above the fetlock and the second loop immediately below the fetlock. Brinsko *et al.* (2001). Reproduced with permission of Elsevier.

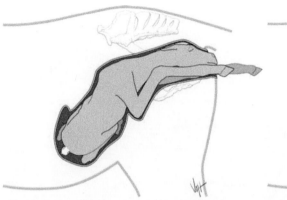

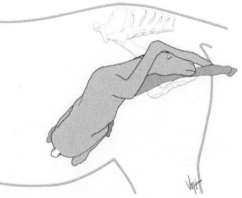

Figure 40.7 Incomplete extension of a forelimb (unilateral elbow lock). McKinnon *et al.* (2011). Reproduced with permission of John Wiley & Sons, Inc.

Figure 40.8 Foot nape posture. McKinnon *et al.* (2011). Reproduced with permission of John Wiley & Sons, Inc.

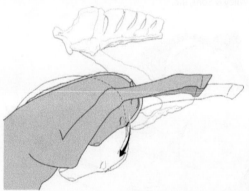

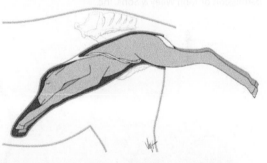

Figure 40.9 Vertex or pool posture. This is relatively easy to correct. Nape posture (arrow) is more difficult to correct and may be referred. McKinnon *et al.* (2011). Reproduced with permission of John Wiley & Sons, Inc.

Figure 40.10 Posterior presentation, dorso sacral position, and extended hindlimbs. Because of compression of the umbilical cord and the high risk of asphyxia, the fetus should be extracted quickly. McKinnon *et al.* (2011). Reproduced with permission of John Wiley & Sons, Inc.

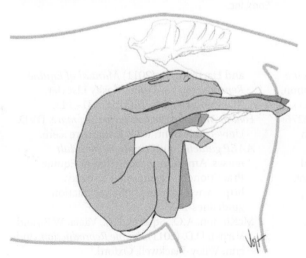

Figure 40.11 Dog-sitting posture (bilateral hip flexion) (as opposed to hurdling posture with unilateral hip flexion). This is very difficult to correct and referral (C-section) is best. McKinnon *et al.* (2011). Reproduced with permission of John Wiley & Sons, Inc.

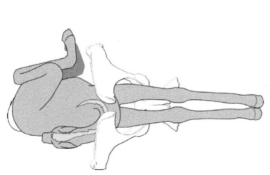

Figure 40.12 Anterior presentation with lateral deviation of the neck and head. This is very difficult to correct, with the possibility of wry neck, and referral is best. McKinnon *et al.* (2011). Reproduced with permission of John Wiley & Sons, Inc.

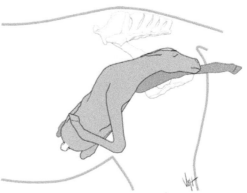

Figure 40.13 Anterior presentation left forelimb extended, right shoulder/elbow/carpus flexed. This is very difficult to correct and referral is best. McKinnon *et al.* (2011). Reproduced with permission of John Wiley & Sons, Inc.

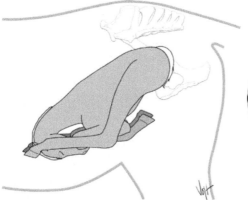

Figure 40.14 Posterior presentation with breech. This is extremely difficult to correct and referral is best. McKinnon *et al.* (2011). Reproduced with permission of John Wiley & Sons, Inc.

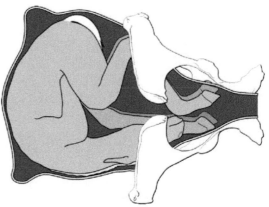

Figure 40.15 Ventro-transverse presentation. This is very difficult to correct and referral is best. McKinnon *et al.* (2011). Reproduced with permission of John Wiley & Sons, Inc.

Bibliography and Further Reading

Christensen, B.W. (2011)Parturition, in *Equine Reproduction*, 2nd edn (eds A.O. McKinnon, E.L. Squires, W.E. Vaala, and D.D. Varner), Wiley Blackwell, Chichester, pp. 2268–2276.

Frazer, G. (2011) Dystocia management, in *Equine Reproduction*, 2nd edn (eds A.O. McKinnon, E.L. Squires, W.E. Vaala, and D.D. Varner), Wiley Blackwell, Chichester, pp. 2479–2496.

Brisko, S.P., Blanchard, T.L., Varner, D.D., Schumacher, J., Love, C.C., Hinrichs, K.,

and Hartman, D. (2011) *Manual of Equine Reproduction*, 3rd edn, Mosby Elsevier, Maryland Heights, MO, pp. 131–142.

Foal in Mare: Insights in the foaling mare. DVD, Universiteit Gent, www.foalinmare .com.

AAEP guidelines vaccinations for adult horses. American Association of Equine Practitioners, Lexington, Kentucky. http://www.aaep.org/info/vaccination-guidelines-265

McKinnon, A.O., Squires, E.L., Vaala, W.E., and Varner, D.D. (2011) *Equine Reproduction*, 2nd edn, Wiley-Blackwell, Oxford.

41

Evaluation and Monitoring of the Post-parturient Mare

Catherine Renaudin

41.1 Purpose

- To describe how to assess a mare and her placenta within 24 hours of foaling (Figure 41.1).
- To describe normal and abnormal placenta appearance.
- To describe how to diagnose the different post-parturient reproductive pathologies for the first week postpartum.
- To describe the guidelines to determine if the mare is a good candidate to be bred at foal heat.
- Evaluation of the post-parturient mare includes:
  - evaluation of the placenta (completeness, abnormalities, weight)
  - evaluation of the umbilical cord
  - general physical examination of the mare
  - examination of the mammary glands
  - examination of the perineum
  - transrectal ultrasound examination (optional)
  - vaginal speculum examination (optional)
  - transvaginal palpation (optional)

41.2 Complications

- Iatrogenic rectal tears (see Table 16.1).

41.3 Equipment Required

- Brown gauze to wrap the tail or a clean neoprene tail wrap

Rectal examination

- Rectal sleeve and lubricant (non-sterile)
- Portable, good-quality ultrasound machine equipped with a 5–7 MHz linear transducer

Speculum examination

- Bucket with a clean plastic liner, cotton, non-residual soap or povidone-iodine
- Clean towel
- Vaginal speculum
- Sterile obstetrical lubricant for vaginal examination
- Flashlight

41.4 Restraint and Positioning

- The evaluation should be conducted with the mare restrained in stocks.
- Additional restraint will depend on the disposition of the mare.

Manual of Clinical Procedures in the Horse, First Edition. Edited by Lais R.R. Costa and Mary Rose Paradis.
© 2018 John Wiley & Sons, Inc. Published 2018 by John Wiley & Sons, Inc.

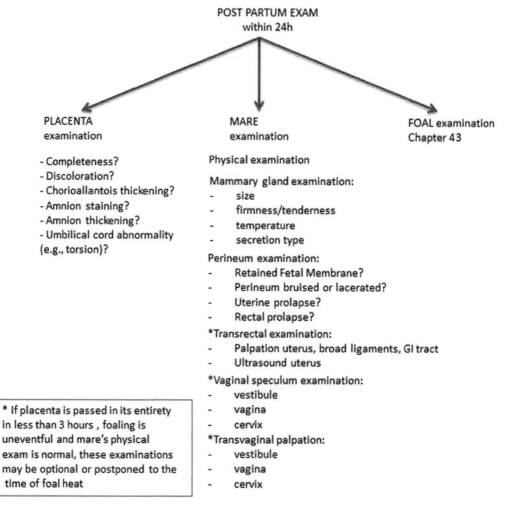

POST PARTUM EXAM
within 24h

PLACENTA
examination

- Completeness?
- Discoloration?
- Chorioallantois thickening?
- Amnion staining?
- Amnion thickening?
- Umbilical cord abnormality
(e.g., torsion)?

MARE
examination

Physical examination

Mammary gland examination:
- size
- firmness/tenderness
- temperature
- secretion type

Perineum examination:
- Retained Fetal Membrane?
- Perineum bruised or lacerated?
- Uterine prolapse?
- Rectal prolapse?

*Transrectal examination:
- Palpation uterus, broad ligaments, GI tract
- Ultrasound uterus

*Vaginal speculum examination:
- vestibule
- vagina
- cervix

*Transvaginal palpation:
- vestibule
- vagina
- cervix

FOAL examination
Chapter 43

* If placenta is passed in its entirety
in less than 3 hours , foaling is
uneventful and mare's physical
exam is normal, these examinations
may be optional or postponed to the
time of foal heat

Figure 41.1 Assessment of the mare and her placenta within 24 hours of foaling.

41.5   Procedure: Evaluation of the Placenta

Technical action	Rationale
First identify the sides of the placenta.	
The placenta is usually expelled inverted with the allantoic surface (smooth, shiny, and whitish) outermost and the chorionic surface (red, velvety) innermost.	
Using non-sterile gloves, place the placenta on a large clean surface that can be thoroughly cleaned and disinfected. The membranes are laid out in an "F" shape (Figures 41.2 and 41.3).	If the placenta is dirty with bedding material, use a hose to gently clean it with water. In cases of abortion it is particularly important not to contaminate the environment.

Technical action	Rationale
Evaluate the Placenta. Placenta should be evaluated for the following:	
• <u>Completeness:</u> The placenta is best observed with the allantoic surface outermost (as it is expelled). The gravid and not gravid horns should be complete. Only one tear is seen at the tip of the body segment at the cervical star (Figure 41.4).	Usually it is the tip of the non-pregnant horn that is retained due to its anatomy (microvilli more branched and thinner chorioallantois than in the pregnant horn) and its slower uterine involution.

• <u>Discoloration and thickening</u> of the chorioallantois (observed on the chorionic side) indicates placentitis (which should be distinguished from autolytic changes) and can occur in the following locations:
   – At the cervical star due to bacterial infection (Figure 41.5a) such as *Strep. equi zooepidemicus*, *Escherichia coli*, *Pseudomonas aeruginosa*, *Klebsiella pneumoniae* or mycotic infection like *Aspergillus fumigatus* (with a leather-like appearance). The placenta is often so thick that it does not break at the cervical star (red bag; see Figure 40.5) (Figure 41.5b). The entire placenta or a piece placed in 10% formalin of a suspicious area should be submitted to a laboratory.
   – In the body or base of the horns due to *Leptospira pomona*, *Salmonella abortus equi*, *Histoplasma*, mare reproductive loss syndrome (MLRS) or nocardia (with a brownish caramel-like and thick discharge). Any suspicious area should be sampled and submitted to a laboratory.
	Autolytic changes will occur with time. It is best to look at a fresh placenta or to store it cool and moist. If placed in a bag, pressure from the weight moves blood in the chorioallantoic, producing discoloration not to be confused with placentitis (discoloration + thickening)
	
	 The placentitis is of ascending origin due to the cervical entrance of germs, which leaves the foal at risk of infection.
	
	 A "red bag" may result in hypoxia and a "dummy foal". The foal should be examined for mental abnormalities.
	
	 It is important to know the cause of abortion in order to treat the mare and foal properly.
	
	 The placentitis that are diffuse or multifocal are often of hematogenic origin. This leaves the foal at risk of infection

• <u>Amnion staining</u> (brown, green) with meconium indicates fetal stress. A normal amnion should be translucent and thin (as shown in Figure 41.3).	Fetal stress will lead to passage of the meconium while in uterus, and thus staining of the amnion.
• <u>Amnion thickened</u> with dilated vessels (amnionitis) indicates an inflammatory response in utero.	The foal should be checked for in utero infections.
Check the Umbilical Cord.	
• <u>Umbilical cord torsion:</u> excessive twists may occur, especially when the cord is long (>80 cm) (Figures 41.6 and 41.7). • <u>Short umbilical cord:</u> may rupture prematurely intrapartum. • <u>Urachal obstruction</u> with umbilical cord distention close to its attachment to the fetal abdominal wall.	The umbilical cord normally has up to 5 or 6 twists. Umbilical cord torsion impairs placental blood flow, leading to placental Insufficiency and abortion. It also leads to fetal asphyxia and stillbirth, may predispose to rupture bladder and patent urachus.
Some structures may look strange but are normal.	
• <u>Hippomanes:</u> soft, flat, spongy brown structure (Figure 41.8).	Hippomanes is a normal finding. It is also called "allantoic calculus".
• <u>Amniotic plaques</u> (yellow hard dots) on the fetal side of the amniotic membrane (Figure 41.9) and the amniotic segment of the umbilical cord.	Amniotic plaques have no clinical significance.
• <u>Chorioallantoic vesicles:</u> focal area of allantoic edema located around vessels (allantoic side of the placenta) (Figure 41.10).	Chorioallantoic vesicles have no clinical significance.
• <u>Chorioallantoic pouches</u> (Figure 41.11): on the allantoic side of the placenta near the base of the gravid horn.	Chorioallantoic pouches are considered a normal finding. They contain necrotic endometrial cup material.

(continued)

Technical action	Rationale

• Normal avillous areas on the chorionic surface:
  – at the cervical star (Figure 41.4)
  – at the base of the gravid horn over endometrial cups
  – over linear areas overlying large vessels
  – on areas of twin placental apposition
  – at the tip of the horn (utero–tubal junction) (Figure 41.12).	

• The ossified remnant of the yolk sac is a bony structure resembling a cranium attached to or within the umbilical cord (Figure 41.13).	The ossified remnant of the yolk sac is a structure that may compromise the umbilical cord blood flow and lead to abortion. The ossified remnant of the yolk sac is generally pedunculated.
Weigh the Placenta. Normal placental weight is 11% of the foal's body weight. • If the placenta is lighter it suggests placental insufficiency. • If the placenta is heavier, it suggests placentitis.	Placenta includes chorioallantois + umbilical cord + amnion. Placental insufficiency is often associated with small newborn foals. Heavier placenta is generally due to edema, inflammation or infection.

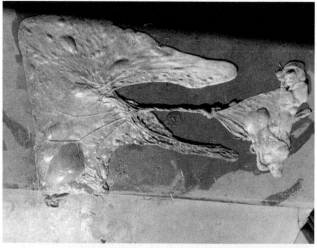

Figure 41.2 Placenta laid out in an "F" shape on its allantoic side. The placenta is complete.

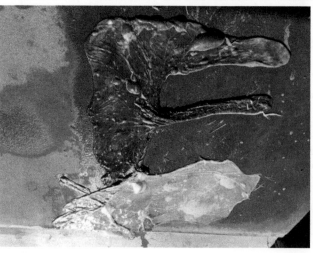

Figure 41.3 Placenta laid out in an "F" shape on its chorionic side.

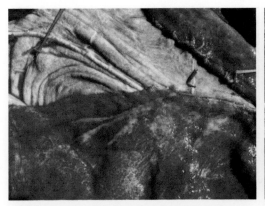

Figure 41.4 Chorionic side of the placenta at the cervical star where the placenta breaks at birth.

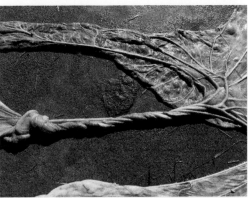

Figure 41.6 Normal twists in a normal umbilical cord.

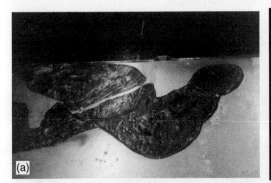

(a)

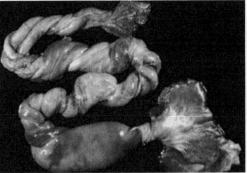

Figure 41.7 Abnormal umbilical cord with excessive torsion. McKinnon *et al.* (2011). Reproduced with permission of John Wiley & Sons, Inc.

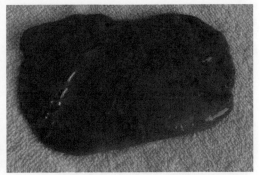

(b)

Figure 41.5 Placentas affected by placentitis break at other parts, not the cervical star. (a) Chorionic side of a placenta broken at the body area due to a placentitis at the cervical star. (b) Close-up of the cervical area showing discoloration and thickening of the placenta. The cervical star did not break: "red bag". Renaudin *et al.* (1999). Reproduced with permission of John Wiley & Sons, Inc.

Figure 41.8 Hippomane: soft, flat, spongy brown structure with no clinical significance. Courtesy of Dr. Ghislaine Dujovne.

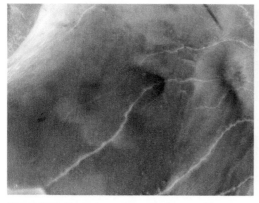

Figure 41.9 Normal amniotic membrane with amniotic plaques. Amniotic plaques have no clinical significance.

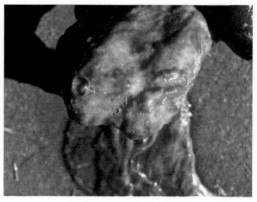

Figure 41.12 Normal avillous area on the chorionic surface at the tip of the horn corresponding to the utero–tubal junction.

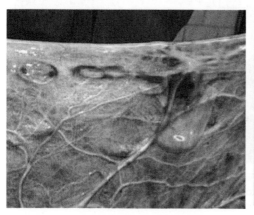

Figure 41.10 Chorioallantoic vesicles seen on the allantoic side of the chorioallantois. They have no clinical significance. McKinnon *et al.* (2011). Reproduced with permission of John Wiley & Sons, Inc.

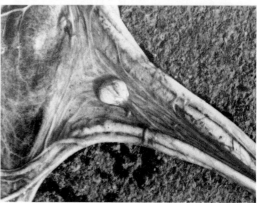

Figure 41.13 Ossified remnant of the yolk sac attached to the umbilical cord. The pedunculated structure may occasionally compromise the umbilical cord blood flow and lead to abortion.

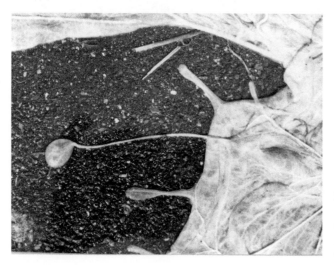

Figure 41.11 Chorioallantoic pouches seen on the allantoic side of the chorioallantois. They have no clinical significance and contain necrotic endometrial cup material.

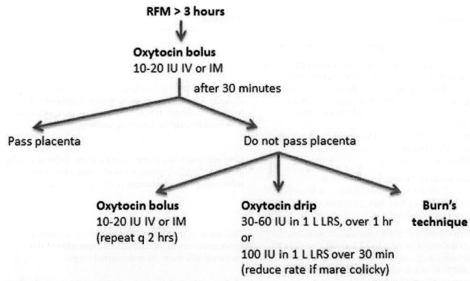

RFM > 3 hours

Oxytocin bolus
10-20 IU IV or IM

after 30 minutes

Pass placenta   Do not pass placenta

Oxytocin bolus	**Oxytocin drip**	**Burn's**
10-20 IU IV or IM	30-60 IU in 1 L LRS, over 1 hr	**technique**
(repeat q 2 hrs)	or	
	100 IU in 1 L LRS over 30 min	
	(reduce rate if mare colicky)	

If placenta retained after dystocia or for > 6 hours or mare has signs of systemic disease:
- Administer systemic antibiotics for 5-7 days
- Administer anti-inflammatory drugs (Flunixin meglumine, pentoxifylline)
- Perform uterine lavage (0.9% saline or LRS or 35 g of table salt in 4L tap or deionized water)
- Cold water hosing or icing of all feet or footpads

Figure 41.14 Decision making for management of retained fetal membranes (RFM).

41.6 Procedure: Evaluation of the Mare in the Immediate Postpartum

Technical action	Rationale
General Physical Examination of the Mare. The general physical examination of the mare is performed with special attention to: • mucous membrane color and moisture • capillary refill time (CRT) • heart rate • respiratory rate • digital pulses and hooves heat • rectal temperature • gut sounds. (See details in Chapter 3.)	Abnormalities may indicate: • anemia, hemorrhage: rupture of the middle uterine artery with or without associated broad ligament hematoma, uterine rupture or tear • infection: postpartum metritis, peritonitis, mastitis • laminitis often associated with retained fetal membranes (RFM) • gastrointestinal pathologies manifested as colic due to large colon volvulus, cecal rupture, small or large intestine trauma, diaphragmatic hernia, evisceration through a vaginal or uterine tear • colic due to non-gastrointestinal pathologies: RFM, rupture of middle uterine artery, uterine rupture or tear, invagination of tip of the horn.
Examination of the Mammary Glands. • <u>Size:</u> should be developed (abnormal: very small or severely enlarged). • <u>Firmness/tenderness:</u> should be soft to moderately firm (depending on time of last nursing) and non-painful (abnormal: firm, painful). • <u>Temperature:</u> should be body temperature (abnormal: hot). • <u>Secretion:</u> milk, colostrum (abnormal: pus or hemorrhage).	Abnormalities include: • agalactia (due to fescue toxicoses, pergolide-treated mare for Cushing disease, post C-section, selenium deficiency, restricted water intake, malnutrition, stress) • hypogalactia (due to systemic disease, malnutrition, restricted water intake, stress) • engorged mammary gland: sign that foal fails to nurse properly (sick, unable to walk), may lead to mastitis • mastitis: complication of lack of hygiene when sampling pre-foaling secretions or failure of the foal to nurse properly.

(continued)

Technical action	Rationale

Examination of Perineum for the Presence of Placenta.

- Placenta hanging for less than 3 hours post parturition: this is normal. There is no need for intervention.
- Placenta not hanging and not passed, or placenta hanging at the vulva for more than 3 hours post parturition indicates retained fetal membranes (RFM).
- Treatment of RFM should be initiated promptly (Figure 41.14) with:
  – Oxytocin injection:

1. bolus 10–20 IU IV or IM q 2 hours, or
2. drip of 30–60 IU in 1 liter of LRS over 1 hour, or
3. drip of 100 IU in 1 liter over 30 minutes (reduce rate if mare becomes colicky).

  – Burn's technique: if the chorioallantois is intact, it is distended with up to 12 liters of a weak (<2%) povidone-iodine solution in water or saline through a sterile stomach tube and held closed with the operator's hand (Figure 41.15).

- If the placenta is retained after a dystocia or for more than 6 hours or the mare has signs of systemic disease, further treatments are necessary, including systemic antibiotics, anti-inflammatories, and uterine lavage.

Incidence of RFM is increased in draft horses, and after dystocia, Caesarean section, prolonged gestation or hydrops condition. It may lead to severe complications, for example metritis, laminitis, and septicemia.

Oxytocin promotes uterine contractions. Bolus is usually given the first 3–6 hours. If not effective, slow drip infusion or Burn's technique is then performed.

Distension of the chorioallantois and uterus induces endogenous oxytocin release, and separation of the chorionic villi from the endometrial crypts.

Additional treatments should be initiated in those cases to prevent the metritis /laminitis/ septicemia complex. Treatment for RFM includes:

- systemic antibiotics for 5–7 days
- systemic anti-inflammatory drugs (flunixin meglumine, pentoxifylline)
- uterine lavage (0.9% saline or lactated Ringer solution or 35 g of table salt in 4 liters of tap water or deionized water)
- cold water hosing or icing of all feet and/or footpads.

Examine the Perineum.
Examination the perineum is performed to ensure that it is intact and note if the perineum is bruised or torn.

- Bruised: no treatment is necessary. May apply ice or phenylephrine ointment (Preparation H).
- First-degree perineal laceration: involves the mucosa, submucosa, and skin of the dorsal aspect of the vestibule. May need a Caslick suture (see Chapter 38) depending on the size of laceration.

- Second-degree perineal laceration: extends through the musculature of the constrictor vulva muscle and the perineal body. Needs vestibuloplasty immediately after parturition or once bruising and swelling have subsided.
- Third-degree perineal laceration (rectovestibular laceration): there is complete disruption of the roof of the vestibule, the floor of the rectum, and the perineal body (Figure 41.16). Surgical repair is performed after 2–3 months or after foal is weaned when tissues are well healed.
- Recto vaginal/vestibular fistula (RVF) is a fistula between the rectum and the vagina/vestibule without perineal involvement. This defect is best located by inserting fingers into it from both the rectal and vaginal side. Surgical repair after 2–3 months.

Mares with second- and third-degree perineal laceration are prone to pneumovagina and urine pooling. Repairing the laceration is crucial for breeding.

Third-degree perineal laceration occurs predominantly in primiparous mares due to their prominent annular fold, which fails to fully dilate.

General health and comfort are hardly affected by RVF. Fecal continuous contamination of the genital tract will cause infertility. If rebreeding, surgical repair is necessary to restore the inter-recto–vestibular barrier.

Technical action	Rationale
If examination of the perineum reveals an engorged, edematous, congested uterus protruding at the vulva, this indicates uterine prolapse.	Uterine prolapse occurs uncommonly post dystocia, RFM or abortion. Uterine prolapse is more likely to occur in older multiparous mares. It is a life-threatening emergency.
Treatment of uterine prolapse is an emergency, and include:	
• Support the uterus at the level of the pelvic brim with a plastic bag or sheet or tray held by two assistants.	Supporting the uterus will prevent uterine artery rupture and congestion of the uterus, and will restore uterine circulation.
• Gently clean the uterus with warm water diluted with povidone-iodine solution.	Metritis is a common complication.
• Evaluate the uterus for tear and repair it if necessary. Identify if the bladder or intestine are involved with the prolapse.	If the urinary bladder is distended, catheterization is necessary for replacement and prevention of ruptured bladder.
• Replacement of the uterus:	
– If possible place the mare with hindquarters elevated.	Gravity will facilitate the replacement of the uterus.
– It is imperative to control straining using sedative (butorphanol and xylazine) or caudal epidural anesthesia, or, as a last resort, general anesthesia.	Straining and pain due to traction on the ovarian and uterine ligaments make it impossible to replace the uterus. Most cases are performed standing.
– Lubricate the uterus with petroleum jelly and gently replace the uterus with the flat of the hands, starting with the ventral aspect.	The uterus is very friable and may tear.
– Make sure the uterus is completely replaced by gently filling it with sterile saline solution.	If uterine horns are not fully replaced (invagination) (Figure 41.17), the uterus will re-prolapse.
	Sterile solution is preferred in case there is a small uterine hole.
– Give low-dose oxytocin (10–20 IU).	Oxytocin increases uterine involution.
– Place the mare on systemic broad-spectrum antibiotics, intravenous fluid, and non-steroidal anti-inflammatory agents for 3–5 days.	Antibiotics prevent metritis and endotoxemia.
If examination of the perineum reveals intestinal involvement the case should be referred to a hospital for evaluation and surgical repair. Intestinal involvement include:	Intestinal involvement carries very poor prognosis if blood supply to the intestinal segment is compromised, leading to bowel necrosis.
– rectal prolapse,	
– intussusception of the rectum,	
– prolapse of the distal small colon.	
Transrectal Palpation.	
Brief transrectal evaluation of the uterus should be performed postpartum.	If the placenta is passed in its entirety in less than 3 hours postpartum, rectal examination may be postponed to the time of foal heat.
During the immediate postpartum, transrectal palpation is aimed to evaluate the uterine shape and the tip of the uterine horns.	
On the first day postpartum, the tip of the horns should be identified, although the uterine bifurcation may not always be reached.	In uterine horn intussusception (Figure 41.17), the tip of the horn is not well defined.
Evaluation of uterine involution:	The uterus may feel smaller than expected for the postpartum stage in case of uterine lacerations.
• For the first few days postpartum the uterus has a high tone and rugal folds can be felt.	
• On day 3 postpartum: the uterine bifurcation should be easily palpated.	
• On day 4 postpartum: the uterus should be half of the size of immediate postpartum.	
• By 2–3 weeks postpartum: uterus should be nearly completely involuted.	

(continued)

Technical action	Rationale
<u>Evaluation of the broad ligament and uterine wall.</u> Pay special attention to the possible presence of hematomas.	Large hematomas located in the uterine wall or in the broad ligaments may be identified. Rectal palpation should be gentle and brief to prevent fatal hemorrhage. It should not be performed if the mare is fractious.
<u>Evaluation of the gastrointestinal tract.</u>	Transrectal palpation is helpful in the diagnosis of large colon volvulus or small intestine abnormalities. In many cases of gastrointestinal trauma, rectal palpation is not diagnostic.
Transrectal Ultrasound Examination of the Uterus. It is normal during the first few days postpartum to see the lumen of the uterus with hyperechoic, hypoechoic or anechoic fluid (lochias). After 5 days postpartum, some anechoic fluid may still be present. Often normal dilated vessels (with anechoic fluid) in the wall of the uterus can also be seen in the first few days postpartum.	If the placenta is passed in its entirety within 3 hours postpartum, and uterine shape and involution are normal, ultrasonographic examination may be optional. Abnormalities: <ul><li>an increase in the diameter of the uterine horn with intraluminal hyperechogenic fluid in case of metritis (pus with or without fetal membranes), urometra (urine), hemometra (blood)</li><li>distinctive hyperechoic areas within the uterine lumen (retained fetal membranes)</li><li>telescoping of concentric rings of soft tissue at the distal tip of a horn (uterine horn intussusception).</li></ul>
Vaginal Speculum Examination.	If the placenta is complete and passed within 3 hours, and the foaling was uneventful, speculum examination may be optional.
• Evaluation of the vestibule and vagina: the wall of the vagina and vestibule should be carefully observed for hematoma/bruises or laceration	Vaginal/vestibular lacerations should be sutured if possible. Rectovaginal/vestibular fistula may be discovered on the dorsal aspect of the vagina or vestibule. They will need to be repaired 2–3 months post foaling if rebreeding is an option.
• Evaluation of accumulation of non-malodorous lochias (red to reddish brown discharge): small to moderate amount of lochias in commonly seen in the vaginal cavity	An abnormal amount of fluid may accumulate in the fornix (anterior portion) vagina: malodorous pus (metritis), urine (urovagina/ urometra), or blood (hemometra, vaginal varicosities). Treatment should be initiated.
• Presence of fetal membranes: fetal membranes should be passed by 3 hours postpartum	If fetal membranes are seen, treatment should be initiated.
• Evaluation of the cervix (external cervical os): – will be opened – lochia may be seen coming out of the cervical os – should be intact, sometimes bruised.	A large amount of blood (hemometra, uterine laceration/ rupture) or the presence of malodorous purulent material (metritis) or the presence of urine (urometra) coming out of the cervical os is abnormal. Cervical lacerations may occur, especially after difficult foaling. The extend of the lesions should be reassessed when the mare is in diestrus to decide whether or not surgical repair is necessary.

Technical action	Rationale
Transvaginal Palpation. Transvaginal palpation is performed with a sterile sleeve or a rectal sleeve turned inside out, with a sterile glove on top, and lubricated with sterile water-soluble lubricant. It should include palpation of:	The use of a sterile surgical glove to perform the transvaginal palpation improves the ability to identify subtle abnormalities.
• the vestibule/vagina, especially areas that looked abnormal on speculum examination (hematoma, tear, RVF) to better evaluate their size and extent	Superficial tears do not need to be repaired.
• the cervix: the entire wall of the external os is assessed between the index finger and the thumb to detect any defect/laceration.	Cervical defects that progresses cranially to involve the junction of the external os with the vagina are candidates for surgery. It is wise to re-evaluate the mare during diestrus when the cervix is tight to assess cervical competency.
• When RFM or a uterine tear is suspected, palpation of the body of the uterus may enable the practitioner to locate the uterine tear.	Uterine tears occur more often in the body of the uterus or in the tip of the pregnant horn (due to the forceful process of straightening the hindlimbs at delivery).

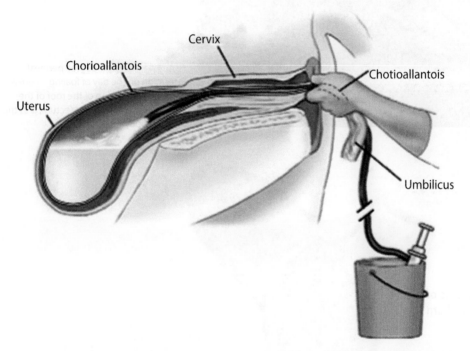

Figure 41.15 Burn's technique is used as a treatment for retained fetal membranes when the chorioallantois is intact. The chorioallantois is distended with a large volume of a weak (<2%) povidone iodine solution in water or saline that is pumped with a sterile stomach tube. The operator's hand holds the chorioallantois and the stomach tube tightly together. Brinsko *et al.* (2011). Reproduced with permission of Elsevier.

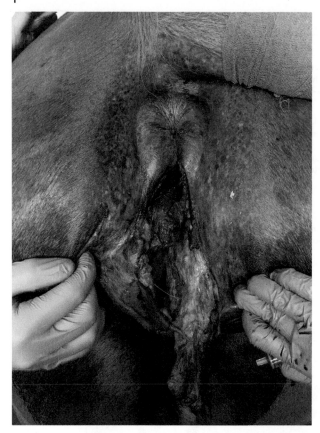

Figure 41.16 Third-degree perineal laceration on the day of foaling. There is complete disruption of the roof of the vestibule, the floor of the rectum, and the perineal body.

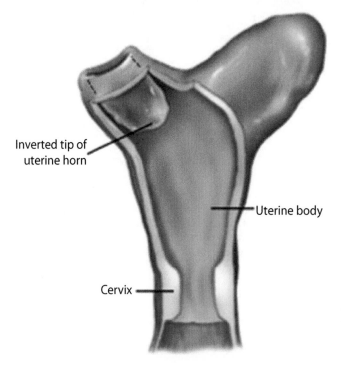

Figure 41.17 Drawing of a uterus with a uterine horn intussusception. The tip of the horn is inverted. Brinsko *et al.* (2011). Reproduced with permission of Elsevier.

41.7 Procedure: Evaluation of the Mare at Foal Heat:

Technical Action	Rationale
Get a complete history of foaling and post-foaling event: • normal foaling/assisted foaling/dystocia • if fetal membranes passed within 3 hours • age of the mare at foaling and number of last consecutive foaling	Any obstetric manipulation predisposes to infection and trauma so the mare is not a good candidate for foal heat breeding. RFM often delays uterine involution so the mare is not a good candidate for foal heat breeding. Increased age (>10 years old) and increased number of consecutive foalings decrease pregnancy rate.
Transrectal palpation should be performed to assess uterine involution. • At 8 days, uterine bifurcation and both horns should be entirely felt. The pregnant horn is still bigger than the non-pregnant horn, and rugal folds are still present. These are signs of normal uterine involution. Normal gross involution is complete by day 25–32. • If there is poor gross uterine involution by day 8, the mare is not a good candidate for foal heat breeding. It is best to skip foal heat, document the first ovulation and eventually short cycle the mare 5 days post ovulation or wait for the second cycle.	 Good uterine involution by day 8 is the result of proper uterine contractility leading to evacuation of lochia. Poor gross uterine involution is associated with decreased pregnancy rate and increased pregnancy losses compared to the second heat cycle.

Tranrectal ultrasound should be performed to assess the following:
 	
• The presence of uterine fluid:
  – at day 8 postpartum - the absence or presence of a minimal amount of anechoic fluid is considered normal.
  – at foal heat - the presence of a moderate to large amount of echogenic fluid (which might be lochia, inflammatory fluid, pus, urine or blood) is abnormal and should be treated. The mare is not a good candidate for breeding at foal heat.
• Follicular activity: if before day 10 post foaling, the follicular activity indicates that the mare is ready to ovulate, then the mare is not a good candidate for breeding at foal heat.
 	
Decision to bred at foal heat:
 	
• A mare is a good candidate for breeding at foal heat, if the following conditions are met:
  – it was an uncomplicated birth, with no or minimal genital tract trauma, with prompt passage of fetal membranes, and good uterine involution;
  – at foal heat there is no or little anechoic uterine fluid;
  – the mare is not ready to ovulate before day 10.
	Important consideration concerning breeding at foal heat:
	
	– Mares with ultrasonographically detectable uterine fluid accumulations during the foal heat ovulatory period have significantly lower pregnancy rates and higher pregnancy loss than mares without fluid.
	– Mares have a higher pregnancy rate if ovulation in the postpartum estrus occurs after day 10.
	– If the uterus is fully involuted by day 14, and the mare ovulates at or after day 10, the embryo will enter the uterus after day 14.

(continued)

Technical Action	Rationale
<u>Vaginal speculum examination and transvaginal palpation</u> should be perform to determine the presence of the following conditions:	

• Urovagina/urometra:
  – This condition is most often seen in older, multiparous mares following normal deliveries or dystocia due to the stretching and relaxation of the caudal reproductive tract.
  – Foal heat should be skipped and the mare should be treated.
  – Treatment include: daily uterine lavages, oxytocin therapy, exercise until foal heat ovulation occurs.
  – These mares should be re-examined on their second cycle. If urovagina persists, surgical correction may be indicated.
	Urovagina often leads to urometra, secondary endometritis, cervicitis, and vaginitis, and results in reduced fertility. Most mares will self-correct once they come under the influence of progesterone (foal heat ovulation).

• Cervical defect/laceration:
  – If present and extensive, foal heat should be skipped.
  – The mare should be re-evaluated later in diestrus.
  – Adhesions may be prevented by applying corticosteroid ointment on the cervical defect.
	Cervical defects/lacerations may result in cervical incompetency and adhesions that could lead to secondary pyometra. When in diestrus, the cervix should become competent and free of adhesions. If not, surgical repair may be indicated for future reproductive success.

Bibliography and Further Reading

Blanchard, T.L. (2011) Postpartum metritis, in *Equine Reproduction*, 2nd edn (eds A.O. McKinnon, E.L. Squires, W.E. Vaala, and D.D.Varner), Wiley Blackwell, Chichester, pp. 2521–2529.

Brinsko S.P., Blanchard, T.L., Varner, D.D., Schumacher, J., Love, C.C., Hinrichs, K., Hartman, D. (2011) Dystocia and postpartum disease. *Manual of Equine Reproduction*. Mosby Elsevier, Maryland Heights, Missouri, pp.131-159.

Byars, T.D. and Divers, T.J. (2011) Periparturient hemorrhage, in *Equine Reproduction*, 2nd edn (eds A.O. McKinnon, E.L. Squires, W.E. Vaala, and D.D. Varner), Wiley Blackwell, Chichester, pp. 2517–2519.

Christensen, B.W. (2011) Partuition, in *Equine Reproduction*, 2nd edn (eds A.O. McKinnon, E.L. Squires, W.E. Vaala, and D.D. Varner), Wiley Blackwell, Chichester, pp. 2268–2276.

McCue, P.M. (1993) Lactation, in *Equine Reproduction* (eds A.O. McKinnon and Voss, J.L.), Lea and Febiger, Philadelphia, pp.588–595.

Pollock, P.J. and Russell, T.M. (2011) Cervical surgery, in *Equine Reproduction*, 2nd edn (eds A.O. McKinnon, E.L. Squires, W.E. Vaala, and D.D. Varner), Wiley Blackwell, Chichester, pp. 2559–2563.

Renaudin, C.D., Liu, I.K.M., Troedsson, M.H.T., and Schrenzel, M.D. (1999) Transrectal ultrasonographic diagnosis of ascending placentitis in the mare: a report of two cases. *Equine Veterinary Education*, **11**, 69–74.

Sprito, M.A. and Sprayberry, K.A. (2011) Uterine prolapse, in *Equine Reproduction*, 2nd edn (eds A.O. McKinnon, E.L. Squires, W.E. Vaala, and D.D. Varner), Wiley Blackwell, Chichester, pp. 2431–2434.

Threlfall, W.R. (2011) Retained fetal membranes, in *Equine Reproduction*, 2nd edn (eds A.O. McKinnon, E.L. Squires, W.E. Vaala, and D.D. Varner), Wiley Blackwell, Chichester, pp. 2521–2529.

Turner, R.M. (2013) Maladies of the post partum mare. *Proceedings of the Annual Resort Symposium of the AAEP*, Jan 27–29, www.IVIS.org.

Part VI

Clinical Procedures in Neonatal Medicine

A Clinical Assessment and Resuscitation of the Neonatal Foal

42

Restraining the Neonatal Foal

Nóra Nógrádi and K. Gary Magdesian

42.1 Purpose

- Proper restraint allows the veterinarian to perform a safe and thorough assessment of the neonatal foal, and minor procedures that do not require sedation.

42.2 Complications

- Injury to the handler or veterinarian
- Injury to the foal (e.g., broken tail)

42.3 Equipment Required

- Large-size adult horse halter
- Soft lead rope

42.4 Procedure: Standing Restraint

Technical action	Rationale
Standing restraint is useful for performing physical examination (e.g., wellness post-foaling examination, sick foal assessment) or for procedures that do not require sedation. For proper restraint of the neonatal foal in a standing position, the handler should stand on one side of the foal with one arm wrapped around the upper neck gently holding the head and another arm around the buttocks (Figure 42.1).	Some foals will sink or collapse in the handler's arms when they are restrained. The initial reaction may be to apply more restraint, but this is counter-productive as increasing pressure will stimulate a sleep-type response in foals. Reduction of restraint will usually result in the foal regaining its composure and standing again.
Additional restraint of the foal can be accomplished by holding the tail head with one hand, while the other hand continues to restrain the front of the foal (Figure 42.2). The tail can be gently but firmly held to the side.	Do not crank the tail straight up over the foal's croup or manipulate it with marked force, as this can result in serious injury to the foal's tail.
An appropriately sized harness is also effective in restraining a neonatal foal for many circumstances. For example, it can help to control the foal during movement of the mare and foal.	A large-size adult horse halter can be used as a harness around the foal's trunk for light restraint (Figure 42.3).
A soft rope around the buttocks should be used to restraint larger foals (Figure 42.4a).	The rope will provide gentle restraint of movement and will help lead the foal.

(continued)

Manual of Clinical Procedures in the Horse, First Edition. Edited by Lais R.R. Costa and Mary Rose Paradis.
© 2018 John Wiley & Sons, Inc. Published 2018 by John Wiley & Sons, Inc.

Technical action	Rationale
Do not utilize a halter on the foal's head for restraint until the foal is halter trained. Even then the buttocks should be supported (Figure 42.4b).	Neonatal foals rarely tolerate halter restraint without training. The untrained foal tends to oppose the direction of pressure, often resulting in the foal pulling against the halter, and sometimes resulting in the foal flipping over backwards.

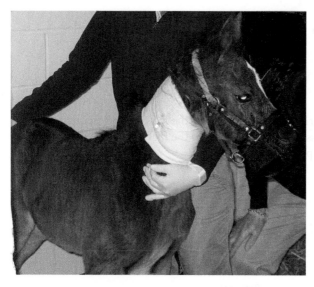

Figure 42.1 The standing foal can be held by placing one arm around the foal's chest and the other behind the foal's rump. Courtesy of Dr. Lais R.R. Costa.

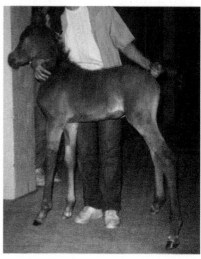

Figure 42.2 Additional restraint can be performed by holding the tail head, while the other arm is wrapped around the upper neck, gently holding the head. Courtesy of Dr. Lais R.R. Costa.

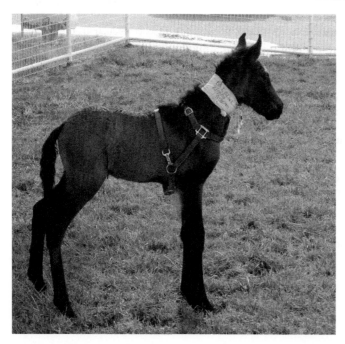

Figure 42.3 A large-size adult horse halter can be used as a harness to restrain the neonatal foal.

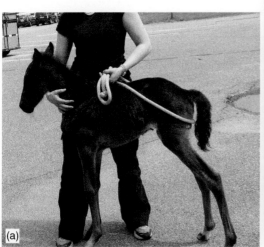
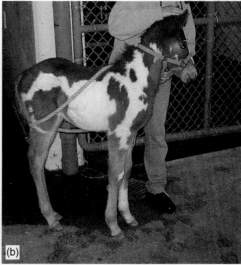

Figure 42.4 Restraint of larger foals. (a) A soft rope around the buttocks is used to provide gentle restraint of movement and will help lead the foal. (b) Because foals rarely tolerate halter restraint without training, the buttocks rope should always be applied until the foal is completely halter trained. Courtesy of Dr. Lais R.R. Costa.

42.5 Procedure: Placing the Foal in Lateral Recumbency ("Folding")

Technical action	Rationale/amplification
Hold the foal in the standing position by gently holding the head with one hand and placing the other hand around the buttocks.	Alternatively, gently hold the tail instead of wrapping the arm around the buttocks.
Slowly but firmly turn the foal's head and neck to the side away from you, curling the head back towards the chest (Figure 42.5a).	The neonate will slowly start to sink. The handler then kneels along with the foal until the foal sinks down into lateral recumbency (Figure 42.5b).

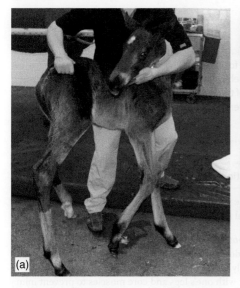
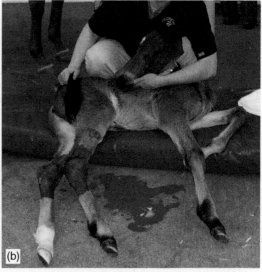

Figure 42.5 "Folding" the foal is a simple method of placing a foal in lateral recumbency. (a) Turn the foal's head toward its chest and grasp the tail. (b) As the foal collapses the handler gently lowers it to the floor.

42.6 Procedure: Restraining the Foal in Lateral Recumbency

Technical action	Rationale/amplification
Once the foal is in lateral recumbency, it will need to be restrained until the desired procedure is completed.	If not restrained immediately after being "folded" to lateral recumbency (see above), the foal will immediately struggle to get up.
There are multiple techniques for restraining a foal in lateral recumbency.	The technique selected depends on the goal of restraint. If foal is restrained in lateral recumbency, ensure that appropriate padding is provided. Avoid lateral recumbency on the same side for more than 2 hours.
Technique 1: The handler holds the foal's head and neck over one of the handler's legs and lap, while the handler's other leg is gently placed over the foal's trunk, all the while being careful not to interfere with the foal's ventilation.	This is a gentle technique that is useful for keeping the foal lightly restrained, especially for quiet or obtunded foals.
Technique 2: The handler kneels down behind the foal's back and holds the limbs using one hand for the front limbs and, if needed, one for the back limbs (Figure 42.6).	Alternatively, the handler holds the recumbent limbs, front and back, with each hand, while applying gentle pressure on the shoulder and the hip with the handler's elbows. This technique provides more control of the struggling foal.
Technique 3: The Madigan Foal Squeeze Procedure can also be used to place and restrain the foal in lateral recumbency.	Details about Madigan Foal Squeeze Procedure can be found in reference listed under further reading.

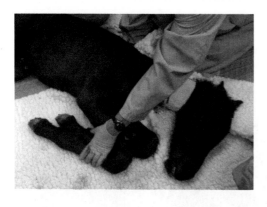

Figure 42.6 An alternative method of restraining a foal in lateral recumbency. The handler kneels behind the foal's back, securing the cannon bone of the down limbs, while using the elbow to apply gentle pressure on the foal's shoulder.

42.7 Procedure: Lifting and Carrying the Neonatal Foal

Technical action	Rationale/amplification
There are multiple techniques for lifting and carrying a foal.	The procedure selected depends on the size of the foal and the strength of the handler.
For a small foal that can be lifted and carried by one handler, wrap one arm around the foal's buttocks under the tuber ischia. The handler's other arm should be wrapped around the foal's chest, just under the manubrium of the sternum (Figure 42.7).	*Note*: Pressure should not be placed on the foal's abdomen directly. This technique is indicated when only one person is available. Care must be taken to lift with one's legs and core muscles to prevent injury to the handler.

Technical action	Rationale/amplification
Lifting and carrying a large foal generally requires two people. The foal can be placed on a stretcher or a blanket and the handlers lift the foal by holding on to the edge of the stretcher or blanket.	This method provides general support of the foal's entire body without putting abnormal pressure on the abdomen or thorax. Handlers should be careful to avoid injuring their own backs.
Another method of lifting a large foal with two handlers is to have one handler positioned at the head and shoulder while the second is positioned by the hips. The foal should be in the sternal position with the legs flexed. Each handler will reach over the foal's either front or hind limbs, and lift the foal up.	Do not lift the foal by the thorax or abdomen. Increased pressure on the thorax may displace fractured ribs if they are present. Lifting by the abdomen may produce enough pressure to rupture a compromised bladder.

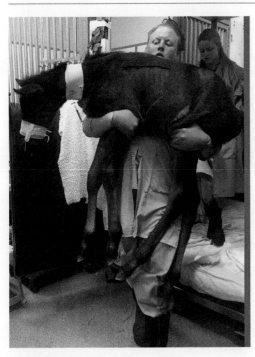

Figure 42.7 Small foals can be lifted and carried by one handler, by wrapping one arm around the foal's buttocks under the tuber ischi and the other arm under the manubrium of the sternum.

Bibliography and Further Reading

Knottenbelt, D., Holdstock, N., and Madigan, J. (2004) *Equine Neonatology Medicine and Surgery*, W.B. Saunders, Edinburgh.

Koterba, A.M., Drummond, W.H., and Kosch, P.C. (1990) *Equine Clinical Neonatology*, Lea and Febiger, Philadelphia.

McAuliffe, S.B. and Slovis, N.M. (2008) *Color Atlas of Disease and Disorders of the Foal*, W.B. Saunders, Edinburgh.

McKinnon, A.O., Squires, E.L., Vaala, W.E. and Varner, D.D. (2011) *Equine Reproduction*, 2nd edn, Wiley-Blackwell, Oxford.

Orsisni, J.A. and Divers, T.J. (2007) *Equine Emergencies: Treatments and Procedures*, 3rd edn, W.B. Saunders, St. Louis.

Sanchez, L.C. (2005) *Veterinary Clinics of North America Equine Practice – Neonatal Medicine and Surgery*, W.B. Saunders, Edinburgh.

Madigan, J.E. (2016) *Manual of Equine Neonatal Medicine*, Live Oak Publishing, Woodland CA.

Toth B, Aleman M, Brosnan RJ, Dickinson PJ, Conley AJ, Stanley SD, Nogradi N, Williams CD, Madigan JE. Evaluation of squeeze-induced somnolence in neonatal foals. *Am J Vet Res. 2012 Dec; 73(12):1881-9.* doi: 10.2460/ajvr.73.12.1881.

www.equineneonatalmanual.com/foalsqueezing

43

Physical Examination of the Neonatal Foal

Nóra Nógrádi and K. Gary Magdesian

43.1 Purpose

- A thorough physical examination is the initial and most important part of assessment of the neonatal foal. The information gained from the examination will allow the veterinarian to formulate a problem list and differential diagnoses. It also allows the appropriate tests to be ordered in pursuit of a definitive diagnosis and therapeutic plan.
- A physical examination is generally performed on the newborn foal after birth (postpartum wellness examination) and for evaluation of the sick neonatal foal.

43.2 Complications

- Injury to the examiner or foal with improper restraint.

43.3 Equipment Required

- Examination gloves
- Watch with a second hand
- Stethoscope
- Thermometer
- Pen light or ophthalmoscope

43.4 Restraint and Positioning

- An active and ambulatory foal can be evaluated in a standing position with application of one of the restraint techniques described in Chapter 42.
- A weak, recumbent neonate should be examined in lateral recumbency.
- Sedatives should not be used to perform a physical examination as they can alter the vital signs and further compromise the critically ill foal's hemodynamic and/or respiratory status.

43.5 Procedure: Physical Examination

Technical action	Rationale
Perform the physical examination in a systematic order.	This way no important detail is missed.
Wash hands and wear examination gloves.	Hand washing and gloves are an important means of infection control by preventing exposure of the foal to infectious agents from other animals or the handler.
If the foal is ambulatory, initially it should be observed from a distance: the body condition, mentation, gait, maternal interaction and nursing behavior can be evaluated.	Healthy foals are interested in the environment and nurse frequently.

Manual of Clinical Procedures in the Horse, First Edition. Edited by Lais R.R. Costa and Mary Rose Paradis.
© 2018 John Wiley & Sons, Inc. Published 2018 by John Wiley & Sons, Inc.

Technical action	Rationale
The respiratory rate and character should be assessed prior to handling.	Handling can falsely alter the respiratory rate and character.
Evaluate the foal for size, body condition, and maturity. The newborn foal should be approximately 10% of its dam's weight (in Thoroughbred horses) (Figure 43.1a).	Signs of prematurity include small size, fine and silky hair coat (or areas with no hair), limb laxity, and domed forehead (Figure 43.1b). A term foal may be small because of placental dysfunction or insufficiency (Figure 43.1c).
Evaluate stance, and check for symmetry, abnormal conformation, and congenital deformations (Figures 43.2 and 43.3).	The presence of angular or flexural limb deformities and spine abnormalities should be noted.
Take vital values (heart rate, respiratory rate and temperature) at the beginning of the examination.	This is done to avoid falsely increasing the values associated with the stress of handling.
Normal body temperature of the neonatal foal (not including the immediate postpartum period) is 99–101.8 °F. Normal heart rate (HR) is 80–110 beats per minute (bpm), and respiratory rate (RR) is 20–40 breaths per minute (brpm).	These parameters will vary with age, breed, level of excitement or activity, and ambient temperature.
It is important to take into account the age (in hours) of the newborn foal, as the range of normal HR and RR varies significantly during the neonatal period.	HR during the first few minutes post foaling should be near 60 bpm, and it should rapidly increase to ≥80 bpm. After that it should stabilize at approximately 80–130 bpm, then 80–110 bpm for the first couple of weeks of life.
	For the first 30 minutes after foaling RR may be as high as 60 brpm, then it should gradually decrease to below 40. The normal respiratory rate is 20–40 brpm at 12–24 hours of age.
	It should be noted that some dysrhythmias (see Chapter 44) may be present for the initial 15 minutes after birth (associated with transient hypoxemia), but these should not interfere with perfusion and should abate spontaneously.
Begin with examination of the head, and then work caudally and distally.	Perform the examination in an orderly manner to ensure completeness.
Evaluate skin for wounds and imperfections/defects (Figure 43.4).	Note the presence of decubital ulcers, edema, and congenital defects such as epitheliogenesis imperfecta or mechanobullous diseases.
Evaluate mucous membranes, both gingival and nasal (Figure 43.5a). They should be pink with a capillary refill time of 1–2 seconds.	Check color, moisture, and for presence of injected vessels or petechiation (Figure 43.5b,c).
Inspect the oral cavity for cleft palate, prognathism, or brachygnathism	
Evaluate the inside of the pinnae for icterus or petechiation.	In the foal with sepsis, petechiation, or even ecchymosis, can be present in this area (Figure 43.6)

(continued)

Technical action	Rationale
Ophthalmic evaluation with pen light (or ophthalmoscope).	
• Check lid position, and for the presence of ocular discharge and foreign bodies.	• Entropion (inward inversion of the eyelids) and ectropion (eyelids turning outward) are common defects seen in the foal.
• Globe position should be evaluated.	• A mild ventro-lateral deviation of the eyes may be seen in foals less than 1 month of age.
• Sclera and conjunctiva should be evaluated (Figure 43.7).	• The presence of scleral injection, hemorrhage, and icterus could be indications of sepsis, shock, neonatal isoerythrolysis or birth trauma.
• Evaluate pupil size and pupillary light reflex. Abnormal mydriasis, miosis, or anisocoria should be noted.	• Newborn foals have a pupillary light reflex but it may be sluggish due to excitement.
• Evaluate the anterior chamber for the presence of: – hypopyon (presence of exudate in the anterior chamber) – hyphema (presence of blood in the anterior chamber).	• Hypopyon is a strong indication of sepsis in the neonatal foal. Hyphema can be seen after a traumatic birth.
• Evaluate the texture and smoothness of cornea. The presence of corneal vessels, ulcers, or opacities should be noted.	• Sick foals may have reduced corneal sensitivity, which can lead to incomplete protection of the cornea.
• Perform a fluorescein stain of the cornea. This is particularly important in the sick foal that is recumbent.	• Check for corneal ulcers, as these may be occult in the lethargic foal.
• Menace response is not present for ≥2 weeks in neonatal foals, despite normal vision.	
Palpate the hard palate with a clean, gloved hand to evaluate for a cleft palate.	Wear disposable gloves to prevent exposure to infectious agents.
	Incomplete clefts in the soft palate may be missed with palpation, and endoscopy or the use of a laryngoscope for detection may be required.
Palpate the submandibular lymph nodes and throat latch area.	Note the presence of cysts or swellings.
	Thyroid glands are more obvious and can be more readily palpated in foals than in adult horses.
Check jugular refill time.	Delayed jugular refill is suggestive of hypovolemia. Prominent jugulars with jugular pulses extending above the caudal third of the neck in a standing foal can be indicative of cardiac disease or hypervolemia.
Gently palpate the ribcage.	Note the presence of pain, crepitus, hematomas, or bony enlargements due to rib fractures.
Evaluation of the umbilicus.	
• Visually inspect and palpate the umbilicus with a clean, gloved hand. • Carefully palpate the umbilical stump to evaluate: – umbilical diameter – presence of heat – presence of discharge – presence of moisture (urine) at the tip of the umbilicus – presence of an umbilical hernia (Figure 43.8).	Wear clean gloves to prevent contamination of the umbilicus. The foal can be habituated to umbilical palpation by slowly rubbing the foal's abdomen and gradually honing in on the umbilical stump.

Technical action	Rationale
Evaluation of the axial musculoskeletal system.	
• Foals are often born with mild laxity of the flexor tendons.	• Mild laxity of flexor tendons in newborn foals usually significantly improves with controlled exercise (large stall) within a few days (Figure 43.9).
• Observe the conformation of the foal, looking for angular or flexural limb deformities (Figure 43.2).	• Limb contracture requires medical intervention more often than laxity does.
• Evaluate the foal for signs of lameness.	• Any lameness in a foal should be assumed to be septic arthritis/synovitis until proven otherwise. This is an emergency situation.
• Palpate all joints and tendon sheaths on the thoracic and pelvic limbs for swelling, edema, or pain.	
Palpate distal limbs and evaluate the surface temperature of extremities.	Cold extremities are suggestive of hypoperfusion in the periphery. An ice-cold extremity, particularly if asymmetrical and different than the other limbs, may be suggestive of digital or other vessel thrombosis.
Palpate the arterial pulse quality by gently pressing on the metatarsal artery one-third to halfway down the hind cannon bone on the lateral side.	Peripheral pulse quality is an indicator of peripheral perfusion. Foals with significant hypoperfusion may not have a palpable metatarsal or facial pulse.
Evaluation of the respiratory system.	
• Evaluate breathing character and chest movements.	• Determine if the foal has increased or reduced respiratory effort. Shallow chest excursions or an inconsistent breathing pattern may result in alveolar hypoventilation.
• Check nostrils for the presence of milk regurgitation, particularly after nursing, as an indicator of dysphagia (Figure 43.10).	• Milk noted at the nostrils after nursing can be due to milk streaming from the mare and incidentally spraying the foal ("milk face"). "Milk face" can indicate that the foal is not nursing well. However, milk present in the nares may also be secondary to dysphagia, which could result in aspiration pneumonia. Congenital defects should also be considered.
• Check nasal airflow bilaterally and evaluate for nostril flaring.	• Nostril flaring is a sign of respiratory distress.
• Auscult the trachea with a stethoscope. A tracheal rattle could represent milk or mucus within the trachea.	• Dysphagia results in a tracheal rattle as the foal aspirates milk. This is best ausculted during or immediately after nursing.
• Auscult the lungs bilaterally by dividing up the lung fields into quadrants on each side (cranioventral, craniodorsal, caudoventral, and caudodorsal). Each of these regions should be ausculted during at least three to four breaths in each quadrant.	• Slightly increased bronchovesicular sounds ("harsh") may be normal in neonatal foals. Adventitious sounds such as crackles or wheezes or quiet areas where air movement is absent are abnormal.

(continued)

Technical action	Rationale
Evaluation of the heart. Auscult (with a stethoscope) from the 3rd through 5th intercostal spaces, bilaterally.	
• Evaluate HR, heart sounds, and for presence of murmurs.	• HR in the foal can be variable with different levels of excitement, but in general ranges from 80 to 110 bpm after the immediate postpartum period in most light breed horses.
• Murmurs should be characterized by: – intensity: grade 1–6 – left or right side – location (e.g., base, apex, pulmonic region, aortic region, mitral region, tricuspid region) – timing or phase of cardiac cycle (systolic, diastolic) – duration (e.g., holosystolic) – quality (e.g., blowing, harsh, rumbling, musical) – shape (e.g., crescendo, decrescendo).	• If murmurs are identified, carefully characterize them. See Table 43.1 for causes and significance of heart murmurs ausculted during the neonatal period.
Evaluation of the gastrointestinal system.	
• Observe the foal for passage of feces. – Excessive straining in a foal during the first day of life may indicate a meconium impaction (Figure 43.11). – Evaluate tail and hind legs for the presence of fecal staining.	• It may be difficult for owners to determine if a foal is straining to defecate or urinate. A foal straining to defecate will dorsally flex its spine. • Foals with diarrhea or meconium staining will have evidence of wetness or pasty to loose feces under the tail and down the hind legs.
• Evaluate the shape and size of the abdomen. Palpate the abdomen for distention. If distention is present, attempt to determine if it is caused by fluid or gas by ultrasound or radiology. – Distention can also be evaluated over time by periodic measurement of the abdominal diameter at the same spot. The same spot can be marked on the coat with a clipper or tape.	• Distention of the abdomen due to gas accumulation is usually secondary to meconium impaction, other form of obstruction, or enteritis. Fluid distension may be secondary to uroperitoneum (e.g., ruptured bladder) or other effusion (chylous, peritonitis, etc.).
• Auscult the abdomen by dividing it into four quadrants (left and right, ventral and dorsal).	• Overtly gassy or "fluidy" sounds, as well as absent borborygmi, are abnormal.
• Palpate the inguinal area, checking for inguinal or scrotal (in colts) hernias (Figure 43.12).	
Evaluation of the urogenital system.	
• Observe urination. – If possible obtain a urine sample for measurement of specific gravity and urine dipstick analysis. – Make sure the foal is not posturing without successful urine elimination or straining to urinate.	• Healthy foals normally begin urinating at an average of 6 hours (colts) and 10 hours (fillies) of age. • It is normal for male foals to either exteriorize their penis during urination or to urinate within the sheath (due to persistent frenulum, which usually breaks down spontaneously within a few days).
• Observe if there is any leakage of urine from the umbilicus during urination.	• Foals may develop a patent urachus.
• Evaluate external urogenital anatomy.	
• Evaluate perineum for edema.	• Perianal edema can be suggestive of straining or ureteral rupture.

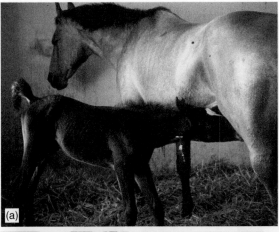

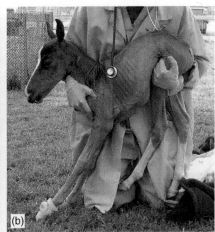

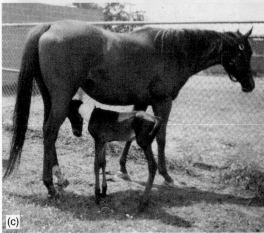

Figure 43.1 Evaluate the foal for size, body condition, and maturity. (a) Normal newborn foal with normal body condition, size approximately 10% of its dam's weight, and no features of prematurity. Courtesy of Dr. Lais R.R. Costa. (b) Newborn foal showing signs of prematurity, including small size/low weight, fine and silky hair coat, and domed forehead. (c) Small-size term foal because of placental dysfunction. Courtesy of Dr. Lais R.R. Costa.

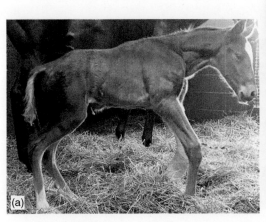

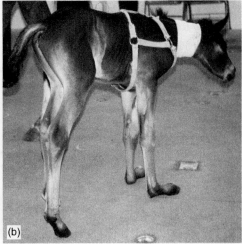

Figure 43.2 Evaluate the foal's stance, and check for deviations of symmetry and abnormal conformational of the limbs. (a) Neonatal foal with bilateral contracted flexor tendons. (b) Neonatal foal with excessive laxity of the flexor tendons on the front limbs bilaterally. Courtesy of Dr. Lais R.R. Costa. (c) Neonatal foal with angular limb deformities called "wind swept". Courtesy of Dr. Lais R.R. Costa. (d) Newborn foal with angular limb deformities called "carpus valgus".

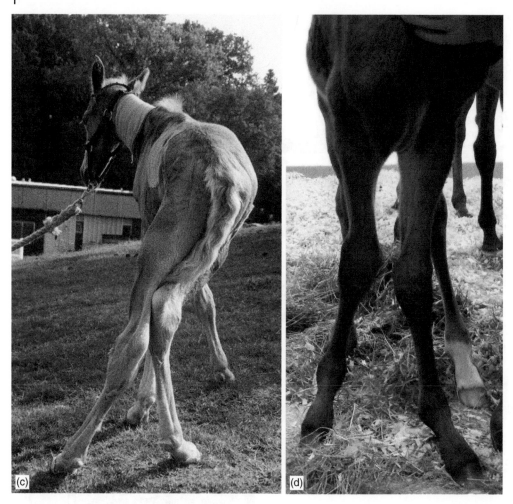

Figure 43.2 (*continued*)

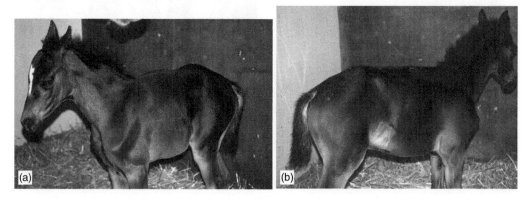

Figure 43.3 Evaluate for the presence of spine deformations. Foal with scoliosis. Courtesy of Dr. Lais R.R. Costa.

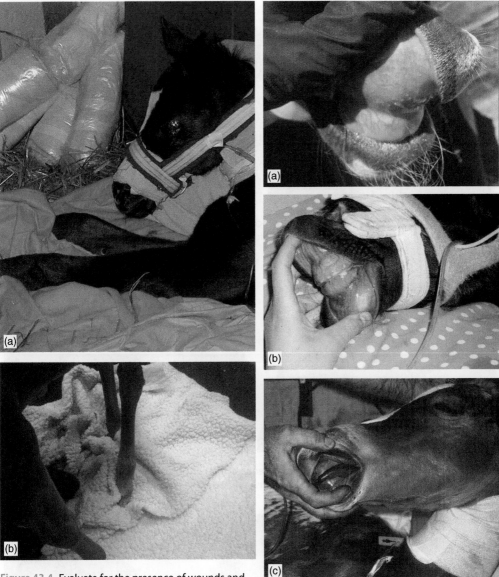

Figure 43.4 Evaluate for the presence of wounds and other abnormalities. (a) Newborn foal with decubital ulcers Courtesy of Dr. Lais R.R. Costa. (b) Foal with edema of the hind left limb extending from the hock to the pastern.

Figure 43.5 Evaluate mucous membranes. Note the color, moisture, capillary refill time. (a) Normal appearance of the mucous membranes of a neonate. (b) Dark pink and injected mucous membrane in a septic neonate. Courtesy of Dr. Lais R.R. Costa. (c) Dark purple (cyanotic) mucous membrane in a neonate with severe hypoxemia. Courtesy of Dr. Lais R.R. Costa.

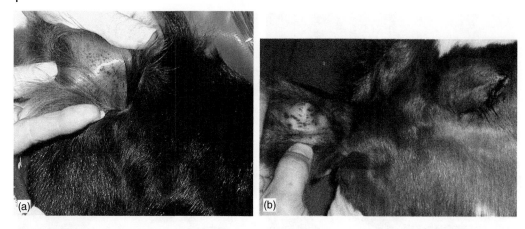

Figure 43.6 Evaluate the inside of the pinnae for petechiation. Note the (a) petechial and (b) ecchymotic hemorrhage inside the pinnae of two septic neonatal foals. Courtesy of Dr. Lais R.R. Costa.

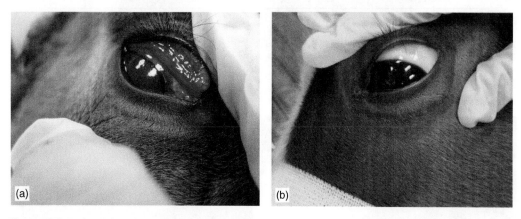

Figure 43.7 Evaluate the sclera and conjunctiva. (a) Neonatal foal with injected sclera and edematous conjunctiva may be early indicators of sepsis. (b) Icterus of the sclera in a foal with neonatal isoerythrolysis.

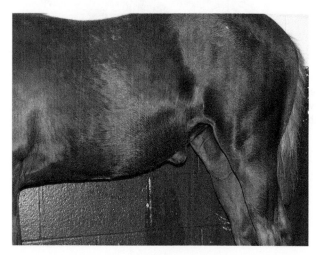

Figure 43.8 Swellings in the umbilical area need to be evaluated to determine if they are due to umbilical herniation or umbilical infection.

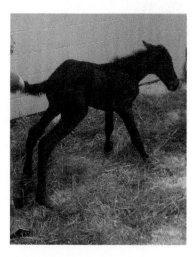

Figure 43.9 Note the mild laxity of flexor tendons in a newborn foal. Courtesy of Dr. Lais R.R. Costa.

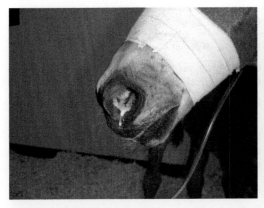

Figure 43.10 The presence of milk on the nostrils of a neonatal foal after nursing. Courtesy of Dr. Mary Rose Paradis.

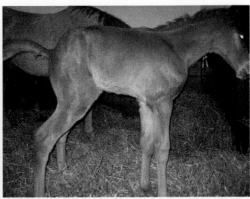

Figure 43.11 Unproductive straining in a neonatal foal with meconium impaction.

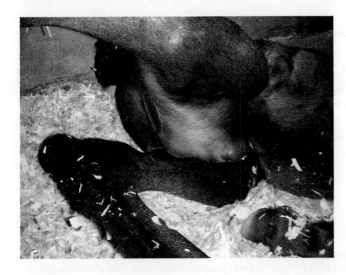

Figure 43.12 A swelling located behind the sheath of male foals should be palpated to determine the presence of an inguinal hernia, as see in this foal.

Table 43.1 Identification of heart murmurs during the neonatal period

Heart murmur	Causes and significance
Soft, systolic, left-sided murmurs of grade 1-3/6 (low-grade murmurs) are common in neonatal foals	Many of these are physiological or functional flow murmurs and occur on the left side in the aortic to mitral valve region
	Some murmurs are associated with increased sympathetic tone and are present only during stress, such as that associated with catching for restraint
	Incomplete closure of the ductus arteriosus (see below)
	Anemia
	Congenital cardiac defects (see below)

(continued)

Heart murmur	Causes and significance
Continuous machinery murmurs, left side, over the pulmonic valve region or holosystolic murmurs, sometimes combined with early diastolic murmurs	Indicative of patent ductus arteriosus (PDA) Closure of ductus arteriosus is part of the transition from fetal circulation PDA may persist for a few days after birth (usually 4–5 days) Incomplete closure, though functionally closed, is thought to result in low-grade systolic murmurs due to small leaks that gradually resolve over time
Systolic murmur, best ausculted on the right side over the apex area, often concurrent with a quieter systolic murmur on the left side over the pulmonic valve area	Indicative of ventricular septal defect (VSD) Further investigation with echocardiography is recommended VSDs are congenital heart abnormalities associated with left to right shunt, unless they are associated with complex defects or pulmonary hypertension
Systolic murmurs that are grade ≥ 4 (have a palpable thrill) Loud murmurs located on the right side Murmurs associated with persistent tachycardia or tachypnea, cyanotic mucous membranes, hypoxemia, or exercise intolerance Loud murmurs that do not decrease in intensity over time Diastolic murmurs	Murmurs that warrant further investigation with echocardiography for potential cardiac defects or pathology

Bibliography and Further Reading

Acworth, N.R.J. (2004) The healthy neonatal foal: routine examination and preventative medicine. *Equine Veterinary Education*, **15**, 207–211.

Koterba, A.M., Drummond, W.H., and Kosch, P.C. (1990) *Equine Clinical Neonatology*, Lea and Febiger, Philadelphia.

McAuliffe, S.B. and Slovis, N.M. (2008) *Color Atlas of Disease and Disorders of the Foal*, W.B. Saunders, Philadelphia.

McKinnon, A.O., Squires, E.L., Vaala, W.E., and Varner, D.D. (2011) *Equine Reproduction*, 2nd edn, Wiley-Blackwell, Oxford.

Madigan, J.E. (2016) *Manual of Equine Neonatal Medicine*, Live Oak Publishing, Woodland CA

Orsini, J.A. and Divers T.J. (2007) *Equine Emergencies: Treatments and Procedures*, 3rd edn, W.B. Saunders, Philadelphia.

Sanchez, L.C. (2005) *Veterinary Clinics of North America Equine Practice – Neonatal Medicine and Surgery*, W.B. Saunders, Philadelphia.

Stoneham, S. (2006) Assessing the newborn foal, in *Equine Neonatal Medicine: a Case-based Approach* (ed. M.R. Paradis), Elsevier, Philadelphia, pp. 1-11.

44

Electrocardiography in the Neonatal Foal

Nóra Nógrádi and K. Gary Magdesian

44.1 Purpose

- To diagnose cardiac rhythm disturbances.
- For continuous heart rate monitoring in critically ill foals.
- For monitoring heart rate during cardio-pulmonary resuscitation.

44.2 Complications

- Insufficient contact with skin or movement/tremors can result in non-diagnostic recordings.

44.3 Equipment Required

- ECG monitor with leads
- ECG clip or adhesive electrodes
- Rubbing alcohol solution or ECG conductive gel
- Clippers

44.4 Restraint and Positioning

- Recordings can be obtained with the foal standing or in lateral recumbency as long as movement is minimized. See Chapter 42 for methods for restraining foals.

44.5 Procedure: Base-apex Lead for ECG in Neonates

Technical action	Rationale
Three electrodes are used for the application of a base-apex lead, which is the lead system used most commonly in foals. • The left arm electrode (positive lead) should be placed on the left side at the apex of the heart (6th intercostal space), just caudal to and level with the point of the elbow (olecranon). • The right arm electrode (negative lead) should be placed at the top of the right scapular spine, or two-thirds of the way down the right jugular groove. • The left leg or ground electrode can be placed anywhere on the body, often near the left shoulder where abundant loose skin is available. Alternatively, the right neck or left stifle areas can be used (Figure 44.1).	• Left arm electrode (positive lead): commonly colored black (as per the American Heart Association). • Right arm electrode (negative lead): commonly colored white. • Left leg or ground electrode: commonly colored red.

(continued)

Manual of Clinical Procedures in the Horse, First Edition. Edited by Lais R.R. Costa and Mary Rose Paradis.
© 2018 John Wiley & Sons, Inc. Published 2018 by John Wiley & Sons, Inc.

Technical action	Rationale
The ECG machine should be set to lead I for recording a base-apex lead system. A paper speed of 25 mm/second is typically used.	This will make the left arm electrode positive and the right arm negative. The "base" electrode (top of right heart) is negative and the "apex" electrode (apex of left heart) is positive.
Clip hair at the sites of electrode placement.	Clipping the hair improves adequate electrical contact.
Apply alcohol or conducting gel over the clipped skin and electrodes.	Alcohol or conducting gel ensures adequate electrical contact.
Obtain an ECG reading and print a representative sample of the tracing.	Continuous ECG may be indicated in foals with dysrhythmias or cardiovascular disease, using a telemetry unit or Holter monitor.
During the first 15 minutes postpartum transient cardiac arrhythmias are common in foals. These include atrial fibrillation and ventricular and atrial premature contractions. These disappear without treatment.	

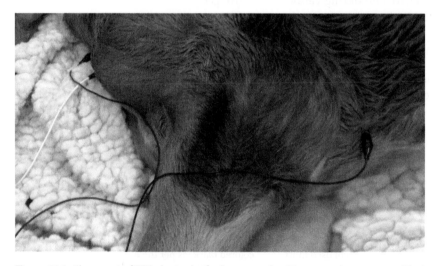

Figure 44.1 Placement of ECG electrodes for base-apex lead in a recumbent neonatal foal.

Bibliography and Further Reading

Koterba, A.M., Drummond, W.H., and Kosch, P.C. (1990) *Equine Clinical Neonatology*, Lea and Febiger, Philadelphia.

Madigan, J.E. (2016) *Manual of Equine Neonatal Medicine*, Live Oak Publishing, Woodland CA

McAuliffe, S.B. and Slovis, N.M. (2008) *Color Atlas of Disease and Disorders of the Foal*, W.B. Saunders, Philadelphia.

McKinnon, A.O., Squires, E.L., Vaala, W.E., and Varner, D.D. (2011) *Equine Reproduction*, 2nd edn, Wiley-Blackwell, Oxford.

Orsisni, J.A. and Divers, T.J. (2007) *Equine Emergencies: Treatments and Procedures*, 3rd edn, W.B. Saunders, Philadelphia.

Rossdale, P. (1967) Clinical studies on the newborn thoroughbred foal. II Heart rate, auscultation and electrocardiogram. *British Veterinary Journal*, **123**, 521–532.

Sanchez, L.C. (2005) *Veterinary Clinics of North America Equine Practice – Neonatal Medicine and Surgery*, W.B. Saunders, Philadelphia.

45

Arterial Blood Pressure Measurement in the Neonatal Foal

Nóra Nógrádi and K. Gary Magdesian

45.1 Purpose

- To indirectly evaluate the potential for end organ perfusion in compromised foals.
- To assess ongoing cardiovascular derangements that can lead to hypoperfusion and secondary organ failure, especially in foals with septic shock.
- To formulate a treatment plan for fluid, inotrope, and vasopressor therapy.
- To evaluate the response to these therapies in intensive care patients.
- To measure arterial blood pressure by direct or indirect methods:
  - indirect blood pressure measurements are practical, relatively accurate in most circumstances, and an easy means of monitoring arterial pressures in foals
  - direct blood pressure measurement requires the maintenance of a catheter in a peripheral artery, such as the great metatarsal, transverse facial, radial, or caudal auricular artery. This is usually reserved for critically ill foals that are recumbent, experiencing shock, or hospitalized in an intensive care unit.

45.2 Complications

- *Indirect blood pressure measurement:* Accuracy is reduced in markedly hypotensive foals. Measurements are inaccurate if the tail cuff size is too large or too small.
- *Direct blood pressure measurement:* Arteritis, cellulitis at insertion site, hematoma,

embolus formation within the intra-arterial catheter, kinking of catheter.

45.3 Equipment Required

Indirect blood pressure measurement
- Automated oscillometric blood pressure monitor
- Size #3–5 neonatal cuff.
  - Internal bladder width of 20–25% of tail circumference
  - Internal bladder length of 80% of tail circumference
  - A tail cuff with a bladder width of 52 mm has been found to be accurate for mean and diastolic, but not necessarily systolic, pressures in foals weighing 44–69 kg

Direct blood pressure measurement
- Clippers
- Sterile preparation material
- 2% lidocaine injectable solution
- #11 or #15 scalpel blade
- Sterile gloves
- 20–22 gauge 1.5″ IV catheter
- Surgical skin glue
- Suture and bandage material
- Heparinized saline (free of benzyl alcohol)
- Direct blood pressure monitor

45.4 Restraint and Positioning

Indirect blood pressure measurement
- Ambulatory foals can be examined standing with minimal restraint. In standing

Manual of Clinical Procedures in the Horse, First Edition. Edited by Lais R.R. Costa and Mary Rose Paradis.
© 2018 John Wiley & Sons, Inc. Published 2018 by John Wiley & Sons, Inc.

foals the head should be in a resting neutral position and at the same level for every measurement.

- Recumbent foals can be examined in sternal or lateral recumbency.
- For consistency of readings the foal should be in the same position for every measurement.

Direct blood pressure measurement

- Placement of an intra-arterial catheter can be performed with the foal in lateral recumbency.

- Most foals that require continuous direct blood pressure monitoring are weak and quiet, therefore sedation is usually not required in most cases.
- One assistant can stabilize the head and thoracic limbs of the neonate, while another can stabilize the pelvic limb by placing one hand over the calcaneal tuber and holding the fetlock with the other hand.

45.5 Procedure: Indirect Blood Pressure Measurement

Technical action	Rationale
Measurement over the coccygeal artery provides the most accurate and consistent readings.	The dorsal metatarsal arteries can also be used.
Clean the tail and the perineal region of the foal.	This ensures good contact for accurate reading.
Place the cuff around the tail head. Make sure to correctly position the occlusion cuff over the coccygeal artery (Figure 45.1).	Ensure the correct cuff size is used for accurate readings.
Turn on the blood pressure monitor and determine systolic, diastolic, and mean blood pressure values (Figure 45.2). A general goal is to maintain mean pressures above 60–65 mmHg in the compromised neonate in the context of perfusion parameters, with normal mean blood pressure ranging between 65 and 110 mmHg in healthy foals.	Arterial pressures must be interpreted in the context of clinical, laboratory, and other monitoring indicators of perfusion status. It is difficult to provide a specific blood pressure target for all foals because "normal" blood pressure varies considerably with gestational age, breed, and size. Some foals appear to have adequate perfusion with mean arterial blood pressures <60 mmHg.
Repeat measurements sequentially three times, then calculate the average. The accuracy of readings can be trusted if the displayed heart rate is correct and the three sequential readings are close in magnitude.	Coupling the blood pressure readings with clinical data, such as urine output and plasma lactate, is critical. Serial blood pressure measurements are more useful than a onetime measurement.

45.6 Procedure: Direct Blood Pressure Measurement

Technical action	Rationale
Clip a 3″ × 3″ area on the lateral side of the third metatarsal bone, directly over the metatarsal artery.	Alternative sites include the facial, transverse facial or caudal auricular arteries. Catheterization of these arteries may be more challenging.
Following sterile preparation of the site, inject 0.25–0.5 ml 2% lidocaine under the skin just proximal to the catheterization site.	The local block aids placement by reducing movement. A large bleb placed at the immediate site of placement can obscure the artery.

Technical action	Rationale
The skin should be tented and incised with a stab incision to make an insertion hole.	A small stab incision will prevent skin dragging on the catheter during placements.
Insert the catheter using sterile technique.	This technique is similar to insertion of intravenous catheterization (see Chapter 53).
Anchor the catheter to the skin with tape in a "butterfly" pattern, with surgical glue anchoring each tab to the skin. Alternatively, sutures can also be placed and the site should be bandaged, leaving the hub with the injection port exposed.	Because of the location, the catheter can dislodge easily if it is not anchored properly.
Connect the catheter to a pressure transducer to acquire direct blood pressure measurements.	The electronic pressure transducer should be positioned and zeroed at the level of the sternal manubrium.
Maintenance of the arterial catheter requires frequent (every 2–3 hours) flushing with heparinized saline solution.	Frequent flushing with heparinized saline will prevent clot formation. Use heparinized saline free of preservatives for foals.

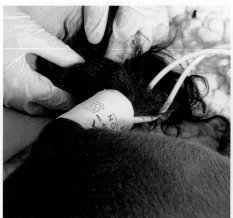

Figure 45.1 Placement of a cuff on the tail of a neonatal foal for measurement of indirect blood pressure.

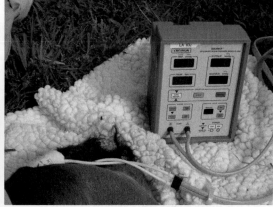

Figure 45.2 Indirect blood pressure monitor.

Bibliography and Further Reading

Koterba, A.M., Drummond, W.H., and Kosch, P.C. (1990) *Equine Clinical Neonatology*, Lea and Febiger, Philadelphia.

Madigan, J.E. (2016) *Manual of Equine Neonatal Medicine*, Live Oak Publishing, Woodland CA

McAuliffe, S.B. and Slovis, N.M. (2008) *Color Atlas of Disease and Disorders of the Foal*, W.B. Saunders, Philadelphia.

McKinnon, A.O., Squires, E.L., Vaala, W.E., and Varner, D.D. (2011) *Equine Reproduction*, 2nd edn, Wiley-Blackwell, Oxford.

Orsini, J.A. and Divers T.J. (2007) *Equine Emergencies: Treatments and Procedures*, 3rd edn, W.B. Saunders, Philadelphia.

Palmer, J. (2006) Recognition and resuscitation of the critically ill foal, in *Equine Neonatal Medicine: a Case-based Approach* (ed. M.R.Paradis), Elsevier, Philadelphia, pp. 121–134.

Sanchez, L.C. (2005) *Veterinary Clinics of North America Equine Practice – Neonatal Medicine and Surgery*, W.B. Saunders, Philadelphia.

46

Measurement of Central Venous Pressure in the Neonatal Foal

Nóra Nógrádi and K. Gary Magdesian

46.1 Purpose

- To determine the pressure in the vena cava (usually measured in the cranial vena cava), which reflects the amount of blood returning to the heart (venous return), cardiac function (the heart's ability to effectively pump blood forward), and venous tone. Central venous pressure (CVP) can also be affected by pleural pressures and pulmonary hypertension.
- CVP is an estimate of preload and right ventricular filling pressure, and indirectly relates to blood volume.
- The trends in CVP can be utilized to guide fluid replacement in cases of altered blood volume. CVP trends and serial changes are more informative than single measurements.
- CVP is more an accurate ceiling or limit to fluid therapy than a marker of adequacy.
- CVP measurements have value in the medical assessment and management of neonatal foals, but over-interpretation of single CVP measurements should be avoided:
  - Normal CVP in foals is 2.1–8.9 mmHg (2.9–12.1 cm H_2O).
  - A subnormal CVP can be indicative of hypovolemia, although it is not specific. Venodilation may also cause a reduction in CVP.
  - An increased CVP may be due to hypervolemia, cardiac dysfunction, venoconstriction, increased pleural pressures, cardiac tamponade, or pulmonary hypertension.

- CVP monitoring during fluid resuscitation can provide guidance to fluid bolus administration. If maximum normal CVP is reached, then bolus administration should be discontinued.

46.2 Complications

- No major complications are expected other than those associated with IV catheterization.
- Inaccuracies in measurement of CVP due to body and head position will make results unreliable.

46.3 Equipment Required

- Central venous catheter placed in the jugular vein:
  - 20 cm length for most standard size foals
  - 30 cm length for large or older foals
- Sterile bag of isotonic fluids (250 ml)
- Fluid administration set.
- IV extension set
- Three-way stopcock
- Manometer (intermittent measurement) or electronic pressure transducer (continuous monitoring). If using an electronic pressure transducer, an electrocardiogram is important (see Chapter 44).

46.4 Restraint and Positioning

- Measurements can be taken with the foal standing or in sternal recumbency but should be consistent among measurements.

Manual of Clinical Procedures in the Horse, First Edition. Edited by Lais R.R. Costa and Mary Rose Paradis.
© 2018 John Wiley & Sons, Inc. Published 2018 by John Wiley & Sons, Inc.

46.5 Procedure: Preparation CVP Measurement

Technical action	Rationale
Choose the appropriate length of IV catheter by measuring the distance from the anticipated catheter insertion site to the approximate location of the cranial vena cava (just cranial to elbow).	The length of the catheter depends on the size of the foal. For term neonates of standard size breeds, the length of the catheter should be approximately 20 cm, and for larger size foals the length of the catheter should be approximately 30 cm. The entirety of the length of the 30 cm catheter does not need to be utilized. Shorter lengths can be used, with butterfly stabilizers used to suture the catheter in place at the desired length.
Place an over-the-wire polyurethane catheter of appropriate length in the jugular vein.	See Chapter 53 for intravenous catheter placement. The same catheter that is used for IV fluid administration can be used for CVP measurement. If a multi-lumen catheter is used, the distal-most port should be used for CVP monitoring. Fluid administration should temporarily cease during CVP measurement.
Ideally, verify the position of the catheter by imaging the thoracic inlet.	If possible, check the location of the catheter tip by taking radiographs of the thoracic inlet as most are radiopaque (Figure 46.1).

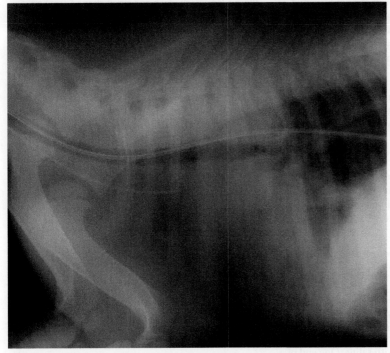

Figure 46.1 Thoracic radiograph taken in a foal to confirm the presence of the central venous catheter tip in the cranial vena cava. Note the feeding tube placed in the esophagus.

46.6 Procedure: CVP Measurement with Water Manometer

Technical action	Rationale
Use the central venous catheter of appropriate length in the jugular vein.	This catheter can be the same catheter that is used for IV fluid administration. CVP can be intermittently measured with a water manometer.

(continued)

Technical action	Rationale
Attach the fluid administration set to the sterile fluid bag. The end of the administration set should then be connected a three-way stopcock.	Be careful to maintain aseptic technique when handling the connection that will be in contact with the IV catheter line.
Attach the manometer to the top port on the three-way stopcock (Figure 46.2).	The knob on the manometer indicates the direction towards the port that is closed.
An extension set or two should be placed on the third port of the stop cock. The entirety of the system should be flushed with saline so that no air bubbles enter the foal. This extension set should be connected to the foal's IV catheter with the stopcock in the closed position towards the manometer. Confirm free fluid flow through the catheter from the fluid bag.	There must be a continuous line of fluid from the pressure transducer or manometer through to the vena cava.
Close the stopcock towards the IV catheter and allow the manometer to partially fill with fluid from the bag.	
Make sure no air bubbles are present in the manometer.	If bubbles are present, allow the fluid to overflow to eliminate the bubbles.
Close the manometer towards the fluid bag and place the bottom of the manometer at the level of the right atrium of the heart. The sternal manubrium can be used as a landmark for the 0 mark (this approximates the level of the cranial vena cava) (Figure 46.3).	Place a landmark (such as a small clipped area) on the foal's chest at the level of the right atrium or sternal manubrium. This allows for measurements to be made at the same level for continuous or intermittent serial monitoring.
The fluid column in the manometer oscillates with the respiratory cycle, rising with expiration and dropping during inspiration. The water pressure reading on the manometer corresponding to end-expiration represents the patient's CVP.	
Reaching a maximum normal CVP (12 cm H_2O) in foals during fluid resuscitation warrants discontinuation of bolus administration, otherwise the risk of edema is high if CVP continues to rise.	CVP is useful as a limit to fluid therapy by providing a "ceiling" to rapid bolus administration along with clinical parameters.

46.7 Procedure: CVP Measured with an Electronic Blood Pressure Transducer

Technical action	Rationale
Place an over-the-wire polyurethane catheter of appropriate length in the jugular vein.	Electronic blood pressure monitors allow for continuous monitoring of CVP in intensive care patients.
An extension set is filled with saline. One end of the extension set is attached to the port on the catheter, while the other end is attached to the pressure transducer.	
The transducer should be positioned and zeroed at the level of the sternal manubrium (right atrium).	It is important to measure CVP with the transducer at the same level during the entire course of measurement.

Technical action	Rationale
On an electronic monitor, simultaneous ECG recording will allow for accurate interpretation of CVP.	The CVP should be measured as the mean of the a-wave at the end of expiration (i.e., just prior to the marked decrease in pressure).

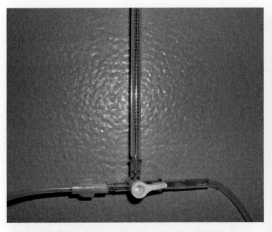

Figure 46.2 Attachment of the water manometer to the fluid set via a three-way stopcock.

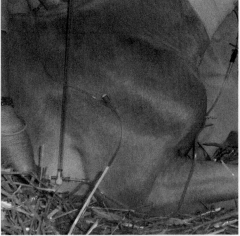

Figure 46.3 Placement of a water manometer at the level of the heart in a recumbent foal.

Bibliography and Further Reading

Koterba, A.M., Drummond, W.H., and Kosch, P.C. (1990) *Equine Clinical Neonatology*, Lea and Febiger, Philadelphia.

Madigan, J.E. (2016) *Manual of Equine Neonatal Medicine*, Live Oak Publishing, Woodland CA

McAuliffe, S.B. and Slovis, N.M. (2008) *Color Atlas of Disease and Disorders of the Foal*, W.B. Saunders, Philadelphia.

McKinnon, A.O., Squires, E.L., Vaala, W.E., and Varner, D.D. (2011) *Equine Reproduction*, 2nd edn, Wiley-Blackwell, Oxford.

Orsini, J.A. and Divers, T.J. (2007) *Equine Emergencies: Treatments and Procedures*, 3rd edn, W.B. Saunders, Philadelphia.

Sanchez, L.C. (2005) *Veterinary Clinics of North America Equine Practice – Neonatal Medicine and Surgery*, W.B. Saunders, Philadelphia.

Wilkins, P. (2009) Central venous pressure monitoring in adults and foals: meaning and confouders. *Large animal proceedings of the International veterinary Emergency and Critical Care Society*, Chicago, IL, January 9-13, p. 293

Wilkins, P. (2009) How to measure central venous pressure. *Large animal proceedings of the North American Veterinary Conference*, Orlando, Florida, January 17-21, North American Veterinary Conference, Orlando, P. 293.

47

Pulse Oximetry in the Neonatal Foal

Nóra Nógrádi and K. Gary Magdesian

47.1 Purpose

- To obtain rapid, continuous, and non-invasive determination of oxygen saturation of arterial blood (SpO_2).
- To assess the need for supplemental oxygen therapy.

47.2 Complications

- Hypovolemia, hypoperfusion, movement or dark skin can result in non-diagnostic recordings.

47.3 Equipment Required

- Pulse oximeter with clamp type attachment. Human finger transducers do not conform to foal anatomy.

47.4 Restraint and Positioning

- Recordings can be obtained with the foal standing or in lateral recumbency.
- No specific restraint is necessary other than keeping the foal still, as movement interferes with readings.
- See Chapter 42 for foal restraint.

47.5 Procedure: Determination of Oxygen Saturation

Technical action	Rationale
The sites commonly used in neonatal foals to obtain pulse oxymetric measurements include the lips, ears, tongue, prepuce, umbilicus, and vulva. The ears, tongue, and lips have been demonstrated to be accurate as compared to co-oximetry. A reflectance probe can also be used at the base of the tail or on the tongue with good agreement with arterial oxygen saturation (SaO_2) obtained by arterial blood gas analysis.	Pulse oximetry detects oxygenation by absorption characteristics of red and infrared lights through a reasonably translucent body site with adequate blood flow. It allows rapid, real-time determination of SpO_2, but its accuracy may lag behind values measured by arterial blood gas analysis depending on location.
Clean the area before application of the transducer.	This ensures adequate contact.
Apply the transducer at the chosen site as depicted: • probe applied to the lip (Figure 47.1) • probe applied to the prepuce (Figure 47.2). Check if able to obtain pulse oxymetric measurements. Re-adjust the positioning of the probe if necessary.	Dark pigment and movement interfere with measurements.

Manual of Clinical Procedures in the Horse, First Edition. Edited by Lais R.R. Costa and Mary Rose Paradis.
© 2018 John Wiley & Sons, Inc. Published 2018 by John Wiley & Sons, Inc.

Technical action	Rationale
Obtain serial measurements to evaluate for consistent results.	The recorded pulse rate should be compared to the foal's actual heart or pulse rate, as another indicator of accuracy.
Measurements should be ≥94% while breathing room air by 24 hours of age (even in lateral recumbency), while lower values indicate a need for oxygen therapy.	It should be noted that the SaO_2 varies with foal positioning, being lower in laterally recumbent foals compared to those in sternal recumbency.

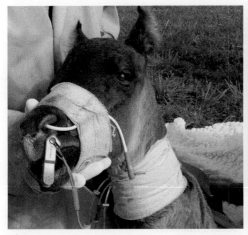

Figure 47.1 Placement of pulse oximetry probe on upper lip.

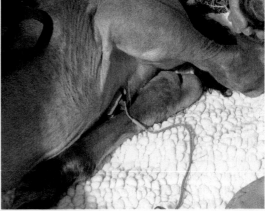

Figure 47.2 Placement of pulse oximetry probe on the prepuce in a colt.

Bibliography and Further Reading

Koterba, A.M., Drummond, W.H., and Kosch, P.C. (1990) *Equine Clinical Neonatology*, Lea and Febiger, Philadelphia.

Madigan, J.E. (2016) *Manual of Equine Neonatal Medicine*, Live Oak Publishing, Woodland CA

McAuliffe, S.B. and Slovis, N.M. (2008) *Color Atlas of Disease and Disorders of the Foal*, W.B. Saunders, Philadelphia.

McKinnon, A.O., Squires, E.L., Vaala, W.E., and Varner, D.D. (2011) *Equine Reproduction*, 2nd edn, Wiley-Blackwell, Oxford.

Orsini, J.A. and Divers, T.J. (2007) *Equine Emergencies: Treatments and Procedures*, 3rd edn, W.B. Saunders, Philadelphia.

Sanchez, L.C. (2005) *Veterinary Clinics of North America Equine Practice – Neonatal Medicine and Surgery*, W.B. Saunders, Philadelphia.

Wong, D.M., Alcott, C.J., and Wang, C. (2011) Agreement between arterial partial pressure of carbon dioxide and saturation of hemoglobin with oxygen values obtained by direct arterial blood measurements versus noninvasive methods in conscious healthy and ill foals. *Journal of the American Veterinary Medical Association*, **239** (10), 1341–1347.

48

Cardiopulmonary Cerebral Resuscitation of the Neonatal Foal

Nóra Nógrádi and K. Gary Magdesian

48.1 Purpose

- Cardiopulmonary cerebral resuscitation (CPCR) is an emergency procedure performed in cases of cardiac and/or respiratory arrest
- It is performed in an effort to restore the flow of oxygenated blood to the brain, heart, and vital organs.
- Other goals include return of spontaneous circulation and respiration, minimization of delayed tissue injury, and prevention of death during cardiopulmonary arrest.
- Foals at risk of cardiopulmonary arrest include newborn foals born as a result of dystocia or caesarean section, foals with evidence of hypoxic brain injury, and foals with septic shock or severe metabolic or electrolyte derangements.

48.2 Complications

- Placement of the nasotracheal tube into the esophagus and iatrogenic gastric tympani.
- Lack of effective ventilation or chest compressions.

48.3 Equipment Required

A basic crash kit should be readily available in the hospital or the ambulatory vehicle. It should contain the following:

- nasotracheal or endotracheal tubes: sizes 7–10 mm internal diameter, 55 cm length

for foals of average to large breeds, and a variety (3–6 mm) for foals of miniature or pony breeds
- self-inflating resuscitation bag (1000–1500 ml volume)
- syringes (3, 5, 12 ml) to inflate the cuff of the nasotracheal tube and administer medications
- needles (20 gauge, 1″)
- razor or electronic clippers
- 14-gauge intravenous catheter
- suture material
- fluid administration set
- crystalloid fluids: 1 liter bags of polyionic fluids (lactated Ringer's solution, Normosol R or Plasmalyte A or 148)
- dry towels
- medications (Table 48.1)
- foal resuscitator (for on-the-farm use by clients)
- tubing attached to a syringe to suction fluids from nasal passage and trachea
- end-tidal CO_2 monitor or disposable CO_2 sensor
- oxygen cylinder with flow meter and humidifier
- electrical defibrillator.

Manual of Clinical Procedures in the Horse, First Edition. Edited by Lais R.R. Costa and Mary Rose Paradis.

Table 48.1 Resuscitation drugs and doses.

Drug	Concentration	Route	Dose	Recommendation for a 50 kg foal	Indication
Epinephrine (low dose)	1 mg/ml (1:1000)	IV, IO, IT	0.01–0.02 mg/kg for IV, IO routes Double to ten times this dose if administered IT	0.5–1 ml, IV, IO can be repeated in 3–5 minutes	Cardiac arrest or heart rate <50 bpm and not increasing with oxygen and CPCR
Vasopressin	20 units/ml	IV, IO, IT	0.3–0.6 units/kg once	0.75–1.5 ml	If no response to epinephrine
Plasma-Lyte A, Normosol-R or lactated Ringer's solution	–	IV	10–20 ml/kg bolus	1 liter for most resuscitation attempts, but 500 ml may be adequate for birth resuscitation where primary hypovolemia is not present	Hypovolemia, hypoperfusion, vasodilation
Sodium bicarbonate	8.5% (1 mEq/ml)	IV, IO	0.5–1 mEq/kg	25–50 ml of the 1 mEq/ml strength, administered slowly over ≥5 minutes	Use after the first 5 minutes of CPCR or as dictated by blood gases
Atropine	1 mg/ml	IV, IO, IT	0.02 mg/kg	1 ml, can be repeated once	Do not use early in birth resuscitation (hypoxemia-induced arrest) Use if no response to oxygenation, ventilation, chest compressions, and epinephrine in foals with sepsis or metabolic derangement-induced arrest Note: Atropine increases myocardial oxygen consumption Stagger with epinephrine by 30 seconds to minimize development of dysrhythmias
Lidocaine	20 mg/ml (2%)	IV, IO, IT	1–1.5 mg/kg slow bolus loading dose, then 0.03–0.05 mg/kg/min	2.5–3.75 ml of 2% lidocaine, as a slow bolus	Indicated for ventricular tachycardia

IV, intravenous; IO, intraosseous; IT, intratracheal.

48.4 Restraint and Positioning

- Place the foal in lateral recumbency on a hard, flat surface (use a firm wooden board if needed, as in the case of a bedded stall).
- If there are fractured ribs, place the side with the fractures down on the ground.
- If bilateral fractures are present, place the side with fractures furthest from the heart up.

- Extend the head and neck of the foal.
- CPCR is best performed with three or more personnel, with one person performing ventilation and two or more people alternating in providing chest compressions and administering medications. This procedure can be initiated with the foal in the birth canal during a dystocia if the head and neck are accessible.

48.5 Procedure: Recognition and Monitoring of Impending Cardiopulmonary Failure

Technical action	Rationale
Clinical signs of impending cardiopulmonary failure: - unconsciousness and/or unresponsiveness - apnea or bradypnea(<10 breaths per minute), gasping, attempts at open-mouth breathing - heart rate <50 bpm and continuing to decrease - absent peripheral pulses, signs of severe shock - non-perfusing tachyarrhythmias such as rapid ventricular tachycardia or ventricular fibrillation - bilateral mydriasis with poorly responsive pupillary light reflex (PLR) - severe hypoxemia, severe hypercapnia - poor muscle tone.	These clinical signs can be seen in the foal in the immediate postpartum period, especially to a dystocia. Foals that are potential candidates for resuscitation include those with bradycardia or very recent asystole, even if they are not currently breathing. Cloudy corneas in a newly delivered foal that has no heart beat or respiration indicates that the foal has been dead for some time and is not a good resuscitation candidate.
Monitoring parameters indicative of impending or present cardiopulmonary failure: - ECG abnormalities such as asystole, bradycardia, ventricular tachycardia or ventricular fibrillation - blood pressure: mean arterial pressure <40 mmHg in combination with clinical signs of severe hypoperfusion - plasma pH of <7.1–7.2 with marked metabolic or respiratory acidosis (or both).	Foals with septic shock are also at high risk for cardiopulmonary arrest. Monitoring the foal with ECG, blood pressure, and blood gas analysis will aid in identifying those foals at risk for arrest. These foals may respond to CPCR but are likely to arrest again if the underlying cause is not correctable. In contrast, foals with arrest due to hypoxemia associated with transient oxygen deprivation have a better prognosis if intervention is early enough to prevent irreversible injury. Examples include foals with prolonged dystocia, airway obstruction from fetal membranes, or premature placental separation.

The ABC sequence of resuscitation procedures of CPCR in a foal: A for Airway, B for Breathing, C for Circulatory, D for drugs and fluid therapy.

48.6 Procedure: A, Establish an Airway

Technical action	Rationale
In newborn foals, during the first 20 seconds of assessment, manually clear the mouth and nasal passages with towels. The foal should be vigorously rubbed with towels to stimulate ventilation. Gentle suction (no more than 15 seconds at a time) of nasal passages and nasopharynx should occur if meconium staining is present.	This will prepare the foal for intubation should that be necessary. Towel drying may act as a strong stimulus for the foal to begin breathing. Vigorous suction of fluids may decrease oxygenation and induce bradycardia, so vigorous suction is not recommended.
Once the airways are cleared, intubate the foal if indicated (i.e., if foal is not breathing spontaneously), using a nasotracheal tube of appropriate size. Most 45–60 kg foals require a 9–10 mm internal diameter tube, whereas smaller foals may require a 7–9 mm diameter tube.	Nasotracheal intubation is preferred over orotracheal intubation because the tube is less likely to be damaged or become dislodged as the foal recovers. However, when nasotracheal intubation is unsuccessful after one or two attempts, the endotracheal tube should be placed through the mouth without delay.
With the foal in lateral recumbency, extend its head and neck so that the nose is in a straight line with the trachea.	This position facilitates placement of the endotracheal tube into the trachea.
Apply sterile lubricating jelly to the tip of the tube.	Lubrication will facilitate the passage of the tube. The tube should be sterile to avoid contamination of the airways.
Advance the tube into the nasal cavity, with one hand pushing the tube ventromedially into the ventral meatus, while the other hand gently advances the tube.	If resistance is encountered at the level of the larynx, the tube should be withdrawn slightly and rotated 90° while advancing slowly. The tube should always be rotated in the same direction, otherwise the tip will end up in the same prior position.
The person performing intubation or an assistant can apply gentle pressure over the left side of the pharynx to occlude the esophagus. This is accomplished by cupping the hand ventrally around the throatlatch, with gentle pressure applied at the left side in the location of the proximal esophagus.	This will aid in prevention of tube placement into the esophagus. This will also allow recognition of inadvertent intraesophageal placement.
Confirm location of the tube by compressing the thorax and listening/feeling for air movement through the tube.	CO_2 detectors (capnograph or disposable CO_2 detector) can also be used to confirm correct placement.
If two attempts fail to successfully pass the tube into the trachea through the nasal cavity, the tube should be placed through the oral cavity. The tongue should be extended and held to the side with one hand, while the other hand is used to gently advance the tube.	Time should not be wasted in repeated attempts at nasotracheal intubation. Although a slightly less preferred route, orotracheal intubation is easier than nasotracheal intubation.
Once placement is confirmed, the cuff should be inflated.	Make sure to inflate the cuff with the appropriate volume to avoid over- or under-inflation of the cuff.

48.7 Procedure: B, Initiate Breathing

Technical action	Rationale
Attach the self-inflating resuscitation bag to the adaptor on the end of the endotracheal tube (Figure 48.1) and begin positive pressure manual ventilation at a rate of 20–30 breaths per minute.	Ideally, the rate of ventilation should be dictated by blood gas analysis (to maintain a normal $PaCO_2$). Avoid using a demand valve for the resuscitation of a foal, as it can cause significant barotrauma.
Attach the oxygen line to the self-inflating bag and set the rate to 15 liters/minute in order to enrich inspired oxygen content.	Periodically check for spontaneous respiratory movements.
Obtain an arterial blood gas sample to evaluate the effectiveness of the ventilation (see Chapter 49).	Change the rate according to $PaCO_2$.

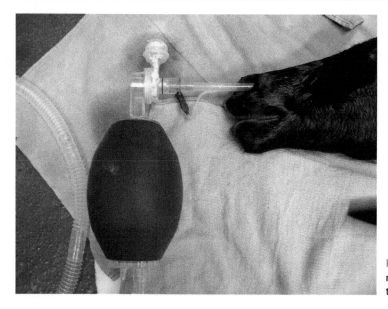

Figure 48.1 Self-inflating resuscitation bag attached to the endotracheal tube.

48.8 Procedure: C, Provide Circulatory Support

Technical action	Rationale
Begin closed chest compressions if asystole is present or if heart rate <50 bpm and not increasing after 30 seconds of initiating A and B.	The person performing cardiac compressions should be positioned at the foal's withers, on the back side of the foal (Figure 48.2a).
The resuscitator's hands should be placed on top of each other, just caudal to the foal's triceps (Figure 48.2b). The resuscitator's shoulders should be directly above the hands.	Keep the elbows locked and use the upper body to perform the compressions with the majority of the movement occurring at the waist. Begin with a rate of 80–120 bpm with a compression/decompression (relaxation) ratio of between 1:1 and 1:2.
For maximal effectiveness, the personnel providing compressions should alternate approximately every couple of minutes if qualified personnel are available.	Chest compressions easily fatigue the compressor, so the performance of the person providing compressions will decline with time. Alternating people frequently will ensure adequate chest compressions.

Technical action	Rationale
Monitor forward flow and the efficacy of cardiac compressions by checking the end-tidal CO_2, quality of peripheral pulse, and pupil size/PLR.	End-tidal CO_2 measurements >10-15 mmHg are suggestive of effective compressions. $ETCO_2$ < 10 mmHg is an indicator of ineffective CPCR.
	Palpation of a peripheral pulse (dorsal metatarsal, femoral or facial arteries) is a positive indicator of the effectiveness of CPCR. It can be difficult to feel the pulse with the movement associated with continuous cardiac compressions.
	Monitor pupil size: This is an indirect reflection of oxygen delivery to the brain. The pupils will dilate with decreased oxygen delivery and will begin to demonstrate a PLR when perfusion improves.

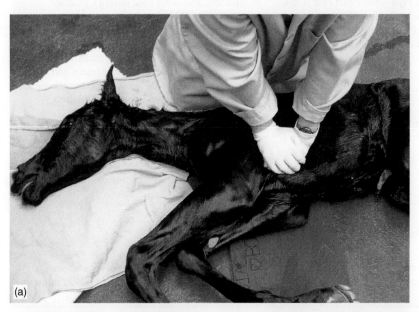

(a)

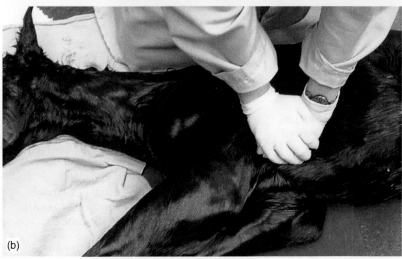

(b)

Figure 48.2 Proper positioning for performing chest compressions in a foal. (a) The person performing cardiac compressions should be positioned at the foal's withers, on the back side of the foal, with the shoulders directly above the hands. (b) The resuscitator's hands should be placed on top of each other, just caudal to the foal's triceps.

48.9 Procedure: D, Drugs and Fluids

Technical action	Rationale
Obtain circulatory access, optimally through venous access, once ventilation and cardiac compressions are initiated.	It is important to establish IV access by placement of an IV catheter to administer medications and fluid.
If placement of an IV catheter is not possible due to circulatory shock, medications can be administered using other routes: intraosseous (IO; see Chapter 54) or intratracheal (IT).	For medications administered IT, the dose should be 2 to 2.5 times greater than the dose recommended for IV administration, up to 10 times for epinephrine administered IT. For medications administered through the IO route, the dose is the same as for IV administration. Fluids can also be administered through the IO route.
If the foal remains in asystole or heart rate is <50 bpm within 30–60 seconds of chest compressions, begin epinephrine 0.01–0.02 mg/kg IV (0.5–1 ml of 1:1000 strength of epinephrine for a 50 kg foal).	Medications and doses used during CPCR are summarized in Table 48.1. The IO or IT routes can also be used. Note: Do not perform intracardiac sticks. The risks of lacerations, coronary artery injury, and arrhythmogenic potential outweigh potential benefits, particularly when alternate routes are available.
Foals with ventricular fibrillation or pulseless ventricular tachycardia are candidates for electrical defibrillation.	The first defibrillation should consist of up to three consecutive discharges: 2 J/kg followed by 4 J/kg followed by 4 J/kg. All subsequent defibrillations should be at 4 J/kg and should take place 1 minute after treatment with epinephrine or an anti-arrhythmic drug.

48.10 Procedure: Discontinuation of CPCR

CPCR can be discontinued when heart rate is >50 bpm and spontaneous breathing is accomplished.	Alternately, if successful return of spontaneous circulation has not been achieved by 10–12 minutes, CPCR attempt should be discontinued.

Further Reading and Bibliography

Corley, K. (2008) Procedures in the neonatal foal, in *The Equine Hospital Manual* (eds K. Corley and J. Stephen), Blackwell, Oxford, pp. 120–146.

Knottenbelt, D., Holdstock, N., and Madigan, J. (2004) *Equine Neonatology Medicine and Surgery*, W.B. Saunders, Edinburgh.

Koterba, A.M., Drummond, W.H., and Kosch, P.C. (1990) *Equine Clinical Neonatology*, Lea and Febiger, Philadelphia.

Madigan, J.E. (2016) *Manual of Equine Neonatal Medicine*, Live Oak Publishing, Woodland CA

McAuliffe, S.B. and Slovis, N.M. (2008) *Color Atlas of Disease and Disorders of the Foal*, W.B. Saunders, Philadelphia.

McKinnon, A.O., Squires, E.L., Vaala, W.E., and Varner, D.D. (2011) *Equine Reproduction*, 2nd edn, Wiley-Blackwell, Oxford.

Orsini, J.A. and Divers, T.J. (2007) *Equine Emergencies: Treatments and Procedures*, 3rd edn, W.B. Saunders, Philadelphia.

Sanchez, L.C. (2005) *Veterinary Clinics of North America Equine Practice – Neonatal Medicine and Surgery*, W.B. Saunders, Philadelphia.

49

Arterial Blood Sampling in the Neonatal Foal

Nóra Nógrádi and K. Gary Magdesian

49.1 Purpose

- Arterial blood gas (ABG) analysis should be performed in any neonate with respiratory compromise and those with suspected hypoventilation. ABG analysis provides the most accurate assessment of oxygenation, gas exchange, pulmonary function, and ventilation in the compromised neonate.
- The arterial oxygen tension (or partial pressure of oxygen, PaO_2) evaluates the oxygenating capacity of the lung. It should be noted that PaO_2 is age dependent. For example, in the healthy immediately postpartum foal PaO_2 may be in the range 40–50 mmHg while in lateral recumbency. By 24 hours of age, the PaO_2 should be >70 mmHg. In general terms, except for the immediately postpartum period, a PaO_2 <71–80 mmHg (sample obtained in lateral recumbency) should be considered hypoxemia in neonatal foals, indicating the need for oxygen supplementation.
- The arterial carbon dioxide tension ($PaCO_2$) assesses ventilatory status, with normal values ranging between 38 and 50 mmHg in the neonate. A $PaCO_2$ value >60 mmHg is associated with clinically significant hypoventilation, indicating the potential need for chemical or mechanical ventilatory support, if the arterial pH or mentation is significantly affected. Treatment of hypoventilation in the newborn is often dictated by the effects on mentation and overall pH status. If mentation is appropriate and arterial pH is >7.25, then permissive hypercapnia may be tolerated.
- Daily evaluation of ABG is indicated to monitor patients receiving intranasal oxygen insufflation to treat hypoxemia. If more frequent evaluation is necessary, an arterial catheter should be placed in a caudal auricular, facial or metatarsal artery. This is indicated in neonates on a mechanical ventilator when ABG analysis is generally performed three to four times daily.

49.2 Complications

- Hematoma formation
- Excessive bleeding
- Air embolization
- Arteritis
- Septic thrombus formation

49.3 Equipment Required

- Examination gloves
- Sterile gloves
- Clippers
- Sterile preparation material
- Topical anesthetic cream or 1 ml 2% lidocaine injection
- 1 ml syringe coated with heparin or specific arterial blood sampling syringe (Figure 49.1)
- 25-gauge ¾″ hypodermic needles
- Rubber stopper
- Blood gas analyzer

Manual of Clinical Procedures in the Horse, First Edition. Edited by Lais R.R. Costa and Mary Rose Paradis.
© 2018 John Wiley & Sons, Inc. Published 2018 by John Wiley & Sons, Inc.

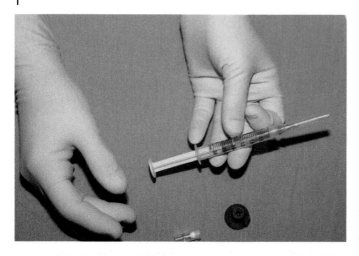

Figure 49.1 Commercial arterial collection syringe and needle system. Courtesy of Dr. Lais R.R. Costa.

49.4 Restraint and Positioning

- The most common sites for arterial blood sample collection in the foal are the metatarsal, brachial and the transverse facial arteries. These can be sampled with the foal in lateral recumbency.
- Positioning for collection from the metatarsal artery requires two assistants: one assistant should stabilize the head and thoracic limbs of the neonate, while another assistant should stabilize the pelvic limb. Movement causes significant interference with arterial sample collection, and therefore the pelvic limb should be restrained using one hand on the calcaneal tuber and the other holding the fetlock. In addition, the person drawing the sample should sit with the foal's hind foot secured between the knees.
- Positioning for collection from the brachial artery requires at least one assistant, who should stabilize the head and neck. The upper leg should be pulled forward, while the down leg should be stabilized by holding on to the carpus.

49.5 Procedure: Arterial Blood Sampling

Technical action	Rationale
Gently palpate for a pulse at the chosen site: • dorsal metatarsal artery (Figure 49.2) • brachial artery (Figure 49.3) • transverse facial artery.	The dorsal metatarsal artery is best felt between the third metatarsal bone and the cranial ridge of the fourth (lateral splint) metatarsal bone of the hind limb. A brachial arterial pulse can be felt on the medial aspect of the elbow, where it crosses the proximal forearm. The transverse arterial pulse can be felt caudal to the lateral canthus of the eye.
Clip a 2″ × 2″ area and inject 2% lidocaine subcutaneously (0.1–0.3 ml) just proximal to the clipped area (proximal to needle insertion site).	Desensitization of the skin will decrease the reaction of the foal to the sample collection. The authors prefer to inject lidocaine just proximal to the needle insertion site rather than directly at the site to avoid obscuring the artery and making it more difficult to palpate.
Apply sterile preparation to the clipped area.	See Chapter 10.
Make sure the needle and syringe are properly connected.	It is very important that the needle and syringe do not come apart during the sample collection to avoid contamination with room air.

Technical action	Rationale
Inserted the needle through the skin at a 30–45° angle.	The arterial blood pressure fills up the syringe once the artery is penetrated, with gentle aspiration. Alternatively, if a commercial arterial collection syringe and needle system is used, then manual aspiration is not required.
Collect a minimum of 0.5 ml of blood in a 1 ml syringe.	Most ABG analyzers require at least 0.5 ml of blood.
Apply pressure to the needle insertion site for at least 5 minutes to avoid hematoma formation and bleeding.	Hematomas will make subsequent samplings from this site more difficult and more painful.
Evacuate all of the air from the syringe and seal the needle with a rubber stopper.	It is important to prevent exposure of the arterial sample to room air. Room air will falsely increase the PaO_2 and pH, and decrease the $PaCO_2$.
Perform ABG analysis immediately.	If the sample will not be analyzed immediately, it must be kept on ice and analyzed within 2 hours of collection.

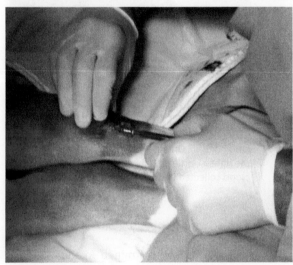
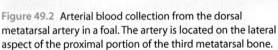

Figure 49.2 Arterial blood collection from the dorsal metatarsal artery in a foal. The artery is located on the lateral aspect of the proximal portion of the third metatarsal bone.

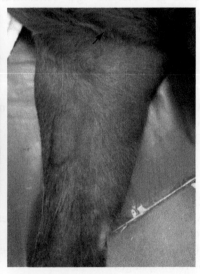

Figure 49.3 Location of the brachial artery in a foal. The artery can be palpated as it crosses the medial aspect of the forearm, near the pectoral muscles (black arrow).

Bibliography and Further Reading

Bedenice, D. (2006) Foal with septic pneumonia, in *Equine Neonatal Medicine: a Case-based Approach* (ed. M.R. Paradis), Elsevier, Philadelphia, pp. 1-11.

Koterba, A.M., Drummond, W.H., and Kosch, P.C. (1990) *Equine Clinical Neonatology*, Lea and Febiger, Philadelphia.

Madigan, J.E. (2016) *Manual of Equine Neonatal Medicine*, Live Oak Publishing, Woodland CA

McAuliffe, S.B. and Slovis, N.M. (2008) *Color Atlas of Disease and Disorders of the Foal*, W.B. Saunders, Philadelphia.

McKinnon, A.O., Squires, E.L., Vaala, W.E., and Varner, D.D. (2011) *Equine Reproduction*, 2nd edn, Wiley-Blackwell, Oxford.

Orsini, J.A. and Divers, T.J. (2007) *Equine Emergencies: Treatments and Procedures*, 3rd edn, W.B. Saunders, Philadelphia.

Sanchez, L.C. (2005) *Veterinary Clinics of North America Equine Practice – Neonatal Medicine and Surgery*, W.B. Saunders, Philadelphia.

50

Venous Blood Sampling in the Neonatal Foal

Nóra Nógrádi and K. Gary Magdesian

50.1 Purpose

- To collect blood samples for complete blood count, biochemistry panel, venous blood gas analysis, IgG concentration, coagulation profiles, blood cultures, and other blood or plasma analyses.

50.2 Complications

- Hematoma formation at injection site.
- Arterial hematoma formation due to inadvertent puncture of the carotid artery.
- Thrombophlebitis.

50.3 Equipment Required

- Examination gloves
- Alcohol-soaked 4″ × 4″ gauze sponges or cotton
- 20- or 21-gauge 1–1.5″ hypodermic needle.
- 3–10 ml syringes
- Blood tubes

For blood culture sample collection

- Sterile gloves
- Clippers
- Antiseptics materials for sterile preparation
- Blood culture bottles, with or without antibiotic resin binding (Figure 50.1)

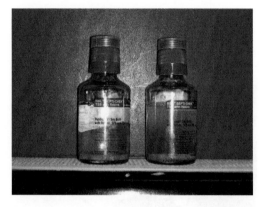

Figure 50.1 Blood culture bottles with antimicrobial binding resin. On the left is an unused bottle and on the right a bottle after injection of 5 ml of venous blood collected under sterile technique.

50.4 Restraint and Positioning

The foal can be restrained in the standing position for venipuncture. In most instances the foal should be restrained in lateral recumbency for cephalic venipuncture (see Chapter 42).

Manual of Clinical Procedures in the Horse, First Edition. Edited by Lais R.R. Costa and Mary Rose Paradis.

50.5 Procedure: Venous Blood Collection for Whole Blood or Plasma Analyses

Technical action	Rationale
The jugular vein is the most common site for venipuncture in the ambulatory, active foal. The cephalic vein can also be used in the recumbent or weak foal.	Ensure that the blood is placed in the correct tube (i.e., correct additive or no additive) for the test requested. Also ensure that enough blood is collected for the requested tests.

Blood collection from the jugular vein

Locate the jugular furrow and identify the jugular vein.	For blood collection, use the site at the junction of the upper and mid third of the neck (Figure 50.2).
Hold off the vein with digital pressure distal to the site of intended puncture.	Distending the vein allows improved visualization.
Use examination gloves and clean the hair and skin over the venipuncture site with alcohol-soaked 4″ × 4″ gauze sponges or cotton.	Perform the venipuncture carefully to prevent contamination or excessive tissue trauma.
The vein lies superficially under the skin. The needle should be inserted through the skin at a shallow angle.	The carotid artery is deep to the jugular vein and can be inadvertently punctured if the foal struggles.

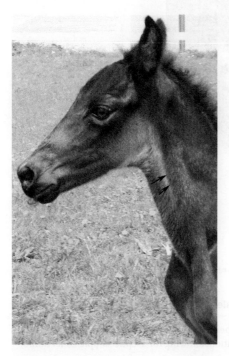

Figure 50.2 Site for blood collection from the jugular vein at the junction of the upper and mid third of the neck (black arrows).

Technical action	Rationale
Blood collection from the cephalic vein	
Identify the site for blood collection on the craniomedial aspect of the radius.	The ideal site for venipuncture is approximately halfway between the elbow and the carpus (Figure 50.3).
Examination gloves should be used to wipe the overlying hair and skin with alcohol-soaked 4″ × 4″ gauze sponges or cotton.	

Technical action	Rationale
The vein lies superficially, just under the skin. Stabilize the vein and allow it to distend by holding it off with a finger just proximal to the cleaned site.	This vein tends to roll easily under the skin.
The needle should be attached to the syringe, inserted at a shallow angle, and aspirated slowly.	Care should be taken to apply only minimal suction on the syringe to prevent collapse of the vein.
Aspirate the appropriate amount of blood steadily.	Do not aspirate too fast to avoid collapsing or damaging the vein.
Apply pressure to the venipuncture site.	Applying pressure after venipuncture prevents hematoma formation at the site.

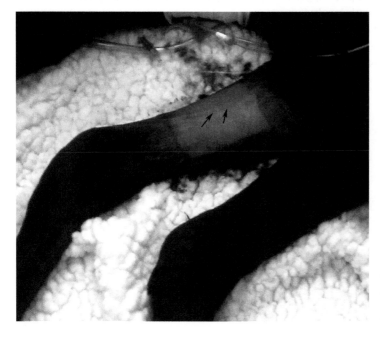

Figure 50.3 Site for blood collection from the cephalic vein at the craniomedial aspect of the radius, halfway between the elbow and the carpus (black arrows).

50.6 Procedure: Venous Blood Collection for Blood Culture

Technical action	Rationale
Identify the sites for blood collection as previously described.	Any superficial vein can be use after sterile preparation, allowing for aseptic sample collection.
Perform a sterile preparation (see Chapter 10): • Clip a 2″ × 2″ area, • Perform aseptic scrub: betadine or chlorhexidine, followed by alcohol (Figure 50.4).	Sterile preparation decreases the chance of culturing a skin contaminant such as *Bacillus sp.*
Use sterile gloves. Use strict sterile technique for collection of the blood sample.	Sterile technique decreases the chance of culturing a skin contaminant.

Technical action	Rationale
Aspirate 3 to 5 ml of blood from the site.	Check the instructions on the bottle to determine the volume of blood required to inoculate the blood culture bottle. Depending on the size and condition of the foal, collect enough blood to inoculate two blood culture bottles.
Change needles on the syringe after the sample has been collected and wipe the rubber top of the blood culture bottle with alcohol before it is filled, unless it has a sterile cap that is removed just prior to filling.	Changing the needle before injecting into culture media decreases the chance of culturing an environmental contaminant.
Apply pressure to the venipuncture site.	Applying pressure after venipuncture prevents hematoma formation at the site.
Repeat the procedure of venous blood collection under sterile technique at an additional site and/or additional time point.	Ideally a total of three blood culture bottles should be inoculated to increase the chance of a successful culture.

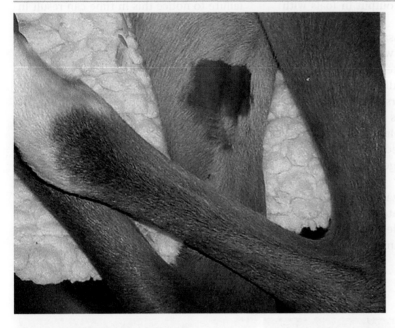

Figure 50.4 The cephalic vein prepared for collection of blood for culture after the area has been clipped and scrubbed with antiseptics.

Bibliography and Further Reading

Knottenbelt, D., Holdstock, N., and Madigan, J. (2004) *Equine Neonatology Medicine and Surgery*, W.B. Saunders, Edinburgh.

Koterba, A.M., Drummond, W.H., and Kosch, P.C. (1990) *Equine Clinical Neonatology*, Lea and Febiger, Philadelphia.

Madigan, J.E. (2016) *Manual of Equine Neonatal Medicine*, Live Oak Publishing, Woodland CA

McAuliffe, S.B. and Slovis, N.M. (2008) *Color Atlas of Disease and Disorders of the Foal*, W.B. Saunders, Philadelphia.

McKinnon, A.O., Squires, E.L., Vaala, W.E., and Varner, D.D. (2011) *Equine Reproduction*, 2nd edn, Wiley-Blackwell, Oxford.

Orsini, J.A. and Divers, T.J. (2007) *Equine Emergencies: Treatments and Procedures*, 3rd edn, W.B. Saunders, Philadelphia.

Sanchez, L.C. (2005) *Veterinary Clinics of North America Equine Practice – Neonatal Medicine and Surgery*, W.B. Saunders, Philadelphia.

51

Urinary Catheter Placement in the Neonatal Foal

Nóra Nógrádi and K. Gary Magdesian

51.1 Purpose

- Indwelling urine catheters are indicated in foals with hypoperfusion to monitor urine output. They are particularly important in monitoring urine output in foals with oliguria or anuria.
- They are often necessary in hospitalized, recumbent neonates with inability to urinate, as these neonates often cannot urinate despite a markedly enlarged bladder. This sometimes occurs as a primary entity in ambulatory foals as well.
- Catheters should be placed in a post-surgical repair of a ruptured bladder to prevent distension and leakage from the bladder repair.
- A onetime catheterization of the urinary bladder is also indicated for collection of a sterile urine sample in foals with suspected urinary tract infection.

51.2 Complications

- Urinary tract infections.
- The urinary catheter can become obstructed with sediment and mucus, and failure to notice this in time can result in obstruction to urine flow.

51.3 Equipment Required

- For Colts: Soft catheter 5–7 mm in diameter and at least 26" (54 cm) in length. Options include soft infant feeding tubes such as: 5 Fr (36", 90 cm) or 8 Fr (42", 105 cm) Kangaroo Feeding Tube (Covidien, Mansfield, MA), or 5 Fr (36", 90 cm) or 8 Fr (42", 105 cm) Kendall Argyle Feeding Tube (Tyco Health Care, Mansfield, MA) (Figure 51.1a)
- For Fillies: Soft catheter 1–1.5 cm in diameter and around 13" (33 cm) in length. Typically a Foley catheter 8–12 Fr, 33 cm (e.g, Dover, Covidien, Mansfield, MA) (Figure 51.1b) with an optional semi-rigid stylet to facilitate catheter placement.

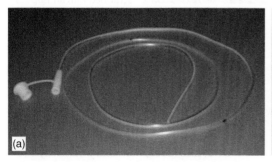
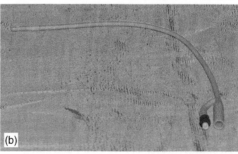

Figure 51.1 Catheters for urinary placement in foals. (a) An infant feeding tube can be used as a urinary catheter. (b) A Foley catheter with a self-retaining balloon. Courtesy of Dr. Lais R.R. Costa.

Manual of Clinical Procedures in the Horse, First Edition. Edited by Lais R.R. Costa and Mary Rose Paradis.
© 2018 John Wiley & Sons, Inc. Published 2018 by John Wiley & Sons, Inc.

- Sterile water-soluble lubricant
- Sterile saline (if using a Foley catheter with an inflatable balloon)
- Sterile gloves
- Gentle soap such as Ivory soap (Proctor & Gamble)
- Chlorhexidine scrub, sterile water, and cotton
- Suture material (2-0 Prolene)
- Sterile instruments (needle driver, scissors)
- Sterile 60 cc catheter tip syringe
- Sterile 20 cc syringe to inflate the cuff, if using a Foley catheter with an inflatable balloon

51.4 Restraint and Positioning

- Some foals may require sedation for this procedure. In such cases diazepam at a dose of 0.05–0.2 mg/kg IV can be administered.
- If additional sedation is required, butorphanol can be administered at 0.01–0.02 mg/kg IV.
- Maintenance of the foal in lateral recumbency for catheter placement is ideal.

51.5 Procedure: Urinary Catheterization of the Colt

Technical action	Rationale
The assistant should exteriorize the penis from the sheath.	This is often the most difficult part of the procedure. Many colt foals have a persistent penile frenulum at birth that usually resolves within a few days. These frenula may prevent exteriorization of the penis, in which case the penis can be held within the prepuce such that the urethral orifice is visualized.
Once the glans penis is exteriorized, it is necessary to firmly hold the penis throughout the procedure (Figure 51.2).	This will prevent retraction into the sheath.
Clean the urethral opening and glans penis with gentle soap (meant for mucous membranes), followed by chlorhexidine-soaked cotton, and ending with a rinse using sterile water.	Maintenance of sterile technique will help prevent iatrogenic urinary tract infections.
Remove the catheter from the sterile package.	Wear sterile gloves when handling the sterile tube.
Apply sterile water-soluble lubricant to the tip of the catheter.	This will prevent trauma to the urethra and mucosa.
Attach a sterile syringe at the end of the catheter.	This will prevent the inadvertent introduction of air into the bladder and will allow collection of a sterile sample.
Gently insert the catheter through the urethral opening.	Mild resistance can be felt while passing through the pelvic brim in colts.
Gentle suction should be applied to the syringe to confirm proper placement by aspiration of urine (Figure 51.3).	
Urine may start spontaneously flowing once the tip reaches the bladder.	

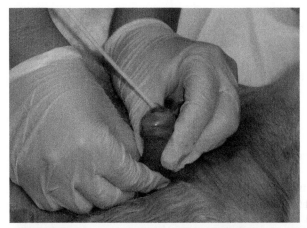

Figure 51.2 Stabilization of the penis during urinary catheter placement in a colt.

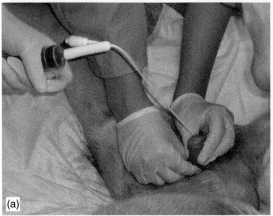
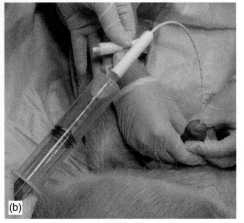

Figure 51.3 Gentle aspiration using a catheter tip syringe to verify the catheter's placement and patency. (a) Negative pressure indicates that the catheter is not patent (either kinked or plugged). (b) If the bladder is distended urine will start to flow easily once the tip of the catheter reaches the bladder.

51.6 Procedure: Urinary Catheterization of the Filly

Technical action	Rationale
Catheterization of fillies is generally more difficult and requires experience.	This is because the urethral opening cannot be visualized and the catheter is advanced blindly.
Clean the perineum and the vulvar lips with gentle soap followed by chlorhexidine-soaked cotton, and finish by wiping the area with sterile water-soaked cotton as a rinse.	Maintenance of sterile technique will help to prevent urinary tract infections.
Remove the catheter from the sterile package. If using a Foley catheter, check the integrity of the balloon.	Wear sterile gloves and maintain aseptic technique to prevent iatrogenic urinary tract infections.
Apply sterile lubricant to the tip of the catheter.	This will minimize trauma to the urethra.
Attach a sterile syringe at the end of the catheter.	This will prevent the inadvertent introduction of air into the bladder and will allow for collection of a sterile sample.

Technical action	Rationale
With one hand advancing the catheter through the vulvar opening, the fingertips of the other hand (gloved, sterile, and well lubricated) should gently push the tip of the catheter towards the vestibular floor.	The urethral opening is approximately 5 cm from the vulvar lips directly on midline in average-sized foals.Ensure that the vestibule is well lubricated with sterile lubricant.
Carefully advance the catheter.	The total length of catheter to be inserted should be around 10-12 cm.
Urine usually flows spontaneously once the tip reaches the bladder.	Gentle suction can be applied with the syringe to confirm proper placement if urine does not flow spontaneously.
A small laryngoscope (sterilized) with a light can be used to attempt visualization of the urethral orifice.	This can facilitate placement in cases in which catheterization proves difficult.

51.7 Procedure: Stabilization and Maintenance of Indwelling Catheter

Technical action	Rationale/amplification
Inflate the balloon of the Foley catheter with sterile saline (volume as directed on the Foley catheter) to secure the catheter in the bladder (Figure 51.4).	Very gentle traction on the catheter should meet with resistance as the balloon occludes the opening of beginning of the urethra.
Alternatively, if you are using an infant feeding tube as an indwelling catheter, it needs to be sutured to the glans or prepuce of colts, or the vulvar lips of fillies after topical and local blocks with 2% lidocaine.	The Chinese finger trap suture pattern provides a stable hold that prevents displacement of the urinary catheter. Two of these, one in either side, are often needed. If the glans is used for stay sutures, extreme caution should be used to avoid suturing the urethra.
The end of the catheter should be connected to a closed urinary system (Figure 51.5).	This will prevent contamination and ascending infections.
For ambulatory foals, a one-way valve (small Heimlich) can be placed on the end of the catheter (Figure 51.6). Alternatively, the urinary collection bag can be secured to the abdomen or hind leg with adhesive bandage material. The foal will need to be kept in a foal box, separated from its dam except when supervised.	This will allow the catheter to drip while maintaining asepsis. Securing a collection bag to the ambulatory foal allows for asepsis as well as monitoring the amount of urine produced.
Clean any ends that are opened at least once daily with chlorhexidine or betadine solution, being careful not to introduce these into the catheter.	To help prevent contamination of the catheter.
Monitor continuously for urine flow. If urine flow abruptly stops or decreases, the bladder should be evaluated by ultrasound.	Perform ultrasonographic evaluation of the bladder to determine whether the urinary catheter is plugged or kinked or whether urine production has truly ceased.
Pull or replace the catheter if an obstruction is suspected.	Mucous plugs can obstruct the catheter. If these plugs can't be dislodged through aspiration and flushing with a syringe, the catheter should be replaced.
Periodic urinalysis should be performed to evaluate for development of cystitis.	A sample should be submitted for culture and susceptibility testing if there is any indication of cystitis.
Foals with an indwelling urinary catheter should be maintained on broad-spectrum antimicrobials for at least 1 week after removal of the urinary catheter.	Longer duration of antimicrobial therapy is indicated if a urinary tract infection is present.

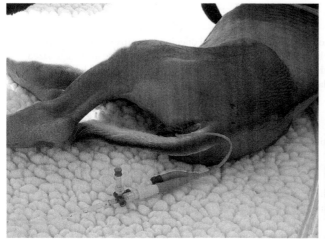

Figure 51.4 Connection of the urinary catheter to a closed urinary collection system in a filly.

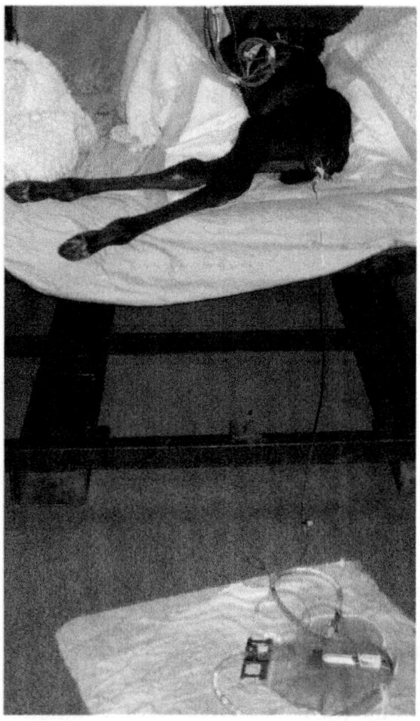

Figure 51.5 A closed urinary catheter system in the neonatal intensive care unit.

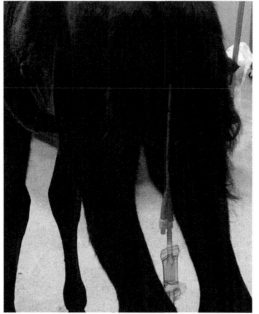

Figure 51.6 One-way valve placed on the end of the urinary Foley catheter in a filly. (Courtesy of Dr. Lais R.R. Costa)

Bibliography and Further Reading

Knottenbelt, D., Holdstock, N., and Madigan, J. (2004) *Equine Neonatology Medicine and Surgery*, W.B. Saunders, Edinburgh.

Koterba, A.M., Drummond, W.H., and Kosch, P.C. (1990) *Equine Clinical Neonatology*, Lea and Febiger, Philadelphia.

Madigan, J.E. (2016) *Manual of Equine Neonatal Medicine*, Live Oak Publishing, Woodland CA

McAuliffe, S.B. and Slovis, N.M. (2008) *Color Atlas of Disease and Disorders of the Foal*, W.B. Saunders, Philadelphia.

McKinnon, A.O., Squires, E.L., Vaala, W.E., and Varner, D.D. (2011) *Equine Reproduction*, 2nd edn, Wiley-Blackwell, Oxford.

Orsini, J.A. and Divers, T.J. (2007) *Equine Emergencies: Treatments and Procedures*, 3rd edn, W.B. Saunders, Philadelphia.

Sanchez, L.C. (2005) *Veterinary Clinics of North America Equine Practice – Neonatal Medicine and Surgery*, W.B. Saunders, Philadelphia.

52

Cerebral Spinal Fluid Collection in the Neonatal Foal

Nóra Nógrádi and K. Gary Magdesian

52.1 Purpose

- To collect cerebrospinal fluid (CSF) sample for fluid analysis, including cytology and microbial (aerobic/anaerobic) culture in foals with suspected septic meningitis.

52.2 Complications

- Rare complication of cellulitis or meningitis at the tap site.
- Hemorrhage into the subarachnoid space or hematoma formation.
- Brain herniation and subsequent death, especially during atlanto-occipital (AO) taps when the intracranial pressure (ICP) is high. It is therefore contraindicated to perform an AO CSF collection when high ICP is suspected.
- Inadvertent penetration of the spinal cord parenchyma during spinal fluid collection from the AO space can lead to signs of brainstem or spinal cord disease. These can vary from temporary vestibular abnormalities to cessation of respiration and death.

52.3 Equipment Required

- Clippers
- Sterile preparation materials

- Sterile gloves
- 2% lidocaine injectable
- 20-gauge 1.5" (3.75 cm) hypodermic needle (for AO tap)
- 20-gauge 2.5–3.5" (6.4–8.9 cm) spinal needle (for lumbosacral (LS) tap)
- 10 ml syringe
- Blood collection tubes

52.4 Restraint and Positioning

- CSF can be collected from two locations, the AO space and the LS space, each with separate restraint and positioning requirements.
- CSF collection from the AO space requires general anesthesia. The patient is placed in lateral recumbency with the head and neck flexed by an assistant.
- CSF collection from the LS space requires heavy sedation. This can be performed in a standing, sedated or recumbent foal. For recumbent procedures, the foal is usually placed in sternal recumbency with both legs tucked under the abdomen, maintaining a straight torso. Alternatively, the foal can be positioned in lateral recumbency with hindlimbs pulled slightly forward to flex the vertebral column. LS puncture is more readily achieved in the sternal position.

Manual of Clinical Procedures in the Horse, First Edition. Edited by Lais R.R. Costa and Mary Rose Paradis.
© 2018 John Wiley & Sons, Inc. Published 2018 by John Wiley & Sons, Inc.

52.5 Procedure: CSF Collection from the AO Space

Technical action	Rationale
The AO space can be located by drawing a line between the cranial edges of the transverse processes ("wings") of the first cervical vertebra, the atlas.	The AO space is where this line crosses the dorsal midline, up to 0.5–1 cm caudal to this intersection (Figure 52.1).
Once the site is located, clip the area and apply sterile preparation (see Chapter 10).	It is important to maintain strict asepsis during the procedure.
While the assistant is flexing the head and neck, the needle is inserted through the skin.	Aim the needle toward the mandibular symphysis.
By stabilizing the needle with the index finger and thumb of one hand, while resting the wrist against the foal's skin, the other hand slowly advances the needle by pointing towards the foal's lower lip.	The stylet should be removed every 1–2 mm to check for the flow of CSF once the needle has been inserted approximately 0.5–1 cm deep.
A "popping" sensation may be felt while advancing the needle, and is suggestive of penetrating the dura mater, indicating that CSF flow can be expected.	This sudden decrease in resistance may not always be felt and should not be relied upon.
The subarachnoid space is fairly shallow, therefore caution should be applied while advancing the needle.	To prevent inadvertent puncture of the spinal cord.
Once CSF is flowing, stabilize the needle against the foal's neck with one hand.	The assistant can collect the freely flowing fluid. Collection of passively flowing CSF is safer than aspiration, especially when increased intracranial pressure may be present.
Samples should be examined for color and transparency. Analysis of the fluid should be done within 30 minutes, or the sample should be placed into an EDTA-containing tube and refrigerated if analysis will be delayed.	Normal CSF in foals is clear and colorless. The number of nucleated cells should be <5 cells/μl (there should be only mononuclear cells) and the total protein content should be 100 ± 50 mg/dl. The glucose concentration should be within 80% of the plasma or blood glucose concentration.
If the CSF has increased protein and cell count, particularly if neutrophils are present, aliquots of the sample should be submitted for bacterial and/or fungal cultures.	An aliquot of the sample can be placed in a blood culture media bottle to enhance growth of bacteria.

52.6 Procedure: CSF Collection from the LS Space

Technical action	Rationale
The LS space can be palpated as a depression located in the dorsal midline behind the last lumbar vertebra (L6). It is bordered laterally by the cranial aspect of the tuber sacrale and caudally by the sacral spine.	To find the LS depression, draw a line between the caudal borders of both tuber coxae, and find the intersection point with the dorsal midline (Figure 52.2).
Once the site has been located, clip the area and apply sterile preparation. Apply a bleb of 2% lidocaine under the skin.	It is important to maintain strict asepsis during the procedure.

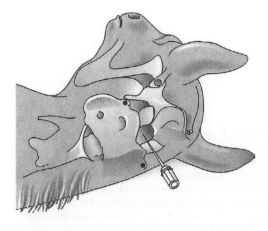

Figure 52.1 Landmarks for collection of CSF from the AO space. To locate the AO space, draw an imaginary line between the cranial edges of the transverse processes ("wings") of the first cervical vertebrae (atlas), and the point where this line (up to 0.5–1 cm caudal to this line) crosses the dorsal midline running between the occipital protuberances is the foramen magnum. Knottenbelt *et al.* (2004). Reproduced with permission of Elsevier.

Technical action	Rationale
Maintaining strict sterile technique, palpate the depression behind the last lumbar vertebra on the midline (Figure 52.3).	Make sure the foal is standing with both pelvic limbs placed symmetrically.
Insert the 20-gauge 3.5″ needle through the skin and direct the needle perpendicular to the spinal cord, through the lidocaine bleb.	The assistant should make sure the foal is still and in a balanced position, not leaning to either side during this procedure.
With your dominant hand, slowly advance the needle directly perpendicular to the spine, while stabilizing the needle with the index finger and thumb of the other hand (Figure 52.4).	To keep the needle steady and ensure it stays perpendicular to the spine, place the pinky finger of the hand holding the needle on the foal's back.
If the foal is not amenable to having the procedure performed in a standing position after sedation, the LS tap can be performed in sternal recumbency or lateral recumbency.	The assistant should make sure that: • if in sternal recumbency the foal is lying in a balanced position, not leaning to either side • if in lateral recumbency the pelvic limbs are brought forward slightly • the foal's back is straight.
A "popping" sensation may be felt while advancing the needle, and is suggestive of penetrating the dura mater.	This sudden decrease in resistance may not always be felt.
With one hand stabilizing the needle, attach a 3 ml syringe and aspirate the CSF.	Free flowing CSF can be expected only when the procedure is performed in lateral recumbency, and is not always present.
Samples should be examined for color and transparency. Analysis of the fluid should be done within 30 minutes of collection. If it must be sent out for analysis, it should be placed into EDTA collection vials and refrigerated.	Normal CSF in foals is clear and colorless, with <5 mononuclear cells/µl and a total protein content of 100 ± 50 mg/dl. The glucose concentration should be within 80% of the plasma or blood glucose concentration.
A sample can be placed in a blood culture media bottle to enhance growth of bacteria.	Cultures should be performed on CSF that has increased protein and cell count, particularly if neutrophils are present.

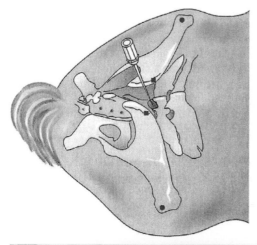

Figure 52.2 Landmarks for collection of CSF from the LS space. To locate the LS space, draw a line between the caudal borders of both tuber coxae, and find the intersection point of this line and the dorsal midline. Palpate the depression located at the dorsal midline behind the sixth lumbar vertebra, between the caudal aspect of both tuber sacrale and cranial to the spinous process of the second sacral vertebrae. Knottenbelt *et al.* (2004). Reproduced with permission of Elsevier.

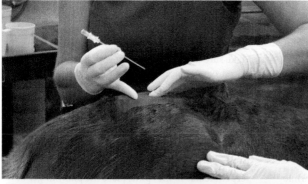

Figure 52.3 Palpation of the LS space for CSF collection right before the insertion of the spinal needle.

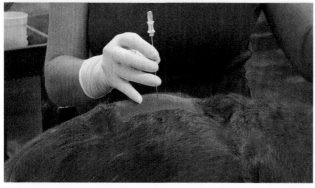

Figure 52.4 Placement of the spinal needle into the LS space for CSF collection. Note the non-dominant hand stabilizing the needle in a perpendicular position in relation to the spinal column.

Bibliography and Further Reading

Knottenbelt, D., Holdstock, N., and Madigan, J. (2004) *Equine Neonatology Medicine and Surgery*, W.B. Saunders, Edinburgh.

Koterba, A.M., Drummond, W.H., and Kosch, P.C. (1990) *Equine Clinical Neonatology*, Lea and Febiger, Philadelphia.

Madigan, J.E. (2016) *Manual of Equine Neonatal Medicine*, Live Oak Publishing, Woodland CA

McAuliffe, S.B. and Slovis, N.M. (2008) *Color Atlas of Disease and Disorders of the Foal*, W.B. Saunders, Philadelphia.

McKinnon, A.O., Squires, E.L., Vaala, W.E., and Varner, D.D. (2011) *Equine Reproduction*, 2nd edn, Wiley-Blackwell, Oxford.

Orsini, J.A. and Divers, T.J. (2007) *Equine Emergencies: Treatments and Procedures*, 3rd edn, W.B. Saunders, Philadelphia.

Sanchez, L.C. (2005) *Veterinary Clinics of North America Equine Practice – Neonatal Medicine and Surgery*, W.B. Saunders, Philadelphia.

B Instrumentation in the Neonatal Foal

53

Intravenous Catheter Placement in the Neonatal Foal

Nóra Nógrádi and K. Gary Magdesian

53.1 Purpose

- To provide venous access for intravenous medications, fluid therapy, and parenteral nutrition.
- To provide venous access for monitoring central venous pressure.

53.2 Complications

- Hematoma formation at catheter insertion site
- Infection or abscess formation at catheter insertion site
- Thrombophlebitis
- Bacterial endocarditis secondary to thrombophlebitis
- Septicemia
- Embolism (air, thrombus, part of the catheter)
- Catheter misplacement (subcutaneous, arterial)
- Catheter occlusion
- Catheter breakage and dislodgement

53.3 Equipment Required

- Clippers
- Sterile preparation material (povidone-iodine or chlorhexidine and alcohol (70% isopropyl alcohol)
- 2 ml 2% lidocaine injection
- Sterile gloves
- Sterile instruments (scissors, needle driver)
- #15 scalpel blade (for over-the-wire catheter)
- Suture material (2-0 Prolene or nylon).
- Catheter and the introduction system (see Table 53.1)
- Heparinized saline (1 IU of heparin per ml of preservative-free saline)
- T-port and injection ports
- Bandage material (sterile gauze, elastic adhesive tape)

Table 53.1 Types of catheters used in neonatal foals

Method of placement	Catheter material	Size	Length (" or cm)	Lumen
Over the needle	FEP polymer[1]	16–20 gauge	2–5"	Single
	Teflon[2,3a]	16–22 gauge	2–6"	Single
	Polyurethane[3b]	16–20 gauge	2.5–5"	Single
Through needle	Polyurethane[3c]	18–20 gauge	18 and 36"[B]	Single
	Polyurethane[3d]	20 gauge	12"	Single

(continued)

Manual of Clinical Procedures in the Horse, First Edition. Edited by Lais R.R. Costa and Mary Rose Paradis.
© 2018 John Wiley & Sons, Inc. Published 2018 by John Wiley & Sons, Inc.

Method of placement	Catheter material	Size	Length (" or cm)	Lumen
Over the wire[A]	Polyurethane[3e]	16, 19 gauge	3.25–24"	Single
		4, 5, 5.5, 7, and 8 Fr	3.25, 5.25, 8, 10, 12, and 24"	Multi-lumen
	Polyurethane[4a]	14–24 gauge	3.5–8"	Single and multi-lumen
	Silicone[6a]	4 and 5 Fr	42 cm[B]	Single
		7 Fr	42 cm[B]	Double
Peel-away over-the-needle introducer	Polyurethane[3f]	16–19 gauge	3.5, 6, 10, and 24"[B]	Single
		4 or 5.5 Fr	3.5, 5.25, and 10"[B]	Multi-lumen
Peel-away over-the-needle introducer with wire stylet	Silicone[3g]	16, 18, 20, and 23 gauge	40 and 60 cm[B]	Single
		5 Fr	60 cm[B]	Double
	Silicone[5a 4b]	4 and 5 Fr	12 and 25 cm	Single
		7, 8, and 12.5 Fr	13, 20, and 25 cm	Multiple

FEP, fluorinated ethylene propylene; ", inches; cm, centimeter; Fr, French.

[A] Seldinger (needle introducer) or modified Seldinger (catheter-over-needle introducer) technique for placement of central venous catheter.

[B] Peripherally introduced central catheter (PICC), can be cut to size.

Products and manufacturers:

[1] BD Angiocath, (Becton, Dickinson);

[2] Abbo-cath® (Abbott);

[3a] Short-term (MILA®);

[3b] Extended-use Milacath (MILA®);

[3c] Long-line catheter (MILA®);

[3d] Veincath (MILA®);

[3e] Long-term Milacath (MILA®);

[3f] Long-term Milacath using peel-away introduction (MILA®);

[3g] PICC silicone catheter (MILA®);

[4a] Arrow central venous catheters (Teleflex®);

[4b] Arrow PICC (Teleflex®);

[5a] Long-term central venous catheters (Cook Medical®);

[6a] Hohn central venous catheters (Bard Access Systems).

53.4 Restraint and Positioning

- Restraining the foal in lateral recumbency allows the clinician to maintain asepsis during the procedure. In fractious (otherwise healthy) foals this may require sedation.
- Sick foals usually can be restrained in lateral recumbency without sedation.
- If sedation is required foals under 10–14 days of age can be sedated with diazepam (0.05–0.2 mg/kg IV), while older foals (>14 days) that are hemodynamically stable can be sedated with xylazine (0.2–0.5 mg/kg IV) (see Chapter 9).
- Catheters can be placed while the foal is restrained standing, but it can be relatively more difficult to maintain aseptic technique if the foal is allowed to move.

53.5 Procedure: Choosing the Appropriate Catheter Type

Technical action	Rationale
There are a number of catheter options for use in foals. The material composition, expected length of use, technique used for placement, and purpose should dictate catheter selection.	The type of case and intended use should be considered when selecting catheter type. For example, foals with sepsis are at risk for coagulopathies and therefore catheters with minimal thrombogenicity should be used.

Aspects to consider:
 	
• material composition types available for catheters:
  – Teflon
  – polyurethane
  – silicone
• expected length of use and thrombogenic potential of the foal.
	Teflon catheters are the most thrombogenic and should not be kept in place for more than 3 days. They are indicated for short-term use such as for general anesthesia or administration of a single unit of plasma in otherwise healthy neonates.
	
	Polyurethane or silicone catheters are preferred for compromised foals. These have the advantage of being relatively less thrombogenic and can remain in the vein for 7–21 days if no heat or swelling is noted.

Consider the method of placement: • over-the-needle • over-the-wire • through a peel-away introducer with wire stylet.	Over-the-needle and over-the-wire catheters are used most commonly. See below for placement.
Depending on the expected level of care, consider the purpose to decide if a single, double, triple or quadruple lumen catheter is required.	Double, triple or quadruple lumen catheters should be utilized when parenteral nutrition (PN) is expected because PN optimally should have dedicated lines to minimize the risks of sepsis.

53.6 Procedure: Catheter Sites and Preparation

Technical action	Rationale
The site preparation is the same regardless of type of intravenous catheter to be used (Figure 53.1).	The jugular vein is the most common site for catheterization but the cephalic and saphenous veins can also be used.
The jugular vein is best catheterized at the junction of the upper and middle third of the neck (Figure 53.1a).	The vein can be located in the jugular furrow. Distending the vein by occluding it distally will allow better visualization.
Clip a 4″ × 4″ area over the vein intended for catheterization.	Make sure that the site for introduction of the catheter is in the middle of the prepared area.
Apply sterile preparation (see Chapter 10).	Rigorous aseptic techniques should be applied in preparation for and during catheter placement.
Inject 0.5–1 ml of 2% local anesthetic under the skin directly overlying the jugular vein.	Desensitization of the area will help to decrease movement in the foal and facilitate placement.
Inject 0.5–1 ml of 2% local anesthetic under the skin at the place where the catheter extension set is to be sutured to the skin.	Desensitization of the area will also facilitate the placement of sutures.

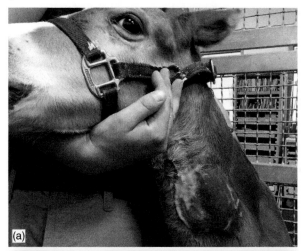

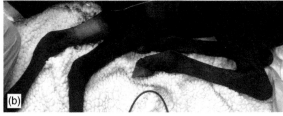

Figure 53.1 Site of venous catheterization in the neonatal foal: (a) jugular vein (Courtesy of Dr. Aloisio Bueno) and (b) cephalic vein. The area is prepared by clipping the hair and performing a thorough surgical scrub with antiseptic and alcohol.

53.7 Procedure: Placement of an Over-the-needle Catheter

Technical action	Rationale
Place sterile gloves on both hands.	The sterility of gloved hands should be maintained by following strict aseptic techniques.
Connect the injection port to the T-port and preload them with heparinized saline.	Only saline without preservatives should be used in neonatal foals.
Partially remove the stylet from the catheter, then replace it.	Make sure the stylet slides easily in and out of the catheter.
Flush the catheter/stylet with heparinized saline.	Having heparinized saline in the lumen of the stylet will allow easy observation of blood flashback during placement of the catheter.
Hold the catheter with the dominant hand, while using the back of the contralateral hand to hold off the vein caudal to the insertion site.	Use the knuckles and the back of the hand to occlude the vein, so that the fingertips can remain sterile.
Once the vein is filled and visualized, the catheter should be firmly introduced through the skin with the bevel facing the operator.	Alternatively, a small stab incision can be made through the skin to facilitate penetration through the skin (i.e., to avoid skin drag or resistance).
Advance the catheter into the vein at a 30–45° angle (Figure 53.2).	Wait for appearance of blood flashback and then slowly advance the catheter while the stylet remains stationary in place. Once the catheter is completely inserted into the vein, remove and discard the stylet.
Attach the T-port to the catheter. Aspirate blood for confirmation of placement within the vein and flush the catheter with heparinized saline, then clamp off the T-port.	To confirm correct placement, aspirate the blood back with a syringe.

Technical action	Rationale
Suture the catheter to the skin.	It is important to securely anchor the catheter to the skin to prevent movement or dislodgement of catheter.
Once the catheter and extension set are secured, cover the catheter with a sterile bandage if the catheter will be used for more than a few hours.	The bandage will protect the catheter and keep the site clean. Note that some types of bedding (shavings, rice hulls, etc.) may get under the bandage if it is not stuck to the skin with an adhesive-type bandage. Note that the neck bandage should not be tight and should not bunch up under the throat latch.
Proper catheter care is essential in the neonatal foals.	For proper catheter care see section 53.9 (page 471).

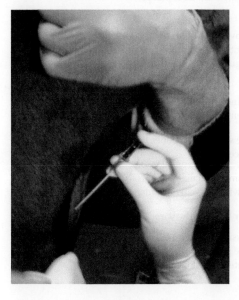

Figure 53.2 Placement of an over-the-needle catheter into the jugular vein of a neonatal foal.

53.8 Procedure: Placement of an Over-the-wire Catheter

Technical action	Rationale
Set up an area to open the sterile materials, including sterile gloves, scalpel blade (#15), sterile 4″ × 4″ gauze, and the catheter kit. Ensure that all materials are kept under strict sterile technique.	The components for an over-the-wire catheter are depicted in Figure 53.3.
Put on two pairs of sterile gloves. Double gloving allows for removal of exterior gloves after placement of the introducer needle or introducer catheter, and prior to placement of the wire and the actual over-the-wire catheter.	Double gloving will allow the catheter and all components to be placed aseptically.
Use a #15 scalpel blade to make a stab incision through skin at the site where the local anesthetic block was placed. The skin should be tented for the stab incision, to prevent inadvertent damage to the underlying vein.	A stab incision through the skin will prevent the catheter from dragging through the skin and will facilitate catheter placement.
Flush the introducer needle/catheter (included in the catheter kit) with heparinized saline.	Only saline without preservatives should be used in neonatal foals.

(continued)

Technical action	Rationale
Hold the introducer needle/catheter in the dominant hand while using the contralateral hand to occlude the vein caudal to the insertion site.	Use the knuckles and the back of the hand to occlude the vein so that the fingertips can remain sterile.
Once the vein is filled and visualized, advance the introducer needle/catheter through the stab incision and pierce through the vein wall with the bevel facing the operator (Figure 53.4).	The stab incision through the skin facilitates penetration of the catheter into the vein so much less force is necessary for introduction of the catheter. Short, guarded movements should be used for catheter insertion into vein.
Advance the introducer needle/catheter into the vein at a 30–45° angle with the bevel facing the operator, and wait for blood flashback.	If using an introduction catheter, remove the stylet once the catheter is placed.
Once the introducer needle or catheter is placed, remove the outer pair of sterile gloves (after the vein is held off). Care should be taken to not allow air to enter the introducer needle or catheter.	Removal of the outer gloves will decrease the chance of contamination during the placement of the J-wire (i.e., guide wire) and the catheter.
Advance the J-wire through the introducer needle/catheter into the vein (Figure 53.5).	One hand should always hold onto the wire to prevent it from escaping into the vein.
Remove the introducer needle/catheter from the vein while leaving the wire in place.	Make sure the wire does not touch any non-sterile surface.
Advance the vein expander over the wire and into the vein (Figure 53.6).	Use small, circular motions to penetrate the skin and vein with the vein expander.
Once the vein expander has entered the vein it should be removed. After removal of the vein expander, the catheter should be threaded over the wire and advanced into the vein while the wire is held in place (Figure 53.7). Note: To feed the catheter over the guide wire, first advance the wire up to the hub of the catheter. Next, while continuing to hold onto the guide wire with one hand, the other hand advances the catheter into the vein.	Never let go of the wire. If possible and necessary, an assistant, wearing sterile gloves, can help the advancement of the catheter over the guide wire.
Once the hub of the catheter is snug against the skin the wire should be withdrawn.	
To confirm correct placement, aspirate blood back with a syringe. Attach the injection port and flush the catheter with heparinized saline.	If using a double or triple lumen catheter, remember to aspirate and flush all lumens. Make sure air bubbles are not introduced when flushing the catheter.
Clamp the T-port and suture the catheter to the skin (Figure 53.8).	It is important to securely anchor the catheter to the skin to avoid any movement or dislodgement of the catheter.
Once the catheter and extension set are secured, cover the catheter with a bandage. Sterile gauze should be placed over the catheter site and an elastic adherent bandage applied over the site (Figure 53.9).	This can add protection to the catheter site and will aid in keeping it clean. Note that some types of bedding (shavings, rice hulls, etc.) may get under the bandage if it is not stuck to the skin.
Proper catheter care is essential in the critically ill foal.	Compromised neonates are more likely to encounter catheter-related problems. For proper catheter care see section 53.9 (page 471).

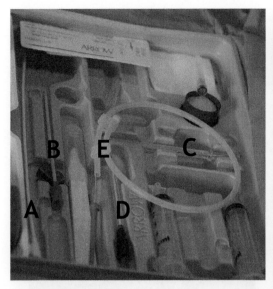

Figure 53.3 Components for an over-the-wire catheter.

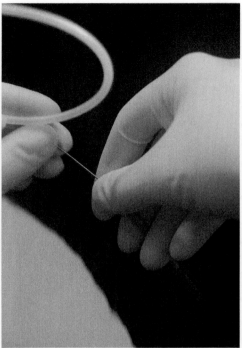

Figure 53.5 After retracting the guidewire into the plastic housing to straighten the tip, attach the plastic housing of the "J" guidewire to the hub of the introducer, and pass the guidewire into the vein.

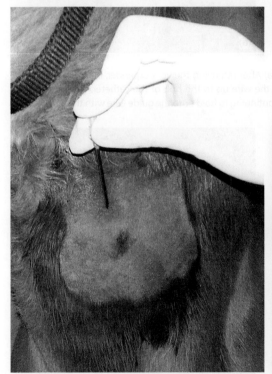

Figure 53.4 Placement of the over-the-wire catheter into the left jugular vein: at the site of the insertion a bleb of local anesthetic was placed subcutaneously, followed by a stab incision with #15 scalpel blade, and the introducer is about to be inserted through the stab incision. Note the bevel of the introducer facing the operator. Courtesy of Dr. Aloisio Bueno.

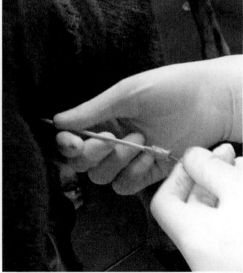

Figure 53.6 After removing the introducer from the vein, remove the plastic housing from the guidewire, leaving out at least 10 cm of guidewire. Insert the vein expander over the wire and advance it into the vein, using gentle, small circular motions.

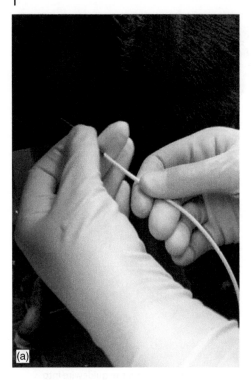
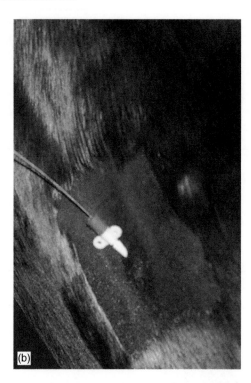

Figure 53.7 Placement of the catheter over the wire: (a) After removing the vein expander, insert the tip of the catheter over the end of the guidewire, and pull back the wire up to the hub of the catheter. (b) Advance the catheter all the way into the vein with one hand, while continuing to hold onto the guide wire with the other hand.

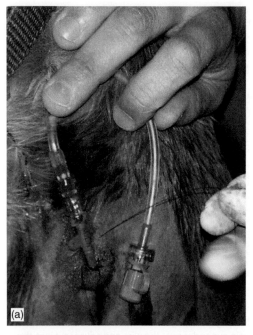
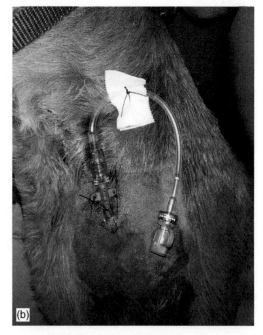

Figure 53.8 Secure the intravenous catheter. (a) Place skin sutures at the appropriate sites (on each wing and an additional suture below the wings of the catheter around the hub and position it in the little grove midway along the hub of the catheter). (b) Catheter completely secured to the skin. Courtesy of Dr. Aloisio Bueno.

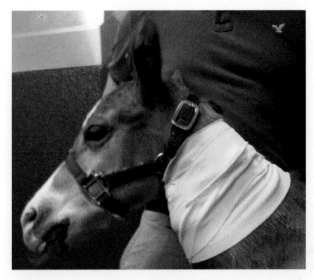

Figure 53.9 Place a bandage over the catheter site. The bandage consists of sterile gauze and an elastic adherent tape (e.g., Elastikon). Courtesy of Dr. Aloisio Bueno.

53.9 Procedure: Catheter Care and Maintenance

Technical action	Rationale
1. Wipe the injection cap with a disinfectant (e.g., 70% alcohol) prior to injecting any solution.	1. Disinfection of the injection port is recommended to minimize bacterial contamination.
2. Flush the indwelling catheter every 6 hours with heparinized saline (the volume of heparinized saline flush will depend on the size of the extension set and number of ports).	2. Flushing the catheter periodically with heparinized saline is necessary to prevent the formation of a clot in the catheter. If solutions do not flow through the catheter easily, do not force them. Check for possible mechanical damage to the catheter (twisting, bending, etc.) or evidence of thrombus formation.
3. Change the injection cap every 24–48 hours.	3. Replacing the injection cap on a regular basis helps to reduce the introduction of bacteria into the catheter and extension set.
4. The catheter site should be checked frequently (preferably twice daily) for swelling and heat.	4. If swelling of the vein or subcutaneous tissues or heat at the insertion site is noted, the catheter should be removed.
5. Proper catheter care is essential in the critically ill foal. The catheter should be checked daily for swelling, thrombi formation, and infection.	5. Compromised neonates are more likely to encounter catheter-related problems, especially if they are septic and hypercoagulable.
6. If infection, phlebitis, or thrombosis is suspected, the catheter should be removed.	6. If the catheter is removed using sterile technique, the tip can be cut with sterile scissors and placed into a sterile container for culture.

Bibliography Further Reading

Corley, K. (2008) Procedures in the neonatal foal, in *The Equine Hospital Manual* (eds K.Corley and J.Stephen), Blackwell, Oxford, pp. 120–146.

Knottenbelt, D., Holdstock, N., and Madigan, J. (2004) *Equine Neonatology Medicine and Surgery*, W.B. Saunders, Edinburgh.

Koterba, A.M., Drummond, W.H., and Kosch, P.C. (1990) *Equine Clinical Neonatology*, Lea and Febiger, Philadelphia.

Madigan, J.E. (2016) *Manual of Equine Neonatal Medicine*, Live Oak Publishing, Woodland CA

Orsisni, J.A. and Divers T.J. (2014) *Equine Emergencies: Treatments and Procedures*, 4th edn, Elsevier, St. Louis.

54

Intraosseus Needle Placement in the Neonatal Foal

Nóra Nógrádi and K. Gary Magdesian

54.1 Purpose

- Placement of an intraosseus (IO) needle or catheter can provide a non-collapsible entry point into the venous system when venous access is impossible. The IO route may be used for fluid therapy or administration of intravenous medications when venous access is unavailable.
- IO fluid administration is an alternative to the intravascular route and is usually reserved for emergency situations (severe dehydration, hypovolemic shock) when attempts at venous catheterization have been unsuccessful.

54.2 Complications

- Failure to follow aseptic technique can result in local infection.
- Extravasation of fluid into the interstitium can ensue if the needle is misplaced or becomes dislodged. This can occur during needle placement or even with a properly placed needle due to excessive movement of the foal, with subsequent dislodgement.
- Hemorrhage
- Periosteal reaction

54.3 Equipment Required

- Clippers
- Antiseptics (disinfectants) for surgical preparation
- Local anesthetic solution (e.g., 2% lidocaine or 1% mepivacaine)
- #15 scalpel blade
- Heparinized saline (without preservatives)
- Bone insertion device: #4 Steinman pin with a Jacob chuck (Figure 54.1)
- Insertion/infusion device: bone marrow aspiration needle (e.g., Jamshidi bone marrow needle, GPC Medical Limited, or illinois sternal/iliac aspiration needle, Monojet) (Figure 54.2)
- 14- or 16-gauge 1.5″ needle
- IO catheter kit (e.g., 15-gauge 1.5″ (MILA International, Inc.) (Figure 54.3)
- IO infusion ports: IO infusion needle (e.g., 16-gauge 3 cm) or IO cannulated screw (Cook Medical) (Figure 54.4)
- Sterile bandage material

Manual of Clinical Procedures in the Horse, First Edition. Edited by Lais R.R. Costa and Mary Rose Paradis.
© 2018 John Wiley & Sons, Inc. Published 2018 by John Wiley & Sons, Inc.

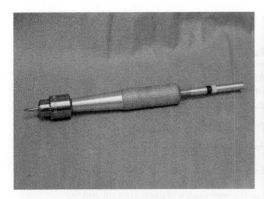

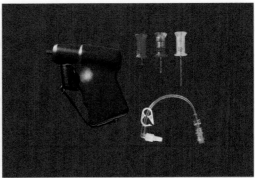

Figure 54.1 Steinmann pin #4 placed in the Jacob chuck. Courtesy of Dr. Lais R.R. Costa.

Figure 54.3 Example of an IO catheter kit, including stainless steel luer-lock catheters of various sizes. Courtesy of M. Zumdick, MILA International, Inc.

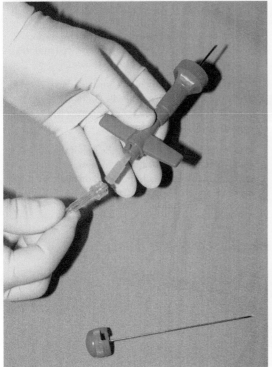

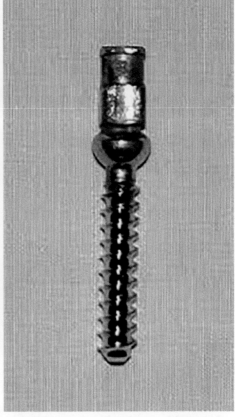

Figure 54.2 A bone marrow needle can be used for the IO infusion procedure. Illinois sternal/iliac aspiration needle with a Luer lock adapter included to facilitate attachment of fluid administration set. Courtesy of Dr. Lais R.R. Costa.

Figure 54.4 A cannulated screw that can be used for IO administration of fluid. Courtesy of Dr. Aloisio Bueno.

54.4 Restraint and Positioning

- Foals requiring IO fluid administration are usually recumbent and weak, therefore minimal restraint is necessary.

- The procedure is performed with the foal in lateral recumbency.

54.5 Procedure: Intraosseus Needle Placement in a Neonatal Foal

Technical action	Rationale
Choose the site for introduction of the IO infusion port. Medial aspect of the proximal tibia, approximately 3 cm distal to the tendinous band from the semitendinosus muscle.	Any of the long bones can be used, but the preferred site of large volume fluid administration in foals is the proximal tibia (Figure 54.5). Locate where the bone is only covered with skin. Avoid the cranial branch of the saphenous vein.
Clip and surgically prep the site.	Exercise strict aseptic technique for placement.
Inject 1–2 ml local anesthetic subcutaneously.	Local anesthetics will decrease pain and the subsequent movement of the foal during the procedure.
Perform a stab incision, penetrating the skin with a #15 scalpel blade.	This will allow the Steinmann pin or Jamshidi needle to directly contact the bone.
A #4 Steinmann pin and Jacobs chuck can be used to penetrate the cortex and the marrow cavity until a decrease in resistance is felt. The depth of penetration should be guarded so as to not enter the distal cortex. The Steinmann pin is then removed and a 16- or 15-gauge 1.5″ stainless steel IO cannula is placed.	Alternatively, a bone marrow biopsy or aspiration needle (e.g., Jamshidi needle) can be placed into the tibia after skin incision with a #15 blade. In newborn foals, particularly those that are premature, a hypodermic needle (14 or 16 gauge) can often be used to penetrate the cortex and to administer fluids or medications.
The IO infusion port should be flushed with heparinized saline and bandaged if left in place for repeated use.	Under normal circumstances, the use of the IO route of fluid administration is temporary. After initial fluid therapy is administered through the IO infusion, an intravenous catheter is placed and the IO catheter is removed.

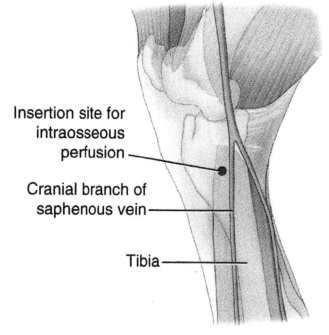

Insertion site for intraosseous perfusion

Cranial branch of saphenous vein

Tibia

Figure 54.5 The preferred site for placement of an IO catheter in the neonatal foal is in the medial side of the proximal tibia, approximately 3 cm distal to the tendinous band from the semitendinosus muscle. Levine (2013). Reproduced with permission of Elsevier.

Bibliography and Further Reading

Renee Golenz, M., Carlson, G.P., Madigan, J.E., and Craychee, T. (1993) Preliminary report: the development of an intraosseous infusion technique for neonatal foals. *Journal of Veterinary Internal Medicine*, 7 (6), 377–382.

Levine, D. (2013) Regional perfusion, intraosseous and resuscitation infusion techniques, in *Equine Emergencies: Treatments and Procedures*, 4th edn (eds Orsisni, J.A. and Divers, T.J.), Elsevier, St. Louis, pp. 16–18.

Madigan, J.E. (2016) *Manual of Equine Neonatal Medicine*, Live Oak Publishing, Woodland CA

55

Placement of a Nasal Insufflation Tube in the Neonatal Foal

Nóra Nógrádi and K. Gary Magdesian

55.1 Purpose

- Nasal insufflation of oxygen is used to treat hypoxemia in the compromised neonate.
- Hypoxemia is defined as a decreased partial pressure of oxygen (PaO_2 < 70–80 mmHg) resulting in decreased oxygen saturation of hemoglobin (SaO_2 < 92–95%).

55.2 Complications

- Inadvertent placement of the nasal cannula into the esophagus can result in severe gastrointestinal distension.
- Prolonged insufflation of high flow rates of 100% oxygen potentially could result in oxygen toxicity to the lungs.
- Lack of provision of humidification of insufflated gas can cause drying of airway mucous membranes.

55.3 Equipment Required

- Nasal cannula: small-diameter soft and smooth tube containing holes on the sides or:
  - a red rubber tube
  or
  - plastic feeding tube (Figure 55.1).
- Tubing with Christmas tree connectors (Figure 55.2)
- Humidifier bottle with sterile water (Figure 55.2)

- Oxygen source with a flowmeter:
  - oxygen tank
  or
  - in-house oxygen source (Figure 55.3).
- Adhesive tape
- Tongue depressor
- Suture material

55.4 Restraint and Positioning

- Standing or sternal recumbency.

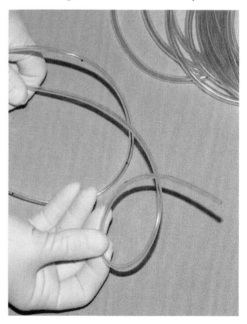

Figure 55.1 A cannula for nasal insufflation of oxygen to neonatal foals is a small-diameter soft, smooth tube such as a human nasogastric tube.

Manual of Clinical Procedures in the Horse, First Edition. Edited by Lais R.R. Costa and Mary Rose Paradis.
© 2018 John Wiley & Sons, Inc. Published 2018 by John Wiley & Sons, Inc.

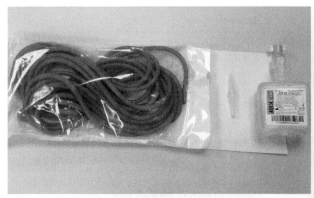

Figure 55.2 Oxygen delivery tubing and Christmas tree connector next to a bottle containing sterile water.

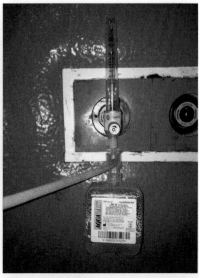

Figure 55.3 Humidifier bottle containing sterile water connected to the flowmeter attached to an oxygen wall unit.

55.5 Procedure: Placement of a Nasal Insufflation Tube

Technical action	Rationale
Before placement, measure the nasal cannula against the side of the face. It should be marked so that the tip of the cannula is at the level of the medial canthus of the eye through the ventral meatus (Figure 55.4).	Apply a ring of adhesive tape at the mark and preload the suture within this tape before placement of the cannula.
The nasal cannula/tube is passed ventrally and slightly medially through the ventral meatus of the nasal passage until the mark on the tube reaches the level of the nares.	This is similar to the passage of a nasogastric tube but the cannula should stop at the level of the nasopharynx.
Once the cannula is in place, attach it to a tape-covered tongue depressor or to elastic adhesive tape (Elastikon[a], Johnson & Johnson, New Brunswick, NJ) placed around the muzzle. Placement of wraps around the muzzle should be done over the level of the cranial aspect of the nasal bones (Figure 55.5).	Alternatively, the nasal insufflation tube can be secured directly to the foal's nostril using a suture. This will ensure that the tube does not slip when the tape becomes wet from nasal secretions.
Attach the cannula, through oxygen tubing, to the humidifier containing sterile water (Figure 55.6). The humidifier is in line with the flowmeter connected to the oxygen source.	Humidification helps to prevent drying of the mucous membranes.
Administer oxygen at a flow rate of 2–10 liters/minute (40-200 ml/kg/minute) depending on the degree of hypoxemia.	The lowest flow rate should be used that results in a PaO_2 of 80–100 mmHg. Higher oxygen tensions are potentially associated with oxygen toxicity if the lungs are exposed to a fraction of inspired oxygen (FIO_2) > 60% for prolonged periods.

(*continued*)

Technical action	Rationale
If hypercapnia is present concurrent to severe hypoxemia (PaO$_2$ < 60 mmHg) then mechanical ventilation with oxygen administration should be considered. An arterial or venous pH < 7.25 or deteriorating mentation is an indication for positive pressure ventilation in hypercapnic foals.	Hypercapnia can be a sign of respiratory distress and is the result of hypoventilation.
Clean the nasal cannula daily as it can become obstructed with mucus and dust.	The terminal end of the nasal cannula can be pulled out and replaced without removing the adhesive tape from the foal. Repetitive removal and reapplication of the adhesive tape is painful and can cause irritation to the foal's skin.

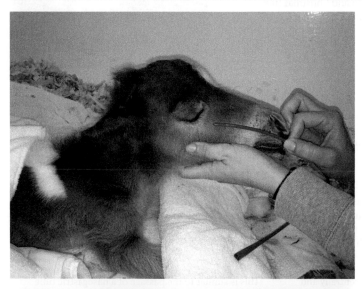

Figure 55.4 Measure the nasal cannula from the medial canthus of the eye to the nares of the foal and mark the tubing prior to inserting it into the nostril.

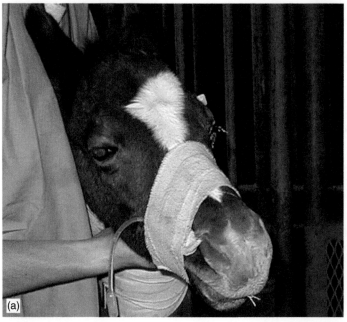

(a)

Figure 55.5 Nasal cannula placement. (a) Note the cannula is not sutured, instead it is anchored to the nostril using elastic adhesive tape and a tongue depressor (Courtesy of Dr. Lais R.R. Costa). (b) Foal receiving nasal oxygen insufflation (Courtesy of Dr. Lais R.R. Costa).

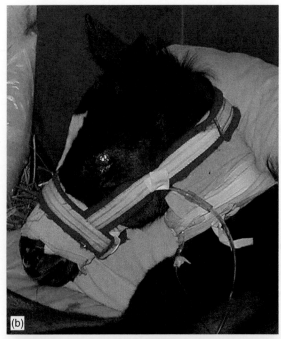

Figure 55.5 (Continued)

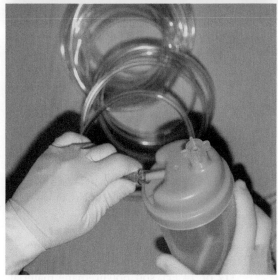

Figure 55.6 Connecting the tubing to the humidifier bottle.

Bibliography and Further Reading

Bedenice, D. (2006) Foal with septic pneumonia, in *Equine Neonatal Medicine: a Case-based Approach* (ed. M.R. Paradis), Elsevier, Philadelphia, pp. 101–111.

Koterba, A.M., Drummond, W.H., and Kosch, P.C. (1990) *Equine Clinical Neonatology*, Lea and Febiger, Philadelphia.

Madigan, J.E. (2016) *Manual of Equine Neonatal Medicine*, Live Oak Publishing, Woodland CA

McAuliffe, S.B. and Slovis, N.M. (2008) *Color Atlas of Disease and Disorders of the Foal*, W.B. Saunders, Edinburgh.

McKinnon, A.O., Squires, E.L., Vaala, W.E. and Varner, D.D. (2011) *Equine Reproduction*, 2nd edn, Wiley-Blackwell, Oxford.

Orsini, J.A. and Divers, T.J. (2007) *Equine Emergencies: Treatments and Procedures*, 3rd edn, W.B. Saunders, St. Louis.

Sanchez, L.C. (2005) *Veterinary Clinics of North America Equine Practice - Neonatal Medicine and Surgery*, W.B. Saunders, Philadelphia.

56

Placement of a Nasogastric Tube in the Neonatal Foal

Nóra Nógrádi and K. Gary Magdesian

56.1 Purpose

- To check for gastroduodenal reflux or residuals in foals with ileus or colic.
- To administer colostrum to foals ≤12 hours of age with failure or partial failure of passive transfer.
- To install an indwelling nasogastric tube for assisted enteral feeding.
- To bypass the pharynx in foals with transient pharyngeal paresis.
  - Nasogastric tube feeding may be required until the dysphagia resolves or the foal learns to pan feed.
  - If allowed to suckle foals with dysphagia can develop aspiration pneumonia.

56.2 Complications

- Nasogastric tube cannot enter the stomach: If severe gastric distension is present or with increased tone at the esophageal cardia, passage of the tube beyond the cardia may be difficult. This should not be mistaken for a lack of gastric reflux. In such cases, a small volume (about 3 ml) of lidocaine can be injected down the nasogastric tube to relax the cardiac sphincter and facilitate entry into the stomach.
- Nasogastric tube inadvertently placed in the trachea: As the coughing reflex is blunted in neonates, confirmation of nasogastric tube placement should always occur with palpation of the tube within the esophagus or radiographic confirmation of intragastric placement.
- Esophageal, nasal or gastric irritation or trauma: Foals in intensive care units may require long-term enteral feeding. In these cases, use of a small diameter and soft, compliant feeding tube can decrease the incidence of complications such irritation or trauma to the nasal passages, pharynx, esophagus, and stomach. Small tubes also allow foals to nurse with tubes in place as they recover and gain the strength and coordination to nurse.

56.3 Equipment Required

- Nasogastric tube for refluxing foal or one-time administration of oral medication or colostrum:
  - 24 Fr Harris flush tube (Covidien)
  - 18 Fr Levin stomach tube (Convidien)
  - Stallion urinary catheter
- Enteral feeding tube to be used as an indwelling stomach tube for frequent enteral feeding of a foal: small-diameter (12 or 14 Fr), soft polyurethane material with a radiopaque stylet and tip. Not practical to relieve large volumes of gastric reflux.
  - veterinary feeding tubes (MILA International, Inc.) (Figure 56.1a)
  - Flexiflo Enteral Feeding Tube (Abbott Laboratories).

Manual of Clinical Procedures in the Horse, First Edition. Edited by Lais R.R. Costa and Mary Rose Paradis.
© 2018 John Wiley & Sons, Inc. Published 2018 by John Wiley & Sons, Inc.

- Examination gloves
- Lubricating jelly
- Adhesive tape
- Suture material
- Gravity feeding set such as Kangaroo®
- Funnel or 60 ml syringe barrel to use as a funnel for fluid/milk administration.

56.4 Restraint and Positioning

- The foal should be restrained in a standing or sternally recumbent position. It is important to flex the neck to facilitate tube placement into the esophagus.
- With the application of proper restraint techniques, sedation is usually unnecessary for tube placement. Administration of light sedation can facilitate the procedure in fractious foals.

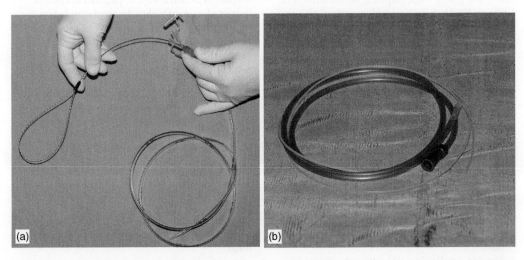

Figure 56.1 Types of tubes that can be used as nasogastric tubes for the foal: (a) veterinary feeding tube (MILA International, Inc.) and (b) stallion urinary catheter.

56.5 Procedure: Nasogastric Tube Placement in Neonatal Foals

Technical action	Rationale
Measure the approximate length required to reach the stomach and mark it on the tube before placement.	The location of the stomach can be estimated to be approximately two hand lengths behind the left elbow.
Apply a small amount of lubricating gel to the tip of the tube.	It is critical to apply lubricant to the stylet wire of the long-term, small-diameter flexible foal feeding tubes prior to insertion, otherwise it may be impossible to remove the stylet wire from the tube lumen once the tube is placed.
Gently advance the tube through the ventral meatus of the nares.	Make sure that the foal's head is in a flexed position.

(continued)

Technical action	Rationale
When using a large tube, resistance can be met at the pharynx.	In this case, wait until the foal swallows the tube, then gently stimulate the back of the pharynx by slowly twisting the tube. The tube should be advanced when the foal swallows.
When using a small-diameter feeding tube no resistance is typically felt. Generally the tube easily slides into the esophagus when the head is in the flexed position and once the foal swallows.	Waiting for the foal to swallow is a key step for successful placement of the nasogastric tube.
Once in the esophagus, continue to advance the tube slowly and gently, while palpating on the left side of lower neck with the other hand to confirm placement. If resistance is met, advancement of the tube should stop until the esophagus relaxes.	When using a large-diameter tube, the cervical esophagus should always be palpated to confirm correct placement within the esophagus before the tube reaches the thoracic inlet. When using a small diameter tube, palpation of the tip can be difficult, therefore additional methods are necessary to confirm proper placement, such as radiography.
If placement in the esophagus is confirmed, continue to advance the tube into the stomach.	It is preferable to place the tube into the stomach rather than the distal esophagus for enteral feeding. While this carries a small risk of gastric irritation, it allows the clinician to check for gastric reflux or residuals before feeding.
Confirmation of correct placement: • Palpation of the tube within the cervical esophagus. • Characteristic gastric smell and bubbling sounds are present on entering the stomach. • Gastric contents can be aspirated via the nasogastric tube. • Blowing (small volumes) on the tube results in bubbling sounds auscultated over the cranial abdomen on the left side. However, this should never be relied on solely to confirm placement. • If aspirating on the tube results in negative pressure the tube is probably in the esophagus, but this should never be relied on solely to confirm placement. A kink in the tube will also produce negative pressure. • The radiopaque stylet and tip of the feeding tube can be visualized caudal to the diaphragm by thoracic radiography (Figure 56.2).	It is critical to confirm the correct location before anything is administered through the nasogastric tube. Intubation of the trachea will result in direct placement of milk or fluid into the trachea and lungs. If blowing on the tube is to be performed, care should be taken to not blow large volumes of air into the stomach. Thoracic radiography and visualization of the tube is the most definitive means of confirming correct tube placement, especially when using small-diameter, soft long-term feeding tubes.
Anchoring the tube to the nose can be done either with adhesive tape (Figure 56.3a) or through suturing the tube to the nostril (Figure 56.3b).	Because there is a potential for the tube to slip through the tape, a Chinese finger trap suture can be used to secure the tube to the nostril as well.
Always check for gastric reflux or residuals before administration of anything through the nasogastric tube.	Neonatal foals, especially those with obtundation, may not exhibit colic signs with accumulation of gastric reflux.
Always use gravity flow when administering liquids through the nasogastric tube (Figure 56.4a,b).	The barrel of a 60 ml syringe can be used as a funnel for administering fluids (Figure 56.4c). For feeding, a "kangaroo bag" is handy and contained, so you don't become covered with milk as the foal moves (Figure 56.4d).
Finish the procedure by rinsing the tube with a small volume of water.	Any residue left in the tube has the potential to plug it, requiring replacement.

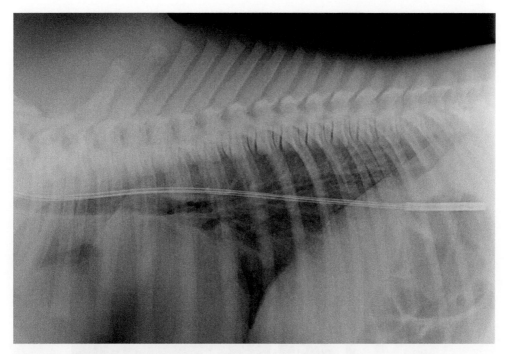

Figure 56.2 Radiographic confirmation of correct positioning of a feeding tube.

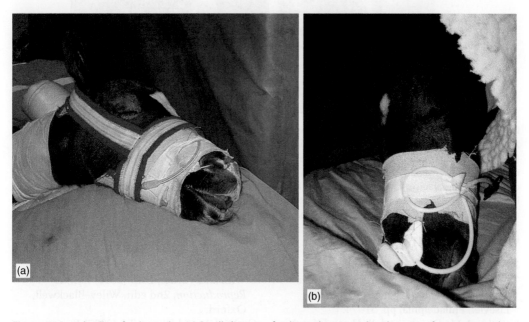

Figure 56.3 Indwelling feeding tube. (a) Small-diameter feeding tube secured to the nose of a neonate with elastic adhesive tape (Courtesy of Dr. Lais R.R. Costa). (b) Small-diameter feeding tube sutured to the nose in a neonate.

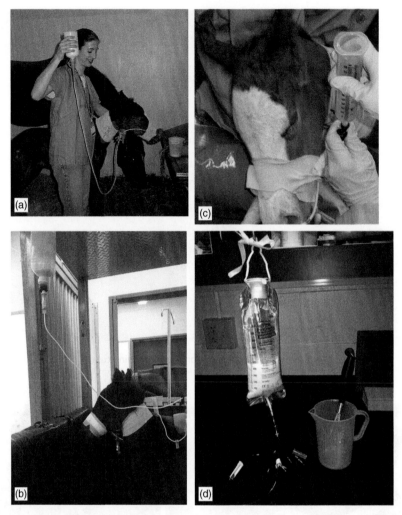

Figure 56.4 When feeding the neonate via the nasogastric tube, administer milk or fluid using gravity flow. (a) Administration of milk to an ambulatory neonate via a feeding tube using a funnel (Courtesy of Dr. Lais R.R. Costa). (b) Administration of milk to an ambulatory neonate via a feeding tube using a closed system. (c) A 60 ml syringe is used as a funnel to administer milk via a feeding tube with gravity flow. (d) "Kangaroo Gravity Set" (Courtesy of Dr. Mary Rose Paradis). Administration using a closed system is handy in foals that are ambulating, especially if feeding larger volumes of milk, because the milk is contained so the feeding can be done easily and without assistance, and the milk will not spill all over the foal and the care taker.

Bibliography and Further Reading

Buechner-Maxwell, V. (2006) Neonatal nutrition, in *Equine Neonatal Medicine: a Case-based Approach* (ed. M.R. Paradis), Elsevier, Philadelphia, pp. 51–74.

Koterba, A.M., Drummond, W.H., and Kosch, P.C. (1990) *Equine Clinical Neonatology*, Lea and Febiger, Philadelphia.

Madigan, J.E. (2016) *Manual of Equine Neonatal Medicine*, Live Oak Publishing, Woodland CA

McAuliffe, S.B. and Slovis, N.M. (2008) *Color Atlas of Disease and Disorders of the Foal*, W.B. Saunders, Edinburgh.

McKinnon, A.O., Squires, E.L., Vaala, W.E. and Varner, D.D. (2011) *Equine Reproduction*, 2nd edn, Wiley-Blackwell, Oxford.

Orsini, J.A. and Divers, T.J. (2007) *Equine Emergencies: Treatments and Procedures*, 3rd edn, W.B. Saunders, St. Louis.

Sanchez, L.C. (2005) *Veterinary Clinics of North America Equine Practice - Neonatal Medicine and Surgery*, W.B. Saunders, Philadelphia.

57

Administration of Enema in the Neonatal Foal

Nóra Nógrádi and K. Gary Magdesian

57.1 Purposes

- To aid in the elimination of meconium and prevention of meconium impaction in high-risk neonatal foals. Meconium is the first fecal material of the neonatal foal, which is normally passed during the first few hours of birth. It is light to dark brown in color and has a firm and tarry consistency.
- To treat meconium impaction. Meconium can be retained in the rectum, small colon or large colon, resulting in signs of straining and abdominal discomfort associated with meconium retention or impaction.
- To maintain regular bowel movements in recumbent, hospitalized neonatal foals. Critically ill foals tend to have decreased gastrointestinal motility and frequently become constipated.

57.2 Complications

- Irritation of the rectal mucosa with repeated enemas
- Perforation of the rectal mucosa with improper technique

57.3 Equipment Required

For single enema
- Soapy water enema using gentle soap such as Ivory soap or commercial pediatric enema (e.g., Fleet enema, CBFleet Co., Lynchburg, VA)
- Soft tube with smooth, rounded, non-traumatic tip. Types of tube commonly used include:

  - red rubber feeding tube, 10–18 Fr (Sovereign Feeding Tube, Tyco Health Care, Kendall, Mansfield, MA)
  - Harris® flush tube (24 Fr), which is usually adequate for neonatal foals of most standard sized breeds
- Lubricating jelly
- 60 ml catheter tip syringe or funnel
- 300–500 ml lukewarm water or physiological saline and Ivory soap (Procter & Gamble, Cincinnati, OH)
- Alternative: enema bag with attached tubing

For retention enema
- 30 Fr Foley® catheter (Figure 57.1).
- 200 ml 4% acetylcysteine solution (e.g., 40 ml Mucomyst 20% acetylcysteine solution added to 160 ml water).
- Syringe to inflate balloon

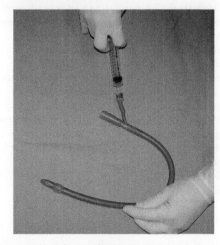

Figure 57.1 Foley® catheter size 30 Fr is adequate for neonates of most standard sized breeds.

Manual of Clinical Procedures in the Horse, First Edition. Edited by Lais R.R. Costa and Mary Rose Paradis.
© 2018 John Wiley & Sons, Inc. Published 2018 by John Wiley & Sons, Inc.

57.4 Restraint and Positioning

- For regular soapy enemas the foal can be restrained either standing or in lateral recumbency.
- For a retention enema, the foal needs to be sedated (diazepam 0.05–0.2 mg/kg IV; in some cases low doses of butorphanol may be necessary in conjunction with diazepam 0.01–0.02 mg/kg, IV; see Chapter 9) and placed in lateral recumbency with the hind end slightly elevated with a pillow or pad.

57.5 Procedure: Administration of Enema in the Neonatal Foal

Technical action	Rationale
Single, standard enema Pediatric human single-use enemas can be used once or twice. Repeated use can result in hyperphosphatemia. The lubricated tip is gently passed into the anus, and half of the volume is administered at a time (for a 45–50 kg foal).	The bottle should be gently squeezed to administer half of the volume to an average-sized foal.
Soapy water enema Lubricate the enema tube with copious amounts of lubricating jelly.	Adequate lubrication is needed to minimize trauma to the rectum.
Slowly and gently advance the enema tube into the rectum to 2–4″ as long as no resistance is met.	Stop if any resistance is met.
Start administration of enema fluid (lukewarm water with Ivory soap) with passive gravity flow, using a funnel, or a 60 ml catheter tip syringe without the plunger (Figure 57.2), or an enema bag. The enema fluid must not be forced into the rectum.	Never force fluid into the rectum with active administration. If the fluid is not flowing with gravity flow the tube is either obstructed or fecal material is present. Reposition or back the tube slightly and try again.
Retention enema - Administer sedation and place the foal in lateral recumbency with the hind end slightly elevated. - Lubricate the Foley catheter and slowly advance as far as possible as long as the catheter is not met with resistance. - Slowly inflate the balloon on the catheter and administer acetylcysteine solution with gravity flow. The balloon should not be overfilled, rather only inject enough air until there is slight back pressure noted. - Maintain enema, with solution inside rectum, for approximately 45 minutes (Figure 57.3). - Before removing the Foley catheter, deflate the balloon. - Remove the catheter. - Recover the foal.	Retention enemas are indicated in foals with meconium impactions that are non-responsive to one or two routine soapy water enemas. Management of a meconium impaction is primarily medical, including the administration of intravenous fluids, soapy and retention enemas, prophylactic antimicrobials, and anti-inflammatory/ analgesic medications. Small volumes of mineral oil can be administered intragastrically long as there is no gastric reflux or residuals. In rare cases where medical management is unrewarding surgical exploration may be necessary.

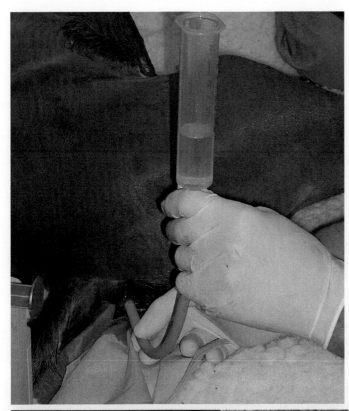

Figure 57.2 A soapy water enema being administered to a neonatal foal. Note that a 60 ml syringe is used as a funnel to administer an enema with gravity flow.

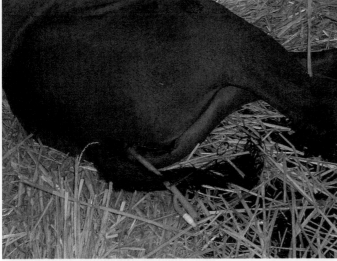

Figure 57.3 Foley® catheter placed into the rectum of a sedated foal for administration of retention enema with 4% acetylcysteine solution.

Bibliography and Further Reading

Knottenbelt, D., Holdstock, N., and Madigan, J. (2004) *Equine Neonatology Medicine and Surgery*, W.B. Saunders, Edinburgh.

Koterba, A.M., Drummond, W.H., and Kosch, P.C. (1990) *Equine Clinical Neonatology*, Lea and Febiger, Philadelphia.

Madigan, J.E. (2016) *Manual of Equine Neonatal Medicine*, Live Oak Publishing, Woodland CA

58

Arthrocentesis and Joint Lavage in the Neonatal Foal

Nóra Nógrádi and K. Gary Magdesian

58.1 Purpose

- To collect synovial fluid for the evaluation of joint effusion in the neonatal foal.
- Septic arthritis is associated with the development of periarticular edema and effusion of the affected joint (Figure 58.1). Septic arthritis, osteomyelitis, or physitis should be ruled out in any foal with joint effusion or lameness.
- Septic arthritis in foals should be considered an emergency. Prognosis depends on timely diagnosis through synovial fluid analysis and institution of a treatment plan consisting of administration of systemic and local broad-spectrum antimicrobials and joint lavage. Arthroscopy may be indicated in joints with large amounts of fibrin.
- To perform joint lavage after diagnosis of septic arthritis.

58.2 Complications

- Displacement of the needle during a joint lavage can result in periarticular fluid accumulation.
- Complications associated with sedation or anesthesia.

58.3 Equipment Required

- Clippers
- Sterile preparation material (disinfectants/antiseptics)
- Sterile gloves
- Sterile needles and syringes:
  - for arthrocentesis: 20-gauge 1″ needle, 3 ml syringes
  - for joint lavage: 14–18-gauge 1-1.5″ needles
- Tubes/vials for collection of joint fluid sample:
  - EDTA evacuated tubes (purple top) for fluid analysis (including total nucleated cell count, protein and cytologic evaluation)
  - heparin evacuated tubes (green top) for chemistry analysis (lactate and glucose concentrations and pH)
  - serum evacuated tubes (red top) for culture and susceptibility testing
  - blood culture vials

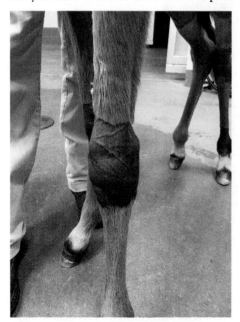

Figure 58.1 Swollen carpal joint in a neonatal foal. Note the periarticular edema and effusion of the radial carpal and intercarpal joints (courtesy of Dr. Lais R.R. Costa).

Manual of Clinical Procedures in the Horse, First Edition. Edited by Lais R.R. Costa and Mary Rose Paradis.

- Lactated Ringer's solution
- Fluid administration set
- Antimicrobial drug to be injected into the joint. Concentration-dependent antimicrobial drugs, such as amikacin, are recommended.
- Sterile gauze and bandage material
- Refractometer (optional)

58.4 Restraint and Positioning

- For both arthrocentesis and joint lavage the foal should be placed in lateral recumbency (Figure 58.2).
- Arthrocentesis can be performed with the foal under heavy sedation and placed in lateral recumbency (see Chapter 9).
- For joint lavage, it is recommended that the foal is placed under short-term general anesthesia (see Chapter 76).

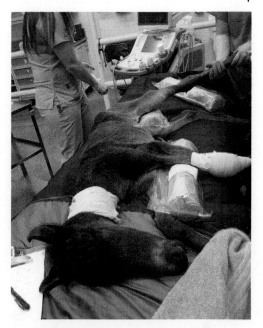

Figure 58.2 A foal is placed in lateral recumbency for arthrocentesis and joint lavage (courtesy of Dr. Lais R.R. Costa).

58.5 Procedure: Arthrocentesis in the Neonatal Foal

Technical action	Rationale
Once joint effusion has been identified, the foal should be prepared for arthrocentesis from each affected joint. Joint fluid should be submitted for cytology and culture.	Restrain the foal (heavy sedation or general anesthesia). Clip and perform aseptic preparation (Figure 58.3). See Chapter 10 for the principles of aseptic technique.
See Chapter 29 for a description of approaches to different joints.	It is fairly easy to perform arthrocentesis in effusive joints.
Collect the synovial fluid using strict sterile technique.	See Figure 58.4.
Once a sample of synovial fluid has been obtained it should be placed into: • an evacuated tube containing EDTA (purple top) • an evacuated tube containing heparin (green top) • an evacuated tube without additive (red top tube) • a blood culture bottle (containing enrichment media).	Make sure you collect enough synovial fluid for the tests needed. Use small evacuated tubes.
Stall side tests that can be performed at the time of arthrocentesis include: • visual inspection for gross turbidity (Figure 58.5a) • total protein measurement using a refractometry (Figure 58.5b) • a viscosity check by testing the "stringiness" of the fluid between two fingers (Figure 58.5c).	These stall side test are helpful to give you an idea if the joint is septic or not: • the fluid should be light amber and clear (no turbidity) • total protein should be less than 2.5 g/dl • When placed between two fingers synovial fluid should string between them as the fingers are separated (increased inflammation in a joint causes the synovial fluid to become less viscous or watery).

(continued)

Technical action	Rationale
The appropriate samples should be submitted for each test: • EDTA (purple top): for fluid analysis (including cell count, total protein, and cytologic evaluation) • heparin (green top): for glucose and lactate concentrations • no additive (red top): for microbial culture and sensitivity • blood culture bottle: for microbial culture and sensitivity	If there is not enough fluid in the EDTA tube, at least a cytologic evaluation should be performed. To improve the likelihood of microbial culture, an aliquot of synovial fluid (typically 3 to 5 ml) should be placed in a blood culture bottle and incubated.
Normal synovial fluid should have (sample submitted in an EDTA tube): • total protein concentration less than 2.5 g/dl • total nucleated cell count of >2,000 cells/μl • cell type predominantly (greater than 90%) mononuclear cells, that is, lymphocytes and macrophages, while neutrophils less than 10%.	Synovial fluid analysis is suggestive of a septic process when: • the total protein concentration is >2.5 g/dl • the total nucleated cell (leukocyte) count is >10,000 cells/μl • cell type distribution is predominantly (greater than 90%) neutrophils. The higher these numbers, the more likely that sepsis is present. Cytologic evidence of degeneration within neutrophils or the presence of bacteria is diagnostic of sepsis.
Normal synovial fluid should have (sample submitted in heparin tube): • glucose: should be similar to that in venous blood sample for that foal at the same sampling time • lactate: is usually similar to that in the venous blood obtained at the same time, however hemoarthrosis can increase the lactate.	Joint fluid with a low glucose and high lactate concentration, as compared to plasma concentrations, is also compatible with sepsis, although hemarthrosis can produce similar results.

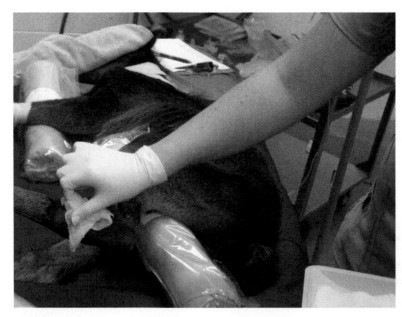

Figure 58.3 Preparation for arthrocentesis: the area is clipped, and an aseptic surgical preparation is performed (courtesy of Dr. Lais R.R. Costa).

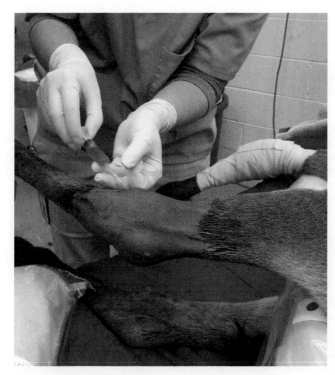

Figure 58.4 Collection of synovial fluid using strict sterile technique. Using a 20-gauge needle the plunger of the syringe is pulled gently (courtesy of Dr. Lais R.R. Costa).

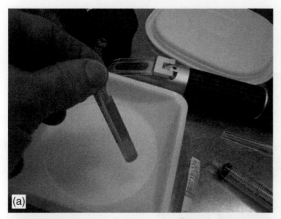

(a)

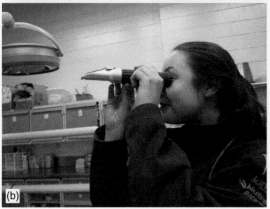

(b)

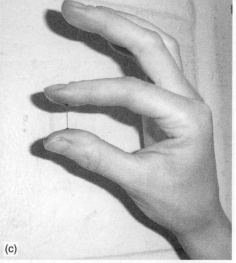

(c)

Figure 58.5 Stall side tests performed at the time of arthrocentesis include: (a) visual inspection for gross turbidity (courtesy of Dr. Lais R.R. Costa), (b) total protein measurement using a refractometry (courtesy of Dr. Lais R.R. Costa), and (c) viscosity of the synovial fluid. Normal synovial fluid should be viscous (courtesy of Dr. Mary Rose Paradis).

58.6 Procedure: Joint Lavage in the Neonatal Foal

Technical action	Rationale
Joint lavage begins with an arthrocentesis of the affected joint(s). Lavage should be performed using 14- or 16-gauge needles.	The large-bore needles allow for lavage using large volumes of fluid through the joint.
Once the joint has been entered, a fluid administration set connected to a bag of sterile lactate Ringer's solution is attached to the entry needle. The fluid should be allowed to flow slowly by gravity, distending the joint more fully. A second needle is then placed on the side opposite the entry point for through and through lavage.	By further distending the joint it is easier to place a second needle. The second needle will become the point for fluid exit to accomplish through and through lavage.
Fluid should flow freely from the exit needle (Figure 58.6).	For large joints a liter or more of fluid should be used to thoroughly lavage the joint. For smaller joints, such as a fetlock, smaller amounts can be used. The joint should be lavaged until the egress fluid is clear.
Intermittent distention of the joint by covering the exit needle hub with a sterile, gloved finger is helpful in ensuring lavage fluid reaches all areas of the joint.	Fibrin accumulation can block the needle and decrease the lavage rate.
Intra-articular antimicrobials can be injected at the end of the lavage before the exit needle is removed.	Intra-articular antibiotics increase the local concentration of antimicrobials.
Following the lavage, the joint should be bandaged with sterile bandage material.	Bandaging will help to prevent joint contamination from the needle holes.

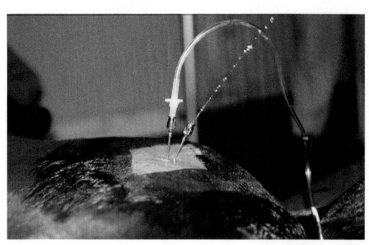

Figure 58.6 Through and through joint lavage of the coxofemoral joint in a neonatal foal. The first needle is used for arthrocentesis of the hip joint, then a fluid administration set is attached to the first needle and a second needle is placed for fluid exit. Note the fluid flowing freely from the exit needle. Courtesy of Dr. Aloisio Bueno.

Bibliography and Further Reading

Paradis, M.R. (2006) Manifestation of sepsis; foal with septic arthritis, in *Equine Neonatal Medicine: a Case-based Approach* (ed. M.R.Paradis), Elsevier, Philadelphia, pp. 112–120.

Madigan, J.E. (2016) *Manual of Equine Neonatal Medicine*, Live Oak Publishing, Woodland CA

59

Regional Limb Perfusion in the Neonatal Foal

Mary Rose Paradis

59.1 Purpose

- Administration of antimicrobial drug to a vein in the distal limb for delivering a high concentration of the antimicrobial to infected synovial lining or bone in the lower limb of foals with septic arthritis/osteomyelitis.

59.2 Complications

- Thrombosis of the vein that is utilized for the administration of the antimicrobial due to multiple applications.

- Subcutaneous leakage of the antimicrobial drug if the catheter is dislodged due to movement.

59.3 Equipment Required

- Supplies for sterile preparation of site of catheter placement.

- Small caliber, short, over-the-needle intravenous catheter (recommended size is 18-gauge, 2").

- Esmarch bandage

- Tourniquet: a pneumatic tourniquet (Figure 59.1) is preferable but a smaller Esmarch bandage can be used.

- Antimicrobial drug diluted in 20–30 ml of sterile saline. Concentration-dependent antimicrobial drugs, such as gentamicin or amikacin, are most effective and, therefore, preferable.

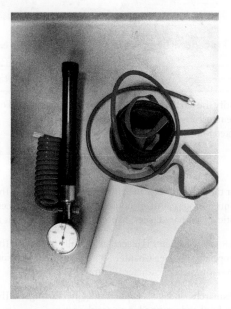

Figure 59.1 Esmarch bandage (light blue) and pneumatic tourniquet (VBM, Germany).

59.4 Restraint and Positioning

- The foal should be anesthetized due to the length of the procedure. This can be accomplished using gas anesthesia or injectable drugs such as valium-ketamine combination or propofol as a constant rate infusion or intermittent injections (Figure 59.2) (see Chapter 76).

- The foal should be placed in lateral recumbency with the affected leg down so that the catheter can be placed in the saphenous or cephalic vein depending on the target joint/bone.

Manual of Clinical Procedures in the Horse, First Edition. Edited by Lais R.R. Costa and Mary Rose Paradis.
© 2018 John Wiley & Sons, Inc. Published 2018 by John Wiley & Sons, Inc.

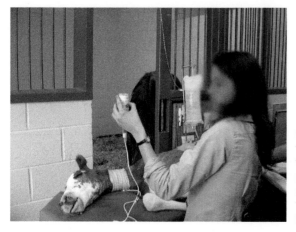

Figure 59.2 Short-term anesthesia is required for regional limb perfusion in foals. Neonatal foal is receiving propofol intravenously in preparation for the regional limb perfusion procedure. Note the placement of a nasal tracheal tube as a precaution for any respiratory problems secondary to anesthesia.

59.5 Procedure: Regional Limb Perfusion in the Neonatal Foal

Technical action	Rationale
Identify the site for the intravenous catheter placement. The catheter is placed above the affected joint.	For instance: • if the hock is affected, the catheter would be placed in the saphenous vein • if the carpus is affected the catheter would be placed in the cephalic vein.
After the foal has been anesthetized, the site for the intravenous catheter should be clipped and aseptically prepared (see Chapter 10).	The site of introduction of the catheter should be in the center of the prepared area. Rigorous aseptic technique is required for catheter placement.
An 18-gauge catheter is placed aseptically in the appropriate vein. See Chapter 53 for placement of an over-the-needle catheter (Figure 59.3).	The catheter should be secured with dental glue or suture material.
An Esmarch bandage is applied snuggly, starting at the hoof and wrapped in an overlapping manner proximally up to the catheter site.	The compressive Esmarch should be tight enough to push the blood from the venous system of the leg.
Apply the tourniquet (either a pneumatic tourniquet or a smaller Esmarch bandage) to the leg just proximal to the catheter.	The tourniquet should be tight enough to abolish the pulse in the lower limb. If using a pneumatic tourniquet, the pressures should be approximately 200–300 mmHg.
The compressive Esmarch bandage is then released to just below the affected joint, for example the tarsus or carpus but left on the remaining lower limb.	By isolating the target joint, the antimicrobial drug delivery can be focused.
The antimicrobial drug of choice is diluted in 20–30 ml of sterile saline and injected into the venous system through the catheter under pressure and left for 20–30 minutes.	The antimicrobial drug delivered under pressure will diffuse from the venous system into the infected synovia or bone during this time and remain at high concentrations for a prolonged period of time. For instance, synovial fluid and bone concentration of gentamicin in post regional limb perfusion remained above minimum inhibitory concentration for 24 and 8 hours, respectively.
At the end of the 20–30 minutes the tourniquet, Esmarch bandage, and catheter are removed. A light bandage can be applied over the catheter site.	This procedure may need to be repeated multiple times and therefore it is important to minimize the trauma to the vein.

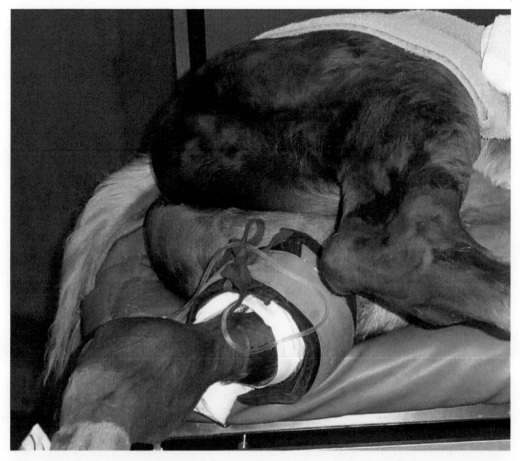

Figure 59.3 The intravenous catheter is placed proximal (above) to the affected joint and the tourniquet is placed proximal to the site of catheter placement.

Bibliography and Further Reading

Knottenbelt, D., Holdstock, N., and Madigan, J. (2004) *Equine Neonatology Medicine and Surgery*, W.B. Saunders, Edinburgh.

Levine, D. (2014) Regional perfusion, intraosseous and resuscitation infusion techniques, in *Equine Emergencies: Treatments and Procedures*, 4th edn (eds J.A. Orsisni and T.J. Divers), Elsevier, Philadelphia, pp. 16–18.

Paradis, M.R. (2006) Manifestations of septicemia: Foal with septic joint, in *Equine Neonatal Medicine: a Case-based Approach* (ed. M.R. Paradis), Elsevier, Philadelphia, pp. 112–120.

Werner, L.A., Hardy, J., and Bertone, A.L. (2003) Bone gentamicin concentration after intra-articular injection or regional intravenous perfusion in the horse. *Veterinary Surgery*, **32**, 559.

Watts, A.E. (2011) How to select cases and perform field technique for regional limb perfusion. *Proceedings of the AAEP Annual Convention*, San Antonio, USA, American Association of Equine Practitioners, Lexington, KY, pp. 385–392.

Part VII

Clinical Procedures by Body Systems: Urinary System

60

Urinary Catheterization of Adult Male Horses

Brett Sponseller and Beatrice Sponseller

60.1 Purpose

- To obtain a urine sample for urinalysis and detection of bacterial and viral pathogens.
- To drain the bladder when the patient is unable to empty its bladder.
- To collect timed volumes of urine for renal function analysis.
- To inject contrast for contrast imaging.
- To assess hydration status, particularly in nursing foals.
- To obtain a minimum database for general health problems such as weight loss and fever of unknown origin.

60.2 Complications

- Bacterial cystitis
- Trauma

60.3 Equipment Required

- To clean the prepuce and penis (Figure 60.1a):
  - mild soap, for example Ivory liquid soap
  - pledgets of rolled cotton
  - bucket of warm water
  - examination gloves.
- To perform catheterization (Figure 60.1b):
  - 60 ml catheter-tip syringe
  - sterile urine specimen cup
  - sterile gloves
  - sterile water-soluble lubricant

  - catheter for males (stallions and geldings): flexible (plastic) stallion urinary catheter, approximately 150 cm in length (diameter 6.6 mm, length 137 cm)

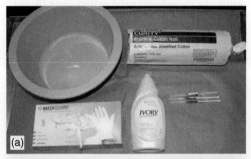

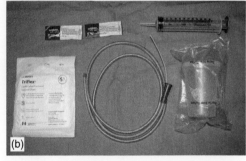

Figure 60.1 Materials necessary for the placement of a urinary catheter in the male adult horse. (a) Small bucket, rolled cotton, examination gloves, mild soap, and sedation. (b) Stallion urinary catheter (flexible and long catheter with diameter 6.6 mm and length 137 cm, and containing a stylet), sterile water-soluble lubricant, sterile gloves, 60 ml catheter-tip syringe, and specimen cup. Courtesy of Dr. Cathleen Mochal-King.

Manual of Clinical Procedures in the Horse, First Edition. Edited by Lais R.R. Costa and Mary Rose Paradis.

60.4 Restraint and Positioning

- The degree of restraint will depend on the age, training, and disposition of the horse.
- Restraint in stocks is optional. For geldings and stallions, in general, moderate sedation with an alpha-2 agonist (xylazine, detomidine, etc.) in combination with butorphanol is effective (see Chapter 9).
- A twitch may be indicated, depending on the horse's demeanor and response to the twitch.

- If urethral obstruction is suspected, administration of alpha-2 agonist drugs, which promote diuresis, may be inappropriate.
- The use of acepromazine in the male results in good relaxation of the penis. Rare side effects of paraphimosis have been reported following use of acepromazine.

60.5 Procedure: Urinary Catheterization of the Male

Technical action	Rationale
Once the horse is properly restrained, while waiting for the sedation to take effect, wrap the tail (optional).	Wrapping the tail with brown gauze (Figure 60.2) is an easy way to avoid the tail interfering with the procedure. Alternatively, have an assistant hold the tail during the entire procedure.
Once the gelding or stallion is relaxed from sedation, it should lower its penis from the sheath (Figure 60.3). At this time, the penis should be gently, but firmly, held to prevent retraction into the sheath.	Be patient in waiting for the relaxation to occur. Male horses have very strong retractor muscles and can retract the penis out of reach unless they are sedated.
Gently hold onto the shaft just behind the glans.	It is extremely important to not let the penis retract once the cleaning has started. An assistant can help with preparation of the glans and to assure that the penis remains exteriorized.
The penis and prepuce must be thoroughly cleaned with cotton pledgets soaked in warm water (Figure 60.4). An assistant can dispense the soap onto the soaked cotton. Use one hand (clean) to transfer the pledget to the other hand (dirty) during cleansing of the penis. The penis can then be rinsed with sterile water.	Use mild soap, for example Ivory liquid. Detergents are too strong. A "clean hand/dirty hand" approach will minimize recontamination of the clean area and the clean bucket of soapy water.
Care must be taken to clean the fossa around the urethral process (Figure 60.5a), paying attention to the diverticulum in the fossa (Figure 60.5b).	Smegma will accumulate in the fossa and diverticulum. This sometimes forms a marble-sized mass commonly known as the "bean".
The person passing the catheter should put on sterile gloves (Figure 60.6).	Sterile surgical gloves are adequate for performance of the procedure; sterile OB sleeves may be used.
Apply sterile water-soluble lubricant to the catheter.	Lubricant mitigates damage to the urethra.
With either the assistant holding the glans or the person passing the catheter stabilizing the penis, the catheter is introduced through the urethral opening and advanced up the penis. The hand holding the penis is not sterile.	Care must be taken to not release the penis as attempts by the horse to retract it are common once catheterization is initiated.

Technical action	Rationale
Resistance may be encountered at the perineal flexure and again at the internal urethral sphincter. Gentle pressure will open this sphincter.	Horses will often wave their tails as the catheter passes over the brim of the pelvis.
Once the catheter has reached the bladder urine should flow freely but sometimes gentle aspiration with a 60 ml catheter-tip syringe is necessary.	Occasionally urine will not flow even with aspiration. In this case the injection of 60 ml of air into the catheter followed by aspiration may help to prime the flow of urine.

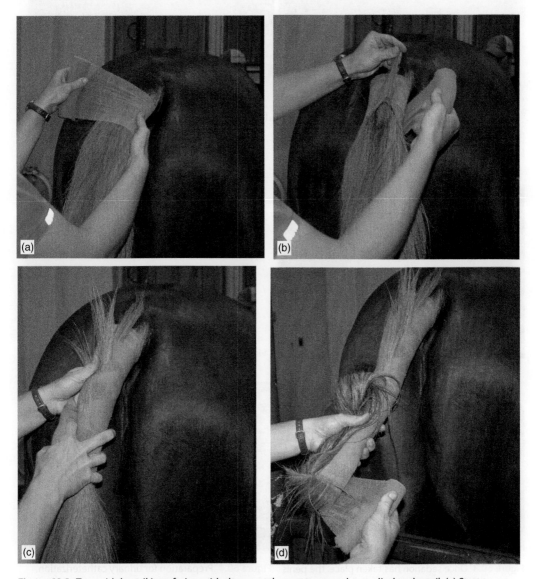

Figure 60.2 To avoid the tail interfering with the procedure, a wrap can be applied to the tail. (a) Start wrapping the base of the tail with the brown gauze. (b) Take a tuft of hair and direct upward, as the tail is wrapped. (c) Repeat in every round of the gauze. (d) Fold the long tail hairs and wrap the folded tail with the gauze. (e) Continue wrapping the brown gauze up to the base of the tail. (f and g) Loosely tie the end of the brown gauze around the base of the tail. Courtesy of Dr. Cathleen Mochal-King.

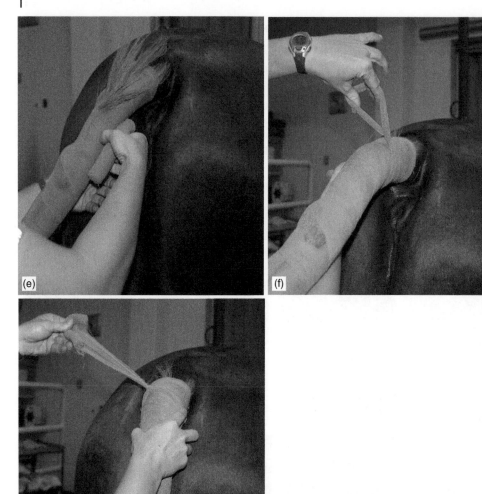

Figure 60.2 (Contiued)

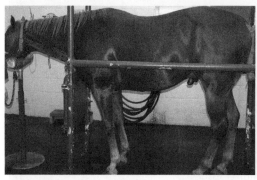

Figure 60.3 Once sedation has taken place, the penis is relaxed and becomes exteriorized. Courtesy of Dr. Cathleen Mochal-King.

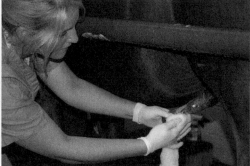

Figure 60.4 Preparation for urinary catheterization. The penis and prepuce must be thoroughly cleaned with cotton pledgets soaked in warm water and mild soap. Courtesy of Dr. Cathleen Mochal-King.

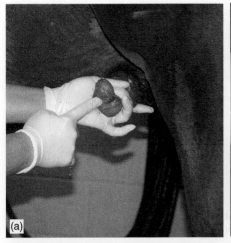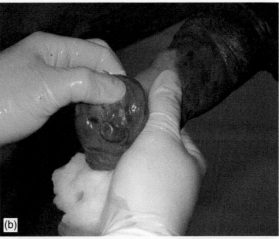

Figure 60.5 Thorough cleaning of the penis glans is important in the preparation for urinary bladder catheterization. (a) Care must be taken to clean the fossa around the urethra. (b) Particular attention should be paid to the diverticulum in the urethral fossa. Courtesy of Dr. Cathleen Mochal-King.

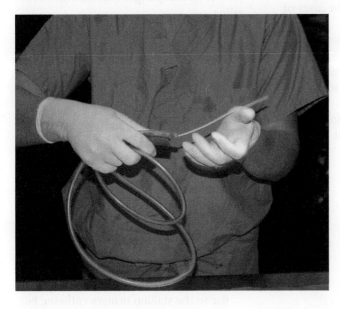

Figure 60.6 The person passing the catheter should put on sterile gloves and apply sterile water-soluble lubricant to the tip of the catheter. Courtesy of Dr. Cathleen Mochal-King.

Bibliography and Further Reading

Divers, T. (2010) Catheterization of the bladder, in Diagnostic Techniques in Equine Medicine, 2nd edn, W.B. Saunders, Philadelphia, pp. 102–104.

Hollis, A. (2008) Urinary catheterization, in The Equine Hospital Manual (eds K. Corley and J. Stephen), Blackwell, Oxford, pp. 84–85.

Schumacher, J. and Moll, H.D. (2006) Collecting urine, in Manual of Equine Diagnostic Procedures, Teton NewMedia, Jackson, WY, pp. 81–87.

61

Urinary Catheterization of Mares

Brett Sponseller and Beatrice Sponseller

61.1 Purpose

- To obtain a urine sample for urinalysis and detection of bacterial and viral pathogens.
- To drain the bladder when the patient is unable to empty its bladder.
- To lavage the bladder, such as in cases of sabulous cystitis.
- To collect timed volumes of urine for renal function analysis.
- To inject contrast for contrast imaging.
- To assess hydration status, particularly in nursing foals.
- To obtain a minimum database for general health problems such as weight loss and fever of unknown origin.

61.2 Complications

- Bacterial cystitis
- Trauma

61.3 Equipment Required

- 60 ml catheter-tip syringe
- Sterile urine specimen cup
- Sterile gloves

- Sterile lubricant
- Pledgets of rolled cotton in a bucket of warm soapy water
- 4″ × 4″ gauze sponges soaked with 2% chlorhexidine scrub
- 4″ × 4″ gauze sponges soaked with sterile saline
- Types of catheter to choose from (Figure 61.1):
  - Foley catheter: range of sizes (26–30 Fr), 16″ in length (which are adequate for average-sized mares of light breed). Foley catheter is cuffed and therefore useful as an indwelling urinary catheter for the mare.
  - mare metal urinary catheter: diameter 8 mm, length 30 cm. It is more traumatic than flexible catheters.
  - a stallion urinary catheter can is flexible and long (diameter 6.6 mm, length 137 cm), and can be used for urinary catheterization of mares.
  - mare flexible plastic urinary catheter (diameter 8.6 mm, length 40 cm) similar to the stallion urinary catheter, but shorter.

Manual of Clinical Procedures in the Horse, First Edition. Edited by Lais R.R. Costa and Mary Rose Paradis.
© 2018 John Wiley & Sons, Inc. Published 2018 by John Wiley & Sons, Inc.

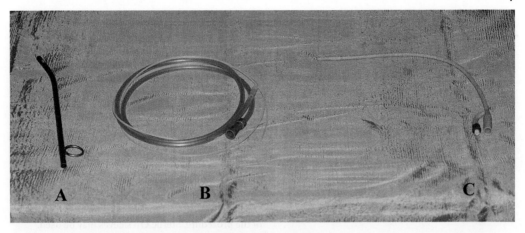

Figure 61.1 Types of urinary catheter used in adult mares. A, The mare metal urinary catheter; B, the stallion urinary catheter; C, the Foley catheter. Courtesy of Dr. Lais R.R. Costa.

61.4 Restraint and Positioning

- The degree of restraint will depend on the age, training, and disposition of the horse.

- For the most part mares do not require sedation prior to urinary catheterization.
- Restraint in stocks is generally recommended.

61.5 Procedure: Urinary Catheterization of the Mare

Technical action	Rationale
The mare's tail is wrapped. The tail is tied around the mare's neck with brown gauze (Figure 61.2a) or other suitable material (Figure 61.2b). The tail should never be tied to any objects.	See detailed instruction for wrapping of the tail with brown gauze in Chapter 60, Figure 60.2a. The mare's tail needs to be kept away from the perineum so that it can be cleaned properly without interference.
The perineal area is thoroughly cleaned with cotton pledgets soaked in water.	Use mild soap, for example Ivory liquid soap. Detergents are too strong.
Use one hand ("clean hand") to pick up the cotton pledget (Figure 61.3a). Transfer the cotton pledget to the other hand (Figure 61.3b), which is referred to as the "dirty hand" (Figure 61.3c) because it will be in contact with the perineum during cleansing. Have an assistant pour a small amount of mild soap onto the pledget of cotton. Scrub the perineum, starting at the center of the vulva and working toward the periphery (Figure 61.3d). Repeat the procedure until the perineum is completely clean.	A "clean hand/dirty hand" approach will minimize recontamination of the clean area and the clean bucket of water.

Technical action	Rationale
After cleansing with soap, disinfect the perineal area with chlorhexidine scrub to provide a sterile site. A rinse with sterile saline or water follows the disinfection.	The procedure requires sterile technique and a sterile field. Chlorhexidine scrub can be irritating to the skin and thus needs to be rinsed.
Choose the type of catheter to be used: flexible catheter, Foley catheter, metal catheter or flexible urinary catheter (Figure 61.1). Prepare your material in a sterile field.	The flexible catheters (the mare flexible urinary catheter, the Foley catheter, and the stallion urinary catheter) are less traumatic than the metal catheters. If there is a need for an indwelling catheter then a Foley catheter should be used. A Foley catheter may need a stylet for ease of introduction.
Put on sterile gloves.	Sterile surgical gloves are adequate for performance of the procedure. Sterile OB sleeves may be used.
Apply sterile water-soluble lubricant to the dorsal aspect of the introducing hand and to the catheter.	Lubricant mitigates damage to the urethra.
One hand is introduced through the vulva lips, guarding the catheter under the fingers (Figure 61.4).	Care must be taken to maintain sterile technique and avoid touching the sterile catheter on the tail and non-sterile areas of the perineum.
The introducing (non-dominant) hand is advanced over the brim of the pelvis (Figure 61.5a), gently palpating the floor of the vagina to find the urethral opening. The urethral orifice is usually found within a hand's length cranial to the brim of the pelvis on the ventral floor of the vagina. Using gentle ventral pressure on the vaginal floor a small depression may be felt.	The urethra lies on the floor of the vagina. Continued gentle digital pressure will cause the urethral sphincter to relax.
Using your other hand, insert the catheter through the vulva under the non-dominant hand and advance it into the urethral opening cautiously to prevent contamination of the catheter during advancement. Advance the catheter under the hand that is in the urethral sphincter and with gentle pressure continue to advance the catheter into the bladder (Figure 61.5b).	Urine will generally flow into the catheter once the bladder is attained. Gentle aspiration with an attached syringe may be required. Maintain the sterility of the catheter exterior to the urethra as the catheter is advanced to avoid a urinary tract infection.
Collect a urine sample into an attached syringe and/or attach a urine collection bag/system.	Maintain sample sterility and catheter sterility should culture of the urine be desired.
Urine samples for urinalysis, culture or examination of sediment should be collected in a sterile leak-proof container.	A sterile specimen cup or a red-top evacuated tube is appropriate for submission.
If an indwelling urinary catheter is to remain in place, the cuff of the Foley catheter should be inflated with the appropriate amount of water (Figure 61.5c).	It is best to inflate the cuff with water rather than air. The catheter should remain in place (Figure 61.5d) until the cuff is deflated.

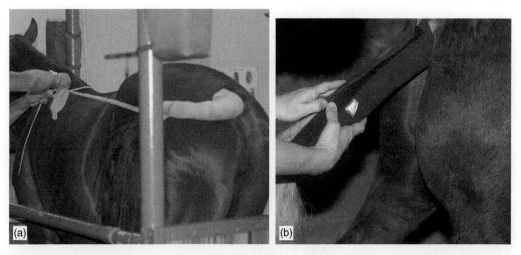

Figure 61.2 The mare's tail should be wrapped, pulled away from the perineal area, and secured by tying around the neck. (a) Brown gauze can be used to wrap and tie the tail around the neck. (b) A neoprene tail wrap can also be used to wrap the tail. In this case a small rope should be used to tie the tail to the mare's neck. Courtesy of Dr. Lais R.R. Costa.

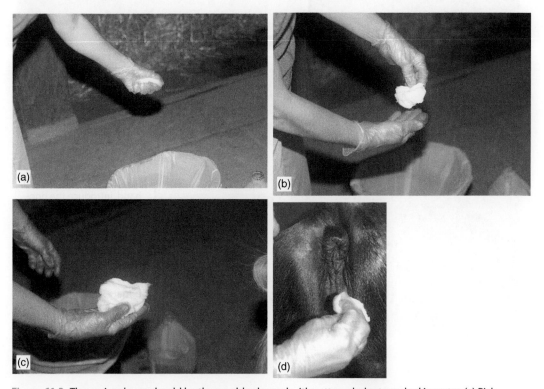

Figure 61.3 The perineal area should be thoroughly cleaned with cotton pledgets soaked in water. (a) Pick up the cotton pledget with one hand (the "clean hand"). (b) Transfer it to the other hand (the "dirty hand"). (c) Have an assistant pour antiseptic scrub onto the cotton pledget. (d) Scrub the perineum, starting at the vulva and working around in a circle towards the periphery. Courtesy of Dr. Lais R.R. Costa.

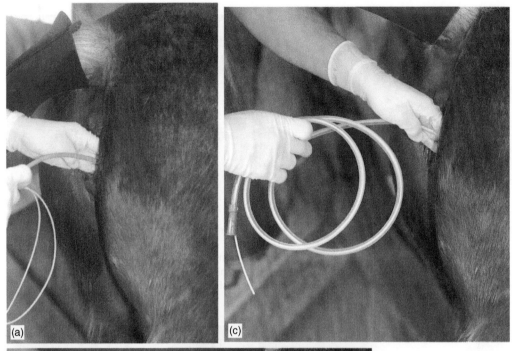

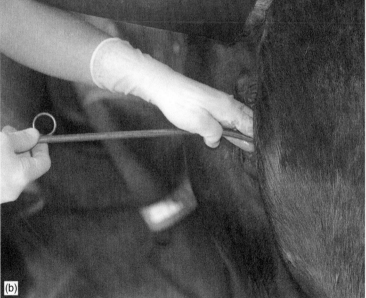

Figure 61.4 Urinary catheterization of the mare. Wearing sterile gloves with sterile water-soluble lubricant applied to the dorsal aspect of the hand and fingers of the introducing hand, introduce the non-dominant hand through the vulva lips, while the other hand holds the catheter. (a) A Foley catheter with a pliable stylet. (b) A metal mare urinary catheter. (c) A stallion urinary catheter. Courtesy of Dr. Lais R.R. Costa.

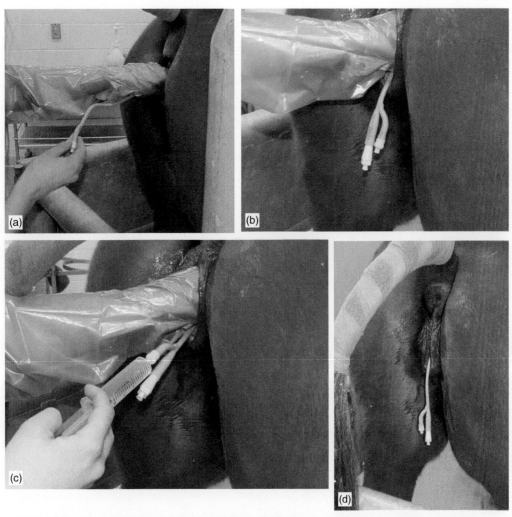

Figure 61.5 Placement of indwelling urinary catheter. (a) While the introducing (non-dominant) hand is advanced over the brim of the pelvis, gently palpate the floor of the vagina to find the urethral opening, which is located about a hand's length cranial to the brim of the pelvis on the ventral floor of the vagina. Use your other hand to guide the catheter through the vulva under the non-dominant hand and advance it into the urethral opening cautiously to prevent contamination of the catheter during advancement. (b) Verify that the catheter is in the urethral sphincter. Palpate rostral to the urethral opening to verify that the catheter is placed through the urethral opening and into the urinary bladder and not into the cervix. (c) Instill the appropriate amount of water in the bulb of the Foley catheter to prevent the catheter from slipping out of the bladder. (d) An indwelling urinary catheter retained in the bladder.

Bibliography and Further Reading

Divers, T. (2010) Catheterization of the bladder, in *Diagnostic Techniques in Equine Medicine*, 2nd edn, W.B. Saunders, Philadelphia, pp. 102–104.

Hollis, A. (2008) Urinary catheterization, in *The Equine Hospital Manual* (eds K. Corley and J. Stephen), Blackwwell, Oxford, pp. 84–85.

Schumacher, J. and Moll, H.D. (2006) Collecting urine, in *Manual of Equine Diagnostic Procedures*, Teton NewMedia, Jackson, WY, pp. 81–87.

Part VIII

Clinical Procedures by Body Systems: Ocular Procedures

62

Equine Ocular Examination

Renee Carter

62.1 Purpose

- To describe the steps taken when conducting a complete equine ophthalmic examination.
- To aid in the recognition of equine ophthalmic disorders.

62.2 Complications

- Ocular trauma.

62.3 Equipment Required

- Sedation (See Chapter 9).
- Local anesthetic may be required for regional nerve block (See chapter 63):
  - 2% lidocaine or mepivacaine
  - 25-gauge needles
  - 1 and 3 ml syringes
- Schirmer Tear Test strips
- Topical ophthalmic anesthetic (0.5% proparacaine HCl)

- Tonometry unit
- Sterile fluorescein stain strips
- Sterile rose Bengal stain strips
- Sterile eyewash
- Gauze
- Light source, transilluminator preferred
- Cobalt blue filter or UV light source
- 1% tropicamide HCl
- Direct ophthalmoscope or Panoptic® ophthalmoscope (monocular indirect)
- Hand-held lens (14 or 20 D)
- Muscle hook or small fixation forceps (optional)

62.4 Restraint and Positioning

- Assistant to restrain the head, standing on the opposite side of the clinician.
- Use of stocks is preferred if available.
- Sedation is often required to obtain a complete examination.
- Use of a nose twitch may be required.

62.5 Procedure: Equine Ocular Examination

Technical action	Rationale
Obtain a complete medical and ophthalmic history.	Some systemic diseases will have ocular manifestations.
	Record all findings in the medical record of the animal.
Evaluate the patient in an environment that is quiet and well-lit for extraocular examination and can be darkened for intraocular examination.	Adequate environment is crucial to perform a thorough ocular examination.

(continued)

Manual of Clinical Procedures in the Horse, First Edition. Edited by Lais R.R. Costa and Mary Rose Paradis.
© 2018 John Wiley & Sons, Inc. Published 2018 by John Wiley & Sons, Inc.

Technical action	Rationale
Standing in front of the patient, start by evaluating for alterations in the normal symmetrical appearance of the eyes and/or periocular regions: • lash height (Figure 62.1a,b) • globe position • periocular bony and soft tissue structures, note abnormalities (Figure 62.1c,d) • pupil size and position: any obvious opacities (Figure 62.1e–h).	Never stand directly over or under the patient's head to avoid injury. Evaluate lash height. Normally lashes are held perpendicular to the cornea (Figure 62.1a). Lashes pointing downward may indicate enophthalmos due to dehydration or malnutrition, primarily foals, or phthisis of the globe (Figure 62.1b), or pain, or ptosis of the lid. Lashes directed upward may indicate exophthalmos (orbital disease) or buphthalmos.
Perform vision testing by evaluating the menace response or maze testing: *Menace response*: Movement of the examiner's hand toward the eye to elicit avoidance behavior or blink reflex. Should be conducted for both eyes (oculi uterque OU), laterally and medially. *Maze testing*: Navigation of a short obstacle course in brightly and dimly lit settings. The obstacle course is created using short, smooth objects such as an over-turned feed bucket. One eye is covered at a time with a towel secured to the halter. The patient is encouraged to maneuver through the course toward a food reward. This procedure is repeated for the second eye.	Vision testing is performed prior to administration of sedation. Avoid generating an air current or hitting hairs (vibrissae and lashes), which could result in a false-positive menace response. The menace response is typically absent until 2 weeks of age. Maze testing is indicated in patients where the results of vision testing are inconclusive. It is often performed in animals with partial or unilateral vision loss.
Evaluate the patient for the presence of palpebral reflexes OU. Digitally tap the periocular skin at both the lateral and medial aspects of the lid margin, stimulating the trigeminal nerve (cranial nerve or CN V).	The patient should respond with a complete blink of the eyelids via the facial nerve (CN VII) to the orbicularis oculi muscle.
Evaluate ocular motility OU (CN III, IV, VI) by moving the animal's head and observing eye movement.	
Evaluate for ocular discharge or discharge from the distal nasolacrimal opening and note the character.	Ocular discharge can be secondary to infection or a blockage of the nasolacrimal duct.
Palpate the periocular structures for bony changes or soft tissue swelling.	This is an important step in horses showing signs of painful conditions or animals with ocular or facial injuries.
Evaluate the size, shape, and symmetry of the pupils by retroillumination using a focal light source (Figure 62.2). To perform retroillumination, stand at an arm's distance in front of the patient and obtain the tapetal reflex.	This evaluation must be performed prior to dilation of the pupils. With equal illumination of the eyes, the examiner can evaluate for changes in pupil symmetry.

Technical action	Rationale
Evaluate both direct and consensual pupillary light reflex (PLR) with a bright, focal light source in a darkened environment (Figure 62.3): • direct PLR: eye that is illuminated constricts • indirect PLR: eye that is not directly illuminated constricts.	This evaluation must be performed prior to dilation of the pupils. Normal PLR responses are slow in equine. Direct PLR responses will be greater than indirect PLR responses. PLR is not a vision test. PLR must be evaluated prior to dilation.
Perform examination of the eyelid position, movement, and conformation before administration of sedation and nerve blocks.	Nerve blocks and sedation will affect eyelid position and movement.
Administer sedation (see Chapter 9) and perform a palpebral nerve block (see Chapter 63 for a detailed description of the procedure).	Sedation and palpebral nerve block facilitate the performance of a complete ophthalmic examination.
Collect samples for microbial culture, if indicated. See Chapter 64 for a detailed description of the procedure.	Collection of a sample for microbial culture should be performed if either ocular discharge or corneal ulceration is present.
If indicated, perform the Schirmer tear test OU. See Chapter 64 for a detailed description of the procedure.	Performed a tear test prior to the application of topical ocular medications or conduction of any diagnostic or therapeutic procedures to avoid affecting test results.
Evaluate corneal reflex (CN V) OU by gently tapping/touching the corneal surface with a small wisp of cotton from a cotton ball or cotton tipped applicator. The horse should blink in response to the mechanical stimulation of the cornea.	This test must be performed prior to application of topical anesthetic. Evaluation of the corneal reflex is indicated in cases with persistent corneal ulceration, suspect neuropathy, decreased Schirmer tear test values, or irregular or lackluster corneal surface.
Administer 0.5 ml of topical anesthetic (proparacaine solution) to each eye by one of two methods: • Instill the anesthetic directly onto the corneal if able to tilt the horse's head such that the corneal surface is nearly parallel to the ground. • Place the solution in a tuberculin syringe and break off a 25-gauge needle manually at the hub prior to application (Figure 62.4a). The solution is squirted onto the eye through the hub of a 25-gauge needle (Figure 62.4b).	Instillation of proparacaine onto the cornea allows the corneal surface to be touched without causing discomfort and eliciting evasive behavior. Direct instillation is not easily performed because of the head position required. When squirting the solution through the hub of a 25-gauge needle, the examiner should be careful not to get too close to the eye, as the hub of the needle is still sharp.
Perform intraocular pressure (IOP) readings OU by touching the cornea with the tonometer. See Chapter 64 for a detailed description of the procedure. Normal values vary depending on whether or not sedation is used. The normal range is approximately 16 and 32 mmHg with an average of 24 mmHg.	Do not apply pressure to the globe if traumatic rupture or deep corneal ulcer is suspected. The head position must be consistent for accurate IOP: • higher IOP readings will be obtained with a low head position or lack of a palpebral nerve block and glaucoma; • lower IOP readings will be obtained in cases with uveitis or phthisis bulbi.
If indicated, collect cytology samples. See Chapter 64 for a detailed description of the procedure.	Collection of a sample for cytologic evaluation is indicated in cases with conjunctivitis or keratitis.

(continued)

Technical action	Rationale
Stain the eye with fluorescein and evaluate stain uptake with a cobalt blue light or UV light source. See Chapter 64 for a detailed description of the procedure.	Fluorescein stain is taken up by the stroma of the cornea when there is disruption of the epithelia (Figure 61.6). Corneal ulcers that progress to desmetocele will no longer uptake stain.
Using a light source, evaluate the lid margins, nasolacrimal system, conjunctiva, and ocular surface for irregularities.	The appearance of fluorescein staining dribbling from the nostril indicates patency of the nasolacrimal duct of that side (Figure 62.5).
Retropulse the globe by gently pressing the globe back into the orbit with a finger placed over the partially closed eyelid. As the globe retropulses, evaluate the third eyelid for any irregularities.	Do not apply pressure to the globe if traumatic rupture or deep corneal ulcer is suspected. Retropulsing the globe allows the examiner to evaluate the third eyelid as well as check for the presence of orbital disease. Evaluate the posterior aspect of the third eyelid if indicated.
Using a focal light source, obtain the tapetal reflex to highlight opacities in the ocular media (aqueous, lens or vitreous).	This must be performed in a darkened environment to maximize visualization. Retroillumination is used to highlight opacities in the ocular media. Opacities will block the tapetal reflex.
Apply a direct light source across the cornea (parallel) (Figure 62.6a). The direct light across the cornea will highlight corneal irregularities (Figure 62.6b).	This must be performed in a darkened environment to maximize visualization.
In a darkened environment, evaluate the anterior chamber using: • the small spot of light or slit-beam on a direct ophthalmoscope or • a hand-held slit lamp (Figure 62.7).	The anterior chamber is the space between the cornea and iris that contains the aqueous humor.
Evaluate for the presence of aqueous flare using a small focal light source directed perpendicular to the cornea.	Breakdown of the blood–ocular barrier (due to anterior uveitis) will result in increased protein in the aqueous humor (referred to as aqueous flare) and can be detected as opacity in the anterior chamber (Figure 62.1h).
Evaluate the depth of the anterior chamber: • Shallow appearance • Greater depth appearance.	Alterations in the depth of the anterior chamber: • The anterior chamber will appear shallow in cases with phthisis bulbi, anterior synechiae, iris bombe, or anterior lens luxation. • The anterior chamber will appear deep in cases with hypermature cataracts, buphthalmia, and posteriorly luxated lenses.
Evaluate the iris, corpora nigra, and pupil for changes in color, size, shape, and position.	

Technical action	Rationale
Dilate pupils with tropicamide. Apply 1% tropicamide solution directly to the corneal surface by instillation or by squirting 0.25 ml of tropicamide solution using a tuberculin syringe (as shown in Figure 62.4).	It will take 10–20 minutes to achieve acceptable dilation. The use of tropicamide is contraindicated in cases with glaucoma. Dilation of the pupil is necessary for full examination of the posterior segment of the eye in cases where it is not contraindicated to do so.
Once the pupils are dilated, repeat retroillumination of the ocular media to evaluate for any major opacities blocking the view of the tapetal reflex.	If a slit lamp is not available the examiner can use an otoscope head or head loupe for magnification. This should be performed in a darkened environment.
Repeat the evaluation of the anterior segment of eye using: • the light from a transilluminator and magnification (as shown in Figure 62.6a) or • a hand-held slit lamp (as shown in Figure 62.7).	
Perform a fundic examination: • directly with a transilluminator (Figure 62.8) • by direct ophthalmoscopy (Figure 62.9) • by indirect ophthalmoscopy (Figure 62.10).	*Transilluminator method*: This is possible in the dilated eyes of large animal patients. The image is upright, requires a close working distance, and provides small fields of view (poor screening tool). *Direct ophthalmoscopy*: This provides an upright image. The instrument should be set at 0 D to bring the fundus into view. It requires a close working distance and provides a small field of view (poor screening tool). *Indirect ophthalmoscopy*: This provides an inverted, virtual image that is less magnified so it is a better screening tool. *Monocular indirect (panoptic) ophthalmoscopy*: This provides an upright image with moderate magnification and field of view.
Record any abnormal findings on the fundic examination. Horses are paurangiotic, meaning that they have vessels that only extend a short distance from the optic nerve head. The optic nerve head lies in the inferior, non-tapetal fundus and is in the shape of a horizontal oval. The dorsal aspect of the fundus contains the tapetum. The Stars of Winslow are a normal anatomical variation of red to dark-colored dots that represent end-on capillaries.	The fundus should be evaluated for: • changes in the size/shape of the optic nerve head • changes in tapetal reflectivity • changes in the appearance of the retinal vessels; • changes in the color of the non-tapetum.

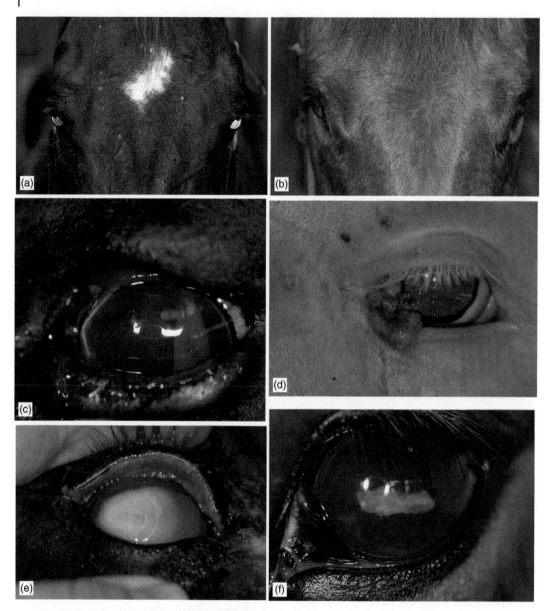

Figure 62.1 On initial examination, while standing in front of the patient evaluate for alterations in the normal symmetry and overall appearance of the eyes and/or periocular regions. (a) Lash height, which normally is perpendicular to the cornea. (b) Lash pointed downward, in this case indicating enophthalmos due to bilateral phthisis of the globe. Courtesy of Dr. Lais R.R. Costa.(c) Full thickness corneal laceration with hyphema, Oculus Sinister (OS, left eye). (d) Periocular growth involving the lower lid, Oculus Dexter (OD, right eye), in this case squamous cell carcinoma. (e) Opacities associated with heavy corneal infiltrate and vascularization due to stromal abscess OD. (f) Chronic cataract and hyperpigmentation of the iris associated chronic uveitis OS. (g) Corneal scar, vascularization, cataract and phthisis associated with chronic uveitis OS. (h) Fibrin in the anterior chamber associated with anterior uveitis OD. (i) Opacities associated with melting corneal ulcer OD. (j) Opacities associated with corneal edema OS. Courtesy of Dr. Lais R.R. Costa.

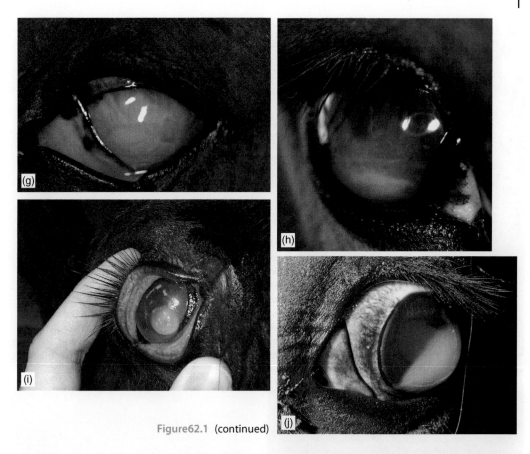

Figure62.1 (continued)

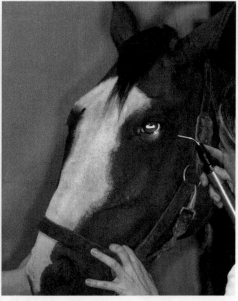

Figure 62.2 Retroillumination is performed using a focal light source to evaluate pupil symmetry and evaluate for opacities of the ocular media.

Figure 62.3 A bright, focal light source is used in a dimly lit environment to evaluate pupillary light reflexes.

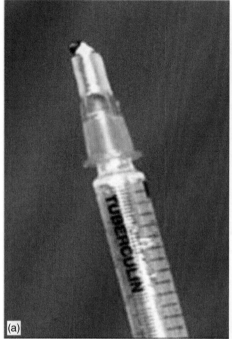

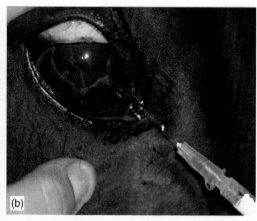

Figure 62.4 Administration of topical medication to the eye, in this case anesthetic proparacaine solution. (a) A tuberculin syringe filled with the medication, with a 25-gauge needle broken off manually at the hub prior to application (the hub of the needle is still sharp). (b) Topical administration by squirting the solution onto the eye through the hub of a broken-off 25-gauge needle. This allows proparacaine to be administered from a short distance from the cornea. (The hub of the needle is still sharp and must not touch the cornea).

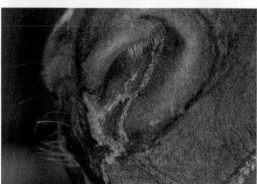

Figure 62.5 As part of the evaluation of the nasolacrimal system, note the appearance of fluorescein staining dribbling from the nostril, indicating patency of the nasolacrimal duct of that side.

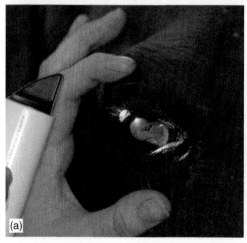

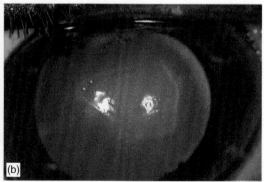

Figure 62.6 Evaluation of the cornea. (a) Applying a light directed across the cornea highlights corneal abnormalities. (b) Uncomplicated corneal ulceration.

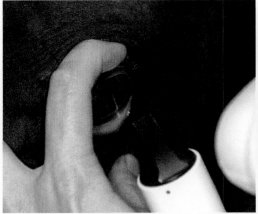

Figure 62.7 A focal light source, in this case a hand-held slit lamp, directed perpendicular to the cornea is used to evaluate the anterior chamber depth and the presence of aqueous flare (see Figure 61.1h).

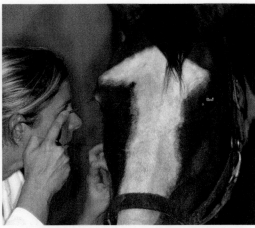

Figure 62.8 The fundus can be directly visualized using a transilluminator.

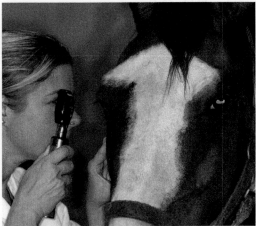

Figure 62.9 Direct ophthalmoscopy performed to evaluate the fundus.

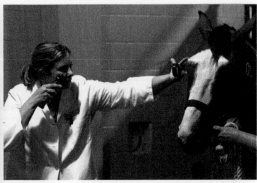

Figure 62.10 Indirect ophthalmoscopy performed to evaluate the fundus.

Bibliography and Further Reading

Dwyer, A.E. (2011) Practical general field ophthalmology, in *Equine Ophthalmology*, 2nd edn (ed. B.C. Gilger), W.B. Saunders, Maryland Heights, pp. 52–92.

Gilger, B.C. and Stoppini, R. (2011) Equine ocular examination: Routine and advanced diagnostic techniques, in *Equine Ophthalmology*, 2nd edn (ed. B.C. Gilger), W.B. Saunders, Maryland Heights, pp. 1–51.

Maggs, D.J. (2008) Basic diagnostic techniques, in *Slatter's Fundamentals of Veterinary Ophthalmology*, 4th edn (eds D.J. Maggs, P.E. Miller, and R. Ofri), W.B. Saunders, St. Louis, pp. 81–106.

63

Ophthalmic Nerve Blocks

Renee Carter

63.1 Purpose

- This chapter describes the procedures for common regional nerve blocks used to facilitate ocular examination, and diagnostic and therapeutic procedures such as eyelid laceration repair or subpalpebral lavage system (SPL) placement in horses (see Table 63.1).

Table 63.1 Description of the nerve blocks and the corresponding areas and structures desensitized

Goal of ocular perineural anesthesia	Name of the nerve block	Landmark and nerve localization
Unable to close the eyelids (akinesia of the orbicularis oculi muscle responsible for eyelids closure)	Auriculopalpebral nerve	Depression anterior to the base of the ear where the caudal border of the coronoid process of the mandible and the zygomatic process of the temporal bone meet
	Palpebral branch of the auriculopalpebral nerve site 1	Strap-like palpable by strumming the index finger over the highest point of the zygomatic arch
	Palpebral branch of the auriculopalpebral nerve site 2	Strap-like palpable along the zygomatic arch, just caudal to the bony process of the frontal bone
Abolish the sensation to the central upper eyelid	Supraorbital (frontal) nerve	Depression in the dorsal orbital rim
Abolish the sensation to the lateral upper lid	Lacrimal nerve	Along the lateral aspect of the dorsal orbital rim
Abolishes the sensation to the lateral lower lid	Zygomatic nerve	Along the lateral aspect of the ventral orbital rim
Abolish the sensation to the medial canthus	Infratrochlear nerve	Trochlear notch, palpated within the dorsal orbital rim at the medial canthus
Temporarily blocks CN II–VI and maxillary and ophthalmic branches of CN V	Retrobulbar nerve	Assessment through the supraorbital fossa perpendicular to the skull just posterior to the posterior aspect of the dorsal orbital rim

Manual of Clinical Procedures in the Horse, First Edition. Edited by Lais R.R. Costa and Mary Rose Paradis.
© 2018 John Wiley & Sons, Inc. Published 2018 by John Wiley & Sons, Inc.

- The following procedures will be discussed:
  - auriculopalpebral nerve block
  - palpebral branch of the auriculopalpebral nerve block
  - supraorbital (frontal) nerve block
  - lacrimal nerve block
  - zygomatic nerve block
  - infratrochlear nerve block
  - retrobulbar nerve block (this procedure is discussed separately because of specific steps and complications).

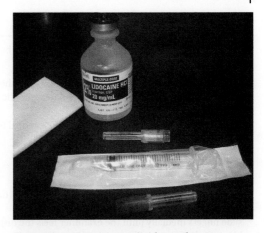

Figure 63.1 Materials needed for performing ariculopalpebral, palpebral branch of the auriculopalpebral, supraorbital, lacrimal, zygomatic, and infratrochlear nerve blocks: local anesthetic (2% lidocaine or mepivacaine), 25-gauge 5/8″ needle, and 3 ml syringe.

63.2 Auriculopalpebral, Palpebral Branch of the Auriculopalpebral, Supraorbital (Frontal), Lacrimal, Zygomatic, and Infratrochlear Nerve Blocks

63.2.1 Complications

- Local irritation, inflammation
- With those blocks that block motor function (akinesia) to the eyelid, exposure keratitis may occur with prolonged akinesia.

63.2.2 Equipment Required (Figure 63.1)

- Local anesthetic (2% lidocaine or mepivacaine)
- 25-gauge 5/8″ needle
- 3 ml syringe

63.2.3 Restraint and Positioning

- An assistant to restrain the head may be required, standing on the opposite side of the clinician or technician.
- Sedation may be required.
- Twitch may be required.

63.2.4 Procedure: Auriculopalpebral, Palpebral Branch of the Auriculopalpebral, Supraorbital (Frontal), Lacrimal, Zygomatic, and Infratrochlear Nerve Blocks

Technical action	Rationale
Perform sedation if deemed necessary (see Chapter 9).	Some horses will resist having work done around their faces. Sedation is often necessary to make the horse lower the head.
Locate the anatomical landmarks for the desired nerve.	
Auriculopalpebral nerve: blocked in the depression anterior to the base of the ear where the caudal border of the coronoid process of the mandible and the zygomatic process of the temporal bone meet.	A block of the auriculopalpebral nerve is motor nerve block (akinesia) of the orbicularis oculi muscle used to close the eyelids.

(continued)

Technical action	Rationale
Palpebral branch of the auriculopalpebral nerve: can be blocked at two locations (Figure 63.2a): • at the site where it can be palpated by strumming the index finger over the highest point of the caudal zygomatic arch (Figure 63.2b) • at a lower site along the zygomatic arch, just caudal to the bony process of the frontal bone (Figure 63.2c)	A block of the palpebral branch of the auriculopalpebral nerve also provides akinesia of the orbicularis oculi muscle used to close the eyelids.
Supraorbital (frontal) nerve: blocked as it exits the supraorbital foramen within the frontal bone: • the examiner should place their thumb and middle finger along both sides of the dorsal orbital rim laterally • slide fingers medially until the examiner feels the distance between the fingers widen • drop the index finger down midway between the thumb and middle finger, palpating for a depression in the dorsal orbital rim, the supraorbital foramen (Figure 63.3a).	A block of the supraorbital (frontal) nerve abolishes sensation to the central upper lid.
Lacrimal nerve: blocked subcutaneously along the lateral aspect of the dorsal orbital rim.	A block of the lacrimal nerve provides anesthesia to the lateral upper lid.
Zygomatic nerve: blocked subcutaneously along the lateral aspect of the ventral orbital rim.	A block of the zygomatic nerve abolishes the sensation to the lateral lower lid.
Infratrochlear nerve: blocked at the trochlear notch, palpated within the dorsal orbital rim at the medial canthus.	A block of the infratrochlear nerve block provides anesthesia to the medial canthus.
Once the region has been identified by palpation, a 25-gauge needle is placed subcutaneously adjacent to the nerve. Use a swift, firm movement (but make sure the horse is not startled). A tentative movement leads to poking the area without proper placement of the needle, requiring several attempts.	
Illustrations of the needle positions for the individual blocks: • palpebral branch of the auriculopalpebral nerve (Figure 63.2e) • supraorbital (frontal) nerve block (Figure 63.3b) • lacrimal nerve block (Figure 63.4) • zygomatic nerve block (Figure 63.5) • infratrochlear nerve block (Figure 63.6).	*Palpebral branch of the auriculopalpebral nerve*: point the needle downward. *Supraorbital (frontal) nerve block*: The needle should not be directed down into the supraorbital foramen to avoid damaging the supraorbital artery and vein. *Lacrimal nerve block*: point the needle from lateral to medial. *Zygomatic nerve block*: point the needle from lateral to medial. *Infratrochlear nerve block*: point the needle downwards.
A syringe of local anesthetic is attached to the hub of the needle.	
Aspiration should be conducted first to ensure the needle is not within a blood vessel.	Avoid injection of anesthetic intravascularly.
Infuse 1–2 ml of anesthetic subcutaneously (Figure 63.2e).	A subcutaneous "bleb" can be felt after injection.
Withdraw the needle and syringe.	
Massage the area and allow the nerve block to take effect before proceeding.	Massage the area to facilitate diffusion of anesthetic.

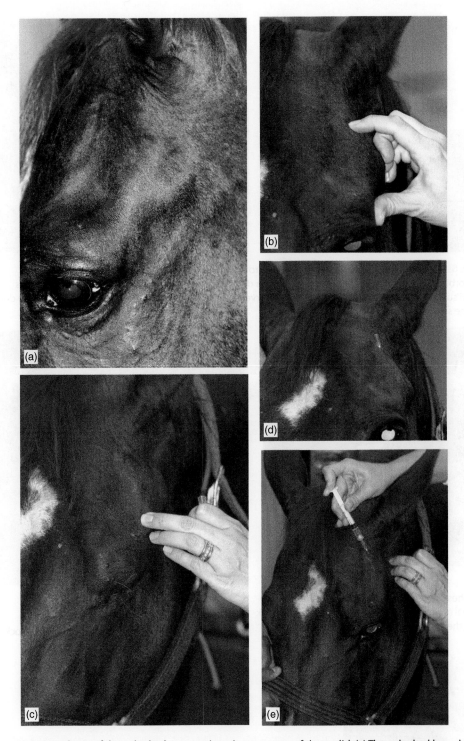

Figure 63.2 Anesthesia of the palpebral nerve to impair movement of the eyelid. (a) The palpebral branch of the auriculopalpebral nerve can be blocked at either of two points as it crosses the zygomatic arch, as marked by the red dots. (b) The palpebral branch can be palpated by strumming the index finger over the highest point of the caudal zygomatic arch. (c) Alternatively, the palpebral branch can be blocked lower along the zygomatic arch, just caudal to the bony process of the frontal bone. (d) The needle is placed downward into the subcutaneous tissue over the palpebral nerve. (e) Anesthetic is infused subcutaneously over the palpebral nerve.

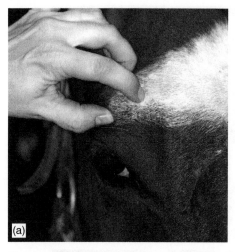

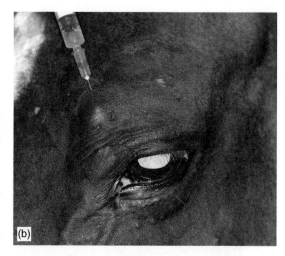

Figure 63.3 Anesthesia of the supraorbital nerve provides analgesia to the central upper eyelid. (a) The supraorbital foramen is identified by palpating for a depression in the dorsal orbital rim. (b) The needle is placed subcutaneously adjacent to supraorbital nerve. Care must be taken to avoid directing the needle down into the supraorbital foramen.

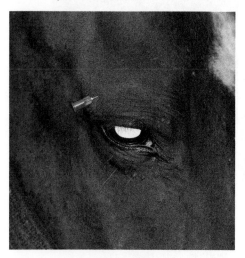

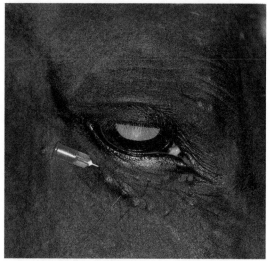

Figure 63.4 Anesthesia of the lacrimal nerve abolishes the sensation to the lateral upper lid. The lacrimal nerve is blocked by performing a line block along the lateral aspect of the dorsal orbital rim.

Figure 63.5 Anesthesia of the zygomatic nerve abolishes the sensation to the lateral lower lid. The zygomatic nerve is blocked by performing a line block along the lateral aspect of the ventral orbital rim.

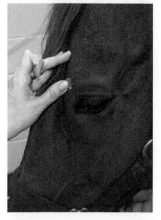

Figure 63.6 Anesthesia of the infratrochlear nerve abolishes the sensation to the medial canthus. The infratrochlear nerve is blocked by infusing anesthetic along the trochlear notch present at the medial canthus.

63.3 Retrobulbar Nerve Block

63.3.1 Purpose

- Temporarily blocks CN II-VI and maxillary and ophthalmic branches of CN V.
- Adjunct to general anesthesia for surgical procedures of the eye.
- Adjunct akinesia and analgesia for standing ocular surgical procedures.

63.3.2 Complications

- Local irritation, inflammation
- Introduction of infectious agents to the orbit
- Laceration to retrobulbar tissues or the globe
- Creation of a retrobulbar hematoma
- Development of optic neuritis
- Development of exposure keratitis
- Induction of an oculocardiac reflex
- Hypersensitivity to lidocaine

63.3.3 Equipment Required

- Local anesthetic (2% lidocaine or mepivacaine)
- 22-gauge, 2.5″ spinal needle
- 12 ml syringe
- Clippers
- Povidone-iodine solution
- Sterile gloves

63.3.4 Restraint and Positioning

- An assistant must restrain the head, standing on the opposite side of the clinician or technician.
- Sedation (prolonged and profound) is required (see Chapter 9).
- A twitch may be required, but profound sedation is recommended to limit any head movement during injection.

63.3.5 Procedure: Retrobulbar Nerve Block

Technical action	Rationale
Administer sedative to ensure a profound level of sedation (see Chapter 9).	Because of possible complications the horse should remain completely still.
Clip and prep the orbital fossa with dilute povidone-iodine solution.	Care should be taken to clean the site of injection to prevent infection. Do not use alcohol.
Place the spinal needle through the skin in the orbital fossa perpendicular to the skull just posterior to the posterior aspect of the dorsal orbital rim.	Placement of the spinal needle is depicted in Figure 63.7.
Advance the needle slowly until it enters the retrobulbar orbital cone, monitoring the eye position during placement.	The clinician should monitor the position of the eye during advancement of the needle.
	The eye will rotate upward when the needle reaches the retrobulbar orbital cone.
	Slow advancement of the needle should proceed until the eye returns to a normal position and a slight "popping" is felt. This indicates placement of the needle within the retrobulbar orbital cone. No further advancement of the spinal needle is recommended.
Remove the stylet of the spinal needle.	

(continued)

Technical action	Rationale
Attach the syringe of local anesthetic to the hub of the spinal needle.	
Aspiration should be conducted to ensure the needle is not within a blood vessel.	
Inject 10–12 ml of local anesthetic.	A mild exophthalmos will be noted following injection of anesthetic. This indicates proper needle placement.
Withdraw the needle and syringe.	
Monitor the effects of the anesthesia and akinesia.	Anesthesia and akinesia should last 1–2 hours.
Apply topical lubricating ointments to the eye because the lack of a palpebral reflex and corneal sensation may cause the eye to dry out due to cessation of blinking.	The lack of palpebral reflex and corneal sensation may last for up to 4 hours post injection.
Monitor activity due to temporary blindness.	Horse will remain blind after sedation has subsided.

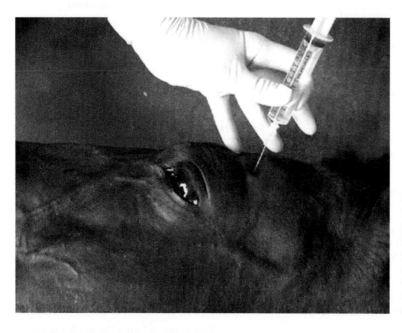

Figure 63.7 A spinal needle is used to perform a retrobulbar block by advancing it perpendicular to the skull in the orbital fossa, caudal to the posterior aspect of the dorsal orbital rim.

Bibliography and Further Reading

Dwyer, A.E. (2011) Practical general field ophthalmology, in *Equine Ophthalmology*, 2nd edn (ed. B.C. Gilger), W.B. Saunders, Maryland Heights, pp. 52–92.

Gilger, B.C. and Stoppini, R. (2011) Equine ocular examination: Routine and advanced diagnostic techniques, in *Equine Ophthalmology*, 2nd edn (ed. B.C. Gilger), W.B. Saunders, Maryland Heights, pp. 1–51.

Maggs, D.J. (2008) Basic diagnostic techniques, in *Slatter's Fundamentals of Veterinary Ophthalmology*, 4th edn (eds D.J. Maggs, P.E. Miller, and R. Ofri), W.B. Saunders, St. Louis, pp 81–106.

64

Ophthalmic Diagnostic Procedures

Renee Carter

This chapter describes a number of diagnostic ophthalmic procedures that are commonly performed in the course of a complete ophthalmic examination and work-up of a patient presenting with an ophthalmic complaint:

- Schirmer Tear Test I (STT I)
- Corneal or Conjunctival Culture
- Fluorescein Stain and Seidel Test
- Rose Bengal Stain
- Corneal or Conjunctival Cytology
- Intraocular Pressure Measurement

64.1 Schirmer Tear Test I

64.1.1 Purpose

- To determine the amount of aqueous tear production.

64.1.2 Complications

- Local corneal irritation
- Possible introduction of contaminants to the corneoconjunctival surface

64.1.3 Equipment Required

- Commercial Schirmer Tear Test strips (Figure 64.1a)

64.1.4 Restraint and Positioning

- An assistant should restrain the head, typically standing on the opposite side to the eye being evaluated.
- Sedation may be required.

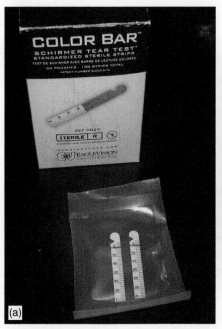

(a)

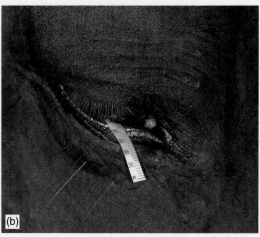

(b)

Figure 64.1 Schirmer tear test I. (a) Schirmer tear test kit. (b) Strip placed in the inferior conjunctival fornix.

Manual of Clinical Procedures in the Horse, First Edition. Edited by Lais R.R. Costa and Mary Rose Paradis.
© 2018 John Wiley & Sons, Inc. Published 2018 by John Wiley & Sons, Inc.

64.1.5 Procedure: Schirmer Tear Test I

Technical action	Rationale
The STT I should be performed prior to any other procedures or application of medication to the eye (especially topical anesthesia).	The STT I measures both basal and reflex tear production. Results will be affected by the application of medications to the eye and also by procedures that stimulate reflex tearing.
	STT I is indicated for cases with unexplained keratitis, ocular discharge, lackluster corneal appearance or when facial or trigeminal nerve dysfunction is suspected.
The notched end of the Schirmer tear test strip should be folded while in the sterile pouch.	Touching the end of the strip may allow contaminants from the examiner's fingers to be introduced to the patient's eye. Bending the end of the test strip makes it easier to place the strip in the lower conjunctival fornix.
The folded end of the test strip is placed in the mid to lateral lower conjunctival fornix (between eyelid and eyeball) (Figure 64.1b).	Placement in this location maximizes corneal contact, ensuring reflex tear production, an important component of the STT I test. If the strip is placed in front of the third eyelid, corneal contact may not occur.
Hold the strip in place for 1 minute. It may be necessary to hold the eyelids closed to prevent the strip from falling out prematurely.	
Remove the strip and immediately measure the distance from the notch on the strip to the end of the watermark that is formed to determine tear production.	Failure to read the result immediately will give the examiner an inaccurate result as tear will continue to wick up the tear test strip.

Normal STT I values for horses are reported as:

- 11 to >30 mm wetting/minute
- 15-20 mm wetting/30 seconds.

64.2 Corneal or Conjunctival Culture and Sensitivity

64.2.1 Purpose

- To aid in the diagnosis of infectious conjunctivitis and/or keratitis.
- To determine the sensitivity of isolated pathogens.

64.2.2 Complications

- Local irritation
- Worsening of a corneal defect if deep/fragile areas are sampled.

64.2.3 Equipment Required

- Sterile swabs with a transport tube for bacterial and fungal cultures

- Local anesthetic (2% lidocaine or mepivacaine)
- 25-gauge 5/8″ needle
- 3 ml syringe

64.2.4 Restraint and Positioning

- An assistant restrains the head, typically standing on the opposite side to the eye being evaluated.
- Sedation may be required.
- Perform palpebral nerve block (see Chapter 63).
- Topical ophthalmic anesthetic (proparacaine) may be required (Figure 64.2a,b).

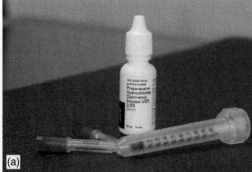

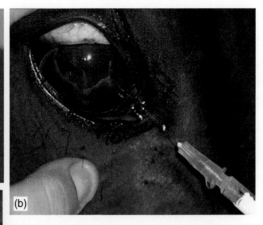

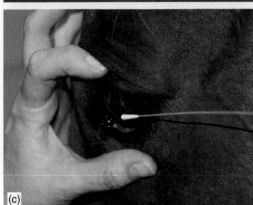

Figure 64.2 Corneal or conjunctival culture and sensitivity. (a) Topical ophthalmic anesthetic (proparacaine). (b) Application of topical ophthalmic anesthetic by squirting the solution through the hub of a 25-gauge needle. (c) The surface of the cornea is swabbed to obtain a corneal culture.

64.2.5 Procedure: Corneal or Conjunctival Culture and Sensitivity

Technical action	Rationale
Obtain samples for culture early in the examination and prior to application of ophthalmic medications.	Culture is indicated in cases with ocular discharge, conjunctivitis or keratitis (especially complex ulcers). The application of stain or medications to the eye may limit growth of microorganisms.
Perform a palpebral nerve block (see Chapter 63).	Performing a palpebral nerve block will facilitate opening the eye and reduce the risk of contamination of the culture by flora from the eyelids (see Chapter 63).
Remove a sterile swab from its packaging.	
Gently part the eyelids with the thumb and index finger.	
Roll or rub the tip of the sterile swab over the affected area to be cultured (cornea or conjunctiva) (Figure 64.2c).	Eyes requiring culture are often painful and ophthalmic anesthetic may be needed to safely collect the culture sample. A single application of proparacaine is unlikely to affect culture results. The edges of a corneal ulcer should be swabbed to avoid the deep aspects of corneal defects.
Open the transport tube and place the swab into the transport tube.	
Cultures should be plated (submitted to a microbiology laboratory) as soon as possible.	Because of the small sample size, a delay in plating cultures may result in a negative culture result. Aerobic culture and sensitivity are recommended. Fungal cultures should be submitted for all complex corneal ulcers, especially in endemic areas.

64.3 Fluorescein Stain

64.3.1 Purpose

- To identify corneal or conjunctival ulceration.
- To determine the patency of the nasolacrimal duct (Jones test): indicated in cases with unexplained epiphora, mucopurulent ocular or nasal discharge.
- To perform a Seidel test: indicated in cases with possible full-thickness corneal injury.

64.3.2 Complications

- Local irritation

64.3.3 Equipment Required

- Sterile fluorescein stain strips (Figure 64.3a)
- Ophthalmic irrigating solution (eye wash)
- Gauze
- Blue or ultraviolet light
- An examination area that can be darkened (required).
- If performing a Seidel test a palpebral nerve block will be required:
  - local anesthetic (2% lidocaine or mepivacaine, see Chapter 63)
  - 25-gauge 5/8″ needle
  - 3 ml syringe
  - topical ophthalmic anesthetic (proparacaine, see Figure 64.2a,b)

64.3.4 Restraint and Positioning

- An assistant restrains the head, typically standing on the opposite side to the eye being evaluated.
- Sedation may be required.

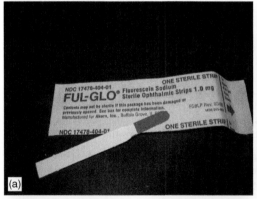

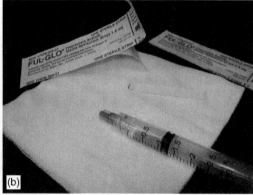

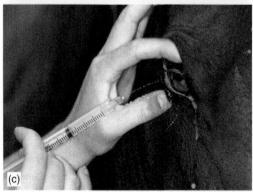

Figure 64.3 The wet fluorescein stain procedure. (a) Fluorescein strip. (b) Sterile fluorescein strip and irrigating solution placed in a 3 ml syringe. The 25-gauge needle is broken off manually at the hub prior to application. (c) Application of fluorescein dye to the corneal surface by squirting the dye solution onto the eye through the hub of a 25-gauge needle, being careful not to get too close to the eye, as the hub of the needle is still sharp.

64.3.5 Procedure: Fluorescein Stain – Wet

Technical action	Rationale
Perform fluorescein staining after the STT I is completed.	To prevent interfering with the results of the STT I. Results are affected by the application of medications or irrigating solutions to the eye.
Remove the fluorescein strip from the packet and place a small amount of irrigating solution on the end of the fluorescein strip.	Only a small amount of irrigating solution is required to wet the strip. Commercial fluorescein solutions are not utilized as they are easily contaminated by bacteria.
	Alternatively, a sterile fluorescein strip may be placed in a 3 ml syringe. The syringe is partially-filled with irrigating solution and the plunger is reinserted (Figure 64.3b).
	The 25-gauge needle is broken off manually at the hub prior to application. The solution is then squirted onto the eye through the hub of the 25-gauge needle (Figure 64.3c).
	The examiner should be careful not to get too close to the eye as the hub of the needle is still sharp.
	Over-dilution of the dye with larger volumes of irrigating solution may result in a false-negative fluorescein test.
Evert the lower eyelid by pulling ventrally on the skin of the lower lid and placing the tip of the moistened fluorescein strip in the inferior conjunctival fornix. Allow a few seconds for the dye to diffuse.	Avoid directly touching the cornea to prevent the creation of an artifact.
Remove the strip and blink the lids to ensure distribution over the entire ocular surface.	
Rinse the eye with irrigating solution to flush away excess fluorescein, and wipe the face with gauze	
Examine the cornea in a darkened environment with a blue light from a cobalt filter or an ultraviolet light source.	The stain will be picked up by exposed corneal stroma and will be bright green when evaluated by a blue or ultraviolet light source. An ulcer with a descemetocele will look clear in the area that the ulcer is down to Descemet's membrane. Melting ulcers have a soft look and will have indistinct stain uptake.
To determine the patency of the nasolacrimal duct, evaluate the distal puncta (in the nares) for the presence of green dye (See Figure 62.5, page 520). This may take up to 20 minutes.	

64.3.6 Procedure: Seidel Test – Fluorescein Dye

Technical actions	Rationale
Perform a palpebral nerve block.	Facilitates performance of the Seidel test as the lids must be held open to prevent blinking across the area being evaluated. This also reduces the amount of force being placed on a potentially compromised eye.
Apply topical ophthalmic anesthetic to the corneal surface.	The Seidel test is used to evaluate corneal injuries to aid in determining if they are full-thickness and leaking. Topical ophthalmic anesthetic reduces the pain associated with a corneal injury, facilitating the examination.
Part the eyelids and keep them open.	The corneal surface must be kept dry. Parting the eyelids prevents blinking of tear film across the cornea.
Gently dry the affected corneal surface with a sterile cotton-tipped applicator.	The surface of the lesion being examined must be dried of tear film.
Utilizing a dry fluorescein strip, paint the surface of the corneal defect being investigated.	Dry fluorescein dye is painted onto the surface of the corneal defect. If the lesion is not leaking aqueous, the dye will remain bright orange.
Observe the corneal defect for a change in the color of the dye from orange to green.	If the lesion is leaking aqueous, the dye will run green. This will also occur if the animal is allowed to blink over the defect or if the wound was not dried prior to application of fluorescein.

64.4 Rose Bengal Stain

64.4.1 Purpose

- To identify dead or devitalized corneal epithelial cells associated with keratitis, keratoconjunctivitis sicca or pre-corneal tear film abnormalities.

64.4.2 Complications

- Local irritation

64.4.3 Equipment Required

- Rose Bengal stain strips (Figure 64.4)
- Ophthalmic irrigating solution (eye wash)
- Gauze
- White light

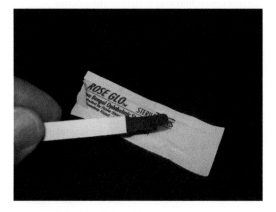

Figure 64.4 Rose Bengal stain strip.

64.4.4 Procedure: Rose Bengal Stain

Technical action	Rationale
Remove the strip from the sterile package.	Rose Bengal strips are preferred over commercial solutions.
Moisten the end of the strip with ophthalmic irrigating solution.	Avoid touching the cornea directly with the strip to avoid creating an artifact.
	Alternatively, the syringe technique could be utilized as described in the section on fluorescein stain.
Place dye in the lower conjunctival fornix (as described for fluorescein stain).	
Blink lids fully over the eye.	Ensures even distribution over the cornea.
Rinse the eye with irrigating solution and wipe any excess with gauze.	
Examine the eye with white light.	Uptake will appear pink with white light.

64.5 Corneal or Conjunctival Cytology

64.5.1 Purpose

- To collect a sample that will aid in the diagnosis of corneal or conjunctival disorders.
- To aid the clinician in the development of a diagnostic and/or treatment plan.

64.5.2 Complications

- Local irritation
- Worsening of a corneal defect if deep/ fragile areas are sampled.
- Non-diagnostic sample is possible given small sample sizes or if inadequate sampling techniques are utilized.

64.5.3 Equipment Required

- Topical ophthalmic anesthetic (proparacaine) (see Figure 64.2a,b)
- Sterile surgical blade, Kimura spatula or cytology brush
- Slides
- Slide stain
- Microscope
- Local anesthetic (2% lidocaine or mepivacaine)
- 25-gauge 5/8″ needle
- 3 ml syringe

64.5.4 Restraint and Positioning

- An assistant restrains the head, typically standing on the opposite side to the eye being evaluated.
- Sedation may be required.
- Perform palpebral nerve block (see Chapter 63).
- Apply topical ophthalmic anesthetic (see Figure 64.2a,b).

64.5.5 Procedure: Corneal or Conjunctival Cytology

Technical action	Rationale
After performing a palpebral nerve block, apply ophthalmic anesthetic to the corneal/conjunctival surface.	This is a painful procedure that will require the use of topical ophthalmic anesthetic.
Peel the foil pouch of a sterile surgical blade back to expose the blunt end. Alternatively, remove a cytology brush from the sterile packaging or use a Kimura spatula.	Any of these sampling methods should result in adequate exfoliation of cells for evaluation.
Gently part the eyelids with the thumb and index finger.	
Scrape the edges of the corneal ulcer (Figure 64.5a) or conjunctiva to exfoliate cells (Figure 64.5b).	The edges of a corneal ulcer should be sampled to avoid deep corneal defects.
Transfer the sample to microscope slides.	Roll the cytology brush onto the slide or tap the sample onto the slide from the blade or spatula. Carefully smear the sample to create a monolayer.
Stain slides and evaluate under a light microscope.	Romanowsky-type stains such as Diff-Quick are often used for initial screening of cytology samples. Further staining by Gram stain may be required.

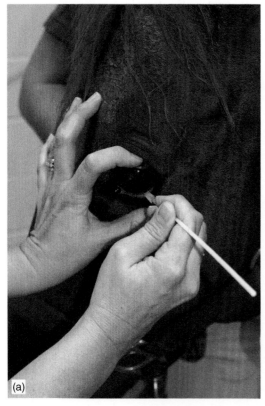

(a)

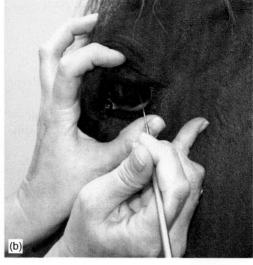

(b)

Figure 64.5 Obtaining a sample for cytologic evaluation. (a) Conjunctival cytology is obtained from the inferior conjunctival fornix using a cytology brush. (b) Corneal cytology is obtained using a Kimura spatula.

64.6 Intraocular Pressure Measurement

64.6.1 Purpose

- To determine the intraocular pressure (IOP).

64.6.2 Complications

- Local corneal irritation or trauma
- Worsening of a corneal defect if pressure is placed on a compromised globe.

64.6.3 Equipment Required

- Commercial hand-held tonometer:
  - digital applanation tonometer (TonoPen)
  - rebound tonometer (TonoVet)

- Local anesthetic (2% lidocaine or mepivacaine)
- 25-gauge 5/8″ needle
- 3 ml syringe
- Topical ophthalmic anesthetic (proparacaine) for performing applanation tonometry (see Figure 63.2a,b).

64.6.4 Restraint and Positioning

- An assistant restrains the head, typically standing on the opposite side to the eye being evaluated.
- Sedation may be required.

64.6.5 Procedure: Intraocular Pressure Measurement

Technical action	Rationale
Perform a palpebral nerve block.	Measurement of IOP is indicated for cases with diffuse corneal edema, redness, a painful globe, pupillary light reflex abnormalities, vision loss, lens subluxation/luxation, or cases with a history uveitis or glaucoma. Higher IOP readings may be seen in cases without a palpebral nerve block, sedation or when the patient's head is maintained in a lowered position.
Apply proparacaine if using a TonoPen unit.	Topical ophthalmic anesthetic is required for the TonoPen unit, but is not required for the TonoVet unit.
Ensure the tonometry unit is calibrated according to manufacturer's instructions.	If using a TonoVet, ensure that the equine mode is selected.
Apply a clean TonoPen cover to the tip of the unit or load a new TonoVet probe.	Minimizes the risk of passing contaminants/infectious agents from patient to patient.
Gently part the eyelids with the thumb and index finger of the non-dominant hand.	
Turn the tonometry unit on.	
Hold the tonometry unit in the dominant hand and maintain the probe or tip of the unit in a position that is perpendicular to the corneal surface.	To ensure accurate readings, the tip of the unit should be kept perpendicular and flat against the corneal surface.

(continued)

Technical action	Rationale
Obtain IOP readings by: • performing applanation tonometry: gently tapping the central cornea with the TonoPen (Figure 64.6a) or • rebound tonometry: clicking the button on the handle of the TonoVet unit to obtain the reading (Figure 64.6b).	The unit should be applied to the central corneal surface, but the position should be adjusted to avoid obvious corneal irregularities. Avoid forcefully tapping the cornea with the TonoPen unit.
The unit will beep when it has obtained enough readings and will display the average IOP in mmHg with a standard error bar.	The units take an average of 6 to 8 readings to give a value. Readings with high standard error should be repeated.
If high error is encountered, as indicated by unit, reading should be repeated.	Reading will vary depending on the device used. Normal IOP for the horse is reported as ranging between 16 and 32 mmHg with an average of 24 mmHg. Sedatives (e.g., xylazine and detomidine) and tranquilizers (e.g., acepromazine) can affect IOP.

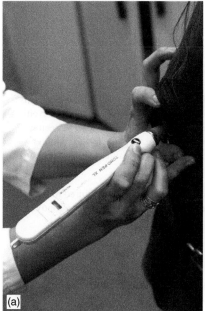

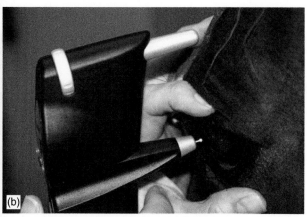

(a)

(b)

Figure 64.6 Obtaining IOP in a horse. (a) Using a TonoPen applanation tonometer. (b) Using a TonoVet rebound tonometer.

Bibliography and Further Reading

Gilger, B.C. and Stoppini, R. (2011) Equine ocular examination: Routine and advanced diagnostic techniques, in *Equine Ophthalmology*, 2nd edn (ed. B.C. Gilger), W.B. Saunders, Maryland Heights, pp. 1–51.

Maggs, D.J. (2008) Basic diagnostic techniques, in *Slatter's Fundamentals of Veterinary Ophthalmology*, 4th edn (eds D.J. Maggs, P.E. Miller, and R. Ofri), W.B. Saunders, St. Louis, pp. 81–106.

Martin, C.L. (2005) Anamnesis and the ophthalmic examination, in *Ophthalmic Disease in Veterinary Medicine* (ed. C.L. Martin) Manson Publishing, London, pp. 1–40.

65

Ophthalmic Therapeutic Procedures

Renee Carter

This chapter discusses some of the common procedures utilized when treating horses for various ophthalmic disorders, including:

- Administering Ocular Medications
- Retrograde Nasolacrimal Flush
- Normograde Nasolacrimal Flush
- Subconjunctival Injection
- Subpalpebral Lavage System Placement
- Cannulation of the Nasolacrimal Duct

65.1 Administering Ocular Medications

65.1.1 Purpose

- To apply ophthalmic medications to the ocular surface for the treatment of infectious or inflammatory conditions of the eye.

65.1.2 Complications

- Iatrogenic trauma to the ocular surface
- Local irritation

65.1.3 Equipment Required

- Ophthalmic medications

65.1.4 Restraint and Positioning

- Assistant to restrain the head may be required, standing on the opposite side of the clinician or technician.
- A twitch may be required to immobilize the head during placement.

65.1.5 Procedure: Administering Ophthalmic Ointments

Technical action	Rationale
Place the index finger within the crease of the upper lid and thumb along the lower lid. Part the lids with thumb and index finger (non-dominant hand in Figure 65.1).	Fingers should be resting along the orbital rim when the lids are fully parted.
With the other hand place a ¼″ strip of ointment along the inferior lid margin in front of the third eyelid (dominant hand in Figure 65.1).	Placing medication in front of the third eyelid minimizes the risk of damage to the corneal surface. *Warning*: Extreme care should be taken, not to touch the cornea.
Blink lids to distribute medication.	

Manual of Clinical Procedures in the Horse, First Edition. Edited by Lais R.R. Costa and Mary Rose Paradis.
© 2018 John Wiley & Sons, Inc. Published 2018 by John Wiley & Sons, Inc.

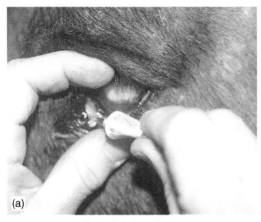
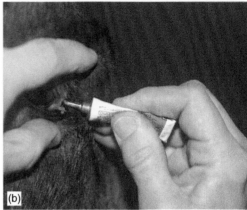

Figure 65.1 Administration of ophthalmic ointment medication. Place the index finger within the crease of the upper lid and thumb along the lower lid. Part the lids with the thumb and index finger, such that the fingers are resting on the orbital rim when the lids are fully parted. With the other hand place a ¼″ strip of ointment along the inferior lid margin in front of the third eyelid: (a) oculus sinister (OS, left eye) and (b) oculus dexter (OD, right eye). Tip of the tube must not touch the cornea.

65.1.6 Procedure: Administering Ophthalmic Drops

Technical action	Rationale/amplification
Part lids with thumb and index finger.	
With the other hand place one to two drops of medication into the lower conjunctival fornix.	Placing medication in front of the third eyelid minimizes the risk of damage to the corneal surface.
	Alternatively, 0.1 ml of medication can be drawn up with a 25-gauge needle and a 1 ml syringe. With the needle removed, the medication is delivered to the lower conjunctival surface with the syringe.
Blink lids to distribute medication.	

65.2 Retrograde Nasolacrimal Flush

65.2.1 Purpose

- To clear blockage from the nasolacrimal duct.
- Indicated in patients with mucopurulent ocular or nasal discharge or in patients with unexplained epiphora.

65.2.2 Complications

- An inability to clear the blockage.
- Local irritation.
- Introduction of contaminants, resulting in infection

65.2.3 Equipment Required

- An appropriate catheter can be any of the following:
  - tomcat catheter, 3.5 - 5 Fr (Figure 65.2a, A)
  - nasolacrimal duct catheter (MILA International, Inc)
  - 3.5 - 5 Fr polyethylene tubing (Figure 65.2a, B and C)
  - 5 Fr feeding tube
- Lidocaine gel
- 12–20 ml syringe
- Saline or eyewash
- Gloves

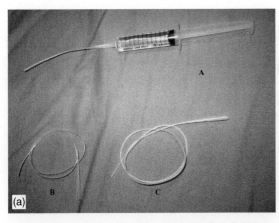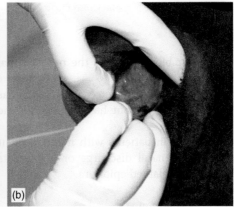

Figure 65.2 (a) Materials for performing a retrograde nasolacrimal flush: A, 4.5 Fr Tomcat catheter; B, 3.5 Fr polyethylene tubing; C, 5 Fr polyethylene tubing. (b) Once the tip of the catheter/tubing is at the distal nasolacrimal opening, advance the tubing into the duct.

65.2.4 Restraint and Positioning

- Place patient in stocks if available.
- An assistant should restrain the head, standing on the opposite side of the clinician.

- Sedation will be required.
- A twitch may be required to immobilize the head during placement.

65.2.5 Procedure: Retrograde Nasolacrimal Flush

Technical action	Rationale
Administer sedation.	See Chapter 9 for details.
Identify the distal nasolacrimal opening on the ventral floor of the nasal vestibule.	
Coat the end of the tubing with lidocaine gel and apply lidocaine gel to the distal nasolacrimal opening.	Alternatively, topical ophthalmic anesthetic can be applied to the distal nasolacrimal opening.
Advance the tubing into the nasolacrimal opening up to approximately 5 cm (Figure 65.2b).	Do not force the catheter to avoid damage to the nasolacrimal duct.
Digitally occlude the opening of the duct to prevent normograde loss of fluid during irrigation.	
Attach the syringe to the end of the tubing and flush with saline or eyewash.	Gently pulse the flush to clear the duct. Excessive force will damage the duct.
Fluid should appear at the medial canthus.	The horse will start blinking prior to the appearance of the fluid at the medial canthus.

65.3 Normograde Nasolacrimal Flush

65.3.1 Purpose

- To clear blockage from the nasolacrimal duct.
- Often used after retrograde flush has been attempted but has not cleared the obstruction.
- Indicated in patients with mucopurulent ocular or nasal discharge or in patients with unexplained epiphora.

65.3.2 Complications

- An inability to clear the blockage
- Local irritation
- Iatrogenic trauma to the ocular surface.
- Introduction of contaminants, resulting in infection

65.3.3 Equipment Required

- Small diameter atraumatic catheter, either:
  - Tomcat catheter (open end; MILA International, Inc) (Figure 64.3a)

or

- 20-gauge intravenous catheter without the stylet
- Topical ophthalmic anesthetic (e.g., proparacaine)
- Local anesthetic (2% lidocaine or mepivacaine)
- 25-gauge needle (for palpebral block, see Chapter 63)
- 3 ml syringe (for palpebral block, see Chapter 63)
- 12 ml syringe
- Saline or eyewash

65.3.4 Restraint and Positioning

- Place the patient in stocks if available.
- An assistant should restrain the head, standing on the opposite side of the clinician.
- Sedation will be required.
- A twitch may be required to immobilize the head during placement.

65.3.5 Procedure: Normograde Nasolacrimal Flush

Technical action	Rationale
Administer sedation.	Sedation is required to minimize movement of the head, as most horses will resent the procedure.
Perform palpebral block of the upper lid.	See the detailed procedure in Chapter 63.
Apply topical ophthalmic anesthetic to the eye.	This will prevent evasive motion if the cornea is touched by the Tomcat catheter.
Identify the inferior punctal opening at the medial canthus just inside the lid margin.	The lower punctum is easier to cannulate.
Remove the Tomcat catheter or intravenous catheter from the packaging.	If using an intravenous catheter, remove the stylet.
Feed the catheter into the inferior punctum by directing the catheter horizontally (or in a parallel direction to the lid margin opening) and toward the medial canthus (Figure 65.3).	Do not force the catheter to avoid damage to the inferior canaliculus. Passing in a horizontal direction will follow the normal path of the inferior canaliculus.
Digitally occlude the opening of the superior punctum to prevent loss of fluid from the superior punctum during irrigation.	Digital occlusion improves flush of the nasolacrimal duct by preventing fluid from escaping through the superior punctum.
Attach the syringe to the end of the tubing and flush with saline or eyewash.	Gently pulse the flush to clear the duct. Excessive force will damage the duct.

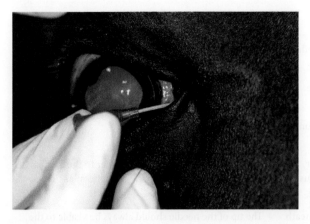

Figure 65.3 Normograde nasolacrimal flush is performed by feeding the catheter into the inferior punctum.

65.4 Subconjunctival Injection

65.4.1 Purpose

- To provide a high concentration depot of medicine to the ocular surface.
- Used for treatment of infectious or inflammatory conditions of the eye.

65.4.2 Complications

- Local swelling, irritation
- Iatrogenic trauma to the ocular surface or deeper ocular tissues
- Introduction of contaminants, resulting in infection
- Unable to withdraw the medication if there is a complication/reaction.

65.4.3 Equipment Required

- Topical ophthalmic anesthetic (e.g., proparacaine)

- Local anesthetic (2% lidocaine or mepivacaine)
- 25–27-gauge 5/8″ needles
- Syringes: 1 and 3 ml
- Povidone-iodine solution
- Small forceps
- Medication to be injected (drawn up in a 1 ml syringe)

65.4.4 Restraint and Positioning

- Place the patient in stocks if available.
- An assistant should restrain the head, standing on the opposite side of the clinician.
- Sedation is required.
- A head rest is recommended to immobilize and support the head.
- A twitch may be required.

65.4.5 Procedure: Subconjunctival Injection

Technical action	Rationale
Administer sedation.	Sedation is required to minimize movement of the head, as most horse will resent the procedure.
Perform a palpebral block of the upper lid.	See the detailed procedure in Chapter 63.
Clean the periocular region with dilute povidone-iodine solution.	To reduce the risk of contamination.
Apply topical ophthalmic anesthetic to the eye.	This will prevent evasive motion if the cornea is touched.

(continued)

Technical action	Rationale
Gently part the eyelids with the thumb and index finger.	To improve exposure.
Stabilize the hand that will be used to give the injection on the patient's head.	Resting the hand on the animal during injection will reduce the risk of inadvertent trauma to the eye.
Lift the conjunctiva with a small pair of fixation forceps.	
Advance the needle tip underneath the bulbar conjunctiva in a direction parallel to the limbus (Figure 65.4)	Advancing the needle perpendicular to the limbus could result in damage to the deeper ocular tissues.
Once the tip of the needle is advanced underneath the conjunctiva, deliver the medication.	The tip of the needle should always be visible to the clinician to avoid injury to deeper ocular tissues.
The administered medication should create a bleb in the conjunctiva.	No more than 1 ml volume of drug should be delivered.

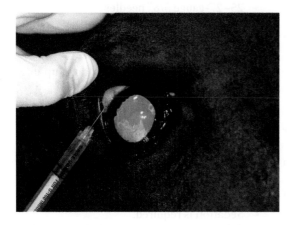

Figure 65.4 A subconjunctival injection is performed to administer a depot of medication underneath the bulbar conjunctiva.

65.5 Subpalpebral Lavage System Placement

65.5.1 Purpose

- Facilitates the administration of ophthalmic medications.
- Commonly used when frequent medical therapy is indicated for treatment of painful ocular conditions or patients who are difficult to treat.

65.5.2 Complications

- Iatrogenic trauma to the ocular surface.
- Development of a corneal ulcer with improper placement of the lavage system.
- Development of localized swelling or infection.

65.5.3 Equipment Required

- Commercial subpalpebral lavage system kit (MILA International, Inc.) (Figure 65.5)
- Local anesthetic (2% lidocaine or mepivacaine)
- Topical ophthalmic anesthetic (e.g., proparacaine)
- 25-gauge needles
- 3 ml syringes
- Povidone-iodine solution
- Sterile gloves
- Sterile, water-soluble lubricant
- Clippers
- Tape
- Tongue depressor
- Non-absorbable suture (2-0 nylon)

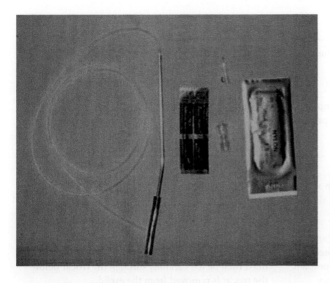

Figure 65.5 Materials needed for placement of a sub-palpebral lavage system: trocar, tubing, catheter or needle to be placed into the free end of the tubing, injection cap to be screwed into the hub of the catheter, suture material, blade or scissors to cut the suture material.

65.5.4 Restraint and Positioning

- Place patient in stocks if available.
- An assistant should restrain the head, standing on the opposite side of the clinician.
- Sedation is required.
- A twitch may be required to immobilize the head during placement.

65.5.5 Procedure: Subpalpebral Lavage System Placement

Technical actions	Rationale
Administer sedation.	Sedation is required to minimize movement of the head, as most horses will resent the procedure.
Perform a palpebral lid block.	Blocking motor to the upper lid will facilitate safe placement of the lavage system. See the detailed procedure in Chapter 63.
Clip hair along the dorsal orbital rim.	Removal of the hair will reduce the risk of infection developing around the tube site.
Clean the region with 1:50 diluted povidone-iodine solution.	Cleaning the region prior to lavage placement will reduce the risk of infection developing around the tube site.
Perform supraorbital nerve block or line block of the central upper lid with local anesthetic (Figure 63.3, page 526).	Sensory block is required for placement of the trocar through the upper lid.
Apply topical ophthalmic anesthetic to the cornea and superior conjunctival surfaces.	Topical ophthalmic anesthetic reduces corneal reflex, decreasing the pain response during placement.
Locate the highest point underneath the upper eyelid proximal to the superior orbital rim (Figure 65.5a). Peel open the commercial lavage kit.	Placement at the highest point underneath the upper eyelid proximal to the superior orbital rim will ensure the lavage system is sitting at the superior conjunctival fornix.
Using a gloved hand, grasp the trocar of the lavage kit so that the trocar lies along the inner aspect of the palm and index finger (Figure 65.6b).	The index finger is used to guide the trocar during placement and protect the eye from iatrogenic trauma to the eye during placement (Figure 65.6c). Alternatively, the lubricated end of a tongue depressor can be used as a guard.

(continued)

Technical actions	Rationale
Place a small amount of sterile lubricant along the outer aspect of the index finger.	A small amount of lubricant is applied to the back of the index finger to make it easier to guide the trocar underneath the eyelid.
Guide the needle (trocar) underneath the upper eyelid to the superior conjunctival fornix (proximal to the superior orbital rim).	To minimize the risk of corneal ulcer development that occurs when the footplate of the lavage comes into direct contact with the cornea, the lavage should enter the conjunctival fornix of the central upper lid just in front of the superior orbital rim.
Insert the trocar from the inner conjunctival surface, exiting full thickness through the skin of the central upper eyelid (Figure 65.6d,e).	
Carefully complete the passage of the trocar through the skin of the upper eyelid and feed the attached tubing through the lid until the footplate of the lavage system is seated in the superior conjunctival fornix (Figure 65.6f).	With some lavage systems the tubing is not directly connected to the end of the trocar and the tubing must then be fed carefully through the trocar before the trocar is removed from the eyelid.
Alternatively, the SPL may be placed in inferomedial lid. The lavage system is placed through the inferior lid in front of the third eyelid after performing a local line block of the lower lid with lidocaine.	Placement in front of the third eyelid minimizes the risk of the SPL footplate contacting the corneal surface.
Palpate the footplate to ensure that it is seated properly.	The footplate should be sitting flush with the conjunctival surface.
Apply a butterfly of duct tape or white tape to the proximal aspect of the lavage at the point that it exits the upper eyelid.	For inferomedial SPL placement, the first butterfly will be placed below the lower eyelid (Figure 65.8).
Place a simple interrupted suture through each wing of the butterfly (tape–skin–tape) on either side of the lavage system (Figure 65.7a,b).	This helps to secure the lavage and prevent slippage. Leave enough slack in the lavage between the first and second tacking sutures so that the horse may move its head without putting tension on the lavage line.
Place a second securing butterfly of tape and suture just below the forelock.	Alternatively, the second butterfly of tape may be sutured toward the base of the ear (Figure 65.7c).
Create several interrupted braids in the mane. Feed lavage tubing through the braids.	
Detach the trocar from the distal end of the tubing.	
Carefully feed the accompanying 20-gauge intravenous catheter into the distal end of the lavage tubing and remove the stylet (Figure 65.9a).	Pull the tip of the stylet back into the catheter so that the tip is not exposed when feeding the catheter into the distal lavage tubing. This makes it easier to feed the catheter (more rigid), but decreases the risk of perforating the lavage line with the stylet.
Attach the injection port to the hub of a 20-gauge catheter (Figure 65.9b).	

Technical actions	Rationale
Tape the catheter/injection port to a tongue depressor and tape it to the final braid (Figure 65.9c).	For added security, this prevents kinking of the catheter.
Treat as directed. Wipe the end of the injection port prior to injecting through the port.	All medications should be followed by 1 ml of air flush to facilitate delivery to the eye. Wait 5 minutes between medications. Not for use with ophthalmic ointments. Use of clear shield, such as Equivizor Multipurpose Helmet (by Provizor International) may prevent the horse from rubbing the eye and SPL.

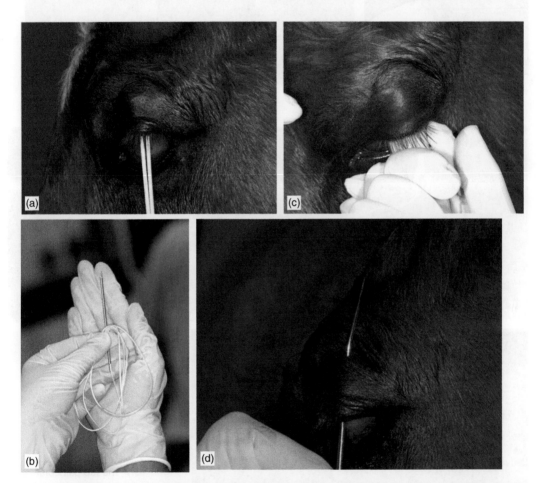

Figure 65.6 Placement of sub-palpebral lavage system through the upper eyelid. (a) Locate the highest point underneath the upper eyelid proximal to the superior orbital rim to ensure the placement of the lavage in the superior conjunctival fornix. (b) Hold the trocar of the sub-palpebral lavage system so that it lies along the inner aspect of the palm and index finger. (c) Use the index finger to guide the trocar during placement and to protect the eye from iatrogenic trauma. (d) The trocar should exit through the central aspect of the upper eyelid. (e) Make sure the trocar exits proximal to the superior orbital rim. (f) After passing the trocar through the skin of the upper eyelid, advance the attached tubing through the lid until the footplate of the lavage system is seated in the superior conjunctival fornix.

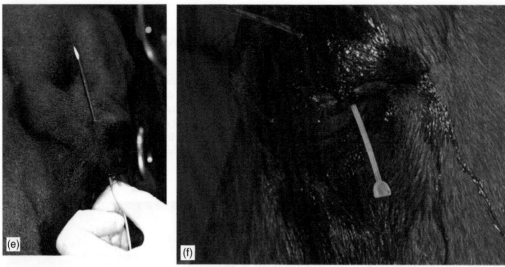

Figure 65.6 (Continued)

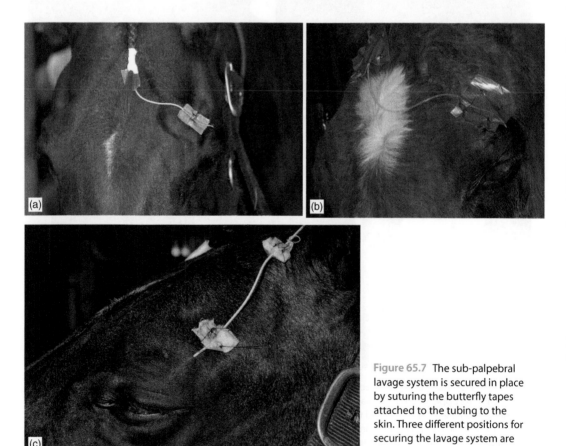

Figure 65.7 The sub-palpebral lavage system is secured in place by suturing the butterfly tapes attached to the tubing to the skin. Three different positions for securing the lavage system are shown.

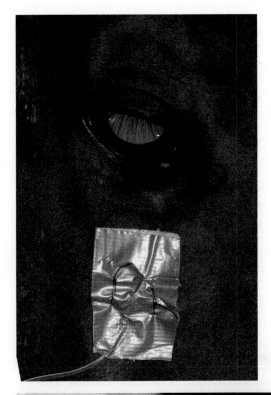

Figure 65.8 Placement of sub-palpebral lavage system through the lower lid.

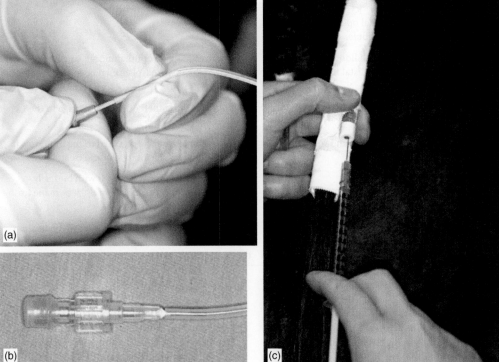

Figure 65.9 Attaching the injection port to the free end of the tubing. (a) A catheter is fed onto the distal end of the lavage line. (b) An injection cap is screwed into the hub of the catheter. (c) The injection port is secured to a tongue depressor taped to a braid in the mane and used for the administration of medication into the eye.

65.6 Cannulation of the Nasolacrimal Duct

65.6.1 Purpose

- An alternative to the placement of a sub-palpebral lavage system.

65.6.2 Complications

- Local irritation
- Introduction of infectious agents
- Premature removal by the patient, not well-tolerated

65.6.3 Equipment Required

- Topical ophthalmic anesthetic or lidocaine gel
- 4–6 Fr polyethylene tubing or 5 Fr feeding tube
- White tape
- Non-absorbable suture (2-0 nylon)

65.6.4 Restraint

- Place the patient in stocks if available.
- An assistant should restrain the head, standing on the opposite side of the clinician.
- Sedation is required.
- A twitch may be required to immobilize the head during placement.

65.6.5 Procedure: Cannulation of the Nasolacrimal Duct

Technical action	Rationale
Administer sedation.	Sedation is required to minimize movement of the head, as most horse will resent the procedure.
Identify the distal nasolacrimal opening on the ventral floor of the nasal vestibule.	
Coat the end of the tubing with lidocaine gel and apply lidocaine gel to the distal nasolacrimal opening.	Alternatively, topical ophthalmic anesthetic can be applied to the distal nasolacrimal opening.
Feed tubing into the nasolacrimal opening up to approximately 5 cm.	Do not force the catheter to avoid damage to the nasolacrimal duct.
Apply butterfly tape to the tubing and suture in place.	An extension set may be attached to the tubing and sutured in place to facilitate medical treatment. The extension set may be sutured with butterfly tape, and taped to the braided forelock or mane for additional security.
Treat as directed.	Not for use with ointments. Follow each medication with an air flush to facilitate delivery medication to the eye.

Bibliography and Further Reading

Dwyer, A.E. (2011) Practical general field ophthalmology, in *Equine Ophthalmology*, 2nd edn (ed. B.C. Gilger), W.B. Saunders, Maryland Heights, pp. 52–92.

Gilger, B.C. and Stoppini, R. (2011) Equine ocular examination: Routine and advanced diagnostic techniques, in *Equine Ophthalmology*, 2nd edn (ed. B.C. Gilger), W.B. Saunders, Maryland Heights, pp. 1–51.

Maggs, D.J. (2008) Ocular pharmacology and therapeutics, in *Slatter's Fundamentals of Veterinary Ophthalmology*, 4th edn (eds D.J. Maggs, P.E. Miller, and R. Ofri), W.B. Saunders, St. Louis, pp. 33–61.

Part IX

Clinical Procedures by Body Systems: Dermatological Procedures

66

Brushing/grooming

Michelle Woodward and Cherie Pucheu-Haston

66.1 Purpose

- Brushing/grooming is a simple diagnostic procedure involving gross examination of hair and skin surface debris.
- It facilitates the detection of lice, other large ectoparasites, and surface feeding mites (such as *Chorioptes equi*) in pruritic horses. Ticks are not removed with brushing, but are detected by careful inspection, especially of the ears.
- Common parasites and their preferred body locations are presented in Table 66.1.

66.2 Equipment Required

- Stiff brush or denture-type toothbrush
- Flea comb
- Petri dish (or cardboard, paper, dustpan)
- Dark surface
- Dissecting microscope (optional)

Table 66.1 Large ectoparasites found on hair or attached to the skin of horses (courtesy of Dr. Lais R.R. Costa)

Type	Common name	Scientific name	Preferred body location
Pediculosis	Chewing lice	*Damalinia* (aka *Werneckiella, Bovicola*) *equi* (Figure 66.a,c)	Head, mane, base of tail
	Sucking lice	*Haematopinus asini* (Figure 66.b,c,d)	Head, neck, back, thighs, fetlocks
Tick	Ixodid	*Dermacentor* spp, *Amblyomma* spp, *Rhipicephalus* spp, *Ixodes* spp.	Ear, false nostril, face, neck, mane, axillae, groin, distal limbs, tail
	Argasid	*Otobius megnini, Ornithodorus* spp	Ear
Trombiculiasis	Trombiculid (chigger)	*Trombicula (Eutrombicula) alfreddugesi, Trombicula splendens, Trombicula (Neotrombicula) autumnalis*	Muzzle, nares, distal limbs, face
Chorioptic mange	Chorioptic mite	*Chorioptes* spp. (Figure 68.3, page 561)	Limbs, foot, tail

Manual of Clinical Procedures in the Horse, First Edition. Edited by Lais R.R. Costa and Mary Rose Paradis.
© 2018 John Wiley & Sons, Inc. Published 2018 by John Wiley & Sons, Inc.

66.3 Procedure: Brushing/grooming

Technical action	Rationale
Select the sites to be sampled.	Choose sites based on location of pruritus or lesions.
Use a brush to sweep dander, hair, and other debris onto a petri dish (Figure 66.1).	A flea comb to collect dander and other debris might improve recovery of ectoparasites such as mites. Any collection container can be used.
Place the collected material on a dark surface.	The dark surface increases the chances of seeing ectoparasites such as lice.
Examine the material for the presence of large ectoparasites (Table 66.1).	Examination is best done with a dissecting microscope.
If available, use a dissecting microscope to check for the presence of smaller parasites (Figure 66.2).	Movement of ectoparasites may be the easiest thing to visualize.

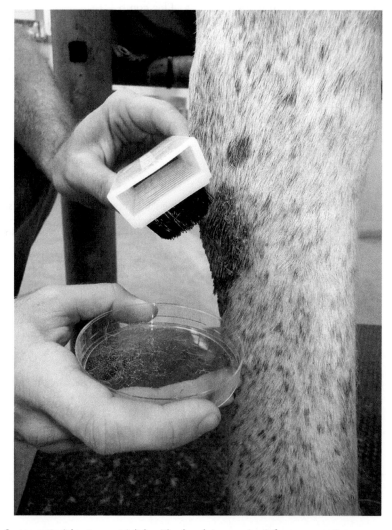

Figure 66.1 Sweep material onto a petri dish with a brush to examine it for any parasites.

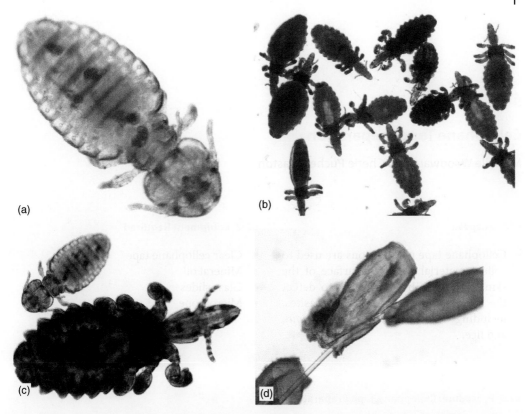

Figure 66.2 Examination of the material under a dissecting microscope for the presence of large ectoparasites: (a) adult chewing louse *Werneckiella (Damalinia) equi* (courtesy of Dr. Eileen Johnson), (b) adult sucking lice (*Haematopinus asini,* (courtesy of Dr. Eileen Johnson), (c) one adult chewing louse *Werneckiella (Damalinia) equi* next to an adult sucking louse (*Haematopinus asini*), and (d) nits of *Haematopinus asini,* attached to a hair (courtesy of Dr. Eileen Johnson).

Bibliography and Further Reading

Bergvall, K. (2005) Advances in acquisition, identification and treatment of equine ectoparasites. *Clinical Techniques in Equine Practice,* **4**, 296–301.

Bowman, D.D. (2009) *Arthropods, in Georgi's Parasitology for Veterinarians,* 9th edn (ed. D.D. Bowman), Elsevier, St. Louis, pp. 4–82.

Evans, A.G. and Stannard, A.A. (1986) Diagnostic approach to equine skin disease. *Compendium Equine,* **8**, 652–660.

Littlewood, J.D. (1997) Diagnostic procedures in equine skin disease. *Equine Veterinary Education,* **3**, 174–176.

Pascoe, R.R. and Knottenbelt, D.C. (1999) *Manual of Equine Dermatology,* W.B. Saunders, London.

Scott, D.W. and Miller, W.H. (2011) *Equine Dermatology,* 2nd edn, W.B. Saunders, St. Louis.

Sorrell, M.S., Fish, R.E., and Taylor, K.H. (2010) Pediculosis in two research ponies (*Equus caballus*). *Journal of the American Association of Laboratory Animal Science,* **49**, 487–490.

67

Cellophane Tape Preparation

Michelle Woodward and Cherie Pucheu-Haston

67.1 Purpose

- Cellophane tape preparations are used to collect material from the surface of the skin and coat. The purpose is to detect the presence of certain skin parasites, including *Oxyuris equi, Chorioptes equi*, and lice.

67.2 Equipment Required

- Clear cellophane tape
- Mineral oil
- Glass slides
- Microscope

67.3 Procedure: Cellophane Tape Preparation

Technical action	Rationale
Select sites for sampling.	If looking for *Oxyuris equi* eggs, the sample should be collected from several areas around the anal and perianal regions. If looking for other parasites, choose an area of scaling or alopecia.
Using a 3–5 cm piece of cellophane tape, press the sticky side of tape to the hair and skin of the selected area (Figure 67.1).	Cellophane tape preparation is particularly useful in obtaining *Oxyuris equi* eggs, and for trapping ectoparasites such as *Chorioptes equi* and lice, which otherwise move around during superficial skin sampling.
Coat a glass slide with mineral oil.	The mineral oil helps to clear debris and facilitate visualization of ova, mites, and lice.
Place the tape adhesive side down onto the glass slide.	Eliminate air bubbles.
Examine the slide microscopically for evidence of ova (Figure 67.2) or other parasites such as mites (see Figure 68.3, page 561) and lice (see Figure 66.2, page 555).	

Manual of Clinical Procedures in the Horse, First Edition. Edited by Lais R.R. Costa and Mary Rose Paradis.
© 2018 John Wiley & Sons, Inc. Published 2018 by John Wiley & Sons, Inc.

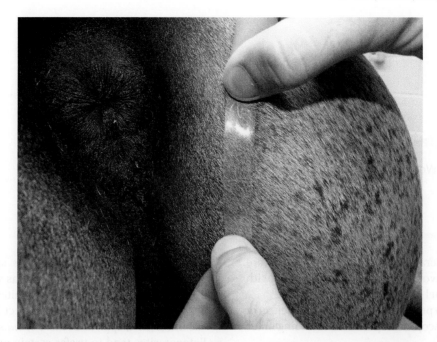

Figure 67.1 Press the sticky side of the cellophane tape to the hair and skin of the selected area.

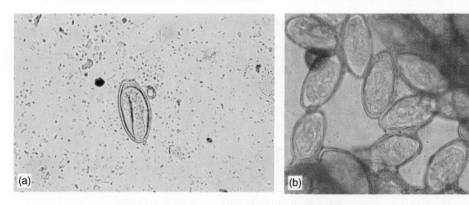

Figure 67.2 Cellophane tape collection at the perineum allows the detection of *Oxyuris equi* ova. (a) The ova have an operculum, or cap, located on one end and measure 90 × 40 μm. Courtesy of Thomas Klei. (b) Egg mass of *Oxyuris equi*. Courtesy of Dr. Eileen Johnson.

Bibliography and Further Reading

Bergvall, K. (2005) Advances in acquisition, identification and treatment of equine ectoparasites. *Clinical Techniques in Equine Practice*, **4**, 296–301.

Evans, A.G. and Stannard, A.A. (1986) Diagnostic approach to equine skin disease. *Compendium Equine*, **8**, 652–660.

Littlewood, J.D. (1997) Diagnostic procedures in equine skin disease. *Equine Veterinary Education*, **3**, 174–176.

Pascoe, R.R. and Knottenbelt, D.C. (1999) *Manual of Equine Dermatology*, W.B. Saunders, London.

Scott, D.W. and Miller, W.H. (2011) *Equine Dermatology*, 2nd edn, W.B. Saunders, St. Louis.

68

Skin Scraping

Michelle Woodward and Cherie Pucheu-Haston

68.1 Purpose

- Skin scraping is a diagnostic procedure that involves abrasion of skin lesions with a scalpel blade or curette.
- Its purpose is to detect the presence of microscopic ectoparasites, including mites such as *Chorioptes* spp., *Psoroptes* spp., *Sarcoptes* spp., and *Demodex* spp., as well as larval stages of the trombiculid mites.
- Scrapings may also be used to detect larvae of *Pelodera* spp., and *Habronema* spp.
- Ectoparasites tend to prefer certain areas of the body (see Table 68.1).

Table 68.1 Ectoparasites identified by skin scraping of horses (courtesy of Dr. Lais R.R. Costa)

Type	Common name	Scientific name	Preferred body location
Mange	Chorioptic mange	*Chorioptes* spp.	Limbs, feet, tail
	Psoroptic mange	*Psoroptes* spp.	Ears, head, mane, tail, trunk
	Sarcoptic mange[a]	*Sarcoptes* spp.	Begins at head, ears, and neck, and spreads caudally
	Demodectic mange	*Demodex caballi*	Eyelids, muzzle
		Demodex equi	Any haired area in the body
Trombiculid mite	Trombiculiasis or chiggers	*Trombicula* (*Eutrombicula* spp.), *Neotrombicula* spp.)	Muzzle, nares, false nostril, face, ears, neck, distal limbs
Other mites	Forage mites	*Pediculoides ventricosus, Pyemotes tritici, Acarus farinae*	Areas in contact with contaminated foodstuff (e.g., muzzle, head, neck, limbs, topline)
	Bird mites	*Dermanyssus gallinae, Ornithonyssus sylviarium*	Areas exposed to contaminated materials (e.g., muzzle, limbs, topline)
Nematodes	Pelodera or rhabditic dermatitis	*Pelodera strongyloides*	Areas in contact with contaminated environment (limbs, ventral thorax, abdomen)
	Habronemiasis	*Habronema* spp.	Ulcerated lesions typically on the eye (medial canthus, conjunctiva, third eyelid), commissure of the lips, prepuce and penis, limbs, ventral thorax, abdomen

[a]Sarcoptic mange is now uncommon throughout the world and considered eradicated in the USA.

Manual of Clinical Procedures in the Horse, First Edition. Edited by Lais R.R. Costa and Mary Rose Paradis.
© 2018 John Wiley & Sons, Inc. Published 2018 by John Wiley & Sons, Inc.

68.2 Complications

No complications.

68.3 Equipment Required

- Clippers
- Dull #10 scalpel blade or curette

- Sterile container (optional)
- Mineral oil
- Glass slides
- Coverslips
- Light microscope

68.4 Procedure: Skin Scraping

Technical action	Rationale
Gently clip the hair in area for sampling.	This may be necessary for lesions in areas such as the fetlock. Hair removal facilities visualization of mites on the microscope slide.
Select the area to be scraped.	Superficial scrapings can be useful for identifying *Chorioptes* spp., *Sarcoptes* spp., *Psoroptes* spp., and larval *Trombicula* spp.
Place a drop of mineral oil on the blade. Another drop can also be placed on the area of skin to be sampled.	Some mite species (notably *Chorioptes* spp.) are very motile and hard to "trap" during scraping. In this case, a drop or two of pyrethrin insecticide (or similar product) may be added to the mineral oil before scraping.
Scrape with the scalpel blade (keeping the blade perpendicular to the skin) in the direction of hair growth several times until a small amount of skin surface debris is obtained (Figure 68.1).	Alternatively, a curette might be used to perform the scrapping in the same fashion.
If demodectic mange is suspected, a deeper skin scrape is necessary. Pinch the area of skin before scraping. The lesion should be scraped until easily visible drops of blood appear.	Pinching the skin may force deeper mites, such as *Demodex* spp., out of the follicles, facilitating collection. Demodex mites are not always of concern in horses. Deep scrapings may also permit the detection of *Pelodera* spp, and occasionally *Habronema* spp. larvae.
Transfer hair and debris onto a drop of mineral oil on a slide and swirl the material to disperse the debris evenly over the slide (Figure 68.2).	Alternatively, if sample collection is being performed in the field, deposit hair and debris that is collected into a sterile container until it can be examined.
Place a coverslip on the slide and examine on 10× objective (Figure 68.3). Evaluate the entire area with the coverslip.	A 40× objective can be used for more detail if something of interest is noted.
Repeat the procedure for several different areas/lesions.	If multiple areas are to be sampled, clean the blade thoroughly between sites to prevent cross-contamination of the samples.

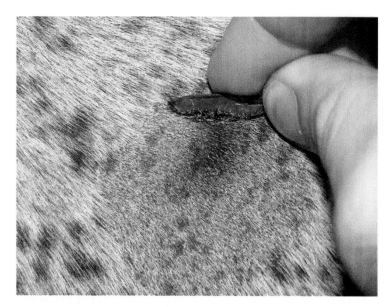

Figure 68.1 Skin scraping technique.

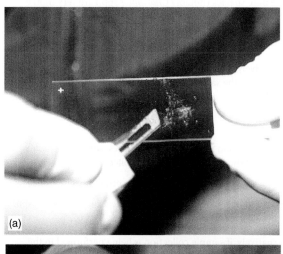

(a)

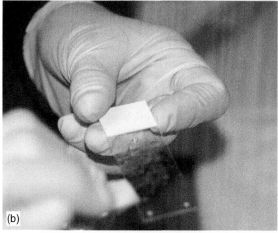

(b)

Figure 68.2 Prepare the slide by (a) transferring hair and debris onto a drop of mineral oil on a slide and (b) swirling the material to disperse debris evenly over the slide. Courtesy of Dr. Lais R.R. Costa.

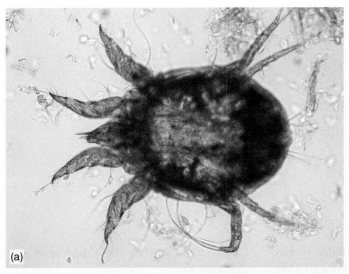

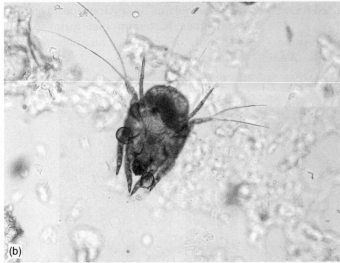

Figure 68.3 Superficial scraping preparations are examined under a light microscope to check for the presence of small parasites: (a) psoroptic mite, and (b) chorioptic mite. Courtesy of Dr. Eileen Johnson.

Bibliography and Further Reading

Bergvall, K. (2005) Advances in acquisition, identification and treatment of equine ectoparasites. *Clinical Techniques in Equine Practice*, **4**, 296–301.

Evans, A.G. and Stannard, A.A. (1986) Diagnostic approach to equine skin disease. *Compendium Equine*, **8**, 652–660.

Littlewood, J.D. (1997) Diagnostic procedures in equine skin disease. *Equine Veterinary Education*, **3**, 174–176.

Pascoe, R.R. and Knottenbelt, D.C. (1999) *Manual of Equine Dermatology*, W.B. Saunders, London.

Scott, D.W. and Miller, W.H. (2011) *Equine Dermatology*, 2nd edn, W.B. Saunders, St. Louis.

69

Dermatophilus Preparation

Michelle Woodward and Cherie Pucheu-Haston

69.1 Purpose

- The purpose of a dermatophilus preparation is to detect the presence of *Dermatophilus congolensis* in crusted lesions (Figure 69.1).
- *Dermatophilus congolensis* is the causative agent of a crusting dermatitis, often referred to as "rain rot", "mud fever", or "rain scald".
- *Dermatophilus* is a Gram-positive, filamentous bacterium that forms parallel rows of cocci that resemble railroad tracks.

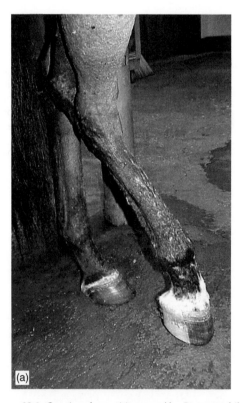 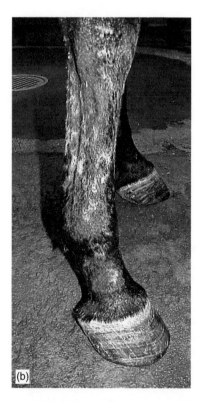

Figure 69.1 Crusting dermatitis caused by *Dermatophilus congolensis*. (a) Crusted lesions on the distal hind limb. (b) Crusted lesions on the distal front limb. (c) Crusted lesions all over the body. (d) A close view of crusted lesions. Courtesy of Dr. Carol Foil.

Manual of Clinical Procedures in the Horse, First Edition. Edited by Lais R.R. Costa and Mary Rose Paradis.
© 2018 John Wiley & Sons, Inc. Published 2018 by John Wiley & Sons, Inc.

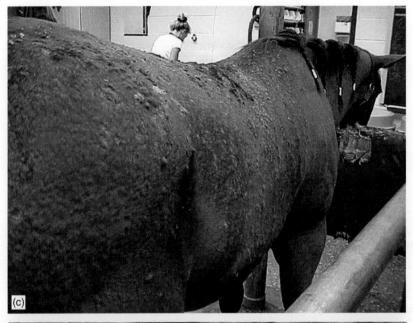

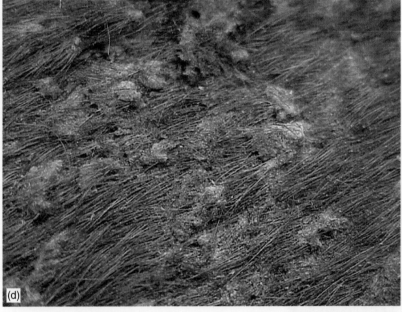

Figure 69.1 (continued)

69.2 Complications

No complications

69.3 Equipment Required

- Small pair of scissors
- Glass slide
- Water
- Optional: covered petri dish with a damp gauze sponge
- Scalpel blade
- Staining techniques:
  - Gram stain
  - Giemsa stain or modified Wright's stain or modified Romanowsky (Diff-Quik)
- Light microscope

69.4 Procedure: Dermatophilus Preparation

Technical action	Rationale
Remove the crust from an affected area on the patient.	If there is suppurative exudate beneath the crust a direct smear of the exudate on a glass slide can be stained and examined for bacteria.
Mince crusts with a small pair of scissors or a scalpel blade (Figure 69.2).	If necessary, trim excess hair from the crust with scissors before mincing the crust.
Mix the crust with several drops of water on a slide (Figure 69.2) and allow the mixture to soften for several minutes.	Alternatively, place the slide and debris in a petri dish containing a dampened gauze sponge. Let it sit for several hours to facilitate softening of the crusts (Figure 69.3). Success may increase if crusts are allowed to soak for longer periods of time.
Mince the crusts with a blade. Press the debris onto the slide with the flat side of the blade.	The crusts should be pressed firmly onto the slide to achieve better results.
Remove excess debris from slide and allow it to air dry.	
Heat-fix and stain the slide.	Heat-fix the slide by gently warming it to 50–60 °C.
Examine for bacteria at 100× objective (Figure 69.4).	If a preparation is negative in a case where *Dermatophilus* is clinically suspected, a sample of crusts should be placed into a sterile vial and submitted for bacterial culture (Figure 69.5).

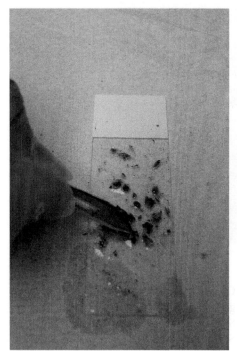

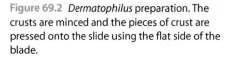

Figure 69.2 *Dermatophilus* preparation. The crusts are minced and the pieces of crust are pressed onto the slide using the flat side of the blade.

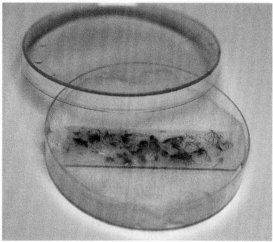

Figure 69.3 Place the slide with the minced crusts in a petri dish containing a dampened gauze sponge, letting it sit for several hours to facilitate softening of the crusts. Courtesy of Dr. Lais R.R. Costa.

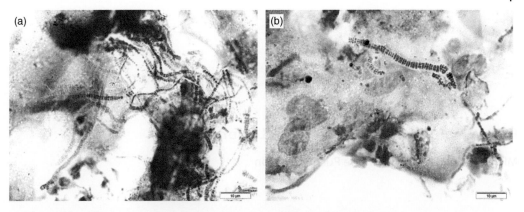

Figure 69.4 Appearance of *Dermatophilus congolensis* from a *Dermatophilus* preparation after Giemsa (Diff-Quik) staining. (a) Note numerous coccoid bacteria forming branching filaments and parallel rows amongst large amount of debris. (b) One individual strand of parallel rows of bacteria, resembling railroad tracks.

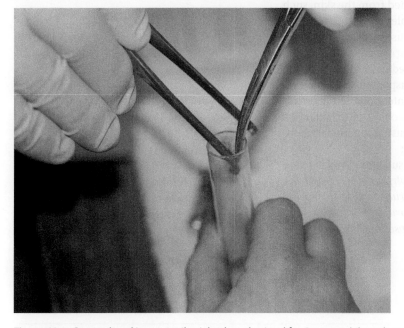

Figure 69.5 Crusts placed into a sterile vial to be submitted for *Dermatophilus* culture. Courtesy of Dr. Lais R.R. Costa.

Bibliography and Further Reading

Bergvall, K. (2005) Advances in acquisition, identification and treatment of equine ectoparasites. *Clinical Techniques in Equine Practice*, **4**, 296–301.

Evans, A.G. and Stannard, A.A. (1986) Diagnostic approach to equine skin disease. *Compendium Equine*, **8**, 652–660.

Littlewood, J.D. (1997) Diagnostic procedures in equine skin disease. *Equine Veterinary Education*, **3**, 174–176.

Pascoe, R.R. and Knottenbelt, D.C. (1999) *Manual of Equine Dermatology*, W.B. Saunders, London.

Scott, D.W. and Miller, W.H. (2011) *Equine Dermatology*, 2nd edn, W.B. Saunders, St. Louis.

70

Fungal Culture of Superficial Skin Lesions

Michelle Woodward and Cherie Pucheu-Haston

70.1 Purpose

- Inoculation of fungal culture medium with material obtained from the skin, such as hair, crusts or scales.
- Types of samples used include plucked hairs within and surrounding the lesion, or skin crust removed from affected areas.
- Fungal culture of suspected subcutaneous and deep mycotic infections requires collection of tissue via biopsy (see Chapter 71).
- Fungal pathogens causing superficial mycosis in horses include:
  - dermatophytes: such as *Trichophyton equinum, Trichophyton mentagrophytes, Trichophyton verrucosum, Microsporum canis, Microsporum equinum,* and *Microsporum gypseum*
  - non-dermatophytes: *Candida, Malassezia,* and *Trichosporum.*

70.2 Complications

No complications.

70.3 Equipment Required

- Clippers
- 70% isopropyl alcohol
- Cotton
- Mosquito forceps
- Scalpel blade
- Toothbrush (optional)
- Dermatophyte test medium (DTM)
- Sabaroud's dextrose agar (optional)

70.4 Procedure: Fungal Culture of Superficial Skin Lesions

Technical action	Rationale
Clip excessive hair (such that the hair length ranges from 0.5 to 1 cm).	This helps to remove surface contaminants and facilitate sampling of broken, infected hairs.
Wipe forceps and gently blot lesions to be sampled with 70% isopropyl alcohol. Allow surface to air dry.	This also helps to remove surface contaminants.
Choose the site of sampling within or around the affected areas.	Note that Wood's lamp examination is rarely helpful in the selection of infected hairs, as the dermatophyte species that infect horses usually do not fluoresce.

Manual of Clinical Procedures in the Horse, First Edition. Edited by Lais R.R. Costa and Mary Rose Paradis.
© 2018 John Wiley & Sons, Inc. Published 2018 by John Wiley & Sons, Inc.

Technical action	Rationale
Collection of the sample. Pluck hairs from the periphery of the lesions using a mosquito forceps (Figure 70.1). If possible, collect hairs from multiple lesions. Obtain scales or crusts (Figure 70.2). Use a new toothbrush to brush over the lesions and hair on the animal.	Hairs from the periphery of the lesions are chosen as areas of active lesion expansion are the most likely to harbor viable fungal elements. Scales and crust are well-defined lesions. A toothbrush can be used when lesions are poorly defined, or if an asymptomatic carrier is suspected.
Inoculate the test medium. Apply the sample to the surface of the test medium(s). The sample should be pressed firmly onto (but not embedded in) the test medium to achieve better results. If a toothbrush was used for collection of the sample, press the toothbrush several times onto the surface of the test medium(s).	DTM is the most commonly used test medium. Prior to inoculation the medium is yellow (Figure 70.3). Fastidious dermatophytes are best isolated by use of Sabaroud's dextrose agar versus DTM.
Place a cover on the culture medium(s), but do not close it too tightly.	Dermatophytes require oxygen to grow.
Incubate in the dark at room temperature.	Fungal growth may be enhanced in the dark.
Check cultures daily for growth. On the DTM, fungal growth should coincide with a red color change in the medium (Figure 70.4).	Cultures should be allowed to grow for at least 3 weeks before being declared negative. Suspected dermatophytes should be identified by microscopic examination for macroconidia formation.
Optional: Collected samples (as described above) may be placed in a sterile container and submitted to a microbiology laboratory for fungal culture and identification (Figure 70.5).	Certain dermatophyte isolates may require specific conditions for growth, for example specific temperatures, media supplementation with amino acids, vitamins, etc. In addition, microscopic identification of macroconidia can be difficult for many *Trichophyton* spp. For this reason, the best results may often be obtained by submitting samples to a veterinary microbiological laboratory.

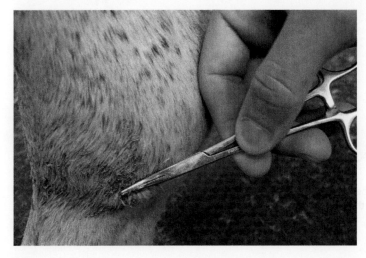

Figure 70.1 Hairs are plucked from the periphery of lesions with mosquito forceps.

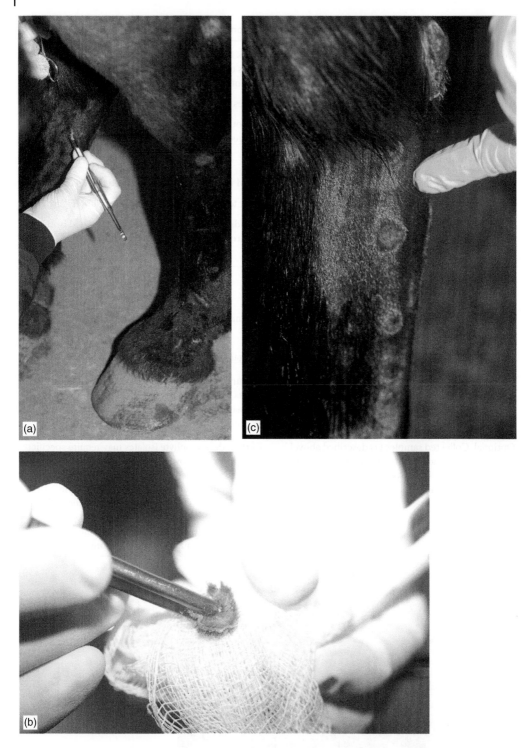

Figure 70.2 Scales or crusts can be used for fungal isolation. (a) Removal of crusts from a horse with suspected dermatophytosis. (b) Close-up of the removed crust. (c) Skin lesions on a horse's leg after removal of the crusts. Courtesy of Dr. Lais R.R. Costa.

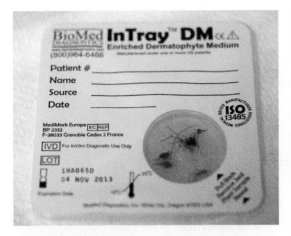

Figure 70.3 Prior to inoculation the DTM is yellow. A sample collected from a horse with multiple lesions suspicious of dermatophytosis was inoculated into the DTM. Courtesy of Dr. Lais R.R. Costa.

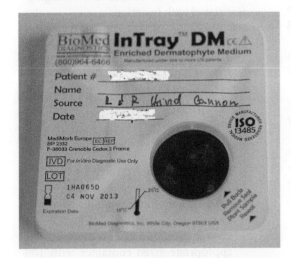

Figure 70.4 The DTM culture should be checked daily for growth. Fungal growth coincides with a red color change in the DTM. Courtesy of Dr. Lais R.R. Costa.

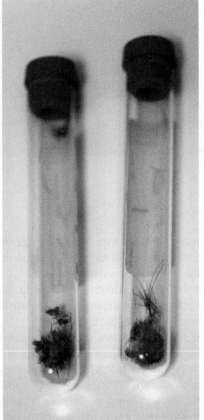

Figure 70.5 Collected samples are placed in a sterile container and submitted to a microbiology laboratory for fungal culture and identification. Courtesy of Dr. Lais R.R. Costa.

Bibliography and Further Reading

Bergvall, K. (2005) Advances in acquisition, identification and treatment of equine ectoparasites. *Clinical Techniques in Equine Practice*, **4**, 296–301.

Chermette, R., Ferreiro, L., and Guillot, J. (2008) Dermatophytoses in animals. *Mycopathologica*, **166**, 385–405.

Evans, A.G. and Stannard, A.A. (1986) Diagnostic approach to equine skin disease. *Compendium Equine*, **8**, 652–660.

Littlewood, J.D. (1997) Diagnostic procedures in equine skin disease. *Equine Veterinary Education*, **3**, 174–176.

Pascoe, R.R. and Knottenbelt, D.C. (1999) *Manual of Equine Dermatology*, W.B. Saunders, London.

Scott, D.W. and Miller, W.H. (2011) *Equine Dermatology*, 2nd edn, W.B. Saunders, St. Louis.

71

Skin Biopsy

Michelle Woodward and Cherie Pucheu-Haston

71.1 Purpose

- Skin biopsy is the removal of a small section of skin for histopathology, culture, and/or impression smear cytology.
- It is helpful in identifying skin tumors and infectious organisms, and diagnosing immune-mediated skin diseases.
- Skin biopsy provides more information about skin lesions than can be obtained by gross examination or aspiration cytology.
- Cutaneous punch biopsies are appropriate for very small nodules that can be removed entirely with the biopsy punch.
- Elliptical incisional biopsies are appropriate for vesicular, bullous, and large ulcerated lesions. They are also used to remove larger nodular lesions.

71.2 Complications

- Hemorrhage (minor)
- Infection
- Scar formation
- Dehiscence of skin suture

71.3 Equipment Required

- Clippers or scissors
- 22- to 25-gauge needle

- 3 ml syringe
- Injectable local anesthetic (e.g., 2% lidocaine): local anesthetic (lidocaine) may be mixed with 8.4% sodium bicarbonate (3:1 dilution) to reduce the "stinging" associated with injection.
- 70% alcohol
- Permanent marker (e.g., Sharpie)
- Materials for cutaneous skin biopsy:
  – 6- or 8-mm biopsy punch
  – #15 scalpel blade
  – forceps
  – tissue scissors
  – gauze sponges
  – needle-holding forceps
  – skin suture material (e.g., 3-0 or 2-0 nylon, polyglyconate, etc.)
- Materials for specimen handling:
  – gauze sponges
  – glass microscope slides (optional)
  – appropriate sized container with 10% buffered formalin
  – tongue depressor or cardboard squares

Manual of Clinical Procedures in the Horse, First Edition. Edited by Lais R.R. Costa and Mary Rose Paradis.
© 2018 John Wiley & Sons, Inc. Published 2018 by John Wiley & Sons, Inc.

71.4 Procedure: Site Preparation and Cutaneous Punch Biopsy

Technical action	Rationale
Select the biopsy site. Circling the area(s) to be biopsied with a permanent marker may facilitate sampling.	Attempt to select more acute, active lesions. Chronic lesions may not provide a good diagnosis. Avoid biopsy of severely traumatized or scarred skin.
Gently clip or cut hair from the biopsy site. Avoid disturbing the skin surface. If necessary, trim the hair with scissors.	Be careful not traumatize the site. Samples to be submitted for histology should not be scrubbed, but the area may be lightly blotted or wiped with alcohol to minimize contamination and infection. Lesions to be cultured can be aseptically prepared by scrubbing with alcohol or chlorhexidine solution.
Using a 3 ml syringe of lidocaine/bicarbonate and a 22- to 25-gauge needle, insert the needle at the margin of the area of interest. Direct the needle toward the area to be biopsied, making sure the needle tip is at a subcutaneous depth (Figure 71.1).	Try not to inject the anesthetic intradermally as this is painful and can distort the structure of the sampled tissue.
Pull back on the syringe to confirm that the needle is not in a vessel.	This confirms that the local anesthetic is not injected intravascularly.
Inject 0.5–1 ml of local anesthetic subcutaneously below each lesion to be biopsied.	Local anesthesia alone is usually sufficient. If restraint is needed, a twitch or sedation can be used.
Wait several minutes for the anesthetic to take effect.	
Place the punch biopsy directly over area to be biopsied.	Consider including a portion of normal skin in the sample.
Rotate the punch biopsy continuously in one direction while simultaneously applying firm pressure (Figure 71.2).	Twisting the punch back and forth introduces shear forces that can alter the tissue architecture.
When the biopsy punch is in skin up to the level of the hub, remove the punch from the site. Apply direct pressure to the area with sterile gauze sponges if needed to control bleeding.	Be careful not to drop the tissue sample if it sticks to the punch and is no longer attached to the subcutaneous tissue.
Using forceps, grasp the subcutaneous portion of the biopsy sample. Curved-tip forceps may facilitate this (Figure 71.3).	Be careful not to traumatize (crush) the dermal or epidermal portions of the sample.
If necessary, cut the sample from the subcutaneous tissue with tissue scissors or a scalpel blade.	
Gently blot the sample on gauze sponges to remove excess blood.	
Make an impression smear of the biopsy sample if desired by blotting or rolling the sample onto a glass microscope slide.	

Technical action	Rationale
Place the sample into 10% buffered formalin and submit it for histopathology.	Make sure that the size of container is adequate for the sample size. The container should allow for 10 parts formalin to every 1 part of tissue. Collecting and submitting multiple samples might be prudent.
Suture the site with non-absorbable suture.	One cruciate or two simple interrupted sutures are often sufficient.

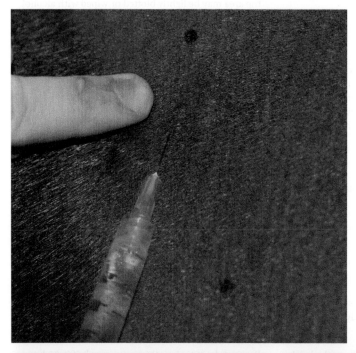

Figure 71.1 Preparation for skin biopsy: local anesthetic is injected subcutaneously to provide analgesia for skin biopsies.

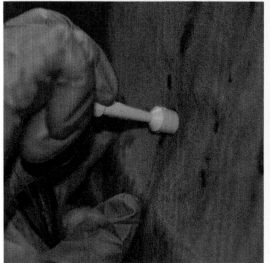

Figure 71.2 The biopsy punch is rotated in one direction until it is fully through the skin.

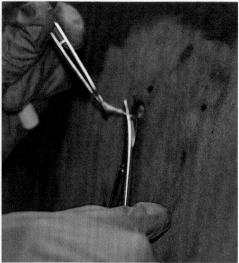

Figure 71.3 The subcutaneous portion of the sample is grasped with forceps.

71.5 Procedure: Elliptical Incisional Biopsy

Technical action	Rationale
Select and prepare the site appropriately as described above.	The sample should include normal tissue, the leading edge of the lesion, and abnormal tissue from the lesion.
Using a 3 ml syringe of lidocaine/bicarbonate and a 22- to 25-gauge needle, insert the needle at the margin of the area of interest. Direct the needle toward the area to be biopsied, making sure the needle tip is at a subcutaneous depth (Figure 70.1).	Try not to inject the anesthetic intradermally as this is painful and can distort the structure of the sampled tissue.
With a scalpel blade, make an elliptical incision extending from normal tissue to the lesion. Make sure the incision is through the full thickness of the skin.	The size of the incision will vary depending on the size of the sample removed.
Remove the biopsy sample, using blunt scissors to gently dissect the subcutaneous portion of the sample from the site. Apply direct pressure with sterile gauze if necessary to control bleeding.	Be careful not to traumatize (crush) the epidermis and dermis of the tissue.
Blot the sample with gauze sponges to remove excess blood.	
Make impression smears if desired by pressing or rolling the sample onto glass microscope slides.	
Mount the biopsy sample on a tongue depressor or cardboard, with the "sticky" subcutaneous portion of the sample down (Figure 71.4).	If not mounted, the sample will curl up in the formalin and may be less diagnostic.
Place the sample (with tongue depressor or cardboard attached) into an appropriately sized container with 10% formalin and submit it for histopathology.	Make sure that the size of the container is adequate for the sample size. The container should allow for 10 parts formalin to every 1 part tissue.
Suture the skin biopsy site using non-absorbable suture material.	Simple interrupted suture is usually adequate. For larger areas, closure of the subcutaneous/subcuticular layer may be necessary to prevent hematoma or seroma formation.

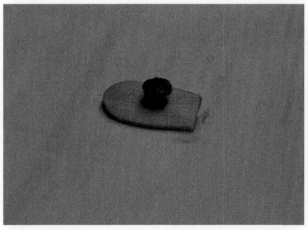

Figure 71.4 The biopsy sample is placed with the subcutaneous side down onto a tongue depressor.

Bibliography and Further Reading

Bergvall, K. (2005) Advances in acquisition, identification and treatment of equine ectoparasites. *Clinical Techniques in Equine Practice*, **4**, 296–301.

Evans, A.G. and Stannard, A.A. (1986) Diagnostic approach to equine skin disease. *Compendium Equine*, **8**, 652–660.

Littlewood, J.D. (1997) Diagnostic procedures in equine skin disease. *Equine Veterinary Education*, **3**, 174–176.

Pascoe, R.R. and Knottenbelt, D.C. (1999) *Manual of Equine Dermatology*, W.B. Saunders, London.

Scott, D.W. and Miller, W.H. (2011) *Equine Dermatology*, 2nd edn, W.B. Saunders, St. Louis.

72

Onchocerca Preparation

Michelle Woodward and Cherie Pucheu-Haston

72.1 Purpose

- Onchocerca preparation is a diagnostic procedure for identifying *Onchocerca cervicalis* microfilariae in the skin of horses.
- The microfilariae of *Onchocerca cervicalis* tend to concentrate in the ventral midline, face, and neck, causing dermatitis and leukoderma (Figure 72.1), whereas the adult worms inhabit the funicular portion of the nuchal ligament.
- Characteristic dermatitis in conjunction with the presence of the microfilariae is supportive of cutaneous onchocerciasis.
- Cutaneous onchocerciasis may be accompanied by ocular onchocerciasis.

72.2 Complications

- Hemorrhage (minor)
- Infection
- Scar formation
- Dehiscence of skin suture

72.3 Equipment Required

- 6 mm biopsy punch
- Saline
- Plain centrifuge tubes or untreated red-topped tubes
- Scalpel blade
- Centrifuge (if not available, see the alternative procedure)
- Glass slide and coverslip
- Microscope
- Petri dish (see the alternative method)
- Tongue depressor (see the alternative method)

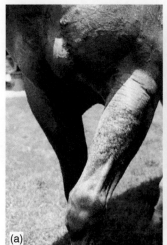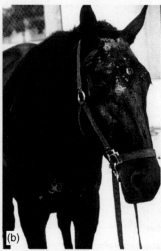

(a)   (b)

Figure 72.1 Cutaneous onchocerciasis manifests as a range of lesions. (a) Focal annular areas of alopecia, scaling, and crusting. (b) Widespread alopecia and ulceration. Courtesy of Dr. Carol Foil.

Manual of Clinical Procedures in the Horse, First Edition. Edited by Lais R.R. Costa and Mary Rose Paradis.
© 2018 John Wiley & Sons, Inc. Published 2018 by John Wiley & Sons, Inc.

72.4 Procedure: Onchocerca Preparation 1 (Centrifuge Available)

Technical action	Rationale
Select the location for sampling.	Preferably sample lesions other than those in the ventral midline.
Follow the procedure for obtaining a skin biopsy using the cutaneous punch biopsy technique.	See Chapter 71.
Once a sample has been obtained, place it in a plain centrifuge tube or petri dish with saline for transport.	Use preservative-free saline to avoid killing the microfilariae.
Mince tissue to 0.5 mm particles with a razor or scalpel blade. Place sample into the centrifuge tube.	This step is important because mincing of the tissue will allow the microfilariae to migrate out of the skin specimen.
Allow tissue to incubate for 4–8 hours at room temperature.	Incubation periods as short as 30 minutes have been described.
Remove the pieces of tissue from the centrifuge tube.	If microfilariae are present in the tissue specimen, they migrate out of the specimen.
Centrifuge the tube at 3000 rpm for 5 minutes.	If a centrifuge is not available, see the alternative method (section 72.5).
Discard the supernatant fluid.	There will be a cell pellet at the bottom of the centrifuge tube.
Remove the pellet from the bottom of the centrifuge tube and place it on a glass slide. Place a cover slip over it.	
Examine the pellet microscopically for microfilariae at 100× magnification. Observe for the presence of movement as well as for still microfilariae (Figure 72.2).	Onchocerca microfilaria are approximately 220 µm in length and 8 µm in diameter (the same as a red blood cell). They have a characteristic "whiplash" movement.

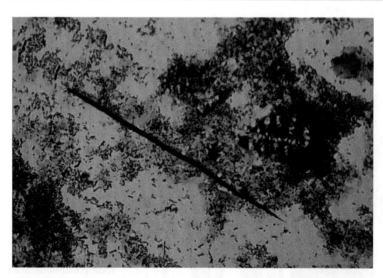

Figure 72.2 Microscopic examination of the sample: microfilaria approximately 8 µm in diameter and 220 µm in length. Courtesy of Dr. Thomas Klei.

72.5 Procedure: Onchocerca Preparation 2 (Alternative Method if Centrifuge not Available)

Technical action	Rationale
Follow the procedure in Chapter 71 for obtaining a cutaneous punch biopsy.	Alternatively, an incisional skin biopsy technique can be obtained (Chapter 71).
Once a sample has been obtained, place it in a petri dish with saline for transport.	Use preservative-free saline to avoid killing the microfilariae.
Place a small piece of tissue that contains the dermis on a glass slide and mince it with a scalpel blade.	The tissue mincing step is important because it will facilitate the migration of the microfilariae out of the skin specimen.
Add a few drops of saline to slide and incubate it at room temperature for 15 minutes. Place a coverslip over the slide before viewing.	Make sure the sample does not dry out.
Scan the slide at 4× magnification along the margins, looking for movement of the parasite.	Movement is indicative of the presence of live microfilariae.
If movement is seen, move to a higher magnification.	Magnification of 100× is generally required for viewing the microfilariae. The microfilariae are approximately 200–240 μm in length (Figure 72.2).
If no movement is seen, place a small amount of water in a petri dish. Elevate the slide above the water on a tongue depressor. Allow the sample to incubate overnight and then reexamine it.	This longer incubation step may be useful when low numbers of microfilaria are suspected as it allows time for more microfilaria to migrate out of the tissue specimen.

Bibliography and Further Reading

Bergvall, K. (2005) Advances in acquisition, identification and treatment of equine ectoparasites. *Clinical Techniques in Equine Practice*, **4**, 296–301.

Evans, A.G. and Stannard, A.A. (1986) Diagnostic approach to equine skin disease. *Compendium Equine*, **8**, 652–660.

Littlewood, J.D. (1997) Diagnostic procedures in equine skin disease. *Equine Veterinary Education*, **3**, 174–176.

Pascoe, R.R. and Knottenbelt, D.C. (1999) *Manual of Equine Dermatology*, W.B. Saunders, London.

Rabalais, F.C. and Votara, C.L. (1974) Cutaneous distribution of microfilariae of *Onchocerca cervicalis* in horses. *American Journal of Veterinary Research*, **35**, 1369–1370.

Scott, D.W. and Miller, W.H. (2011) *Equine Dermatology*, 2nd edn, W.B. Saunders, St. Louis.

73

Intradermal Sweat Testing

Lais R.R. Costa

73.1 Purpose

- To perform a semi-quantitative test, using serial dilutions of a selective β_2-adrenergic receptor agonist drug intradermally, to evaluate the sweating response of the horse when anhidrosis is suspected.
- Anhidrosis, partial or complete inability to sweat, leads to impairment of proper thermoregulation and is manifested by hyperthermia and persistent tachypnea to compensate for the inability to dissipate heat adequately;
  - partial anhidrosis manifests as sweating only in small areas of the body (i.e., under the mane, saddle and halter, axillary, inguinal and perineal regions), whereas other areas do not sweat at all
  - long-standing anhidrosis leads to the development of dry, flaky skin and alopecia, often accompanied by systemic signs of lethargy, anorexia, and decreased water intake (Figure 73.1).
- Secretion by the equine sweat glands is controlled by β_2-adrenergic receptor stimulation, therefore the intradermal injection of selective β_2-adrenergic receptor agonist drug (i.e., terbutaline, salbutamol) should result in stimulation of the sweat gland secretion.

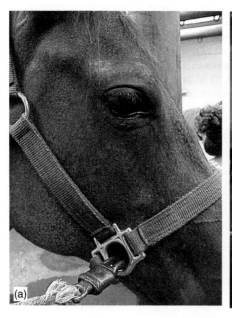
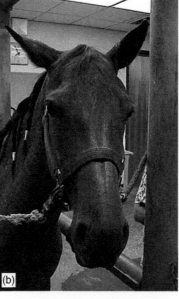

Figure 73.1 Horse with long-standing partial anhidrosis. (a) Note the dry, flaky skin and alopecia over the entire head of the horse. (b) The dry, flaky skin and alopecia extends over the neck and chest of the horse. Courtesy of Dr. Carol Foil.

Manual of Clinical Procedures in the Horse, First Edition. Edited by Lais R.R. Costa and Mary Rose Paradis.
© 2018 John Wiley & Sons, Inc. Published 2018 by John Wiley & Sons, Inc.

73.2 Equipment Required

- Clear sterile test-tubes (e.g., 12×75 mm^2 disposable tubes or small red-top evacuated tubes)
- A rack to hold the tubes
- Pipette system capable of delivering 1.0 ml and 0.1 ml volumes, for example P-100 and P-1000 pipettor and sterile tips (if pipette and sterile pipette tips are not available, an alternative is to use a tuberculin syringe, which will deliver these small volumes with reasonable accuracy).
- Sterile 0.9% NaCl as a diluent for serial dilutions
- Sterile β_2-adrenergic agonist drugs as parenteral preparations solution*:
  - terbutaline sulfate solution (e.g., Breathine 1 mg/ml)

or
  - salbutamol sulfate solution (e.g., Ventolin injection 1 mg/ml)
- 70% alcohol
- Marker or small pieces of adhesive tape
- Sterile syringes (1 ml)
- Sterile 25-gauge needles

*The intradermal sweat test is best performed with terbutaline or salbutamol rather than epinephrine because they are selective β_2-adrenergic receptor agonists, whereas epinephrine has both β_2-adrenergic and α-adrenergic receptor agonist properties. Moreover, intradermal injection of epinephrine may result in leukotrichia at the injection sites.

73.3 Procedure: Intradermal Sweat Test

Technical action	Rationale
Label the tubes: • saline (negative control) • 10^0 to 10^{-6} for the remaining tubes 10^0 is the undiluted solution, 1 mg/ml = 1000 mg/liter	
Add 900 µl of sterile 0.9% saline to each of the serial dilution tubes except the tube labeled 10^0 (undiluted solution) and to the saline tube.	
Prepare the serial dilution ranging from 10^0 to 10^{-6}, using an injectable solution of terbutaline sulfate (e.g., 1 mg/ml) (see Figure 73.2).	To prepare the serial ten-fold dilutions of terbutaline: • Place 0.5 ml or 500 µl of terbutaline solution (1 mg/ml) in the first tube (labeled 10^0). • Add 0.1 ml or 100 µl of terbutaline solution (1 mg/ml) to the second tube (labeled 10^{-1}) containing 0.9 ml of saline. Pipette up and down to mix well. Transfer 0.1 ml (100 µl) of the mixture to the next tube (labeled 10^{-2}), and so on until the tube labeled 10^{-6} is reached.
Clean an area (20×8 cm) of the neck by washing, drying and wiping with alcohol.	Wash and rinse the skin well. Wipe it with 70% alcohol. Allow it to dry completely.
Mark seven points in the prepared area, 2 cm apart, following a straight line.	

(continued)

Technical action	Rationale
Inject 0.1 ml intradermally from each tube below each of the marked points, starting with the saline, and then each dilution from 10^{-6} (the least concentrated) to 10^0 (undiluted, which is the most concentrated) (Figure 73.3).	Some clinicians will only use six concentrations of terbutaline, from 10^{-5} (the lowest dilution) to 10^0 (undiluted, which is the most concentrated).
Allow 20–30 minutes then evaluate the sweat response.	Horses with long-standing severe anhidrosis do not sweat at any of the β_2-adrenergic dilutions.
Normally, the intradermal injection of each dilution should result in focal sweating, except for the saline, within 20 minutes (Figure 73.4).	Partially anhidrotic horses respond to the least diluted injections (Figure 73.5).

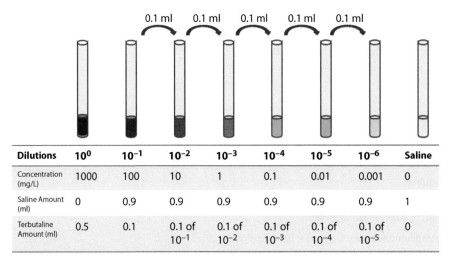

Dilutions	10^0	10^{-1}	10^{-2}	10^{-3}	10^{-4}	10^{-5}	10^{-6}	Saline
Concentration (mg/L)	1000	100	10	1	0.1	0.01	0.001	0
Saline Amount (ml)	0	0.9	0.9	0.9	0.9	0.9	0.9	1
Terbutaline Amount (ml)	0.5	0.1	0.1 of 10^{-1}	0.1 of 10^{-2}	0.1 of 10^{-3}	0.1 of 10^{-4}	0.1 of 10^{-5}	0

Figure 73.2 Preparation of the serial dilution of β_2-adrenergic agonist drug, using an injectable solution of 1 mg/ml (1000 mg/liter) of terbutaline sulfate.

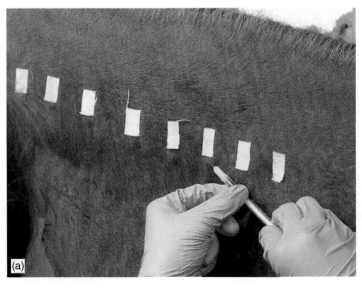

Figure 73.3 Administration of the intradermal sweat test. (a) Intradermal injection of a volume of 0.1 ml of each serial dilution of terbutaline sulfate or saline control below each of the marked points, starting with the saline (left), and then each dilution from 10^{-6} (least concentrated) to 10^0 (undiluted, which is the most concentrated, far right). (b) Note the needle placement intradermally and the small bumps under each mark/tape.

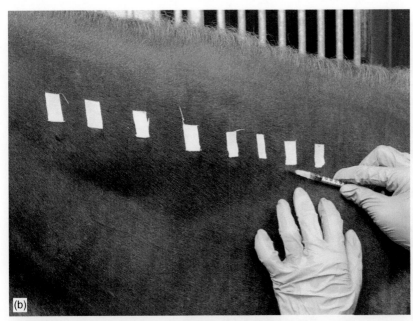

Figure 73.3 *Continued*

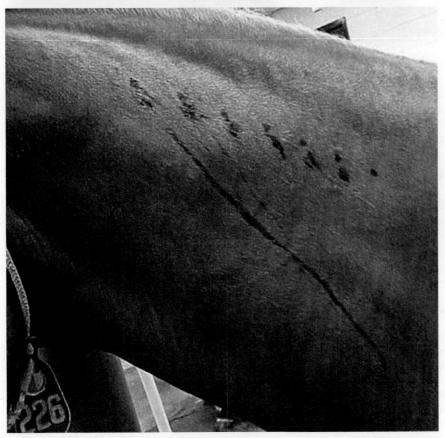

Figure 73.4 Intradermal sweat test showing the intradermal injections below each of the marked points, and the normal response to the intradermal injection of each dilution of β_2-adrenergic agonist drug, resulting in focal sweating after 20 minutes. Saline (first spot on the right) elicited no sweat. Courtesy of Dr. Carol Foil.

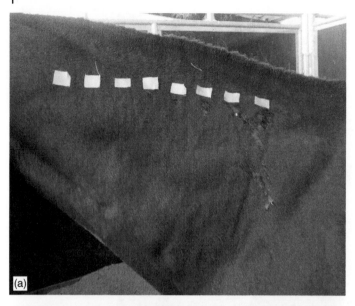

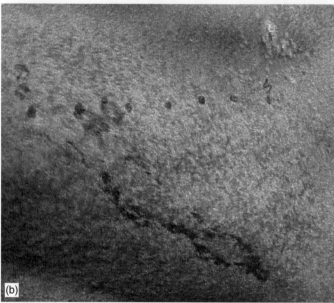

Figure 73.5 Intradermal sweat test of partially anhidrotic horses. (a) Mildly affected horse with sweat response occurring on the intradermal injection of the five most concentrated solutions of terbutaline, that is, the five injections on the right, which correspond to 10^0–10^{-4}. (b) More severely affected horse with sweat response only occurring on the intradermal injection of the two most concentrated solutions of β^2-adrenergic agonist terbutaline, that is, the two injections on the left, which correspond to 10^0 and 10^{-1}. Courtesy of Dr. Carol Foil.

Bibliography and Further Reading

Hubert, J.D., Beadle, R.E., and Norwood, G. (2002) Equine anhidrosis. *Veterinary Clinics of North American, Equine Practice*, **18**, 355–369.

Hubert, J.D., Beadle, R.E., and Norwood, G. (2003) Anhidrosis, in *Current Therapy in Equine Medicine*, 5th edn (ed. N.E. Robinson), Saunders, St. Louis, pp. 816–818.

Hubert, J.D. and Beadle, R.E. (2008) Anhidrosis, in *Blackwell's Five Minute Veterinary Consultant: Equine*, 2nd edn (eds J.P. Lavoie and K.W. Hinchcliff), Wiley-Blackwell, Aimes, pp. 78–79.

MacKay, R.J. (2008) Quantitative intradermal terbutaline sweat test in horses. *Equine Veterinary Journal*, **40** (5), 518–520.

Part X

Clinical Procedures by Body Systems: Neurologic Procedures

74

Neurologic Examination

Mary Rose Paradis

74.1 Purpose

- The first goal of the neurologic examination is to determine if the horse indeed has neurologic deficit(s).
- The next step is to localize where in the nervous system the lesion(s) is/are likely to be. This is accomplished through observation of the horse and its responses to a variety of tests that evaluate various reflexes and reactions, allowing neuroanatomical localization of the neurologic deficits.
- This chapter only describes the neurologic evaluation of the ambulatory horse.

74.2 Complications

- Complications of the neurologic examination are mainly dependent on how severely affected the animal is.
- A horse that is severely ataxic could be in danger of falling when asked to walk or perform tight turns.

- A horse that is at risk of falling may endanger the handler as well as itself when asked to move.

74.3 Equipment Required

- Halter
- Lead shank
- Pen light
- Hemostats
- Pleximeter
- Towel to potentially use as a blindfold

74.4 Restraint and Positioning

- An experienced horse handler is needed to lead the standing neurologic horse through a series of gait evaluations, including walking and trotting in a straight line, circling, backing, leading up and down a hill, and stopping quickly.

74.5 Procedures: Signalment, History, Observation and Palpation

Technical action	Rationale
The signalment of the suspected neurologic horse is sometimes helpful in raising the level of suspicion for certain diseases.	For example, cerebellar abiotrophy and atlantoaxial malformations are seen in Arabian foals. Cervical vertebral malformations are more likely in thoroughbred and standardbred colts <2 years of age.
History should include the following questions: • What is the animal's vaccination history?	A vaccination history should include rabies, Eastern and Western equine encephalitis, and West Nile virus. If other horses are affected on the farm then an infectious cause, such as equine herpes virus 1, or toxic exposure should be considered.

(continued)

Manual of Clinical Procedures in the Horse, First Edition. Edited by Lais R.R. Costa and Mary Rose Paradis.
© 2018 John Wiley & Sons, Inc. Published 2018 by John Wiley & Sons, Inc.

Technical action	Rationale
• Have there been any other horses affected on the farm? • Was there any traumatic injury seen? when? • Is the problem acute or chronic? Recurrent, or intermittent? • Has the problem been progressive or static?	Formulate the questions carefully to avoid leading the respondent to providing an affirmative answer, which might be incorrect.
Suspected neurologic horses should be observed from a distance to assess mentation, evaluate behavior abnormalities, and detect abnormal head posture and stances.	Neurologic horses may exhibit signs of aberrant behavior, mental depression, and severe proprioceptive deficits while standing free in the stall. These signs may be changed with human interference. It is also important to assess whether the horse is safe to handle before proceeding with the rest of the neurologic examination.
Stand the horse square on all four feet and observe for symmetry of the muscle anatomy (Figure 74.1). Horses with lower motor neuron (LMN) lesions often develop neurogenic atrophy of specific muscle groups.	If a specific muscle group is atrophied, diseases causing asymmetrical LMN deficits, such as equine protozoal myelitis, should be placed on the differential diagnosis list.
Spinal flexibility or range of motion can be tested by offering the horse a handful of grass and guiding it to turn the head to the left, to the right, and up and down (Figures 74.2). A decrease in the range of motion may suggest cervical pain.	A normal horse should be able to touch both its flanks, the ground, and extend its head up.
Palpation of the horse's spine should be performed to detect asymmetry of the neck, as well as cervical and back pain (Figure 74.3).	The vertebra and musculature of the neck are the easiest to palpate as they are more prominent. A pain response can be elicited from palpation of the thoracic and lumbar spine but the pain here is usually secondary to muscular, skeletal or ligamentous injury and not neurologic.
Cutaneous sensation and subsequent contraction of subcutaneous muscle can be assessed by eliciting the panniculus (cutaneous trunci) reflex. A firm touch/prick with the end of a mosquito forceps should elicit a skin twitch (Figure 74.4).	Some horses are more sensitive than others so if a decrease in panniculus reflex is the same on both sides of the horse then it may be normal for that horse.
Anal reflex and tail tone should be checked (Figure 74.5). Anal reflex is checked by pinching around the anus and seeing a contracture of the anal sphincter. Tail tone can be assessed by feeling the resistance of the tail to upward movement.	Caution should be taken before approaching the hindquarters of an unfamiliar horse. Sudden pinching in the anal region or grasping of the tail may startle a horse and lead to kicking.

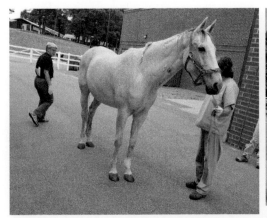

Figure 74.1 The horse should be observed as it is standing squarely with equal weight on each leg. The major muscle groups are evaluated for equal mass and symmetry.

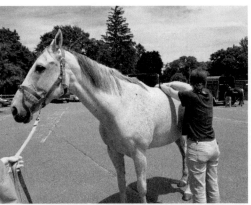

Figure 74.3 The thoracic and lumbar spinal musculature can be palpated gently, squeezing the muscles on either side of the spinous processes. A horse with a painful back may ventroflex away from the pressure.

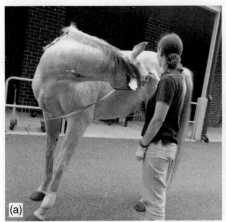

(a)

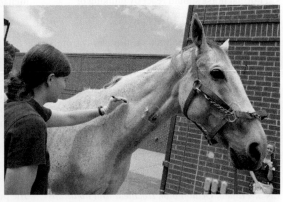

Figure 74.4 A panniculus reflex is being elicited in this horse using the end of a ballpoint pen.

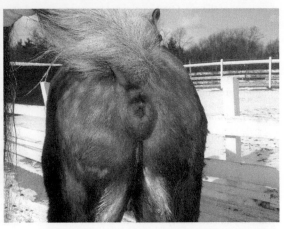

(b)

Figure 74.2 (a) A normal horse will be able to laterally move its head to touch its flank. A decreased range of motion to either side may indicate pain. (b) Likewise, the normal horse should be able to touch the ground with its nose or lift the head up without hesitation.

Figure 74.5 This horse has decreased tail tone and no anal tone. The final diagnosis was polyneuritis equi (neuritis of the cauda equina).

74.6 Procedure: Cranial Nerve Examination

Technical action	Rationale
Cranial nerve examination allows determination of neurologic lesions within or near the brain stem.	Assessment of the function of each cranial nerve examination is performed sequentially from rostral to caudal.
CN 1: Olfactory nerve Assessed by seeing if the horse can smell its feed or detect a noxious scent.	It is rare that an olfactory deficit is noted in the horse.
CN 2: Optic nerve Assessed by evaluating visual perception (Figure 74.6). The visual pathway is evaluated by the menace reflex. To test this reflex a hand is moved quickly toward the horse's eye: • a normal horse should react by blinking or moving its head away from the threatening motion • a blind horse will not blink or move away from the hand.	Some examiners will try to determine if the horse has difficulty with peripheral vision by testing it from the front and back of the eye as well as the side (Figure 74.7). Neurologic blindness can be secondary to lesions in the optic nerve, brainstem or the visual cerebral cortex. Animals with cerebellar disease may lack a menace response but are not blind.
CN 3: Oculomotor nerve Controls the diameter of the pupil of the eye. The pupils should be evaluated for size and symmetry. The pupillary response to a bright pen light should be to constrict. This is a direct response. The contralateral pupil should also constrict (this might be difficult to see in horses with a dark iris).	The eye should be examined closely for other ocular pathology that might affect pupillary constriction, for example the presence of synechia may restrict the pupillary movement.
CN 3, 4 and 6: Oculomotor, trochlear and abducens nerves Innervate the extraocular muscles and control the movement of the eye. Often evaluated together. Lesions in one of these nerves will result in a strabismus of the eye that persists despite the position of the head. The retractor oculi muscle function can be tested by lightly pressing on the closed eyelids.	The pupil orientation of the horse is normally horizontal in the eye. Any deviation of this horizontal plane is considered to be strabismus. Lateral eye deviation is associated with oculomotor lesions. Dorsomedial deviation can be from diffusion brain lesions or trochlear nerve damage. CN 3, 4 and 6 are also involved in eyeball retraction.
CN 5: Trigeminal nerve Associated with motor function to the muscles of mastication and sensory to most parts of the head. Sensory function is evaluated by touching the ears, eyelids, face, and inside of the nares. Motor function is evaluated by observing masseter symmetry and the ability to hold food in the mouth (Figure 74.8).	A lesion in the trigeminal nerve will result in: • loss of the sensory component of CN 5, resulting in decreased sensation to the skin and mucous membranes of the face • loss of motor function of CN 5, resulting in difficulty chewing and a dropped jaw if the lesion is bilateral (may be followed by masseter atrophy after 1–2 weeks).

Technical action	Rationale
CN 7: Facial nerve Provides motor function to the muscles of facial expression, including movement of the ears, eyelid, nostrils, and muzzle/lips. Innervates lacrimal and certain salivary glands. Facial nerve paresis and paralysis is generally unilateral and presents as: • one drooping ear, ptosis of one eyelid, and drooping of the lip and nostril on the same side as the lesion (Figure 73.9) • decreased tear production.	Paresis of the buccal branch of the facial nerve is seen in horses that have been anesthetized without proper padding of the head, or while a halter has been left on. Pressure on the buccal branch of the facial nerve results in drooping lip and nostril (ear and eyelid are normal) on the injured side.
CN 8: Vestibulocochlear nerve Responsible for balance and hearing. Observe the horse's posture and positioning. Deficits in balance might manifest as head tilt, atypical positioning of the limbs, gait abnormalities, and spontaneous nystagmus. Horses recovering from vestibular deficits often learn to compensate with their sight. To determine the degree of compensation versus true recovery, the horse is evaluated after applying a blindfold. Observe the horse's response to auditory stimuli. It is sometime difficult to detect unilateral deafness.	Horses with vestibular deficits will often have a head and body tilt. The degree of vestibular deficit might be so severe that the horse leans on the walls of the stall (Figure 74.10). Placing a blindfold on a horse should be done with caution and the blindfold should be placed so that it can be quickly removed if the animal begins to have a head tilt or loses it stability. Use of brain stem auditory evoked potentials can be helpful in detection of deafness.
CN 9, 10 and 11: Glossopharyngeal, vagus, and accessory nerves Involved in motor and sensory function of the pharynx and larynx. Pharyngeal function is tested by watching the horse swallow. Laryngeal function can be checked with an upper airway endoscopy and/or a slap test. The slap test is performed by gently slapping the horse on the withers while either palpating or visualizing the larynx endoscopically (Figure 74.11). The accessory nerve also provides motor function to the trapezius muscle.	Dysphagia is one of the clinical complaints seen with CN 9 dysfunction. Owners will report seeing food and water coming out of the nostrils when the horse eats or drinks. The most common clinical problem noted with CN 10 dysfunction is unilateral paralysis of the larynx. This creates a "roaring" sound when the animal is exercised. A normal (positive) response is for the contralateral arytenoid to adduct from the midline. Its loss of function may be difficult to detect but has been reported to cause atrophy of the trapezius muscle.
CN 12: Hypoglossal nerve This is the motor nerve to the tongue. It can be tested by pulling the tongue to the outside of the horse's mouth and seeing if it can retract it back into the mouth (Figure 74.12).	A normal horse will have a strong retraction to the pulling of its tongue. In the case of unilateral tongue paralysis that has been present for 1–2 weeks atrophy of the tongue muscle may be seen.

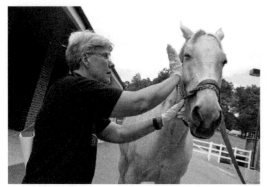

Figure 74.6 This horse is illustrating a positive menace response by closing his eye in response to a threatening gesture.

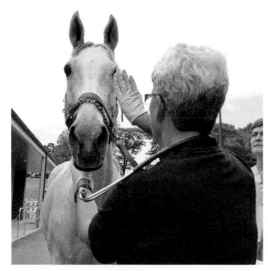

Figure 74.7 Some clinicians feel that they can assess the animal's peripheral vision by menacing from in front of and behind the eye.

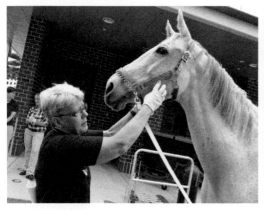

Figure 74.8 Bilateral palpation of the masseter muscle is helpful in determining subtle muscle atrophy.

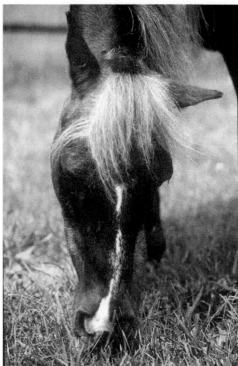

Figure 74.9 This animal has a left facial nerve paralysis. Note the drooping left ear, ptosis of the eyelashes of the left eye, and a deviation of the muzzle to the right.

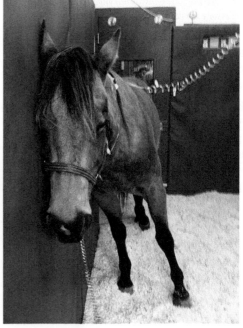

Figure 74.10 This animal has a vestibular lesion. He has a body tilt to the right and can only stand when supported by the wall.

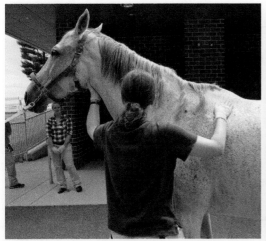

Figure 74.11 The slap test can be performed by palpating the larynx while simultaneously slapping the horse on the withers. A positive response would be feeling a twitch of the arytenoids as they adduct toward the midline.

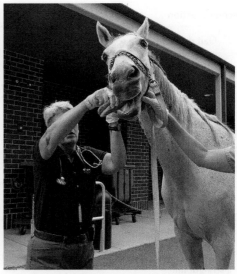

Figure 74.12 A gentle pull to assess the strength of the tongue and inspection of the tongue for any atrophy helps to evaluate the hypoglossal nerve function.

74.7 Procedure: Gait and Postural Evaluation

Technical action	Rationale
Evaluation of the gait and posture of the horse involves a number of maneuvers to highlight deficits. These maneuvers include walking with the head raised, backing, circling, going up and down hills, and blindfolding.	It is important for the veterinarian to become familiar with how a normal horse will respond to these tests. The normal horse does change its gait when these tests are done. Knowing the normal helps you to recognize the abnormal.
When performing a neurologic examination in the standing horse, look for signs of: • weakness • ataxia • hypermetria • spasticity. It is important to determine the symmetry and the limb(s) affected, and to grade the severity of the deficits.	Weakness presents in the horse clinically as dragging the toes, stumbling on a weak limb, and decreased resistance to the tail pull. Ataxia consists of unconscious proprioceptive deficits that clinically present as poor coordination, truncal sway, abnormal stance, and abduction of outside hind leg when circled. Hypermetria is denoted by excessive flexion of joints with a high stepping gait, usually seen in cerebellar disease. Spasticity is seen as decreased flexion of joints such as the carpus and the tarsus.
Grading of deficits: 5 Horse is unable to stand. 4 Gait deficits obvious with the horse within the stall. Horse falls or nearly falls at normal gaits. 3 Gait deficits obvious when the horse is led out of the stall.	It is helpful to establish your own standard for gait evaluation using this grading system as a guideline so that you can re-examine horses for a worsening or improvement in their neurologic deficit. Gait deficits at Grades 2 to 4 are fairly evident.

(continued)

Technical action	Rationale
2 Gait deficits can be seen at normal gaits and when asked to circle. 1 Gait deficits may be difficult to see but are present when the horse is asked to back, circle, negotiate hills, or walk with the head raised. 0 No neurologic deficits seen at the gait.	Grade 1 gait deficits might be challenging, as it is often difficult to differentiate a neurologic deficit or from a subtle lameness. Sometime both may be present.
The gait evaluation should be done in a consistent manner. Start with the horse walking in a straight line away from you and then back. You should view the gait from the side as well as the front (Figure 74.13). The horse should be walked with its head in the normal position and in an elevated position (Figure 74.14).	Ideally, a lameness evaluation should be performed at the same time as the neurologic examination. Elevating the head while walking the horse will decrease his visual compensation for ataxia. This will exaggerate subtle gait abnormalities.
If the horses is stable enough it should be asked to trot in a straight line.	Sometime the deficits are more noticeable at a trot.
After the gait has been evaluated, the horse can be asked to perform tests that may emphasize neurologic gait deficits, such as: • circling • backing (Figure 74.15a) • stepping over elevated object such as a curb (Figure 74.16) • going up and down hills. These tests should not be performed if the horse clearly has a Grade 4 neurologic deficit.	When circling a horse that has proprioceptive deficits, circumduction of the outside hind leg is often, but not always, seen as the circle becomes smaller. Similarly, a horse with neurologic gait deficits when asked to back may be hesitant to step its hind legs back and may slide or drag the front legs (Figure 74.15b). A horse with neurologic gait deficit may stab its feet into the hillside when ascending and stumble when descending.
As stated above, pulling on the horse's tail while standing or walking can test the animal for signs of weakness. A normal horse will be able to brace against the pull (Figure 74.17). The tail pull test when performed at a walk tests strength as well as the ability to recover balance.	The standing tail pull test is performed by grasping the horse's tail and pulling the animal to the side, left, and right. It is normal for the horse's initial reaction to be that the horse steps toward the pull but after this one step the horse should resist further pulling.
Limb placement tests are intended to test the horse's ability to correct an abnormal posture. The limb is manually placed in an awkward position and the amount of time taken to replace the limb to the proper position is evaluated. For instance: • the limb is crossed over the contralateral limb (Figure 74.18) • the limb is placed in a very wide base • the limb is forced to knuckle such that the horse can't bear weight on the limb unless it is repositioned.	Although many clinicians trust the results of limb placement tests, they are often unreliable tests. Some well-trained animals will do what you ask, while some neurologic horses will immediately replace the limb to the normal stance. Limb placement can be evaluated while moving the horse in tight circles slowly and intermittently pausing; this manuever often reveals neurologic deficits evidenced by the horse acquiring abnormal posture.
Once the examination has been completed, the clinician should be able to determine if a neurologic lesion is present and the anatomical localization of the neurologic lesion.	The neuroanatomic localization of the lesion(s) will aid the clinician in the formulation of a list of differential diagnosis and guide the diagnostic plan.

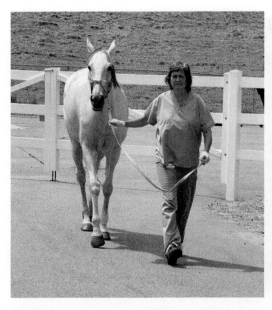

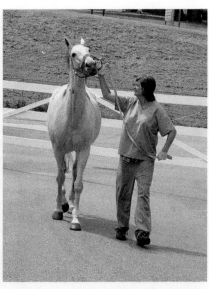

Figure 74.13 The horse's gait should be evaluated at a walk with the head in a normal position.

Figure 74.14 The gait evaluation should be repeated with the head in an elevated position. This decreases the input of sight in the horse's foot placement.

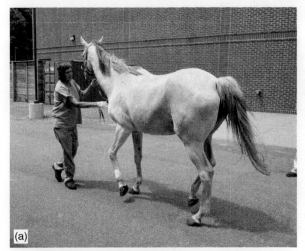

(a)

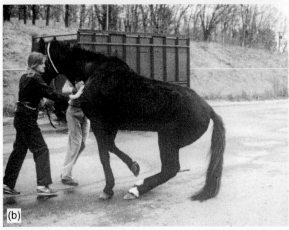

(b)

Figure 74.15 Asking the horse to back is a maneuver that highlights neurologic deficits. (a) A normal horse will back easily when asked by stepping each foot back individually. (b) A horse with proprioceptive deficits may not know where his hind feet are when asked to back. The horse may hesitantly slide the hind legs back or not move them at all.

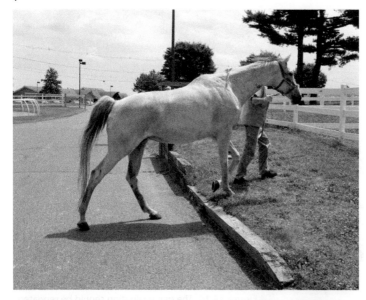

Figure 74.16 A normal horse should be able to place his feet up or down a curb without stumbling.

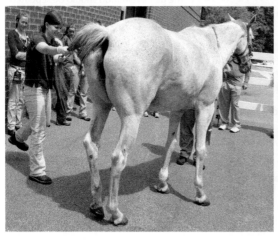

Figure 74.17 When the tail pull test is performed in a horse that is standing still, the horse may give one step back in response to the initial pull but should be able to brace against any further pulling.

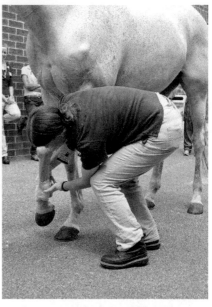

Figure 74.18 Attempting to place a horse's feet in abnormal positions is often futile. A normal "trained" horse may place its feet where you put them and a severely ataxic horse may immediately put the foot in the normal position. It is more important to see if the horse assumes abnormal stances in the stall on its own volition.

Bibliography and Further Reading

Mayhew, I.G. (2009) *Large Animal Neurology*, Wiley-Blackwell, Philadelphia.

Smith, M.O. and George, L.W. (2009) Localization and differentiation of neurologic diseases, in *Large Animal Internal Medicine*, 4th edn (ed. B. Smith), Mosby Elsevier, St. Louis, pp. 117–146.

75

Epidural Anesthesia and Analgesia

Antonio José de Araujo Aguiar

75.1 Purpose

- To administer local anesthetics, alpha-2 agonists, opioids, and other anesthetic agents, or a combination of these drugs, into the epidural space, to produce regional anesthesia or analgesia without the loss of stability and function of the hind limbs.
- To perform clinical examinations, and diagnostic and surgical procedures of the perineum, vulva, vagina, urethra, tail, anus and rectum in horses (e.g., rectal palpation and ultrasonography, obstetric manipulations in difficult labor, fetotomy, repair of rectovaginal fistula or laceration, corrections of uterine torsion and prolapsed uterus, vagina or rectum, urethrostomy, amputation of tail).
- To supply preemptive hind limb and abdominal analgesia to surgical procedures (e.g., perioperative analgesia to orthopedic surgery, standing laparoscopy or laparotomy), management of chronic lameness, trauma and other conditions associated with severe or long-term pain (e.g., fractures, osteomyelitis, arthritis).
- The practice of epidural anesthesia/analgesia requires good knowledge of anatomic references of the sacrum-coccygeal region, as well as previous training in the technique of epidural injection.

75.2 Complications

- Overdose
- Marked ataxia

- Potential to recumbency (e.g., large volume of local anesthetics)
- Infection
- Hypotension
- Bradycardia (e.g., sympathetic blockade with local anesthetics, systemic alpha-2 effects)
- Adverse drug reaction (e.g., urticaria, pruritus)
- Unilateral analgesia (e.g., fibrous adhesions from previous epidural injections)
- Catheter occlusion (e.g., tip clotting, catheter curling or kinking)

75.3 Equipment Required

- Drugs: see Table 75.1 for drug selection and Table 75.2 for drug dosages:
  - local anesthetics: lidocaine, bupivacaine, ropivacaine, mepivacaine
  - sedatives (alpha-2 agonists): xylazine, detomidine
  - opioids: morphine, methadone, buprenorphine, tramadol, meperidine, fentanyl, hydromorphone
  - dissociative anesthetics: ketamine
- Other materials:
  - sterile syringes: 3, 5, and 10 ml
  - sterile needles: 18, 20, 23, and 25 gauge, and 1 and 1½" in length
  - sterile spinal needles (with stylet): 18 or 20 gauge, and 5–9.0 cm in length
  - sterile Tuohy needle for epidural catheter introduction (with stylet and markings): 16 or 18 gauge, 10.5 cm in length
  - sterile surgical gloves

Manual of Clinical Procedures in the Horse, First Edition. Edited by Lais R.R. Costa and Mary Rose Paradis.
© 2018 John Wiley & Sons, Inc. Published 2018 by John Wiley & Sons, Inc.

- Teflon, nylon or spring-wire reinforced epidural catheter (with markings): 18 or 20 gauge, 90 cm in length
- bacterial epidural filter and catheter adaptor port
- sterile adhesive plastic dressing
- cyanoacrylate glue or skin suture material
- hair clippers
- tail bandage
- antiseptic solution (e.g., chlorhexidine and alcohol)
- sterile gauze sponges
- biohazard container
- halter and lead rope
- twitch (rope or chain)
- stock for horses.

Table 75.1 Selection of drugs and doses administered by the epidural route to horses (for detail information see the procedures for each individual drug group)

Drug group	Recommendation	Examples
Local anesthetics: • lidocaine • mepivacaine • bupivacaine • ropivacaine	To allow examination and performance of obstetric manipulations, surgical procedures in the perineum and tail, and control of tenesmus	Rectal palpation Transrectal ultrasonography Corrections of fetal malpresentation Fetotomy Repair of rectovaginal fistula Caslick's surgery for pneumovagina Corrections of uterine torsion and prolapsed uterus, vagina or rectum Correction of postpartum vulva/vagina lacerations Urethrostomy and tail amputation
Alpha-2 agonist agents alone or in combination: • xylazine • xylazine + lidocaine • detomidine	To perform obstetric manipulations and produce perioperative analgesia for surgical procedures in the perineum and tail for longer than 2 hours	Same as for local anesthetics (above)
Opioids alone or in combination: • morphine • morphine + detomidine • morphine + lidocaine • methadone • buprenorphine + detomidine • tramadol • tramadol + lidocaine • meperidine • fentanyl + ropivacaine • hydromorphone	To produce perioperative analgesia for surgical procedures of the pelvic limbs and abdomen, as well as in the perineum and tail Analgesia produced by opioids is particularly suitable for the treatment of painful conditions of the pelvic limbs	Surgical procedures of the pelvic limbs and abdomen, such as orthopedic surgery, arthroscopy, standing laparoscopy and laparotomy Procedures of perineum and tail (as listed above) To provide analgesia of painful injuries involving the pelvic limbs, such as trauma, chronic lameness, or other conditions that cause severe or long-term pain in the pelvic limbs (e.g., fractures, osteomyelitis, arthritis)
Dissociative anesthetic: • ketamine	To produce dose-dependent analgesia in the perineum, tail, and upper pelvic limbs of short duration	Short-term manipulation or surgical procedures in the perineum, rectum, and tail

Table 75.2 Summary of drugs and doses used for epidural anesthesia and analgesia in horses

Drug group	Drug (brand name)	Concentration	Dose range (mg/kg)[a]
Local anesthetics	Lidocaine (Xylocaine)	1% (10 mg/ml)	0.2–0.32
		1.5% (15 mg/ml)	
		2% (20 mg/ml)	
	Bupivacaine (Marcaine, Sensorcaine)	0.25% (2.5 mg/ml)	0.06
		0.5% (5 mg/ml)	
		0.75% (7.5 mg/ml)	
	Ropivacaine (Naropin)	0.2% (2 mg/ml)	0.08
		0.5% (5 mg/ml)	
		0.75% (7.5 mg/ml)	
		1% (10 mg/ml)	
	Mepivacaine (Carbocaine)	1% (10 mg/ml)	0.2–0.32
		1.5% (15 mg/ml)	
		2% (20 mg/ml)	
Alpha-2 agonists	Xylazine (Rompun, Sedazine)	100 mg/ml	0.17–0.25
		20 mg/ml	
	Detomidine (Dormodesan)	10 mg/ml	0.03–0.04
Opioids	Morphine (Duramorph)	0.5 mg/ml	0.05–0.2
		1 mg/ml	
		50 mg/ml	
	Methadone (Heptadon)	10 mg/ml	0.1
	Buprenorphine (Buprenex)	0.324 mg/ml	0.005
	Tramadol (Ultram)	50 mg/ml	0.5–1.0
	Meperidine (Demerol)	50 mg/ml	0.6–0.8
	Fentanyl (Sublimaze)	50 mcg/ml	100 mcg (total dose)
	Hydromorphone (Dilaudid)	1 mg/ml	0.04
		2 mg/ml	
		4 mg/ml	
Dissociative anesthetics	Ketamine (Ketalar)	50 mg/ml	0.5–2.0

Administer only preservative-free formulations of drugs and diluent solutions.

[a] Combinations of drugs are listed in the text.

75.4 Restraint and Positioning

- The horse must be placed into stocks for physical containment prior to administration of premedication and other general preparation procedures.
- The use of halter and lead rope is necessary for the proper positioning and control of the head of the animal and to reduce movements during administration of sedation and execution of epidural anesthesia or analgesia techniques.
- In case of restless, stressed or aggressive horses, it may be necessary to use a twitch or another physical restraint method.
- Chemical restraint is employed as a premedication procedure to perform epidural anesthesia or analgesia techniques.

75.5 Procedure: General Preparation of the Epidural Site

Technical action	Rationale
Ensure proper sedation or tranquilization of the horse.	Immobilization of the horse is mandatory to make the epidural injection procedure smooth and safer for patient and personnel. The selection of sedatives, opioids, and tranquilizers is based on the demeanor, characteristics, and clinical status of the patient. The drugs and doses of sedatives to be administered (ml) are described in Chapter 9.
Clip the hair of a 10 × 10 cm area over the first coccygeal space, on the base of tail.	Hair clipping ensures adequate scrubbing of skin on the area to be punctured by the spinal needle, reducing the risk of infection. Hair clipping facilitates accurate location of the intervertebral space and the exact point for needle insertion.
Bandage the tail.	Tail bandaging keeps the tail hairs off the scrubbed area or the surgical site (e.g., perineum), ensuring that it stays clean. It also facilitates the manipulation of the base of tail to locate the first coccygeal space and the point of puncture accurately.
Scrub the skin with antiseptic, preparing the site as for a surgical procedure (see Chapter 10).	Epidural injection must be performed under strict aseptic conditions. Infection in the spinal canal is one of the most serious complications related to the epidural injection. Surgical scrubbing and aseptic technique must be employed in the epidural anesthesia or analgesia.

75.6 Procedure: Caudal Epidural Anesthesia and Analgesia

Technical action	Rationale/amplification
To locate the point of needle insertion, palpate the first coccygeal space and find the depression between the first and second coccygeal vertebrae (Figure 75.1).	Move the tail up and down (in a pumping movement) slowly, holding firmly onto the base of the tail (Figure 75.2). The second coccygeal vertebrae is moveable, the first one is not. The point of puncture for the epidural is immediately cranial to the second coccygeal vertebrae.

Technical action	Rationale/amplification
Desensitize the point of puncture for the epidural by administering 2–3 ml of 2% lidocaine, subcutaneously using a 23- or 25-gauge needle (Figure 75.3).	The subcutaneous injection should be over and towards the interspinous ligament. The subcutaneous anesthesia will reduce the painful reaction associated with the insertion of the spinal needle.
Insert the spinal needle (18 or 20 gauge, 5–9.0 cm) slowly at a right angle in relation to the skin, with the bevel pointed cranially (Figure 75.4).	The spinal needle should penetrate through the skin, subcutaneous tissue, interspinous and flavum (interarcuate) ligaments. A "popping" sensation is perceived as the needle transpass the flavum ligament, penetrating the epidural space.
Confirm the correct position of the needle by identifying the presence of negative pressure (air rushes into the epidural space or liquid is sucked in). If correct positioning is not confirmed, reposition the spinal needle and repeat the confirmation techniques.	If the spinal needle is positioned correctly, a hissing sound is frequently heard right after the stylet is removed, as air penetrates the needle hub (negative pressure in the epidural space). The hanging-drop technique can be used to confirm the correct position of the needle. When one drop of sterile 0.9% saline is placed on the needle hub it is immediately sucked in (Figure 75.5). Alternatively, injection of a small volume (3–5 ml) of air without resistance to compression is a further technique to confirm the correct position of the spinal needle in the epidural space (Figure 75.6).
Connect the syringe containing the anesthetic or analgesic drug(s) to the spinal needle hub (Figure 75.7). The injection of anesthetic/analgesic drug volume must be performed slowly and steadily (Figure 75.8).	Selection of the drug to be used depends on the effects that are needed. See Tables 75.1 and 75.2 for the classes of drugs, doses, and their effects. Before injection, aspiration should be done with syringe to check that a blood vessel has not accidentally been punctured.
After the injection, remove the spinal needle and place an adhesive plastic dressing on the skin over the site of puncture (Figure 75.9).	
Observe the patient and verify the expected effects following an epidural anesthesia.	Time to onset of effects depends on the anesthetic/analgesic drugs administered. Relaxation of the tail is the first signal to be observed (Figure 75.10), followed by relaxation of the anus sphincter. Some degree of ataxia or incoordination may be observed if a local anesthetic is administered.

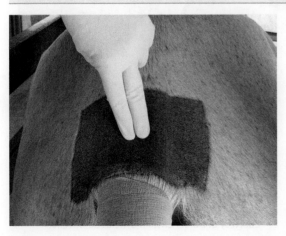

Figure 75.1 The depression between the first and second coccygeal vertebrae can be easily located by applying pressure with the fingertips on the base of the tail. Courtesy of Daniel Cristian Ornelas de Oliveira.

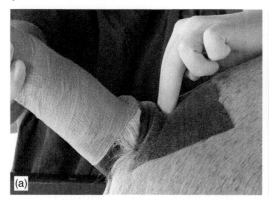
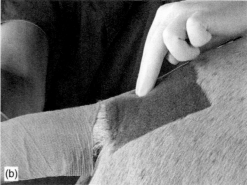

Figure 75.2 Firmly palpating the vertebrae at the base of the tail while slowly moving the tail up (a) and down (b), mimicking a pumping movement, allows detection of the movement of the second coccygeal vertebrae. Courtesy of Daniel Cristian Ornelas de Oliveira.

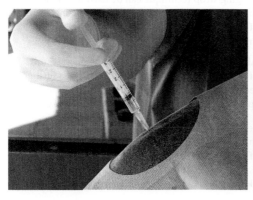
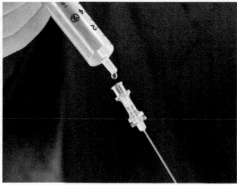

Figure 75.3 Subcutaneous administration of 3 ml of 2% lidocaine using a 25 × 0.6 mm (23-gauge) needle, over and towards to the interspinous ligament, reduces the painful reaction to the insertion of the spinal needle. Courtesy of Daniel Cristian Ornelas de Oliveira.

Figure 75.5 Performing the hanging-drop technique to confirm the correct position of the spinal needle. When one drop of 0.9% saline is placed on the needle hub, it is immediately sucked in. Courtesy of Daniel Cristian Ornelas de Oliveira.

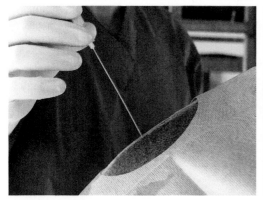
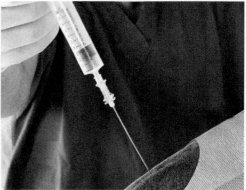

Figure 75.4 Insertion of the spinal needle, 90 × 0.9 mm (20 gauge), at right angles to the skin, with the bevel pointing cranially. Courtesy of Daniel Cristian Ornelas de Oliveira.

Figure 75.6 An additional technique to confirm the correct position of the spinal needle consists of injection of 3 ml of air. The absence of resistance to compression of the plunger confirms the correct position of the spinal needle in the epidural space. Courtesy of Daniel Cristian Ornelas de Oliveira.

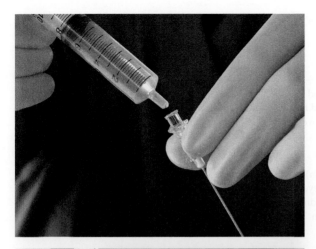

Figure 75.7 A syringe containing the anesthetic/analgesic drugs (e.g., 7 ml of 2% lidocaine) is carefully connected to the spinal needle hub. Courtesy of Daniel Cristian Ornelas de Oliveira.

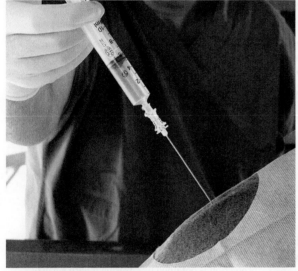

Figure 75.8 The injection of anesthetic/analgesic drugs must be performed slowly and steadily. Courtesy of Daniel Cristian Ornelas de Oliveira.

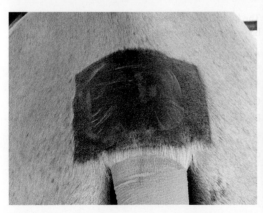

Figure 75.9 After the removal of the spinal needle, an adhesive plastic dressing is placed on the skin over the site of puncture. Courtesy of Daniel Cristian Ornelas de Oliveira.

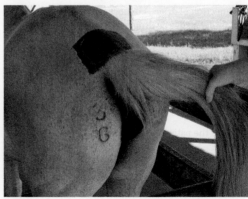

Figure 75.10 Relaxation of the tail is the first signal observed 5–10 minutes after epidural administration of 2% lidocaine. Courtesy of Daniel Cristian Ornelas de Oliveira.

75.7 Procedure: Placement of Epidural Catheter for Continuous Caudal Epidural Anesthesia and Analgesia

Technical action	Rationale
Locate the point of insertion of the needle and desensitize the point of injection as described for caudal epidural anesthesia and analgesia (above).	Long-term epidural analgesia with repeated administration of analgesics is best managed by placing an epidural catheter into the epidural canal. The epidural catheter is introduced into the epidural space using a Tuohy needle (Figure 75.11).
Slowly insert a Tuohy needle (18 gauge, 10 cm) at right angles to the skin, with the curved bevel directed cranially, penetrating through the skin, subcutaneous tissue, interspinous and flavum (interarcuate) ligaments (Figure 75.12).	A "popping" sensation is perceived as the needle pierces the flavum ligament, penetrating the epidural space.
Confirm the correct position of the needle.	Follow the same procedures described for caudal epidural anesthesia and analgesia technique.
Insert the epidural catheter (with markings, 20 gauge and 90 cm in length) into the needle and advance it 4–6 cm beyond the tip of the needle (Figure 75.13).	The catheter length marks guide the operator in calculating how far the catheter has been inserted.
Remove the needle slowly, making sure the catheter is left in place.	Take care when pulling the Tuohy needle. Either hold the catheter in place or push it in slightly while removing the needle, otherwise the catheter will be displaced from the epidural space.
Attach the adaptor port to the free end of the catheter and connect a bacterial epidural filter to it (Figure 75.14).	The adaptor port is necessary to connect the bacterial filter (or a syringe) on the free end of the catheter. Connection of a bacterial filter is a safety procedure to prevent infection in the epidural canal.
Suture the catheter to the skin and cover it with a gauze sponge and a sterile adhesive plastic dressing.	Accidental displacement or migration is avoided if the catheter is sutured to the skin. Further catheter protection is obtained by covering it with a gauze sponge.
For injection of drugs, connect the syringe containing analgesic drugs to the bacterial epidural filter port.	The injection of the entire volume of the drug must be performed slowly and steadily.
	After the injection the catheter is flushed with 0.9% saline solution. Repeat this procedure after each analgesic drug injection.
	Cover the injection port with a sterile adhesive plastic dressing.
Observe the patient to monitor for expected effects.	Time to onset of effects depends on the analgesic drug administered.

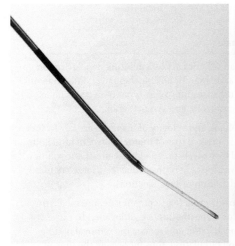

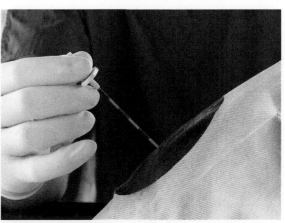

Figure 75.12 Insertion of a Tuohy needle, 105 × 1.6 mm (16 gauge), at right angles to the skin, with the curved bevel directed cranially. Courtesy of Daniel Cristian Ornelas de Oliveira.

Figure 75.11 A Tuohy needle (Huber point, slightly curved, beveled needle) is used to aid the placement of an epidural catheter. Note the catheter tip emerging from the end of the needle. Courtesy of Daniel Cristian Ornelas de Oliveira.

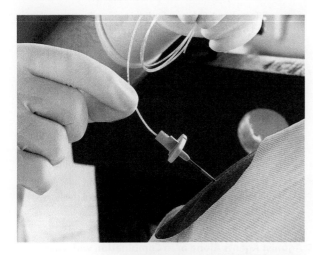

Figure 75.13 A nylon epidural catheter (with markings), 20 gauge and 90 cm in length, is inserted into the Tuohy needle and advanced 4–6 cm beyond the tip (the catheter length marks guide the operator in calculating how far the catheter has penetrated). Courtesy of Daniel Cristian Ornelas de Oliveira.

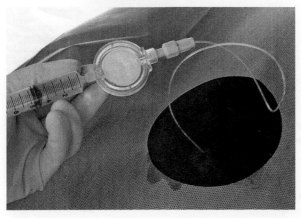

Figure 75.14 The adaptor port (light blue) and bacterial epidural filter are attached to the free end of the catheter. The syringe with analgesic drugs is connected to the bacterial epidural filter port and the injection of the drug must be performed slowly. Courtesy of Daniel Cristian Ornelas de Oliveira.

75.8 Procedure: Administration of Local Anesthetic Drugs by the Epidural Route

Technical action	Rationale

Selection of local anesthetics (preservative-free 0.9% saline is added to the solution to obtain the total volume of the injection, not to exceed 10 ml):
 	
• 2% lidocaine
  – doses: 0.2–0.32 mg/kg
  – volume: 5–8 ml/500 kg horse
• 2% mepivacaine
  – similar to 2% lidocaine
• 0.5% bupivacaine
  – dose: 0.06 mg/kg
  – volume: 6 ml/500 kg horse
• 0.5% ropivacaine
  – dose: 0.08 mg/kg
  – volume: 8 ml/500 kg horse
	Local anesthetics act by inhibiting depolarization of the axon membrane, blocking the conduction of nerve impulse along of all types of nervous fibers (motor, sensory, and sympathetic).
	
	The volume and velocity of injection are key factors. There is a risk of loss of motor control of hind limbs caused by rostral spread of local anesthetic solution, as nerve blockade is unspecific (e.g., large volume administration or fast injection).
	
	Vasoconstrictors (e.g., epinephrine) are mixed to some local anesthetics (e.g., lidocaine) to cause vasoconstriction and reduce the removal of drug by blood circulation, thus increasing the time of anesthetic effect.

Observe the patient for onset of expected effects: • tail and anus relaxation • little ataxia • lack of motor response to pinprick stimuli applied on perineum and tail.	Time of onset of anesthesia is 5–10 minutes for lidocaine and bupivacaine, and 20 minutes for ropivacaine. Time to peak effects is 15–30 minutes. Effects last 1–2 hours for lidocaine and mepivacaine, and 3–4 hours for bupivacaine and ropivacaine.
Monitor the patient for side effects: • hypotension/bradycardia • marked ataxia • excitation • recumbency.	Hypotension and bradycardia are associated with sympathetic blockade.
Take additional care to prevent or handle recumbency of the patient.	In case of marked ataxia with risk of recumbency, the use of the tail-tie method is recommended to support the hindquarters until the horse regains stability. If sudden recumbency occurs, induction of general anesthesia might be necessary to control the horse and avoid accidents.

75.9 Procedure: Administration of Alpha-2 Agonist Agents Alone or in Combination with Local Anesthetics by the Epidural Route

Technical action	Rationale

Selection of alpha-2 agonist agents or a combination:
 	
• xylazine
  – doses: 0.17–0.25 mg/kg
  – preservative-free 0.9% saline is added in a sufficient amount to bring the total volume up to 6 ml/450 kg horse.
• xylazine + 2% lidocaine
  – doses: 0.17 mg/kg + 0.22 mg/kg
  – preservative-free 0.9% saline is added in a sufficient amount to bring the total volume up to 6 ml/450 kg horse.
	Alpha-2 agonists produce analgesia via the epidural route, inhibiting the impulse conduction in primary afferent neurons. This effect is more intense in C-fibers, which are responsible for conducting nociceptive stimuli (pain) and reflex responses. Analgesia is also produced by direct action on alpha-2 receptors in the neurons of the dorsal horn of the spinal cord, inhibiting the release of norepinephrine and substance P neurotransmitters.

Technical action	Rationale

• detomidine
  – doses: 0.03–0.04 mg/kg
  – preservative-free 0.9% saline is added to expand to a maximum volume of 10 ml.
	Typically, proprioception and the motor function of hindlimbs are not compromised to any great extent with epidural administration of alpha-2 agonists, so the risks of hindlimb weakness, marked ataxia, and recumbency are low.
	
	The association of alpha-2 agonists and local anesthetics is synergistic, as it reduces the latency and extends the duration of the analgesic effects compared to either group of drugs administered alone.

Observe the patient for onset of expected effects: • tail, vulva, and anus relaxation • analgesia of tail, perineum, sacral region, and pelvic limbs • sweating.	Time of onset of analgesia 10–15 minutes (detomidine), 20–30 minutes (xylazine), and 5 minutes (xylazine/lidocaine). Duration of analgesia 2.5 hours (detomidine), 3.5 hours (xylazine), and 5.5 hours (xylazine/lidocaine). Analgesia extends from the coccygeal vertebrae to the sacral region and pelvic limbs. The rear abdomen may be blocked depending on the alpha-2 agent (e.g., detomidine), total volume, and the rostral spread of solution administered (e.g., >10 ml).
Monitor the patient for side effects: • hypotension/bradycardia • marked ataxia • recumbency • urination.	The systemic effects of alpha-2 agonists may be observed particularly when detomidine is administered (head lowering, drowsy expression, hypotension, bradycardia, second-degree atrioventricular (AV) block, bradypnea, marked ataxia and incoordination, exteriorization of penis). Recumbency has been reported after epidural analgesia with detomidine, or xylazine associated with lidocaine. Bladder catheterization is recommended when performing genitourinary procedures in a mare to prevent urination during the procedure.
Take additional care to prevent or handle recumbency of the patient.	In the case of marked ataxia or recumbency, proceed as recommended previously for local anesthetics.
The systemic effects of the alpha-2 agonists can be reversed by administration of alpha-2 antagonists intravenously.	Atipamezole (0.1 mg/kg, IV) or yoimbine (0.05 mg/kg, IV) are the reversal drugs that can be used.

75.10 Procedure: Administration of Opioids Alone or in Combination with Other Drugs

Technical action	Rationale

Selection of opioids or combinations:
 	
• morphine
  – dose: 0.05–0.2 mg/kg
  – preservative-free 0.9% saline or sterile water is added, not exceeding 30 ml of the total volume of injection
• morphine + detomidine
  – dose: 0.1–0.2 mg/kg + 0.01–0.03 mg/kg
• morphine + 2% lidocaine
  – dose: 0.1–0.2 mg/kg + 0.2–0.3 mg/kg
• methadone
  – dose: 0.1 mg/kg.
  – preservative-free 0.9% saline is added to bring the total volume up to 20 ml of the total volume
• buprenorphine + detomidine
  – dose: 0.005 + 0.015 mg/kg
  – volume: preservative-free 0.9% saline is added to bring the total volume up to 20 ml of the total volume
• tramadol
  – dose: 1.0 mg/kg
  – sterile water for injection: 20 ml/500 kg horse
• tramadol + 2% lidocaine
  – dose: 0.5 + 0.2 mg/kg
• 5% meperidine
  – dose: 0.6–0.8 mg/kg
• fentanyl + 0.5% ropivacaine
  – dose: 100 µg of fentanyl (total dose) + 0.1 mg/kg of 0.5% ropivacaine
• hydromorphone
  – dose: 0.04 mg/kg
  – volume: sterile water is added in a sufficient amount to bring the total volume up to 20 ml.
	Opioids interact on specific receptors located in the spinal cord, inhibiting the release of substance P and other neurotransmitters related to pain transmission.
	
	Deposition of the opioid must be done as close as possible to the end of the spinal cord by using a larger volume of solution to improve the rostral spread and diffusion of medication, or by using an epidural catheter.
	
	Meperidine is an opioid agonist that also has local anesthetic effects.
	
	Tramadol produces spinal pain modulation as result of its opioid action mixed with inhibition of the reuptake of norepinephrine and serotonin.
	
	Hydrophilic opioids (e.g., morphine) are more suitable for epidural analgesia than lipophilic ones (e.g., fentanyl) as systemic absorption is low, staying at the site of administration, acting on the opioids spinal receptors during prolonged time and leading to analgesia without systemic effects.
	
	Opioids can be associated with alpha-2 agonists (e.g., morphine and detomidine) and local anesthetics (e.g., morphine and lidocaine). These combinations are synergistic as latency is reduced and analgesia is intense and prolonged.
	
	The use of an epidural catheter is essential for long-term analgesia (see the procedure for the placement of an epidural catheter).

Observe the patient for the onset of expected effects: • analgesia of the pelvic limbs, perineum and tail • loss of motor control of the pelvic limbs should not occur • sedation and head drooping can be observed with higher doses of morphine.	Time of onset and duration of epidural analgesia are variable depending on the physicochemical characteristics of the opioid administered. Time of onset of analgesia can be slow (e.g., morphine 0.5–6 hours) or fast (e.g., meperidine 5–15 minutes, tramadol 20 minutes). Epidural administration of morphine must be done a few hours before the surgical procedure to ensure preemptive analgesia. Duration of analgesia is prolonged with morphine (e.g., 6–24 hours), and intermediate with methadone (5 hours), meperidine, and tramadol (4–5 hours).
Monitor the patient for side effects: • pruritis • excitation • increase in spontaneous locomotor activity • intestinal hypomotility.	Side effects are very rare. Cases of pruritus and urticaria have been described, especially after morphine epidural administration.

75.11 Procedure: Administration of a Dissociative Anesthetic Drug by the Epidural Route

Technical action	Rationale

Selection of dissociative anesthetic:
 	
• ketamine
  – dose: 0.5–2.0 mg/kg
  – preservative-free 0.9% saline is added in a sufficient amount to bring the total volume up to 9 ml/400 kg horse.
	Epidural analgesia using ketamine produces dose-dependent analgesia in the perineum, tail, and upper hindlimbs of short duration (latency 10–15 minutes, analgesia duration 30–75 minutes).
	
	Ketamine acts as a non-competitive antagonist on N-methyl-D-aspartate (NMDA) receptors located in the spinal cord. NMDA is related to the processes of acute and chronic pain transmission.
	
	Despite concerns about the low pH of ketamine solution and its possible effects on nervous tissues, studies have demonstrated a lack of neurotoxicity.

Bibliography and Further Reading

Burford, J.H. and Corley, K.T.T. (2006) Morphine-associated pruritus after single extradural administration in a horse. *Veterinary Anaesthesia and Analgesia*, **33** (3), 193–198.

Chopin, J.B. and Wright, J.D. (1995) Complication after the use of a combination of lignocaine and xylazine for epidural anaesthesia in a mare. *Australian Veterinary Journal*, **72** (9), 354–355.

Clarke, K.W., and Trim, C.M., and Hall, L.W. (2014) Anaesthesia of the horse, in *Veterinary Anaesthesia*, W.B. Saunders-Elsevier, London, pp. 245–311.

DeRossi, R., Sampaio, B.F.B., Varela, J.V., and Junqueira, A.L. (2004) Perineal analgesia and hemodynamic effects of the epidural administration of meperidine or hyperbaric bupivacaine in conscious horses. *Canadian Veterinary Journal*, **45** (1), 42–47.

DeRossi, R., Módolo, T.J.C., Maciel, F.B., and Pagliosa, R.C. (2013) Efficacy of epidural lidocaine combined with tramadol or neostigmine on perineal analgesia in the horse. *Equine Veterinary Journal*, **45** (4), 497–502.

Doherty, T. and Valverde, A. (2006) Epidural analgesia and anesthesia, in *Equine Anesthesia and Analgesia*, Blackwell Publishing, Oxford, pp. 275–281.

Fischer, B.L., Ludders, J.W., Asakawa, M., Fortier, L.A., Fubini, S.L., Nixon, A.J., Radcliffe, R.M., and Erb, H.N. (2009) A comparison of epidural buprenorphine plus detomidine with morphine plus detomidine in horses undergoing bilateral stifle arthroscopy. *Veterinary Anaesthesia and Analgesia*, **36** (1), 67–76.

Ganidagli, S., Cetin, H., Biricik, H.S., and Cimtay, I. (2004) Comparison of ropivacaine with a combination of ropivacaine and fentanyl for the caudal epidural anaesthesia of mares. *Veterinary Record*, **154** (11), 329–332.

Gómez de Segura, I.A., DeRossi, R., Santos, M., San-Roman, J.L., and Tendillo, F.J. (1998) Epidural injection of ketamine for perineal analgesia in the horse. *Veterinary Surgery*, **27** (4), 384–391.

Grubb, T.L., Riebold, T.W., and Huber, M.J. (1992) Comparison of lidocaine, xylazine, and xylazine/lidocaine for caudal epidural analgesia in horses. *Journal of the American Veterinary Medical Association*, **201** (8), 1187–1190.

Haitjema, H. and Gibson, K.T. (2001) Severe pruritus associated with epidural morphine and detomidine in a horse. *Australian Veterinary Journal*, **79** (4), 248–250.

LeBlanc, P.H., Caron, J.P., Patterson, J.S., Brown, M., and Matta, M.A. (1988) Epidural injection of xylazine for perineal analgesia in horses. *Journal of the American Veterinary Medical Association*, **193** (11), 1405–1408.

Lerche, P. and Muir, W.W. (2009) Perioperative pain management, in *Equine Anesthesia: Monitoring and emergency therapy*, Saunders Elsevier, St. Louis, pp. 369–380.

Muir, W.W., Hubbell, J.A.E., Bednarski, R.M., and Skarda, R.T. (2007) Local anesthetic drugs and techniques, in *Handbook of Veterinary Anesthesia*, Mosby Elsevier, St. Louis, pp. 51–71.

Natalini, C.C. (2010) Spinal anesthetics and analgesics in the horse. *Veterinary Clinics of North America – Equine Practice*, **26** (3), 551–564.

Natalini, C.C. and Linardi, R.L. (2006) Analgesic effects of epidural administration of hydromorphone in horses. *American Journal of Veterinary Research*, **67** (1), 11–15.

Natalini, C.C. and Robinson, E.P. (2000) Evaluation of the analgesic effects of epidurally administered morphine, alfentanil, butorphanol, tramadol, and U50488H in horses. *American Journal of Veterinary Research*, **61** (12), 1579–1586.

Olbrich, V.H. and Mosing, M. (2003) A comparison of the analgesic effects of caudal epidural methadone and lidocaine in the horse. *Veterinary Anaesthesia and Analgesia*, **30** (3), 156–164.

Skarda, R.T. and Muir III, W.W. (1992) Physiologic responses after caudal epidural administration of detomidine in horses and xylazine in cattle, in *Animal Pain*, Churchill Livingstone, New York, pp. 292–302.

Skarda, R.T. and Muir III, W.W. (1994) Caudal analgesia induced by epidural or subarachnoid administration of detomidine hydrochloride solution in mares. *American Journal of Veterinary Research*, **55** (5), 670–680.

Skarda, R.T. and Muir III, W.W. (1996) Analgesic, hemodynamic, and respiratory effects of caudal epidurally administered xylazine hydrochloride solution in mares. *American Journal of Veterinary Research*, **57** (2), 193–200.

Skarda, R.T. and Muir III, W.W. (1996) Comparison of antinociceptive, cardiovascular, and respiratory effects, head ptosis, and position of pelvic limbs in mares after caudal epidural administration of xylazine and detomidine hydrochloride solution. *American Journal of Veterinary Research*, **57** (9), 1338–1345.

Skarda, R.T. and Muir III, W.W. (1998) Influence of atipamezole on effects of midsacral subarachnoidally administered detomidine in mares. *American Journal of Veterinary Research*, **59** (4), 468–477.

Skarda, R.T. and Muir III, W.W. (1999) Effects of intravenously administered yohimbine on antinociceptive, cardiorespiratory, and postural changes induced by epidural administration of detomidine hydrochloride solution to healthy mares. *American Journal of Veterinary Research*, **60** (10), 1262–1270.

Skarda, R.T. and Muir III, W.W. (2001) Analgesic, hemodynamic, and respiratory effects induced by caudal epidural administration of meperidine hydrochloride in mares. *American Journal of Veterinary Research*, **62** (7), 1001–1007.

Skarda, R.T. and Tranquilli, W.J. (2007) Local and regional anesthetic and analgesic techniques: Horses, in *Lumb & Jones' Veterinary Anesthesia and Analgesia*, Blackwell Publishing, Ames, pp. 605–642.

Sysel, A.M., Pleasant, R.S., Jacobson, J.D., Moll, H.D., Modransky, P.D., Warnick, L.D., Sponenberg, D.P., and Eyre, P. (1996) Efficacy of an epidural combination of morphine and detomidine in alleviating experimentally induced hindlimb lameness in horses. *Veterinary Surgery*, **25** (6), 511–518.

Taylor, P.M. and Clarke, K.W. (2007) Analgesia, in *Handbook of Equine Anaesthesia*, Saunders Elsevier, Edinburgh, pp. 105–122.

Valverde, A., Little, C.B., and Dyson, D.H. (1990) Use of epidural morphine to relieve pain in a horse. *Canadian Veterinary Journal*, **31** (3), 211–212.

Wittern, C., Hendrickson, D.A., Trumble, T., and Wagner, A. (1998) Complications associated with administration of detomidine into the caudal epidural space in a horse. *Journal of the American Veterinary Medical Association*, **213** (4), 516–518.

76

Equine Field Anesthesia

Antonio José de Araujo Aguiar

76.1 Purpose

- To administer intravenous anesthetics, or combinations of these with other drugs (e.g., sedatives, analgesics, and centrally acting muscle relaxants), as protocols for total intravenous anesthesia (TIVA).
- To produce general anesthesia (e.g., unconsciousness, analgesia, and muscle relaxation) to perform surgical procedures under field conditions.
- To perform a major anesthetic procedure in a situation of very limited resources, without life-support apparatus (e.g., large animal anesthesia machine and ventilator, oxygen supply, and monitoring equipment), surgical suite facilities, and trained and experienced personnel. Thus, the risks of accidents, injuries to patient and people, as well as clinical emergencies, are potentially higher.

- Only minor and short-duration surgical procedures should be carried out in horses subjected to intravenous anesthesia in the field, such as castration, tenotomy, desmotomy, wound or laceration repairs, minor orthopedic procedures, dental removals, enucleation, collection of cerebral spinal fluid, or any other procedure that could be completed within 60–90 minutes.
- In adult horses, recumbency is accompanied by significant alterations in cardiovascular and respiratory systems. Thus general anesthesia of a horse under field conditions should be performed in clinically healthy patients.
- The administration of intravenous anesthetics, which are substances that depress the central nervous system, requires much attention and care. Concerns and facts to consider concerning preparation of the patient to be anesthetized under field conditions are highlighted in Table 76.1.

Table 76.1 Concerns and facts to consider on preparation of the patient to be anesthetized under field conditions

Factors that determine a successful anesthesia	Facts to consider
Evaluation of the type of patient	Clinical condition, age, weight, sex, breed, and patient behavior are determinants factors to be considered in the selection of premedication and anesthetic induction drugs, as well as the most adequate doses to be administered

(continued)

Manual of Clinical Procedures in the Horse, First Edition. Edited by Lais R.R. Costa and Mary Rose Paradis.
© 2018 John Wiley & Sons, Inc. Published 2018 by John Wiley & Sons, Inc.

Factors that determine a successful anesthesia	Facts to consider
Fasting	In adult horse food must be withheld for 6–8 hours before the anesthetic procedure
	This ensures the stomach is empty, reducing the abdominal pressure on the diaphragm and the dependent lung when the horse is positioned in lateral recumbency
	Pulmonary ventilation is improved, the functional residual capacity of the lungs is increased up to 30%, and hypoxemia and hypercapnia are reduced
	Nursing foals should not be subjected to Fasting, just apply muzzle to prevent nursing for 1 hour prior to procedure
	Free access to water should be allowed in all cases until just before premedication
	Fasting is not possible before field anesthesia for emergency cases
Weight measurement	Doses of all premedication agents and intravenous anesthetics are established according to body weight in kilograms (kg)
	To avoid overdose and reduce the risks of adverse effects, it is very important to accurately measure or estimate the body weight of the horse
	Body weight can be measured using scales for large animals (may be unavailable in the field conditions) or estimated using weight tapes (commonly used in field practice) (see Chapter 3 for estimation of body weight)
	Weight tapes are not accurate in estimating the weight of foals, ponies, and donkeys.
Clinical examination	A full clinical evaluation of the cardiovascular and respiratory systems is required prior to administration of sedatives and intravenous anesthetics, drugs that depress the central nervous system
Catheterization	Venous catheterization must always be done before anesthetic induction as this ensures reliable delivery of drugs by the intravenous route, avoiding the need for several punctures of the jugular vein, the risk of perivascular administrations of intravenous agents (some irritants in tissues, e.g. guaifenesin, thiopental), and the risk of intra-arterial injection
	Venous access allows the ready administration of anesthetic induction drugs, maintenance doses of anesthetics (e.g. top-up doses or CRIs), and emergency drugs and fluids
	The placement of an intravenous catheter should be performed according to aseptic technique (see Chapter 8).
Environment where the intravenous anesthesia and the surgical procedure are carried out	The selection of the environment is a very important measure for safety reasons
	An open-field flat area, covered by grass with shade available, far from fences, gates or buildings, is a good choice
	Remove rocks or any kind of hazard materials from the area where the horse will lie down
	Weather is a limiting factor when performing field anesthesia
	Rain, snow, wind, and cold temperatures should be avoided
	An alternative could be to perform the anesthetic procedure in a large stall, with the floor covered by a thick layer of hay

Factors that determine a successful anesthesia	Facts to consider
	The administration of premedication agents should preferably be done at the same place as the anesthetic induction and surgical procedure, avoiding unnecessary relocation of the animal, because of the ataxia and reluctance to walk induced by these drugs
Duration of the surgical procedure	Time is a key factor when administering intravenous anesthetics for maintenance of anesthesia in the field
	Some drugs are cumulative (e.g., guaifenesin, thiopental, ketamine) and the total dose administered will influence the duration and quality of recovery from anesthesia
	Only surgical procedures lasting up to 90 minutes should be carried out under field conditions
Preparation of material	All material needed for the anesthesia procedure must be organized, prepared, and ready to be used in advance of the anesthetic induction (e.g., all drugs in labeled syringes, extra drugs vials and other items on hand)

76.2 Complications

- Cardiorespiratory depression
- Cardiac arrhythmias (e.g., alph-2 agonists)
- Bradycardia
- Hypotension
- Upper airway occlusion
- Hypoxemia
- Hypercapnia
- Accidents during anesthetic induction and recovery (e.g., fractures, luxation)
- Adverse drug reaction (e.g., urticaria, anaphylactoid reaction)
- Injuries to patient and support team
- Marked ataxia (e.g., before induction and right after recovery)
- Poor-quality and prolonged recovery from anesthesia
- Accidental perivascular administration of drugs
- Myopathy and neuropathy
- Overdose
- Respiratory arrest (apnea)
- Death

76.3 Equipment Required

- Drugs (depend on the type of anesthesia chosen):
  - sedatives: xylazine, detomidine, romifidine, medetomidine
  - tranquilizers: acepromazine, diazepam, midazolam
  - opioids: butorphanol, morphine, methadone
  - centrally acting muscle relaxant: guaifenesin
  - dissociative anesthetics: ketamine, tiletamine
  - antagonists: atipamezol, yohimbine, flumazenil, naloxone
  - hypnotic: sodium thiopental.
- Other drugs:
  - water-soluble lubricant gel (for orotracheal intubation)
  - eye lubricant (artificial tears)
  - fluids: 0.9% NaCl solution (to dilute TIVA drugs)
  - emergency drugs: atropine (or glycopyrrolate), epinephrine, ephedrine, phenylephrine
- Other materials:
  - sterile syringes of appropriate sizes: 1, 3, 5 or 10 ml
  - syringe: 20 ml (cuff inflation of the intratracheal tube)
  - sterile needles: 18, 20 or 22 gauge 1″ or 1½″ in length
  - over-the-needle catheters: 14 or 16 gauge
  - three-way stopcock or injection port adaptor
  - IV infusion set and fluid pole

- cyanoacrylate glue or skin suture material
- hair clippers
- antiseptic solutions (e.g., chlorhexidine and alcohol)
- sterile gauze sponges
- biohazard and sharps containers
- demand valve
- small O_2 cylinder (e.g., model/type E)
- pulse oximeter
- stethoscope
- Materials for restraint:
  - halter (without metal rings or clips)
  - lead and tail ropes (e.g., cotton ropes)
  - twitch (rope or chain)
  - ropes for physical restraint
  - hobbles
  - foam-rubber pad (large if possible) and cushion
- endotracheal tubes (e.g., 20 and 24 mm internal diameter)
- mouth gag

76.4 Restraint and Positioning

- The use of a halter and lead rope is essential for the proper positioning and control of the head of the animal during administration of premedication and induction drugs. For restless, stressed or aggressive horses it may be necessary to use a twitch or another physical restraint method. Depending on the procedure to be performed, it is preferable to place the horse in stocks for physical containment during placement of an intravenous catheter prior to administration of sedatives or tranquilizers.

76.5 Procedure: Preparation of Patient

Technical action	Rationale
Perform a thorough evaluation of the patient, taking into consideration: • signalment • presence of any clinical condition • animal's demeanor and level of training/handling.	These are important determinant factors to consider when selecting the premedication and anesthetic induction drugs, as well as the most adequate doses to be administered.
Ensure that the patient has been subjected to adequate fasting: • adult horses: 6–8 hours • foals, if nursing: apply muzzle to prevent nursing for 1 hour prior • weanlings and yearlings: similar to adults.	If the patient is an adult food should be withheld for 6–8 hours before an anesthetic procedure to allow gastric emptying and reduce the abdominal pressure on the diaphragm, thus improving pulmonary ventilation and reducing hypoxemia and hypercapnia. Foals that are nursing should not be subjected to fasting. Free access to water should be allowed in all cases until 1 hour prior to premedication. Fasting may not be possible when field anesthesia is performed in an emergency situation.
Make your best effort to obtain an accurate measurement or estimate of the animal's body weight: • measure weight using scales for large animals or • estimate weight using weight tape (see Chapter 3).	Accurately measuring or estimating the body weight of the horse is very important to avoid overdose of drugs and reduce the risks of adverse effects associated with TIVA. In field conditions, body weight is commonly estimated in adult horses using weight tapes, but these tapes do not provide an accurate estimate of weight in foals, ponies, and donkeys.

Technical action	Rationale
Perform a complete physical examination of the patient.	See Chapter 3. Pay special attention to the cardiovascular and respiratory systems.
Place an intravenous catheter according to aseptic technique (see Chapter 8).	Venous catheterization must be done before anesthetic induction to ensure reliable delivery of drugs intravenously, avoiding: • the need for several punctures of the jugular vein • the risk of perivascular administration of intravenous agents (some irritants in tissues, e.g. guaifenesin, thiopental) • the risk of intra-arterial injection: venous access allows the ready administration of anesthetic induction drugs, and maintenance doses of anesthetics (e.g., top-up doses or CRIs), emergency drugs, and fluids. *Exception*: For animals that are too wild, feral or unbroken, a drug may be given intramuscularly to achieve deep sedation to perform the placement of the intravenous catheter.
Choose an appropriate location where the intravenous anesthesia and the surgical procedure are to be held, ideally: • an open-field, flat area, covered by grass • in the shade, if available • far from fences, gates or buildings. Check for the presence of holes, and remove rocks and any hazardous materials from the area.	The selection of a suitable location is a very important measure for safety reasons: • flat area: avoid areas of irregular or sloped footing • grass: helps to limit dust (dirt or sand) and mud (this is particularly important for surgical procedures) • shade is particularly important during hot times of the year so that the patient does not develop hyperthermia while under anesthesia • work away from objects (fences, gates or buildings) to avoid the risk of injury to the animal and personnel on induction and recovery of anesthesia when the patient is the most ataxic (see Figure 76.1). An alternative could be to perform the anesthetic procedure in a large stall, with the floor covered by a thick layer of hay. The administration of premedication agents should preferably be done at the same place as the anesthetic induction and surgical procedure, avoiding unnecessary relocation of the animal, because of the ataxia and reluctance to walk induced by these drugs.
Choose the anesthetic drugs and dosage based on the duration of the surgical procedure.	Time is a key factor when administering intravenous anesthetics for maintenance of anesthesia in the field. Some drugs are cumulative (e.g., guaifenesin, thiopental, ketamine) and the total dose administered will influence the duration and quality of recovery from anesthesia. Only surgical procedures lasting up to 90 minutes should be carried out under field conditions.

(continued)

Technical action	Rationale
All material needed for the anesthesia procedure must be organized, prepared, and ready to be used prior to the anesthetic induction (e.g., all drugs in labeled syringes, extra drugs vials and other items on hand).	Time is of the essence when doing field anesthesia. Each animal's response to the anesthetic will be different so you need to be prepared to handle the horse that is waking up earlier than you thought, or the animal that needs a reversible agent now.

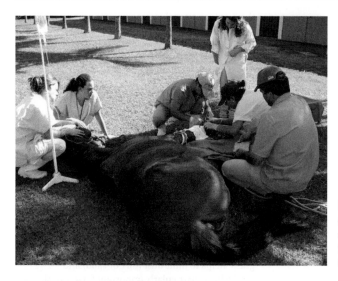

Figure 76.1 An open-field flat area, covered by grass, far from fences, gates or buildings, is a suitable environment for carrying out intravenous anesthesia and surgical procedures.

76.6 Procedure: Premedication

Technical action	Rationale/amplification

Select the premedication drugs:
 	
• acepromazine: 0.03–0.05 mg/kg (IV)
• alpha-2 agonists:
  – xylazine: 0.5–1.0 mg/kg (IV)
  – detomidine: 0.01–0.02 mg/kg (IV)
  – romifidine: 0.08–0.12 mg/kg (IV)
  – medetomidine: 0.0035–0.01 mg/kg (IV).
• Combinations of acepromazine + alpha-2 agonists:
  – acepromazine administered 15–20 minutes (if IV) or 30–40 minutes (if IM) before the alpha-2 agonist: 0.05 mg/kg (IV, IM)
  – xylazine: 0.3–0.5 mg/kg (IV), or
  – detomidine: 0.01 mg/kg (IV), or
  – romifidine: 0.05–0.08 mg/kg (IV).
• Combinations of alpha-2 agonists + opioids:
  – xylazine: 0.5–1.0 mg/kg (IV), or
  – detomidine: 0.02 mg/kg, (IV), or
  – romifidine: 0.08 mg/kg (IV), associated in combination with
  – butorphanol: 0.02–0.04 mg/kg (IV), or
  – methadone: 0.05–0.1 mg/kg (IV).
	Premedication is a very important step in the anesthetic protocol as it prepares the patient to receive the anesthetic drugs, reducing stress and distress. Premedication produces sedation, tranquilization, analgesia, and anxiolysis, making the horse indifferent to the surrounding environment.
	
	Premedication facilitates the preparation of the patient for the induction of anesthesia.
	
	Quality of induction is to a large extent dependent on adequate premedication.
	
	Check the intravenous catheter carefully just before premedication injection.

Technical action	Rationale/amplification
Observe the patient for signs of sedation. Do not induce anesthesia if signs of sedation are not evident. Supplementation may be necessary.	Clear signs of sedation must be observed before the administration of induction anesthetic drugs: • head lowering: 50% of the head height before premedication is the ideal • drowsy expression: ptosis of eyelids and lips, and wide-based stance) (Figure 76.2). Premedication should be supplemented, or even re-administered, if the sedation degree observed is not adequate. Never try to induce anesthesia in a horse without good sedation signs having been clearly observed. Expected and adverse effects of premedication drugs are described in Chapter 9.
Additional points to remember: • administer the premedication at the same place as induction of anesthesia • avoid commotion around the horse • have all drugs and supplies at hand.	Avoid unnecessary locomotion and stimulation of the horse. Try to keep the surroundings as quiet as possible. Check again if all the materials you need for induction of anesthesia are ready to use.

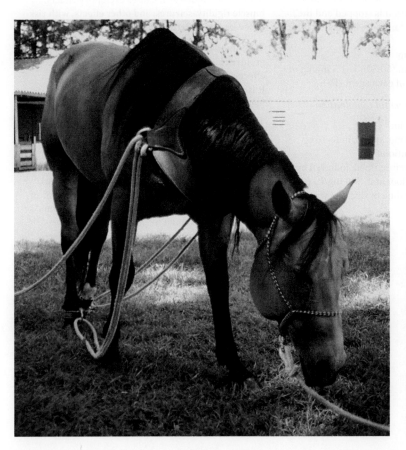

Figure 76.2 This horse was premedicated with xylazine (0.5 mg/kg, IV) before the administration of induction anesthetic drugs. Note the clear signs of sedation (head lowering, drowsy expression, and ptosis of lips). Premedication was performed in an open-field flat area, covered by grass and with shade, far from fences, gates or buildings.

76.7 Procedure: Induction of Anesthesia

Technical action	Rationale
Selection of induction drugs or protocols (Table 76.2). *I. Protocols based on dissociative anesthetics and their combinations* • Ketamine: 2–2.5 mg/kg (IV), administered only after premedication with higher doses of alpha-2 agonists (e.g., xylazine 1.0 mg/kg, detomidine 0.02 mg/kg, or romifidine 0.12 mg/kg, IV), associated or not with opioids (e.g., butorphanol 0.04 mg/kg, IV). • Ketamine + benzodiazepines: – ketamine: 2–2.5 mg/kg (IV), associated with – midazolam: 0.05–0.1 mg/kg (IV), or – diazepam: 0.05–0.1 mg/kg (IV). • Ketamine + benzodiazepines + guaifenesin: – ketamine/midazolam, or – ketamine/diazepam – all doses as previously described, in combination with guaifenesin: 25–50 mg/kg (IV) in 5–10% (50–100 mg/ml) solutions – administered first until the horse becomes ataxic, then the infusion is stopped and the bolus injection of ketamine + benzodiazepine is performed. • Tiletamine + zolazepam: – tiletamine/zolazepam (50:50): 1–1.5 mg/kg of total drug, 0.5–0.75 of each agent (IV). *II. Protocol based on thiopental combination* • Thiopental + guaifenesin: – guaifenesin: 50–100 mg/kg (iv), in 5–10% (50–100 mg/ml) solutions – infused as previously described, followed by a bolus injection of thiopental: 5–6 mg/kg (IV) in 5% (1 g/20 ml of saline or distilled water) solution.	Intravenous anesthetics associated with sedatives and/or central muscle relaxants are the combinations employed to induce anesthesia in horses. The protocols of induction of anesthesia are based on dissociative anesthetics (e.g., ketamine, tiletamine) or hypnotics (e.g., thiopental). Both of these are associated with alpha-2 agonists (e.g., xylazine, detomidine, romifidine), benzodiazepines (e.g., diazepam, midazolam) and/or central muscle relaxants (e.g., guaifenesin). Ketamine is a dissociative anesthetic that presents good analgesic properties and produces minimal cardiorespiratory depression. However, it is a poor muscle relaxant, so it needs to be associated with, or be preceded by, other drugs with muscle relaxant effects, such as benzodiazepines, alpha-2 agonists, and/or guaifenesin. Administration of ketamine as the sole agent for induction of anesthesia (i.e., without premedication with an alpha-2 agonist) is not recommended as it causes excitatory effects, muscle rigidity, seizures, and other effects, with risk of severe injury to the horse and personnel involved. Tiletamine belongs to the same pharmacological group as ketamine, and produces similar effects, but tiletamine is a little longer lasting. It is only recommended in association with the benzodiazepine zolazepam (50:50). Thiopental is an ultrashort-acting barbiturate that produces rapid onset, short-lived hypnosis (unconsciousness), and good muscle relaxation. Adverse effects include dose-dependent cardiovascular and respiratory depression (apnea may occur). Strongly alkaline (pH > 10) solutions of thiopental are irritants to the tissues. Intravenous administration should be performed with care (only through an IV catheter), to avoid accidental perivascular injection. In recent years, the use of this drug for induction of anesthesia in horses has decreased, and it has almost completely been replaced by ketamine-based combinations. Guaifenesin is a centrally acting muscle relaxant used as adjunct to intravenous anesthesia in horses. It produces skeletal muscle relaxation by depressing transmission in the internuncial neurons located on the spinal cord, without interfering with respiratory muscles and diaphragm functions. Clinical doses of

Technical action	Rationale
	guaifenesin that promote recumbency in horses do not cause cardiorespiratory depression. This drug has a wide therapeutic range, and thus is suitable for use under field conditions. It is an irritant to the tissues, causing thrombophlebitis and tissue lesions if accidental perivascular administration occurs (Figure 76.3). Reports of hemolysis and urticaria reactions were described after administration of more concentrated solutions (>15%) of guaifenesin.

The choice of protocol depends on the clinical state of the patient, the expected time to perform the surgical procedure, the premedication previously administered, and personal experience/preference with induction technique. |
| Observe the patient closely and control the head of the horse (Figures 76.4 and 76.5).

An experienced person should take the control of the head of horse during the whole anesthesia induction process.

Induction time is variable according to the premedication and induction protocols administered (e.g., ketamine-based protocols, from 30 to 40 seconds until 1 or 2 minutes after the end of intravenous injection).

The time of anesthesia is very short (e.g., 5–15 minutes for ketamine and ketamine combinations, 15–20 minutes for thiopental/guaifenesin or tiletamine/zolazepam). | It is vital to anticipate and react to the horse' movements immediately after the administration of the induction agents, assisting it at the critical moment of recumbency.

The head should be firmly secured, held by the lead rope, keeping the horse steady and calm, not allowing it to walk.

As soon as the induction drugs begin to take effect, the horse becomes unstable, with signs of muscle weakness and some degree of ataxia (e.g., ketamine-based protocols).

The head should be kept under control (straight in front of the body) then, after a few seconds (or more, possibly 1–2 minutes), the horse starts to flex (buckles) its knees, going slowly into sternal position first or rolling straight to lateral recumbency.

If the lead rope is kept loose, there will be a tendency for the horse to lift its head, and to step back until rolling over backwards. When the horse lifts its head, pull the lead rope firmly down to stop this movement and avoid a potential accident and the injuries associated with it. |
| Be prepared for the induction and avoid complications.

Severe ataxia is noted right after induction drug administration and immediately before recumbency. | Adverse effects/complications:
- accidents during anesthetic induction (e.g., fractures)
- injuries to the support team
- respiratory depression
- bradycardia
- cardiac arrhythmias
- adverse drug reactions (e.g., urticarial, anaphylactoid reaction). |

(continued)

Technical action	Rationale
Additional care is required immediately after lateral recumbency: • position the head over a pillow • remove the halter • protect the eyes • apply cotton ear plugs • pull the dependent leg forward.	Positioning the head over a pillow and removing the halter are important steps to reduce the potential risk of facial neuropathy. Protecting the eyes from injuries is critical. Apply eye lubricant to both eyes and cover the head/eyes with a cloth or a towel for protection against the sunlight and to reduce stimuli. Introducing cotton ear plugs will reduce stimuli from the surroundings. Pulling the dependent foreleg forward will relieve compression over the triceps brachii muscle and radial nerve.

Table 76.2 Drugs, doses, and routes of administration

Drug group	Drug (brand name)	Concentration	Dose (mg/kg)	Route
Phenothiazine	Acepromazine (Promace)	10 mg/ml	0.02–0.05	IV
			0.05–0.1	IM
Alpha-2 agonists	Xylazine (Rompun, Sedazine)	100 mg/ml or 20 mg/ml	0.5–1.0	IV, IM
	Detomidine (Dormodesan)	10 mg/ml	0.01–0.02 0.02–0.04	IV IM
	Romifidine (Sedivet)	10 mg/ml	0.05–0.12	IV, IM
	Medetomidine (Domitor)	1 mg/ml	0.0035–0.01	IV
Alpha-2 antagonists	Atipamezole (Antisedan)	5 mg/ml	0.05–0.2	IV
	Yohimbine (Antagonil, Yocon)	5 mg/ml	0.04–0.15	IV
Opioids	Butorphanol (Torbugesic)	10 mg/ml	0.02–0.04	IV, IM
	Morphine	50 mg/ml	0.05–0.1	IV, IM
	Methadone (Dolophine)	10 mg/ml or 50 mg/ml	0.05–0.15	IV
	Buprenorphine (Buprenex)[a]	0.324 mg/ml	0.006–0.01	IV
Benzodiazepines	Diazepam (Valium)	5 mg/ml	0.1–0.2	IV
	Midazolam (Versed)	5 mg/ml	0.1–0.2	IV

Drug group	Drug (brand name)	Concentration	Dose (mg/kg)	Route
Benzodiazepine antagonist	Flumazenil (Romazicon)	0.1 mg/ml	0.01–0.05	IV
Dissociative anesthetics and associations	Ketamine (Ketalar, Vetalar, Ketaset, Ketaject)	100 mg/ml	2-2.5	IV
	Tiletamine/zolazepam (50:50)	1–1.5 mg/kg of total drug	0.5–0.75 of ea agent	IV
Hypnotics	Thiopental (Pentotal) diluted as 5%	50 mg/ml	5-6 mg/kg	IV
Centrally-acting Relaxant	Guaifenesin (diluted as 5-10%)	50-100 mg/ml	50-100 mg/ml	IV

[a]Buprenorphine should only be administered in conjunction with alpha-2 agonists. The alpha-2 agonist is administered first, and only after signs of sedation become evident should buprenorphine be administered intravenously.

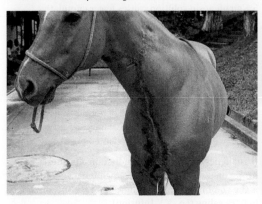

Figure 76.3 Accidental perivascular administration of 10% guaifenesin solution in a horse submitted to a castration procedure. This photograph was taken several months after the drug infusion. This perivascular damage highlights that only a venous catheterization ensures reliable and safe delivery of drugs by the intravenous route.

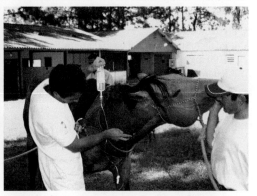

Figure 76.4 Intravenous administration of 10% guaifenesin solution in a horse as part of the anesthetic induction protocol. An experienced person should take control of the horse's head during the whole anesthesia induction process.

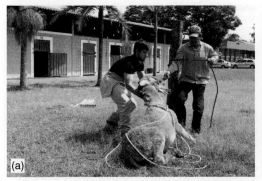
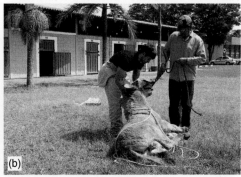

(a) (b)

Figure 76.5 As soon as the induction drugs begin to take effect, the animal becomes unstable, with signs of muscle weakness and some degree of ataxia. (a) While the animal goes down during induction the head is supported by the halter and lead rope, and guided. (b) Once the animal becomes recumbent, the head should be firmly supported to prevent it from hitting the ground.

76.8 Procedure: Maintenance of Anesthesia

Technical action	Rationale
Selection of protocols for the maintenance of anesthesia.	A major concern about TIVA in horses is the cumulative effects of intravenous drugs, resulting in a prolonged and poor-quality recovery of anesthesia.
I. Protocols for maintenance of anesthesia for short-duration surgical/diagnostic procedures (<30 minutes) based on supplementary incremental boluses doses of the induction agents previously administered.	Management of the time of anesthesia and surgical/diagnostic procedures is crucial in determining the total amount of drugs administered, which then have to be biotransformed and eliminated from the horse' body. Administration of larger doses means prolonged recumbency and recovery from anesthesia.
• Ketamine: 1.0–2.0 mg/kg (IV). • Thiopental: 0.5–1.0 mg/kg (IV).	
II. Protocols for maintenance of anesthesia for longer-duration surgical/diagnostic procedures (30–60 minutes) based on continuous infusion administration of two or three agents.	Most intravenous anesthetics and their adjuvants are, or have the potential to be, cumulative, especially long-lasting infusions (e.g., guaifenesin, thiopental, xylazine, detomidine, ketamine).
Combinations of guaifenesin + ketamine + alpha-2 agonists ("triple drip")	5% guaifenesin solution causes fewer cumulative effects than 10%, so is the best choice for field anesthesia procedures.
• Preparations: – guaifenesin: 500 ml of 5% (50 mg/ml) or 10% (100 mg/ml) solution; add – ketamine: 1.0 g (2 mg/ml); and – xylazine (GKX Infusion): 500 mg (1 mg/ml), or – detomidine (GKD Infusion): 10 mg (0.02 mg/ml), or – romifidine (GKR Infusion): 30 mg (0.06 mg/ml), or – medetomidine (GKM Infusion): 10 mg (0.02 mg/ml). • Infusion rates: – rates of 1.0–1.5 ml/kg/h, infused to effect – rates of 2.0 ml/kg/h may be necessary in the first 5–15 minutes of infusion – after 60 minutes of infusion, reduce the rate to 0.6 ml/kg/h – it is not advisable to extend these infusions to more than 90 minutes, otherwise prolonged recovery will be needed.	"Triple drip" maintenance protocols with guaifenesin should not be administered after anesthesia induction regimens including this muscle relaxant agent. If the total dose is larger than 100 mg/kg, anesthesia recovery will be prolonged and of poor quality, with the horse presenting muscle weakness and severe ataxia, with several unsuccessful attempts to get up. If guaifenesin is part of the induction anesthesia protocol, the best choice for a maintenance infusion is the combination of ketamine and xylazine, mixed in 0.9% saline (i.e., KX Infusion). Once a "triple drip" solution has been prepared (i.e., drugs mixed together), it should be used within 48 hours.
Combination of ketamine + xylazine (KX Infusion)	The time of anesthesia produced by these induction protocols is around 10–15 minutes (or 20 minutes with tiletamine/zolazepam). This time can be extended to 30–35 minutes with incremental bolus doses of ketamine or thiopental (small doses).
• Preparations: – 0.9% NaCl solution: 500 ml, to add – ketamine: 2.7 g (5.4 mg/ml), and – xylazine: 2.1 g (4.2 mg/ml). • Infusion rates: 1.0 ml/kg/h.	Thiopental can be administered as long as the total maximum dose is not larger than 10 mg/kg. It is a cumulative agent and anesthesia recovery will be prolonged, with hindlimb weakness and severe ataxia, if larger doses of thiopental are administered.
Combinations of ketamine + alpha-2 agonists + midazolam (KXM and KDM Infusions)	Monitoring of anesthesia is a challenging task as the equipment available is very limited under field conditions.
• Preparations: – 0.9% saline: 500 ml, add – ketamine: 1000 mg (2.0 mg/ml), and – xylazine: 250 mg (0.5 mg/ml), or – detomidine: 1.4 mg (0.0028 mg/ml), and – midazolam: 15 mg (0.03 mg/ml). • Infusion rates: 1.0–1.2 ml/kg/h, infused to effect.	Auscultation of heart and breath sounds, measurement of heart rate, respiratory rate, and body temperature, palpation of the pulse, and observation of capillary refill time and mucous membrane color are the monitoring methods employed.
Consider reversing the effects of midazolam.	

Technical action	Rationale
	These parameters give the veterinarian valuable information about the cardiorespiratory status of the patient and are very important in the early detection of life-threatening complications and the adoption of emergency treatment.
	A portable pulse oximeter is a valuable piece of non-invasive equipment that can be used during equine anesthesia under field conditions. It is not essential, but if available provides significant information about arterial blood oxygenation and the peripheral circulation (e.g., in recumbent horses, breathing air is a very important sign in the early detection of hypoxemia).
	The effects of midazolam can be reversed using the benzodiazepine antagonist, flumazenil (0.01–0.05 mg/kg (IV), given 15 minutes after KXM or KDM infusion is stopped).
Observation of the patient: • eyes: remain opened and in the central position, blinking, with tear production and discrete nystagmus • ocular reflexes present • muscle relaxation • respiratory pattern in response to surgical stimulation	Clinical signs of anesthesia during TIVA administration (e.g., ketamine–based protocols) are markedly different from those classically observed in inhalation anesthesia.
	It is difficult to evaluate the depth of anesthesia by observation of the ocular reflexes. Observation of respiratory pattern and rate in response to surgical stimulation can also be made.
	Typically, good muscle relaxation is achieved with administration of TIVA protocols, including associations of guaifenesin and alpha-2 agonists.
	Profuse urination is a common effect with infusions of alpha-2 agonists. A large volume of urine is produced during the maintenance and recovery phases of the anesthesia. All alpha-2 agonists inhibit insulin secretion by pancreas causing marked hyperglycemia and diuresis.
Recognize the adverse effects and complications of TIVA administration: • cardiovascular • respiratory.	Adverse effects/complications include: • cardiorespiratory depression • bradycardia • cardiac arrhythmias • hypotension (not common in healthy horses and during alpha-2 agonist infusion regimens) • hypoxemia (progressive throughout the time of recumbency) • hypercapnia (progressive throughout the time of recumbency) • apnea • upper airway occlusion • adverse drug reactions (e.g., urticarial, anaphylactoid reaction).

(continued)

Technical action	Rationale
Additional care is required for the adverse effects of TIVA: • oxygen supplementation • tracheal intubation.	In anesthetic procedures lasting more than 30 minutes, respiratory depression and hypoxemia are very common. Oxygen supplementation with a cannula positioned in the nasal cavity or the end of a endotracheal tube (10–15 ml/kg/min), is strongly recommended in all anesthetic procedures lasting more than 30 minutes. In cases of severe respiratory depression or apnea, tracheal intubation should be quickly performed and assistance to ventilation can be carried out using a flushing O_2 demand valve (e.g., JDM-5040 Equine Demand Valve™, JD Medical Inc.). Large horses can be ventilated with this device for 10–20 minutes until spontaneous respiration is restored.

76.9 Procedure: Anesthesia Recovery

Technical action	Rationale
Two experienced attendants should assist in the recovery from anesthesia (Figure 76.6). Put the halter in place and connect a lead rope to it. A cotton rope should be attached to the tail. Avoid any kind of environmental stimuli or attempts to rush the recovery process. Keep ear plugs and blindfold in place. Keep the horse in lateral recumbency until you judge the horse to be coordinated enough to stand up. Restraining the head and neck is an efficient way of doing this.	The recovery from anesthesia is the least controllable phase of general anesthesia. The equine species presents flight behavior. It is common to regain consciousness earlier than motor coordination. Accidents are reported during this time, for example limb fractures, which are the second most common cause of mortality related to anesthesia in horses. Time to recovery is 30–35 minutes after ketamine or ketamine/benzodiazepine induction. Recovery can be prolonged until 40–60 minutes (or more) after the end of administration of protocols with ketamine/alpha-2 agonists/guaifenesin.
The attendant holding the lead rope should be ready to assist the horse's attempt to go into sternal recumbency. The horse should not be stimulated to get up. When the horse attempts to stand up, both attendants should assist the horse at the same time. Remove the ear plugs and endotracheal tube (if intubated during maintenance of anesthesia) immediately after standing.	The horse' first movement is to use the head to roll the body from lateral to sternal recumbency. When the horse stands up, there is a tendency to move its body forward. At this point one of attendants should hold the lead rope closely while the second attendant pulls the tail rope straight backwards. This helps with balance and slows the forward movement. Keep the horse steady and calm. Avoid walking until the horse is completely coordinated.
Observe the patient during the first few minutes after recovery.	Expected effects: • mild ataxia and incoordination • urination.

Technical action	Rationale
Be aware of complications and be prepared to provide additional care. Adverse effects/complications: • prolonged recumbency • poor-quality recovery of anesthesia • respiratory depression • upper airway occlusion • hypoxemia • hypercapnia • post-operative pain • severe ataxia/incoordination • myopathy and neuropathy • accidents during anesthetic recovery (e.g. fractures) • injuries to the support team. Additional care: • oxygen supplementation (nasal cannula) and assistance with ventilation (flushing O_2 demand valve) as previously described to maintain anesthesia • post-operative analgesia.	These complications are not common with TIVA, but they may occur, which is the reason why TIVA is recommended for elective procedures performed in clinically healthy horses.

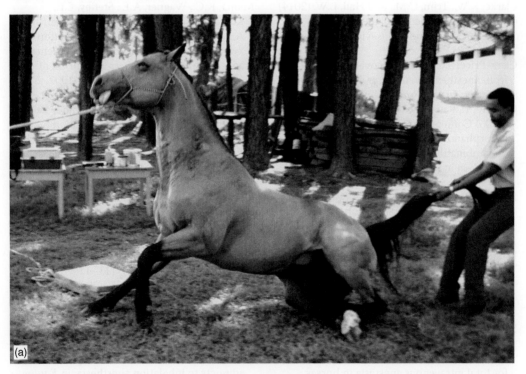

(a)

Figure 76.6 Assistance to the recovery of anesthesia. When the horse stands up, there is a tendency to move its body forward. One of the attendants holds the lead rope while the second attendant pulls the tail straight backwards. (a) The support of the head and tail helps with balance and slows the forward movement. (b) The horse is able to get up and remain stable.

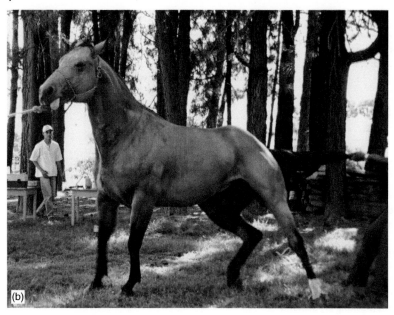

(b)

Figure 76.6 *Continued*

Bibliography and Further Reading

Clarke, K.W., Trim, C.M., and Hall, L.W. (2014) Anaesthesia of the horse, in *Veterinary Anaesthesia*, Saunders Elsevier, London, pp. 245–311.

Clark-Price, S.C. (2013) Recovery of horses from anesthesia. *Veterinary Clinics of North America: Equine Practice*, **29** (3), 223–242.

Corletto, F., Raisis, A.A., and Brearley, J.C. (2005) Comparison of morphine and butorphanol as pre-anaesthetic agentes in combination with romifidine for field castration in ponies. *Veterinary Anaesthesia and Analgesia*, **32** (1), 16–22.

Doherty, T. and Valverde, A. (2006) Management of sedation and anesthesia, in *Equine Anesthesia and Analgesia*, Blackwell Publishing, Oxford, pp. 206–259.

Hubbell, J.A.E. and Muir, W.W. (2009) Considerations for induction, maintenance and recovery, in *Equine Anesthesia: Monitoring and emergency therapy*, Saunders Elsevier, St. Louis, pp. 381–396.

Hubbell, J.A.E., Aarnes, T.K., Lerche, P., and Bednarski, R.M. (2012) Evaluation of midazolam-ketamine-xylazine infusion for total intravenous anestesia in horses. *American Journal of Veterinay Research*, **73** (4), 470–475.

Lerche, P. (2013) Total intravenous anestesia in horses. *Veterinary Clinics of North America: Equine Practice*, **29** (3), 123–129.

Mama, K.C., Wagner, A.E., Steffey, E.P., Kollias-Baker, C., Hellier, P.W., Golden, A.E., and Brevard, L.F. (2005) Evaluation of xylazine and ketamine for total intravenous anestesia in horses. *American Journal of Veterinay Research*, **66** (6), 1002–1007.

Marntell, S., Nyman, G., and Funkquist, P. (2006) Dissociative anaesthesia under field and hospital conditions for castration of colts. *Acta Veterinaria Scandinavica*, **41** (1), 1–11.

Muir, W.W., Hubbell, J.A.E., Bednarski, R.M., and Skarda, R.T. (2007) Anesthetic procedures and techniques in horses, in *Handbook of Veterinary Anesthesia*, Mosby Elsevier, St. Louis, pp. 389–401.

Staffieri, F. and Driessen, B. (2007) Field anesthesia in the equine. *Clinical Techniques in Equine Practice*, **6** (2), 111–119.

Taylor, P.M. and Clarke, K.W. (2007) Intravenous anaesthesia, in *Handbook of Equine Anaesthesia*, Saunders Elsevier, Edinburgh, pp. 33–53.

Yamashita, K. and Muir, W.W. (2009) Intravenous anesthetic and analgesic adjuncts to inhalation anesthesia, in *Equine Anesthesia: Monitoring and emergency therapy*, Saunders Elsevier, St. Louis, pp. 260–276.

Part XI

Clinical Procedures by Body Systems: Miscellaneous Procedures

77

Bone Marrow Aspiration

Alfredo Sanchez Londoño

77.1 Purpose

- To obtain diagnostic and prognostic information from horses with blood cell abnormalities.
  - To investigate causes of cytopenia such as anemia, neutropenia, and thrombocytopenia that cannot be explained by normal blood work.
  - To investigate for neoplasia or infectious disease.
  - To determine if an anemic horse has a good regenerative response in the bone marrow. This is generally determined by the number of myeloid to erythroid precursors (M:E ratio) found in a bone marrow sample by a clinical pathologist.
  - Bone marrow aspiration is used to obtain mesenchymal stem cells in the horse.

77.2 Complications

- Inadvertent puncture of the thoracic cavity when obtaining a sample from the sternum or ribs.
- Pneumopericardium and cardiac laceration can occur, but have been rarely reported.
- Infection of the bone marrow or the aspiration site can occur, but very infrequently.
- Hemorrhage could potentially occur in horses with coagulation disorders such as those affected by severe thrombocytopenia.

77.3 Equipment Required

- Sedation: use of alpha-2 agonist (e.g., xylazine or detomidine) will provide adequate sedation.
- Clippers
- Antiseptic solutions: betadine or chlorhexidine solution and alcohol for sterile preparation of the site (see Chapter 10)
- Sterile surgical gloves
- Local anesthetic: 2% lidocaine, 2–3 ml
- #15 scalpel blade
- Sterile syringe: 6 ml
- EDTA blood tubes
- Bone marrow aspiration needle: Remington or Jamshidi or Illinois sternal iliac bone marrow aspiration needle (choose a size appropriate to the patient), typically 11 gauge 4″ (Figure 77.1).
- Sterile 4″ × 4″ gauze pads
- Skin stapler gun or suture material.
- Ultrasound (optional)

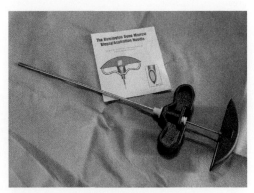

Figure 77.1 Remington bone marrow needle with stylet (Remington Medical, Inc., Alpharetta, GA). Courtesy of Dr. Jose Garcia-Lopez.

Manual of Clinical Procedures in the Horse, First Edition. Edited by Lais R.R. Costa and Mary Rose Paradis.
© 2018 John Wiley & Sons, Inc. Published 2018 by John Wiley & Sons, Inc.

77.4 Restraint

- This procedure can be painful to the horse, therefore the handler and clinician should be cautioned.
- The horse should be adequately restrained using moderate sedation (see Chapter 9) and application of a nose twitch (see Chapter 2).
- If restraining stocks are available, the horse should be placed in them.
- The veterinarian should be positioned in a squatting position at the side of the horse at the level of the front limb.

77.5 Procedure: Bone Marrow Aspiration

Technical action	Rationale
Locate the sternum. The sternum is palpated on the ventral midline of the cranial thorax, caudal to the olecranon. Although bone marrow can be aspirated from the fourth, fifth or sixth sternebrae, the body of the fifth sternebra is preferred.	The sternum is the most common site of bone marrow collection in the adult horse. There are seven sternebrae and the exiphisternum in the horse's chest. The body of the fifth sternebra is the safest aspiration site because it is cranial to the apex of the heart and not between the front limbs of the horse. This can be accurately located using ultrasound (Figure 77.2).
The wing of the ilium can be used as an alternative site when collecting bone marrow from a foal.	The cortex of the wing of the ilium is thinner in the young horse and easily used as a site for bone marrow aspiration. In the adult this bone is thick and often hard to penetrate.
The hair is clipped and the area is prepared with a surgical scrub.	Clipping the hair is important in the sterile technique for this procedure. It is also beneficial if ultrasound imaging is used to locate a specific site for aspiration.
Local anesthetic is injected to desensitize the subcutaneous tissues, the muscle layers, and the periosteum (Figure 77.3). The area is surgically prepped using sterile gloves.	The procedure can be painful and it is important that the animal stands still during the aspiration for animal and clinician safety.
Using sterile gloves, a #15 surgical blade is used to make a small stab incision through the desensitized area.	This allows the needle to penetrate the skin without causing discomfort to the animal due to pressure applied to the surface.
The bone marrow needle is placed through the stab incision and muscle layers until it comes into contact with the ventral surface of the sternebra (Figure 77.4).	The needle will proceed easily to the point where the bone is contacted.
The index finger of the clinician is placed on the needle approximately 2 cm from the skin.	The index finger placement acts as a guide to determine the depth of the needle required.
The needle is rotated and advanced in a clockwise/counterclockwise motion until the index finger is against the skin and the needle is firmly seated in the bone (Figures 77.5 and 77.6).	This may require some force to penetrate the cortex of the bone. Stopping the upward progression of the needle at 2 cm minimizes the chance that the thorax and/or heart will be entered.

Technical action	Rationale
The stylet of the needle is removed and a 6 ml syringe containing EDTA is attached to the hub of the needle (Figures 77.7 and 77.8).	Clotting of the sample can occur quickly, therefore aspirating the EDTA from an evacuated lavender-top (vacuntainer) tube into the collection syringe will prevent coagulation of the sample.
Quick, repeated aspirations need to be performed to dislodge spicules and marrow particles.	This type of aspiration helps to break down some of the trabecular walls in the bone marrow at the needle tip.
Once blood becomes evident at the hub of the syringe and mixes with the EDTA solution, the syringe should be detached from the needle.	The trabecular bone contains a large number of small arteries and veins. Forceful aspiration of a large volume causes hemodilution of the sample.
A drop of the sample can be placed on a clean slide. If an excessive amount of blood is present, tip the slide to drain off the blood. Bone marrow spicules (particles) should adhere to the slide.	The bone marrow spicules are the most important part of the sample for the pathologist to examine. The excess blood is not important.
To further prepare the slide a second slide can be gently placed on top of the first slide and horizontally pulled apart. The preparation can then be air dried.	Do not apply pressure to the slides as this will result in a "squashed" preparation which cannot be interpreted accurately.
The procedure can be repeated if the sample is inadequate or not of diagnostic quality.	If no spicules are seen on the slide, the aspiration should be repeated by advancing the needle another 1 cm or withdrawing the needle and replacing it in another location.
Aspiration site care. Once the needle is removed manual pressure with 4" × 4" gauze pads can be placed on the site to prevent hemorrhage. One or two skin staples may be placed to close the skin where the stab incision was made.	In general, the bleeding should be minimal unless the horse is thrombocytopenic or has other coagulation problems.

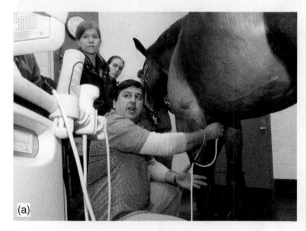
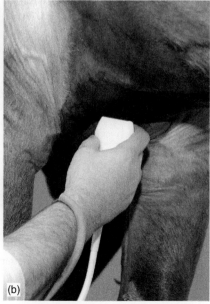

Figure 77.2 (a) Use of ultrasound to determine the location of the body of the fifth sternebra. (b) A 5–10 MHz linear probe is used to locate the fifth sternebra. Courtesy of Dr. Jose Garcia-Lopez.

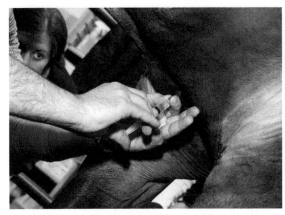

Figure 77.3 2% lidocaine should be injected subcutaneously and into the deeper layers of muscle and periosteum. Courtesy of Dr. Jose Garcia-Lopez.

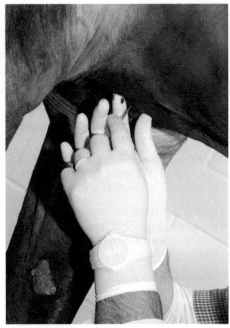

Figure 77.4 A bone marrow needle is advanced through the skin and soft tissue. Courtesy of Dr. Jose Garcia-Lopez.

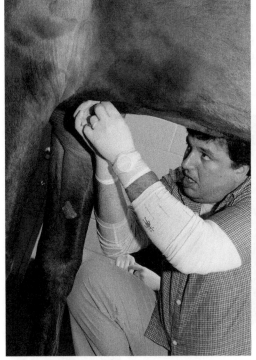

Figure 77.5 Some force is required to penetrate the bone. Courtesy of Dr. Jose Garcia-Lopez.

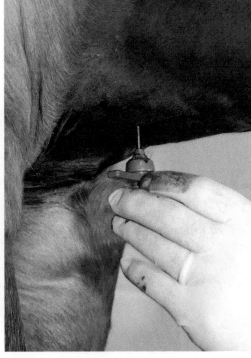

Figure 77.6 Once the needle penetrates the bone it will be firmly seated. Courtesy of Dr. Jose Garcia-Lopez.

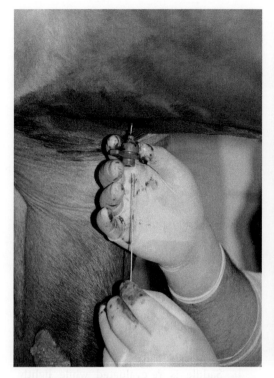

Figure 77.7 The stylet is removed from the needle. Courtesy of Dr. Jose Garcia-Lopez

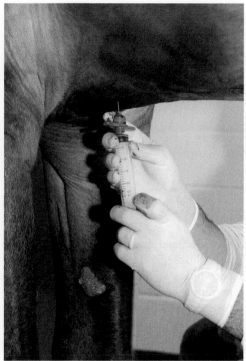

Figure 77.8 A syringe containing a small amount of ETDA can be attached to the needle. The EDTA will prevent clotting of the sample. Courtesy of Dr. Jose Garcia-Lopez

Bibliography and Further Reading

Durando, P., Zarucco, L., Schaer, T.P., Ross, M., and Reef, V.B. (2006) Pneumopericardium in a horse secondary to sternal bone marrow aspiration. *Equine Veterinary Education*, **18** (2), 75–79.

Kasashima, Y., Ueno, T., Tomita, A., Goodship, A.E., and Smith, R.K.W. (2011) Optimisation of bone marrow aspiration from the equine sternum for the safe recovery of mesenchymal stem cells. *Equine Veterinary Journal*, **43** (3), 288–294.

Russell, K.E., Sellon, D.C., and Grindem, C.B. (1994) Bone marrow in horses: Indications, sample handling, and complications. *Compendium of Continuing Education for the Practicing Veterinarian*, **16**, 1359–1366.

Sellon, D.C. (2006) How to obtain a diagnostic bone marrow sample from the sternum of an adult horse. *AAEP Proceedings*, **52**, 621–672.

Smith, R. (2008) Bone marrow biopsy, in *The Equine Hospital Manual* (eds. K. Corley and J. Stephen), Blackwell, Oxford, pp. 89–91.

78

Saddle Evaluation and Fitting

Kerry Ridgeway

78.1 Purpose

- To understand saddle fitting as an important and valuable part of equine practice because poor-fitting saddles create pain and loss of performance ability, and set up pathologic consequences to the horse's muscles, tendons, ligaments, bones, and joints.
- To establish the relationship of equine soundness to saddle fit.
- To educate the rider/client in regard to this issue as an important part of preventative medicine.

A saddle can be considered to be an interface between the horse and the rider. As a metaphor, think of the cartilage/menisci interface between the femur and the tibia. That interface can be functional or it can be essentially a torture device for the horse or the rider or both. Saddle fitting is best learned in a class and laboratory format, so this chapter should be considered introductory.

The goal and function of the evaluation and fit of a saddle is to ensure that the horse has a pain-free and functional interface:

- The saddle fit must allow the horse to easily and athletically perform to its level of training and to meet its genetic potential.
- The saddle fit for the rider must provide an interface that ensures rider security, comfort, and balance, and thereby allows the rider to experience harmony with the movement of the horse.

The evaluation consists of five phases or steps:

1. First phase: Evaluation of the horse.
2. Second phase: Evaluation of the saddle off the horse.
3. Third phase: Evaluation of the saddle placed on the horse:
   a. Saddle placed on the back with no pads (Western saddles may require a 1 cm thick pad).
   b. Saddle is re-evaluated while lightly girthed or cinched.
4. Fourth phase: Evaluation of the fit with the rider up and not in motion:
   a. Evaluate the posture and position of the rider and note the attitude of the horse.
   b. Evaluate without a pad under the saddle.
   c. Evaluate Western saddles with the pad usually used with the saddle.
   d. Evaluate the saddle fit with the rider's weight in the saddle.
5. Fifth phase: Evaluate the horse and rider in motion:
   a. Determine the appropriateness of the saddle, pad(s), and rider in combination.

78.2 Equipment Required

- An adequate space to see the horse walk, trot, and canter in hand and on a lunge line is needed during the first phase of evaluation.
- Flat, firm, level ground is important for the static evaluation because the horse must be able to stand "squarely" during the evaluation.

Manual of Clinical Procedures in the Horse, First Edition. Edited by Lais R.R. Costa and Mary Rose Paradis.
© 2018 John Wiley & Sons, Inc. Published 2018 by John Wiley & Sons, Inc.

- A mounting block or other stable object is needed to stand on when evaluating from above the horse's back, including from above and behind the hindquarters.
- A flashlight is needed to evaluate panel contact and channel clearance of the saddle. LED flashlights are recommended.

- The saddle to be evaluated. See saddle parts for Western saddles (Figure 78.1) and English saddles (Figure 78.2).
- The rider must be present and ready to ride the horse (for Phase 5 of the evaluation).

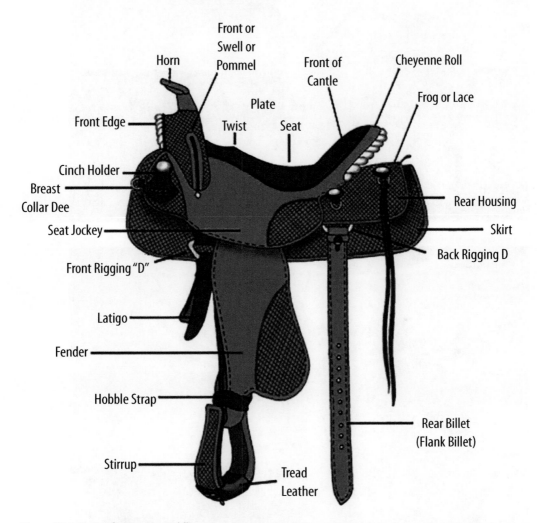

Figure 78.1 Parts of a Western saddle.

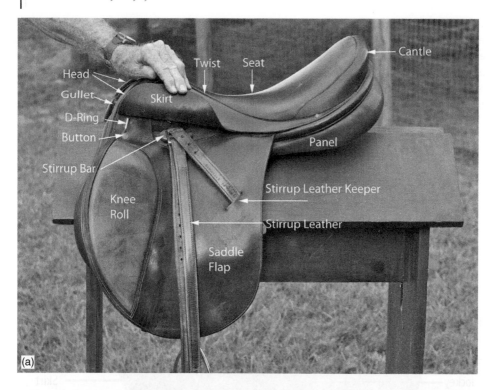

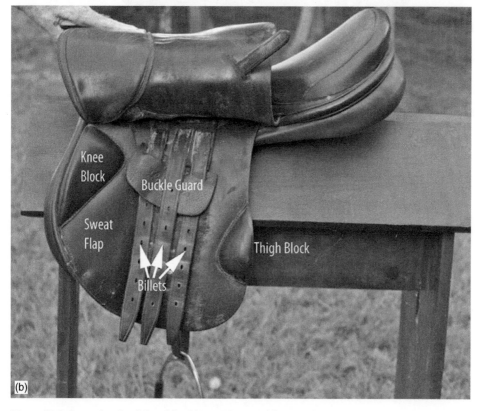

Figure 78.2 Parts of an English saddle: (a) Lauriche 1 and (b) Lauriche 2.

78.3 Procedure: Phase 1 – Evaluation of the Horse

Technical Action	Rationale
Make sure that the horse is in an acceptable state of soundness for its intended use before proceeding with saddle evaluation.	Assess the horse's "attitude" for evidence of general discomfort or pain. Note the horse's manner and symmetry of tracking.
Determine whether the horse is of an appropriate weight and level of condition to properly assess the appropriate fit for the tasks and movements required. Determine whether the horse has musculoskeletal issues present that will affect saddle fit.	Being underweight and/or loss of muscle mass (especially the topline) will affect saddle fitting.
The horse needs to be standing squarely for evaluation (Figure 78.3).	Make sure the ground is flat, firm, and level.
Note head carriage and symmetry of movement.	Rule out any dental problems as this will affect the carriage of the head and back when the horse is in motion.
Confirm bilateral symmetry of the musculature, especially in croup and thighs.	You may have to stand on a stepstool to evaluate the horse thoroughly (Figure 78.3).
Assess conformation and posture, evaluating: • the topline for the presence of lordosis, scoliosis, kyphosis, and levelness • the wither height and shape • the croup height and symmetry	Carefully observe the horse from above and behind: • note any asymmetry of withers, back and spine (Figure 78.4) • assess the horse's musculature and skeleton • palpate the back for evidence of pain or pathology.
Evaluate hoof symmetry and functional limb leg length.	Determine if there is high heel/low heel syndrome present. It is important to remember that asymmetry in heel height is also reflected in the scapula. A low heel causes the scapula to rotate more vertically, thus affecting saddle fit (Figure 78.5a). Identify if there is a club foot present.
Evaluate scapular height, shape and, bilateral symmetry.	Note if the scapula appears bulging or more prominent on left or right side (Figure 78.5b).
Determine if the shoulders and scapulae blend well into the thorax.	Shoulder asymmetry affects saddle fitness by causing the saddle to move diagonally across the back during movement (Figure 78.5c).
Verify if there are galls, scars or brands that will be impacted by saddle pressure or movement.	Make a note of these.

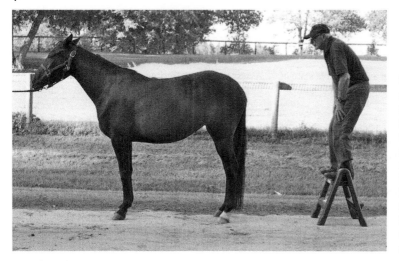

Figure 78.3 Inspection of the conformation and posture of the horse (Phase 1). It is important that the horse is standing squarely and with a normal head posture. Examination should include inspection from above and behind, such that any asymmetry of withers, back, and spine can be observed.

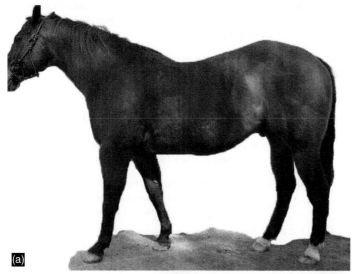

(a)

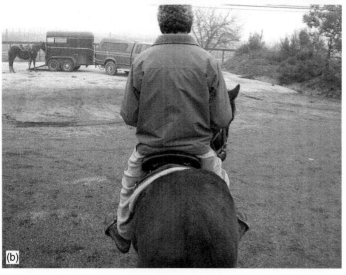

(b)

Figure 78.4 Abnormalities of the croup and pelvis should be noted during observation of the symmetry in the horse. (a) A high croup makes for a difficult saddle fit. The saddle tends to form a "bridge", with no contact at the center of the panels. This creates a "four-legged table" effect with pressure points at both ends of the saddle. The saddle tends to slide into the back edge of the scapulae. (b) Asymmetry of the pelvis is best noted from behind. This horse has marked asymmetry to the pelvic muscles due to long-term poor saddle fit.

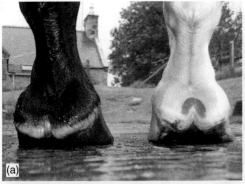

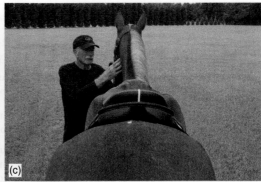

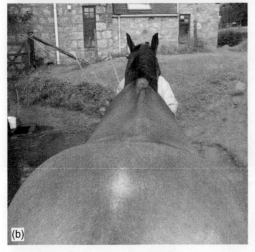

Figure 78.5 Abnormalities that can be noted during observation of the symmetry in the horse. (a) Heel height asymmetry between the right and left front limbs is evident, and is also reflected in the scapula. The low heel will cause the scapula to rotate more vertically, thus affecting saddle fit. (b) Note that the left scapula appears more prominent or "bulged" outward as it rotates more vertically. (c) The shoulder asymmetry causes the saddle to move diagonally across the back. This will be most evident when the horse is moving.

78.4 Procedure: Phase 2 – Evaluation of the Saddle off the Horse

Technical action	Rationale
Evaluate the saddle before it is placed on the horse's back. Note the overall integrity of the saddle.	Note the condition of the leather, stitching quality and integrity, nails or other protrusions that can be palpated.
Evaluate the integrity of the tree for weakness or fracture in its components.	Check for a broken or weak tree (Figure 78.6a).
Evaluate the general symmetry of the saddle, including the: • head (pommel arch) • gullet (the channel formed by the two panels, running the length of the saddle), which should have appropriate width.	The gullet channel should be between 2.5″ and 3″ wide to prevent impingement on the spine during the lateral movement of the saddle while the horse is in motion (Figure 78.6b).
Assess panel symmetry and condition, noting: • the smoothness of the flocking of "flocked saddles" or foam • the condition of the sheepskin on Western saddles.	Note whether panels are attached to the tree in a symmetrical manner. Pay attention to any asymmetry in the shape and angle of the panels (Figure 78.7). Look for abnormal wear patterns.

(continued)

Technical action	Rationale
Note the condition and placement of: • the billets on English saddles, or • the "rigging" on Western saddles.	It is critical that the billets/rigging are placed in exactly the same location bilaterally. Asymmetrical placement of the billets/rigging leads to twisting of the saddle (Figure 78.8).
Note the condition (structural soundness) of the stirrup hangers or stirrup bars.	Ensure that the stirrup bars are in exactly the same location bilaterally. Ensure that they are not placed at a depth at which they could possibly create pressure points for the horse.

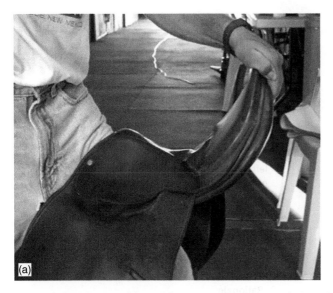 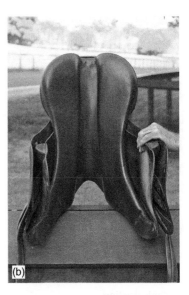

Figure 78.6 Evaluation of the saddle prior to placement on the horse's back (Phase 2). (a) This position demonstrates how one can check for a broken or weak tree in an English saddle. (b) The channel should be between 2½" and 3" wide to prevent impingement on the spine during the lateral movement of the saddle when the horse is in motion.

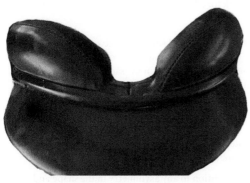

Figure 78.7 Symmetry of the panels is critical to saddle fit. These panels are obviously quite different in both shape and angle.

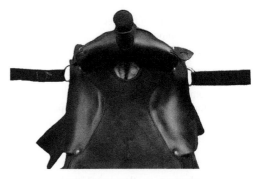

Figure 78.8 Symmetry of placement of the billets or rigging is also critical to saddle fit. When the billets or rigging are not placed exactly the same on both sides, the saddle will twist diagonally across the back when the saddle is secured.

78.5 Procedure: Phase 3 – Evaluation of the Saddle Placed on the Horse

Technical action	Rationale
Place the saddle on the horse's back with no pads. A Western saddle may require a 1 cm thick pad.	Always have the rider place the saddle, so it can be ascertained that the saddle placement is appropriate.
With the saddle not cinched or girthed, ensure that it sits in the natural "sweet spot" where the individual horse's back will best accept it (Figure 78.9).	Place one hand on the pommel and one hand on the cantle to be sure that the saddle will not rock front to rear like a see-saw.
Ensure that the bars and the fork of a Western saddle, or the "points" of an English saddle, do not interfere with the movement of the shoulder.	Typically there should be no pressure applied by the saddle by having clearance for approximately 5 cm (approximately 2"). Interference with shoulder movement causes problems.
Determine if the tree or panel length is appropriate for the horse.	Check that the tree or panel gives maximum support within the space allowed for the saddle.
The bars of a Western saddle or the panels of an English saddle should not make contact (thus not bear any weight) beyond the last rib (Figure 78.9).	If the bars or panels make contact it means that the saddle bears weight beyond the last rib.
Determine if the saddle sits straight on the horse's back before girthing the saddle. This will be rechecked after girthing.	The saddle should sit straight on the horse's back. Note if the saddle sits somewhat diagonally on the horse's back.
Re-evaluate the saddle while lightly girthed or cinched.	Be sure that the saddle does not tend to tip to one side.
Note the balance point after girthing: • For English saddles, the balance point should be in the center. • For Western saddles the balance point varies depending on the purpose. • Some performance modalities/purposes may require the balance point to be shifted further backwards.	The balance point is the lowest point in the seat. This can be found by placing a small tube on the saddle and allowing it to roll to the lowest point (Figure 78.10).
Evaluate pommel clearance. Determine if the head of the saddle is of an appropriate width.	Evaluate both lateral and dorsal aspects.
Determine if the pitch (English saddles) or rafter (Western saddles) is appropriate for the horse.	The angle (pitch/rafter) of the gullet bar/points (fork of a Western saddle) must have the same angle as the horse's wither pocket conformation. The contact must be even throughout.
Determine if the arc (English saddles) or rocker (Western saddles) from front to rear is appropriate.	
Determine if the points of the English saddle are of appropriate length and direction for the horse's discipline or use.	Make sure the saddle is not too narrow at the points (Figure 78.11).
Evaluate the contact surface area of the bars or panels while the horse is not in motion.	Visually, and by palpation, assure that there is adequate surface area (square inches or square centimeters) of the bars or panels contacting the horse's back.

(continued)

Technical action	Rationale
Estimate the contact surface area of the bars or panels while the horse is in motion, recognizing that the horse's back elevates slightly when the horse moves.	There needs to be some room for the back to elevate or the saddle will rock forward and back (see-saw) when the horse is in a forward gait, jumping, sliding, etc.
Palpate for excess bridging (lack of contact) of the saddle's panels or bars between the pommel and the cantle.	Palpate carefully and softly, bringing the fingers upward and under the panels or bars near the center of saddle.
Excessive bridging creates a "four-legged table" on the horses back.	Do not force the hand under the bars or panels.
	The bridge should not exceed 1 cm on English saddles and 1.5 cm on Western saddles.
Palpate the contact of the exterior edges carefully.	
Stand on a mounting block and look front to rear and rear to front with the flashlight illuminating the channel space.	One should not be able to see past the point where the skirts at the cantle end of the Western saddle are laced together.

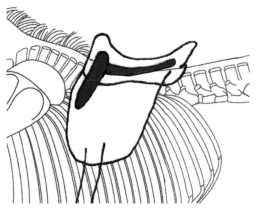

Figure 78.9 Correct saddle placement. The points allow room for shoulder freedom. The saddle does not bear weight behind the last rib.

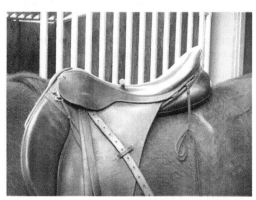

Figure 78.10 Placement of a small tube on the saddle is used to determine the balance point (lowest point) of the saddle. The balance point should be in the center of the saddle. In this case, the yellow long cylinder/tube has rolled forward, indicating that the balance point of the saddle is shifted forward, which will take the rider out of balance.

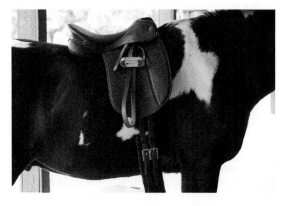

Figure 78.11 A saddle that is too narrow will perch on the withers and the points will dig into the shoulder.

78.6 Procedure: Phase 4 – Evaluation of the Fit with the Rider up and not in Motion (Static Examination)

Technical action	Rationale
Evaluation of the saddle fit with the rider's weight in the saddle: • evaluate without a pad under an English saddle • evaluate with the normal pad used in a Western saddle.	
Observe the horse's reaction as the rider mounts.	Flinching from the horse indicates either back soreness or saddle fit problems.
Saddle fit is dynamic and may change drastically once the rider is mounted.	A perfect fit can turn into a poor fit when the rider is mounted.
The saddle must fit the rider for the horse to be able to perform well with that particular saddle.	If the rider is unbalanced in the saddle, the saddle fitting will reflect this unbalance, leading to or exacerbating the horse's performance problems or musculoskeletal issues.
Observe the rider's posture and position from front, rear, and side views. Determine: 1. if the rider's weight is distributed equally 2. if the rider's shoulders are even 3. if the rider's body/thorax twisted 4. if the rider's head is tilted to one side 5. if the rider sits with one hip cocked, forward or collapsed 6. if the stirrup lengths are the same on both sides 7. if the rider's feet point in the same direction 8. if one of the rider's legs is turned outward more than the other 9. if one foot or leg is further forward than the other 10. where the rider is placed in the saddle.	
Draw an imaginary line vertically through the rider's ear, shoulder, hip, and heel: • determine if the head is jutted forward • determine if the rider appears to be in a chair seat • determine if the rider is upright or slumped in the saddle.	
Compare the saddle fit before and after the rider mounts: • Determine if the saddle has deformed with the rider's weight. • Does the saddle still align with the horse's spine? • Recheck the pommel clearance, both vertically and laterally. • Determine if the channel (on an English saddle) is open through its entire length.	This information will highlight the interaction of rider, saddle, and horse.

(continued)

Technical action	Rationale
Determine if the knee blocks/rolls on an English saddle are placed correctly for the rider's legs. Determine if the flaps are of correct length and dimensions for the rider's legs.	Determine if the thigh blocks (if present) on an English saddle are placed correctly for the rider's legs.

78.7 Procedure: Phase 5 – Evaluate the Horse and Rider in Motion

Technical action	Rationale
Saddle evaluation with the rider up and in motion is the last, but not least, step in the saddle-fit evaluation. The goal is to evaluate the harmony between horse, saddle, and rider when asking the horse to do the movements required of it in its given discipline or sport.	The saddle's balance often changes considerably when the horse is in motion. During motion, a poorly fitting saddle makes abnormalities become evident (Figure 78.12), whereas a well-fitting saddle demonstrates the harmony of the rider and horse during motion (Figure 78.13).
Up to this point the saddle fit may appear to be satisfactory, but the relationship can change markedly when the horse moves with the weight of the saddle plus the rider's weight and balance.	The horse may exhibit discomfort either because of the fit of the saddle or the balance/position of the rider in the saddle during the motion phase.
Make comparisons with the observations from Phase 3 and make the following determinations: • Does the saddle remain aligned with the spine and move laterally back and forth at the cantle by the same amount left and right? • Does the saddle "fishtail" excessively laterally to right and left?	This comparison highlights if/how motion changes the fit of the saddle to the horse. "Fishtailing" is often associated with a saddle that is too wide (open angled at either the pommel or the cantle).
Evaluate the rider's position and balance while the horse moves. Make comparisons with the observations from Phase 4 and try to determine if motion changes the rider's position and balance.	Make the following determinations: • Can the rider post with ease and balance? • Can the rider maintain the ear, shoulder, hip, and heel line? • Has the rider slipped into a "chair" seat once the horse is in gait?
Evaluate the horse's gait and attitude. Make the following determinations: • Is the horse's tracking significantly changed from Phase 1 of the examination? • Does the horse show signs of resistance or discomfort while going through the gaits? • Are these signs exacerbated when going through a tight turn at an arena corner?	Signs to look for while trying to determine resistance or discomfort: • elevated head • ears directed backwards • tail swishing. Signs may be exacerbated during tight turns. The corners of the saddle may dig into the horse's back or on the lateral aspects of the withers and should be checked.

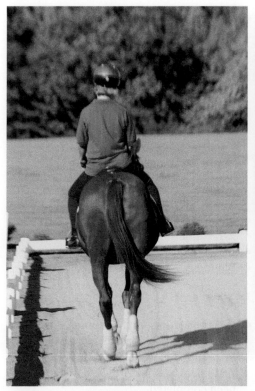

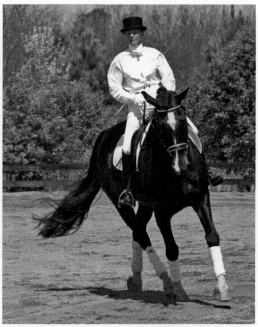

Figure 78.13 A well-fitting saddle goes a long way toward allowing balance and harmony between horse and rider.

Figure 78.12 The saddle may fit, but a crooked rider will create saddle pressure points. A crooked rider will create a crooked horse that will have many musculoskeletal problems, eventually leading to lameness.

78.8 Conclusion

In most cases it is not appropriate to do a saddle evaluation until musculoskeletal issues have been addressed and, if possible, corrected. This is often an area (in the opinion of the author) where integrative medicine and conventional veterinary examination can be complimentary to one another.

Bibliography and Further Reading

Harman, J. (2004) *The Horse's Pain–Free Back and Saddle Fit Book*, Trafalgar Square Publishing, North Pomfret, VT.

Langdon, J.R. and William, G. (1997) *Saddle Fitting – How to select the right saddle to fit you and your horse*, Langdon Enterprises, Hardesty, Colbert, Washington. (This is an excellent reference TEXT, especially for Western saddles.)

Patillo, D. (2012) *Saddle Fitting and Hoof Biomechanics*, course manual for EQ700, Equinology Inc.

Ridgway, K.J. (2006) *Saddle Fitting From A to Z*, DVD, HorseCity.com.

79

Pre-purchase Examination

Daniel J. Burba

79.1 Purpose

- To bring to light to a prospective horse buyer any potential issues that may affect the soundness, present or future of the horse for its intended purpose.

79.2 Complications

- Masking of disorders (i.e., lameness) by present owner.
- Inadvertently overlooking issues that later result in unsoundness.

79.3 Equipment Required

- Stethoscope
- Hoof testers
- Hoof pick
- Lunge rope and whip
- Thermometer
- Ophthalmoscope
- X-ray unit
- Endoscope
- Blood/serum biochemical analysis

79.4 Pertinent Points

- All procedures and examinations performed must be recorded accurately and in detail. This will clarify any controversy that might arise after the examination has been completed.
- It is best not to perform the examination in the presence of the current owner.
- Part of a pre-purchase examination is to be thorough in getting information from the buyer and possibly the owner regarding the horse.
- Talk to the prospective buyer about how extensive an examination they want (based on time and economics).

79.5 Procedure: Obtaining a Complete History and Performing a Complete Physical Examination

Technical action	Rationale
Obtain a history from the prospective buyer.	Questions to ask: • Have they ridden the horse (if applicable)? • Intended use? • What is the horse's insurance status?
Obtain an anamnesis from the current owner or trainer (see Chapter 3).	For example: • What is the horse being fed? • Does the horse have a current Coggins? • Is the horse up to date with its vaccinations?
Observe the horse for any vices or stereotypes (i.e., cribbing, stall weaving).	Investigate the history to determine if the horse has exhibited any vices.

Manual of Clinical Procedures in the Horse, First Edition. Edited by Lais R.R. Costa and Mary Rose Paradis.
© 2018 John Wiley & Sons, Inc. Published 2018 by John Wiley & Sons, Inc.

Technical action	Rationale
Perform a complete physical examination (see Chapter 3).	This includes, but is not limited to: • auscultation of the heart • auscultation of the chest, including using a rebreathing bag • inspection of the genitalia, especially in aged horses, for possible tumor formations (this may require tranquilization in male horses and thus should be reserved for later, after the lameness examination).
In additional to detailed physical examination specifically inspect for surgical scars (Figure 79.1).	For example of the ventral abdomen and palmar digital area.
It is also important to inspect conformation.	Faulty conformation may be a source of unsoundness even if lameness is not currently present.
Perform a lameness examination (see Chapter 27).	If abnormalities (i.e., lameness, enlarged tendons, joint effusion) are found, inform the prospective buyer. They may not want to proceed further.

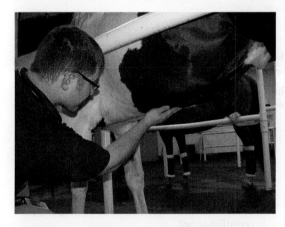

Figure 79.1 Inspection of the ventral abdomen for an incisional scar.

The continuation of the pre-purchase examination is conditional on no abnormalities being found at this point, and therefore the buyer wishes to proceed.

79.6 Procedures: Additional Examinations

Technical action	Rationale
Perform a thorough examination of the eyes.	See Chapter 62.

Obtain radiographs of the limbs.	The author recommends that a series of radiographs is performed on the following as these are the most commonly affected joints:
	
	• forelimbs (bilateral):
	  – navicular bone and P3
	  – fetlock
	• hind limbs (bilateral)
	  – tarsi.
	
	The owner may request additional joints to be evaluated, particularly the stifle and carpi.

(continued)

Technical action	Rationale
Perform upper respiratory tract endoscopy.	See Chapter 20.
If the horse is being sold as a breeding prospect, then a breeding soundness examination (BSE) should be performed.	Please refer to relevant chapters: Chapter 35 for soundness examination of stallions, Chapter 36 for soundness examination of mares.
	Stallions may need blood samples to be collected for equine virus arteritis (EVA) serum neutralization.
Inquire as to whether the prospective buyer wants to have a drug/medication screening performed. (Ask if the horse owner/seller has consented to blood sample collection.)	This is performed to determine if the horse has received any medication that may affect the examination (e.g., phenylbutazone may mask lameness).
Obtain a blood sample and if possible a urine sample for drug screening.	Consider obtaining a blood sample and storing it in case the buyer later decides to have drug screening performed.
Discuss with the buyer if any additional laboratory work might be considered.	Some buyers request additional diagnostic tests, including equine infectious anemia c-ELISA, complete cell count (CBC), biochemistry profile, and fecal egg count.
Review findings with the prospective buyer.	
Write up your findings and present a copy to the prospective buyer.	There are standardized forms to report the findings on the pre-purchase examination (see bibliography).
Obtain permission from the prospective buyer before you share your report with the horse's current owner.	The buyer may request that the results are not made known to the owner.

Bibliography and Further Reading

Mitche ll, R.D. and Dyson, S.J. (2003) Prepurchase examination of the performance horse, in *Diagnosis and Management of Lameness in the Horse* (eds M.W. Ross and S.J. Dyson), W.B. Saunders, Philadelphia.

American Association of Equine Practitioners. *Guideline for Reporting Purchase Examinations*, http://www.aaep.org/info/guidelines.

British Equine Veterinary Association. *Pre-Purchase Examination*: https://www.beva.org.uk/Home/Resources-For-Vets/Guidance/Revised-PPE-Exam-Certificate;

https://www.beva.org.uk/Portals/0/Documents/ResourcesForVets/2sample-ppe-certificate.pdf

https://www.beva.org.uk/Portals/0/Documents/ResourcesForVets/BEVA.RCVS 2 Guidance Notes on Pre-Purchase Examination.amended 2012.pdf

Mair, T.S. (ed.) (1998) *The Pre-Purchase Examination. A British Equine Veterinary Association Manual*, Equine Pre-Purchase Exam Diagnostic Plan, in *Diagnostic Plans/Panels*, Cornell University, Animal Health Diagnostic Center, page 9, https://ahdc.vet.cornell.edu/docs/Equine_Diagnostic_Plans_Panels.pdf.

80

Euthanasia

Mustajab H. Mirza and Lais R.R. Costa

80.1 Purpose

- To achieve rapid loss of consciousness followed by cardiac or respiratory arrest and ultimate loss of brain function. Most importantly, distress and anxiety must be minimized prior to the animal's loss of consciousness. Death should be as painless and free of distress as possible.
- To follow the AVMA Guidelines on Euthanasia, which state that it is the responsibility of the veterinarian to ensure that the death of the animal is brought about with the highest degree of respect. Human safety must be considered because of the risk of injury associated with the horse's reaction when falling and thrashing. Table

80.1 lists methods of euthanasia of horses. Only the acceptable method is described here.

- To follow the AAEP Guidelines for Euthanasia (2011) to assist in making humane decisions regarding euthanasia of horses.

80.2 Complications

- Inability to achieve death.
- Distress prior to or during the procedure culminating with injury to the animal and/or the personnel handling or performing the procedure.
- If euthanasia is to be performed with lethal injection of an agent, perivascular injection may occur.

Table 80.1 Methods of euthanasia of horses

Acceptable	Conditionally acceptable	Acceptable adjunctive	Unacceptable
Barbiturates or barbituric acid derivatives given as a bolus intravenously	Penetrating captive bolt OR Gunshot to the brain (only to be used by well-trained personnel who are regularly monitored to ensure proficiency, and their firearms must be well maintained) *	In conjunction with general anesthesia, potassium chloride given intravenously or intracardially	Chloral hydrate alone; Succinylcholine alone; Potassium chloride alone; Electrocution alone.

Modified from AVMA Guidelines on Euthanasia, *Journal of the American Veterinary Medical Association*, 2013

*Humane euthanasia of sick, injured and/or debilitated livestock. http://vetmed.iastate.edu/HumaneEuthanasia.

Manual of Clinical Procedures in the Horse, First Edition. Edited by Lais R.R. Costa and Mary Rose Paradis.
© 2018 John Wiley & Sons, Inc. Published 2018 by John Wiley & Sons, Inc.

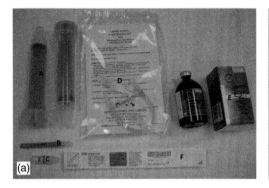 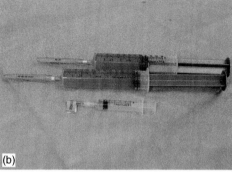

Figure 80.1 Material required for proper euthanasia of a non-anesthetized horse. (a) A, two 60 ml syringes; B, large-gauge needle to aspirate the euthanasia solution from the bottle; C, injection cap; D, extension set; E, barbiturate combination solution for euthanasia; F, short-term catheter to be placed intravenously. (b) Prepare the drugs, drawing up the appropriate amount of pre-euthanasia sedative and euthanasia solution.

80.3 Equipment Required (Figure 80.1)

- Sedation (optional):
  - xylazine (100 mg/ml) at a dose of 1 mg/kg of body weight
  - appropriate size of syringe and needle to administer sedation
- Materials for catheter placement:
  - 14-gauge 3–5″ over-the-needle catheter
  - Luer lock extension set
  - injection cap adaptor
  - suture material: 2-0 nylon on needle
  - heparinized saline (2 units/ml) in a 20 ml syringe
- 14-gauge 1″ needle to aspirate the euthanasia solution from the bottle.
- Euthanasia solution containing pentobarbital to be given at a dose of 100 mg/kg of body weight. Commercial euthanasia solutions are listed in Table 80.2.
- Appropriate sizes of syringes to deliver the total dose of euthanasia solution quickly.
- Stethoscope

Table 80.2 Euthanasia agents containing pentobarbital

Agent	Pentobarbital concentration (mg/ml)	Phenytoin concentration	Examples of commercial names
Class II pentobarbital alone	260	NA	Sleepaway (Pfizer)[a]
	390	NA	Fatal-Plus solution (Vortech)[b]
	392 (after reconstitution of the powder with 250 ml of water)	NA	Pentasol powder (Virbac)[b]
Class III pentobarbital + phenytoin	390	50 mg/ml	Beuthanasia-D Special (Schering-Plough)[a]
			Euthasol (Virbac)[a]
			Euthanasia-III Solution (Henry Schein Animal Health)[a]

NA, not applicable.
[a] labeled for use in dogs or dogs and cats
[b] labeled for use in animals regardless of species

80.4 Other Requirements

- Personnel with training and experience in proper handling and restraint of horses.
- Euthanasia consent form completed and signed by owners. If the horse is to be subjected to a postmortem examination, make the appropriate arrangements.
- Insurance company contacted, if applicable.
- Arrangements made for disposal of the horse's remains. The disposal of the remains must be arranged taking into consideration federal, state, and local regulations.
- If indicated, means to collect mane and tail; and/or clay material to obtain impression of the horse's feet/foot.

80.5 Restraint and Positioning

- The horse should be appropriately restrained for placement of the intravenous catheter.
- The horse should be handled by an experienced person and walked to the chosen area, either an open, leveled grassy area or against a smooth wall with soft footing at a corner (the horse is backend into the corner with the long axis of the horse's body resting against the wall).

80.6 Procedure: Performing Euthanasia by Intravenous Administration of Barbiturate

Technical action	Rationale
Ensure all paperwork is completed appropriately (especially consent form) and that arrangement are made for postmortem examination, if applicable, and for handling of the remains. Select the materials necessary for the procedure (Figure 80.1).	Calculate the total amount of sedation and euthanasia solution required based on the body weight of the animal.
An intravenous catheter (preferably a large-gauge, short-term type of catheter) should be placed in the jugular vein (see instructions for catheter placement in Chapter 8).	Use of an appropriately placed catheter, instead of simply use of a large-gauge needle, is recommended to ensure that all the euthanasia solution is administered intravenously, and not perivascularly. Aseptic technique is not necessary.
The horse should be walked to the chosen area (Figure 80.2). Alternatively, an open, level grassy area may be used (Figure 80.3).	If the horse is unable to walk, it may have to be euthanized at the site.
Administer sedation intravenously, via the catheter, and flush it with heparinized saline.	Heavy sedation is recommended to decrease the risk of injury to personnel. Remember that administration of alpha-2 agonists or acepromazine affects the circulation and therefore prolongs the time for the loss of consciousness.
Position the horse appropriately and coordinate personnel to minimize the risk of injury.	The veterinarian must be in charge of all safety measures.
If the horse is to be positioned against a smooth wall with soft footing, the horse is backed into the corner such that the long axis of the horse's body rests against the wall.	This gives people a chance to push the horse against the wall and therefore slow the descent to the ground instead of the horse falling forward, sideward, or backward.
Warn everyone about the unpredictability of the horse's reaction.	Make sure to point out that it is likely that the horse will experience varying degrees of muscular activity and agonal gasping.

(continued)

Technical action	Rationale
Ensure that the entire amount of the euthanasia solution is ready to be injected.	If the exact weight of the horse is not known, it is best to error by overestimating the horse's weight and administering an excessive dose of euthanasia solution, rather than giving an insufficient amount.
Administer the total amount of euthanasia solution intravenously (preferably via the intravenous catheter) as quickly as possible.	If an intravenous catheter is not placed, the euthanasia solution should be administered through a 14-gauge 2″ needle connected to the extension set after the horse is well sedated.
Once all the solution has been administered and the catheter flushed, minimize the number of people in the vicinity of the horse because of the unpredictable nature of horses when falling down.	If an intravenous catheter was not placed, remove the needle and discard it appropriately.
Allow time for the drug to take effect, then check to make sure the horse's heart is no longer beating. Check the corneal reflex.	Administration of additional euthanasia solution might be necessary. Enter in the medical record the total amount of euthanasia solution administered.
Once you are certain that the horse has died, place a tarp over the body. Take the necessary measures to organize for postmortem examination (if applicable) and for the disposal of the body. Clean up the area.	Remove the catheter and discard it. Make sure no unused euthanasia solution or sedative are left behind.

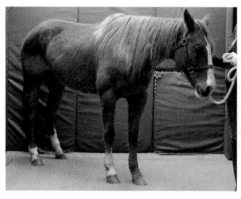

Figure 80.2 Area along a smooth wall and with soft footing for euthanasia of an ambulatory horse. Place the horse against the smooth wall with soft footing at a corner, backed into the corner with the long axis of the horse's body resting against the wall.

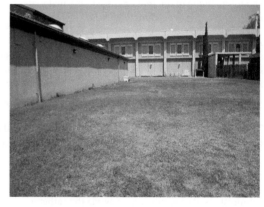

Figure 80.3 An open, level grassy area for euthanasia of an ambulatory horse.

Bibliography and Further Reading

AAEP Guidelines for Euthanasia (2011) https://aaep.org/horsehealth/aaep-guidelines-euthanasia-2011

AVMA Guidelines on Euthanasia of Animals (2013), http://www.avma.org/issues/animal_welfare/euthanasia.pdf. ISBN 978-1-882691-21-0

Ireland, J.L., Clegg, P.D., McGowan, C.M., Platt, L., and Pinchbeck, G.L. (2011) Factors associated with mortality of geriatric horses in the United Kingdom. *Preventative Veterinary Medicine*, **101**, 204–218.

Plumb, D. (2011) Euthanasia agents with pentobarbital, in *Plumb's Veterinary Drug Handbook*, 7th edn, Wiley-Blackwell, Hoboken.

Procedures for Humane Euthanasia: Humane euthanasia of sick, injured and/or debilitated livestock. Shearer JK, Ramirez, A. http://vetmed.iastate.edu/HumaneEuthanasia

Index

Manual of Clinical Procedures in the Horse, First Edition. Edited by Lais R.R. Costa and Mary Rose Paradis.
© 2018 John Wiley & Sons, Inc. Published 2018 by John Wiley & Sons, Inc.